INFECTIOUS DISEASE AND THERAPY

Series Editor

Burke A. Cunha

*Winthrop-University Hospital
Mineola, and
State University of New York School of Medicine
Stony Brook, New York*

Antibiotic Optimization

Concepts and Strategies
In Clinical Practice

Antibiotic Optimization

Concepts and Strategies
In Clinical Practice

edited by

Robert C. Owens, Jr.
*Department of Clinical Pharmacy Services
and Division of Infectious Diseases,
Maine Medical Center, Portland,
and Department of Medicine,
University of Vermont, College of Medicine,
Burlington, Vermont, U.S.A.*

Paul G. Ambrose
*School of Pharmacy and Pharmaceutical Sciences,
University at Buffalo, and Division of Infectious Diseases,
Cognigen Corporation,
Buffalo, New York, U.S.A.*

Charles H. Nightingale
*Hartford Hospital,
Hartford, Connecticut, U.S.A.*

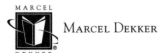

MARCEL DEKKER

NEW YORK

Although great care has been taken to provide accurate and current information, neither the author(s) nor the publisher, nor anyone else associated with this publication, shall be liable for any loss, damage, or liability directly or indirectly caused or alleged to be caused by this book. The material contained herein is not intended to provide specific advice or recommendations for any specific situation.

Trademark notice: Product or corporate names may be trademarks or registered trademarks and are used only for identification and explanation without intent to infringe.

Library of Congress Cataloging-in-Publication Data
A catalog record for this book is available from the Library of Congress.

ISBN: 0-8247-5431-X

This book is printed on acid-free paper.

Headquarters
Marcel Dekker, 270 Madison Avenue, New York, NY 10016, U.S.A.
tel: 212-696-9000; fax: 212-685-4540

Distribution and Customer Service
Marcel Dekker, Cimarron Road, Monticello, New York 12701, U.S.A.
tel: 800-228-1160; fax: 845-796-1772

World Wide Web
http://www.dekker.com

The publisher offers discounts on this book when ordered in bulk quantities. For more information, write to Special Sales/Professional Marketing at the headquarters address above.

Foreword

Among the most critical factors in reducing or reversing the emergence of antimicrobial resistance is the optimization of usage of our highly valuable antimicrobial resources, a concept also known as practicing good antimicrobial stewardship. We squander our antimicrobial resources by using these agents inappropriately for non-bacterial infectious indications, by not dosing them appropriately, and by not using them for the optimal duration to treat infection and avoid unintended consequences of their use. The unintended consequences of antimicrobial use have not been fully appreciated in the past. Certainly immediate adverse events such as rashes and anaphylaxis have long been recognized and have been directly associated with the use of the antibiotic. Other unintended consequences of antimicrobial use are not so readily or immediately recognized. A major unintended consequence of using antimicrobials in hospitals and institutions is *Clostridium difficile* associated disease (CDAD) which most often presents as diarrhea and pseudomembranous colitis. We have long sought to prevent this increasing antibiotic-induced problem by using infection control measures designed to prevent patients from acquiring *C. difficile* spores in the hospital environment. These infection control efforts remain the mainstay of institutional CDAD prevention, but it is now apparent that this problem arises as a direct result of use of specific antimicrobials in the hospital setting, including clindamycin, second and third generation cephalosporins, and newer fluoroquinolone agents. The good news is that controlling or restricting these specific antimicrobials (practicing better antimicrobial stewardship) has resulted in marked decreases in CDAD rates in these institutions.

An unintended consequence of antimicrobial use that is even more difficult to associate directly with usage is the emergence of antimicrobial resistance, one of the most critical current problems in the treatment of many infectious diseases. Considerable new information has been developed to assist the clinician in the practice of good antimicrobial stewardship. This textbook, prepared under the editorship of Robert Owens, Jr., Paul Ambrose, and Charles Nightingale is a compendium of the best practices developed by experts across the U.S. who have extensive experience in the use of data-driven practices that result in fewer unintended consequences without compromising (and often improving) the treatment of infection in the patient. Considerable sources of information for the practice of good antimicrobial stewardship at both the institutional and individual practitioner level have been developed in the past several years. Both types of information are thoroughly assembled, described, and discussed in this text. Infection control professionals, hospital epidemiologists, pharmacists, infectious disease specialists, and all practitioners who utilize antimicrobials or are tasked with managing the ever increasing problems of the unintended consequences of antimicrobial use will find this text an invaluable asset. The editors and authors are to be congratulated on compiling such a thorough approach to improved antimicrobial practice, an approach that if followed will certainly result in fewer unintended consequences and better antimicrobial stewardship by all antimicrobial users.

Dale N. Gerding, MD
Professor of Medicine
Loyola University Chicago Stritch School of Medicine
Associate Chief of Staff for Research and Development
Hines Veterans Affairs Hospital

Preface

Institutionally acquired infections impact approximately 2,000,000 people annually in the United States alone. An increasing percentage of these infections are attributed to antimicrobial resistant organisms. Considering that 25 million pounds of antibiotics are produced yearly for human consumption and are administered to 30–50% of hospitalized patients, the utilization of these miracle drugs is of significant health and economic importance. All the while, studies and surveys suggest that as much as 50% of all antimicrobial use is inappropriate. The problem of increasing antimicrobial resistance, due in part to suboptimal antimicrobial use, coupled with the fact that a growing number of pharmaceutical companies have abandoned anti-infective research and development, has resulted in an emerging public health crisis. As hospitals are characterized by high-density antibiotic use, they are target-rich venues for proactive interventions to improve antimicrobial stewardship. "Antimicrobial stewardship," a term coined by Dale Gerding, describes the optimal selection, dose, and duration of an antimicrobial that results in the best clinical outcome for the treatment or prevention of infection, with minimal toxicity to the patient, and minimal impact on subsequent resistance.

Recognizing the importance of drug resistant organisms, the Infectious Diseases Society of America and the Society for Healthcare Epidemiology of America published recommendations for preventing and reducing antimicrobial resistance in hospitals in 1997. Two years later, the Interagency Task Force on Antimicrobial Resistance, co-chaired by the Centers of Disease Control and Prevention, Food and Drug Administration, and the National Institutes of Health, assembled a more global document addressing the threat of increasing resistance. Both documents stress the importance of improving the use of antimicrobials, or antimicrobial stewardship, at the institutional level in combating antimicrobial resistance.

We have condensed issues stressed by the aforementioned agencies and societies and expanded the content to incorporate emerging data related to the use of antimicrobial agents in the institutional setting. This book is intended to be of relatively broad interest while focusing on contemporary principles essential to optimizing the use of antimicrobial agents. The first section addresses fundamental concepts including the role of the Pharmacy and Therapeutics Committee, antimicrobial resistance, health economics, pharmacodynamics, and benchmarking antimicrobial use, to name a few. The second section reviews practical applications of science, providing examples of programs and strategies designed to foster good antimicrobial stewardship. Issues addressed include antimicrobial stewardship programs, role of computer-assisted decision support, infection control programs, short course therapy, and the institutional use of antifungal agents, among others.

This book is a collaborative effort among recognized authorities in the areas of infectious diseases, hospital epidemiology, medical informatics, clinical pharmacology, and health economics. It is intended to be of interest and value to all clinicians who practice in the institutional setting and prescribe or evaluate antimicrobials. In addition, policy makers and administrators within these institutions will find this book a valuable resource for understanding the crucial interactions of these disciplines, which should help them foster the appropriate development, implementation, and analysis of policies and procedures related to antimicrobial use. While this book is focused on the individual institution, it is hoped that it will encourage the coordination of scientific and practical efforts on regional, national, and global levels that are aimed at the optimal development of current and future antimicrobial strategies.

Robert C. Owens, Jr.
Paul G. Ambrose
Charles H. Nightingale

Contents

Contributors

Paul G. Ambrose School of Pharmacy and Pharmaceutical Sciences, University at Buffalo, and Division of Infectious Diseases Cognigen Corporation, Buffalo, New York, U.S.A.

David Andes Department of Medicine, Section of Infectious Diseases, University of Wisconsin, Madison, Wisconsin, U.S.A.

Elizabeth Dodds Ashley Infectious Diseases Clinical Pharmacy, Duke University Medical Center, Durham, and Campbell University School of Pharmacy, Buies Creek, North Carolina, U.S.A..

Sujata M. Bhavnani School of Pharmacy and Pharmaceutical Sciences, University at Buffalo, and Cognigen Corporation, Buffalo, New York, U.S.A.

Lou Ann Bruno-Murtha Cambridge Health Alliance, Cambridge, and Harvard Medical School, Boston, Massachusetts, U.S.A.

John P. Burke Department of Clinical Epidemiology and Infectious Disease, LDS Hospital, and Department of Medicine, University of Utah School of Medicine, Salt Lake City, Utah, U.S.A.

Ralph Cordell   Centers for Disease Control and Prevention, National Center for Chronic Disease Prevention and Health Promotion, Division of Adolescent and School Health, Atlanta, Georgia, U.S.A.

William A. Craig   Department of Medicine, Section of Infectious Diseases, University of Wisconsin, Madison, Wisconsin, U.S.A.

Debby Ben David   Infectious Diseases Unit, Sheba Medical Center, Tel Aviv University School of Medicine, Tel Hashomer, Israel

Richard H. Drew   Infectious Diseases Clinical Pharmacy, Duke University Medical Center, Duke University School of Medicine, Durham, and Campbell University School of Pharmacy, Buies Creek, North Carolina, U.S.A.

Brian L. Erstad   University of Arizona College of Pharmacy, Tucson, Arizona, U.S.A.

Thomas M. File, Jr   Northeastern Ohio Universities College of Medicine, Rootstown, and Summa Health System, Akron, Ohio, U.S.A.

Gilles Fraser   Department of Critical Care Medicine, Maine Medical Center, Portland, and Department of Medicine, University of Vermont, College of Medicine, Burlington, Vermont, U.S.A.

David Howard   Rollins School of Public Health, Emory University, Atlanta, Georgia, U.S.A.

Melissa D. Johnson   Infectious Diseases Clinical Pharmacy, Duke University Medical Center, Duke University School of Medicine, Durham, and Campbell University School of Pharmacy, Buies Creek, North Carolina, U.S.A.

Ronald N. Jones   The JONES Group/JMI Laboratories, North Liberty, Iowa, and Tufts University School of Medicine, Boston, Massachusetts, U.S.A.

Jetahn Kelley   Consultants in Infectious Diseases, LLP, and Texas Tech University, Lubbock, Texas, U.S.A.

Marin H. Kollef Washington University School of Medicine and Barnes-Jewish Hospital, St. Louis, Missouri, U.S.A.

Joseph L. Kuti Center for Anti-Infective Research and Development, Hartford Hospital, Hartford, Connecticut, U.S.A.

Marianne McCollum School of Pharmacy, University of Colorado Health Sciences Center, Denver, Colorado, U.S.A.

John E. McGowan, Jr. School of Medicine, Emory University, Atlanta, Georgia, U.S.A.

Rajesh R. Mehta Department of Clinical Epidemiology and Infectious Disease, LDS Hospital, and Department of Medicine, University of Utah School of Medicine, Salt Lake City, Utah, U.S.A.

David P. Nicolau Center for Anti-Infective Research and Development, Hartford Hospital, Hartford, Connecticut, U.S.A.

David E. Nix University of Arizona College of Pharmacy, Tucson, Arizona, U.S.A.

Robert C. Owens, Jr. Department of Clinical Pharmacy Services and Division of Infectious Diseases, Maine Medical Center, Portland, and Department of Medicine, University of Vermont, College of Medicine, Burlington, Vermont, U.S.A.

John R. Perfect Division of Infectious Diseases, Duke University School of Medicine, Durham, North Carolina, U.S.A.

Robert A. Quercia Hartford Hospital, Hartford, and University of Connecticut School of Pharmacy, Storrs, Connecticut, U.S.A.

Richard Quintiliani University of Connecticut School of Medicine, Farmington, and University of Connecticut School of Pharmacy, Storrs, Connecticut, U.S.A.

Julio Ramirez Division of Infectious Diseases, Department of Medicine, University of Louisville School of Medicine, Louisville, Kentucky, U.S.A.

Gili Regev-Yochay   Infectious Diseases Unit, Sheba Medical Center, Tel Aviv University School of Medicine, Tel Hashomer, Israel

Rebecca R. Roberts   Department of Emergency Medicine, John H. Stroger Jr. Hospital of Cook County, Chicago, Illinois, U.S.A.

Ethan Rubinstein   Infectious Diseases Unit, Sheba Medical Center, Tel Aviv University School of Medicine, Tel Hashomer, Israel

R. Douglas Scott II   Centers for Disease Control and Prevention, National Center for Infectious Diseases, Division of Healthcare Quality Promotion, Atlanta, Georgia, U.S.A.

Steve L. Solomon   Centers for Disease Control and Prevention, National Center for Infectious Diseases, Division of Healthcare Quality Promotion, Atlanta, Georgia, U.S.A.

Patricia Stogsdill   Division of Infectious Diseases, Maine Medical Center, Portland, and Department of Medicine, University of Vermont, College of Medicine, Burlington, Vermont, U.S.A.

Alan D. Tice   Section of Infectious Diseases, John A Burns School of Medicine, University of Hawaii at Manoa, Honolulu, Hawaii, U.S.A.

August J. Valenti   Department of Epidemiology and Infection Prevention, Maine Medical Center, Portland, Maine, and University of Vermont College of Medicine, Burlington, Vermont, U.S.A.

J. Todd Weber   National Center for Infectious Diseases, Centers for Disease Control and Prevention, Atlanta, Georgia, U.S.A.

1

How to Create a Therapeutics Committee That Is Scientifically and Economically Sound

RICHARD QUINTILIANI

University of Connecticut School of
Medicine, Farmington, and University
of Connecticut School of Pharmacy
Storrs, Connecticut, U.S.A.

ROBERT A. QUERCIA

Hartford Hospital, Hartford, and University of
Connecticut School of Pharmacy
Storrs, Connecticut, U.S.A.

One of the primary challenges in today's medical environment is to find treatments that provide good clinical outcomes but also satisfy pressures on heath care professionals and hospitals to deliver health care as cost effectively as possible. To attain this goal, a hospital must have a therapeutics committee that is both scientifically and economically sound. From the combined experience of more than 25 years as both a chairman of a therapeutics committee (R. Quintiliani) and a director of drug informational services (Robert Quercia) at Hartford Hospital, a large tertiary hospital in New England, we discuss ways to accomplish this goal, with particular attention paid to anti-infective agents.

CONFOUNDING PROBLEMS WITH CONTROLLING DRUG COSTS AND BEST DRUG SELECTION OWING TO PHYSICIAN BEHAVIOR

Unfortunately, physicians often view hospital pharmacies as "candy shops" where everything should be available regardless of its cost and without any restriction as to drug availability. Paradoxically, most physicians in their office practice have become compliant with drug limitations mandated by health maintenance organizations (HMOs) but have much greater trouble accepting this approach regarding their hospitalized patients. Often an adversarial relationship develops between physicians and hospitals that interferes with making cost-effective choices, because the physicians lack sympathy or concern for the economic problems of the hospital. Clinicians are beginning to understand that a hospital that constantly loses money will soon be replaced by a more cost-conscious hospital with even harsher restrictions, or be eliminated altogether.

Once a drug goes off patent, small generic companies typically produce the drug at a much lower cost. Traditionally, physicians have a fear of "generic" products, with concerns about the reliability of their bioavailability and quality control issues in general. This is unfortunate because the Food and Drug Administration (FDA) now scrutinizes generic companies as intensely as it does any major pharmaceutical company. Pharmacy departments, without the approval of any committee in the hospital, including the therapeutics committee, should be allowed to make an automatic substitution of a brand-name drug with a generic equivalent, with the exception of sustained-released medications.

Another disturbing issue is how rapidly clinicians become "obsolete" because they do not keep up with the medical literature and because of infrequent attendance at medical education sessions such as grand rounds and state and national meetings. Because of this obsolescence, clinicians often become easy prey for pharmaceutical representatives, who may provide information that may be overly biased for their product. This problem is now being remedied in many states by requiring physician attendance at a certain number of continuing medical education sessions to maintain medical licensure.

Clinicians are prone to make judgments on anecdotal observations and testimonials rather than from evidence-based medicine. In our therapeutics committee, we try hard to avoid use of any anecdotal or testimonial comments in decision making regarding whether a drug should be added or deleted from the formulary. Once this type of nonquantifiable information is permitted, the entire integrity and effectiveness of the committee is destroyed

Unwillingness to change old prescribing habits has been another dilemma for therapeutics committees. For decades, physicians have adopted the simplistic dosing method often suggested in antibiotic package inserts, i.e., all you have to know is to give a low, moderate, or high dosage of an antibiotic, depending on the severity of the infection. Another mistake is the belief that injectable antibiotics are always more potent than their oral formulations. Dosing in this fashion often results in suboptimal clinical outcomes, increased drug toxicity, and higher costs. The return of dosing beta-lactams by continuous infusion (1), the novel once-daily dosing of aminoglycosides (2), and the growing popularity using oral antibiotics (3) in serious infections are classic examples of using recent pharmacodynamic observations (4, 5) to optimize the best clinical responses and to minimize the emergence of bacterial resistance, toxicity, and increased costs.

To many clinicians, these new dosing methods run such a "collision course" with old dosing methods that they will not accept any changes. To deal with this problem, many hospitals, including ours, have adopted an automatic conversion policy whereby pharmacists are authorized to change dosing methods if there is adequate scientific information to make these conversions and the policy has been approved by the hospital's therapeutics committee and the medical executive committee of the staff. Educational efforts, such as newsletters distributed to the medical staff, are important and serve a beneficial purpose but by themselves are inadequate. For example, we permit our pharmacists to convert an order for intermittent dosing of gentamicin or tobramycin to once-daily dosing—except for some unusual situations, such as endocarditis—and to switch patients from intravenous to oral therapy for antibiotics with over 90% bioavailability, as long as the patient meets the criteria for transitional therapy, which will be elaborated on later.

CONFOUNDING PROBLEMS CONTROLLING DRUG COSTS AND BEST DRUG SELECTION OWING TO PHARMACEUTICAL COMPANY ACTIVITIES

Influencing physician choices can be accomplished by approaches that are disguised as educational support. Probably one of the most inappropriate ways is for a company to provide a large "educational" grant to a member or a department of the hospital. These grants typically have nothing to do with education or research projects that warrant grant support. These "educational" grants become subtle ways to maintain support for their product by creating a close alliance, typically with members of the staff who are on the therapeutics committee. These uncontrolled grants should really be viewed as bribes and not allowed. These educational grants from drug companies should not be accepted unless the funds are given to a general fund available to anyone in the hospital or are used to defray overall hospital operational expenses.

Use of drug samples is another method to undermine a therapeutic committee's decision and becomes a way to "seed" a drug. Sampling should not be allowed unless the drugs are given for specific indications approved by the therapeutics committee. Moreover, there is the potential for serious medico-legal problems for the hospital because the pharmacy is required by law to maintain precise records on samples given to patients in case of a major adverse reaction to the drug. Maintaining records and ensuring compliance to the sampling policy creates considerable labor costs for the pharmacy.

Information presented at national and international meetings sponsored by drug companies should be viewed with great skepticism. Only information from these meetings that has been published in peer review journals should be used in comparing and evaluating agents. It should be underscored that of every three abstracts presented at these meetings, only one ever gets published. Unfortunately, pharmaceutical companies often use these types of meetings to popularize a drug for a non-FDA indication, to avoid the major expense of performing a properly scientifically designed study.

Likewise, information presented at drug company–sponsored grand rounds, focus group meetings, continuing education programs at resorts, and dinner meetings should be carefully scrutinized. These presentations can be a valuable source of information as long as the speaker is a highly recognized authority on the subject matter and provides published references for the information given during the presentation.

These unethical approaches to marketing drugs for non-FDA indications have most recently been a primary tactic used by some pharmaceutical companies. It predicted this method of marketing will be deterred by ongoing investigations of these practices by the federal government and new legislation.

Similar to speakers, pharmaceutical representatives may vary tremendously in their knowledge and integrity. It is typical today for representatives from major pharmaceutical companies to attend in-depth training sessions about their products for months. Many are well informed about their products and can provide valuable, accurate information but seldom provide the downside of their products. Moreover, their information about a competitor's product may be meager. To remedy this situation, one should try to integrate the information provided about a product from competing companies, and then match these comments with data obtained from scientifically designed studies. Unless the therapeutics committee can review so-called data on file from a pharmaceutical company, any information of this type should not be used in determining the merits of a particular drug.

Another important caution of pharmaceutical representatives is their behavior in promoting drugs within the hospital. There needs to be formal policies sanctioned by the therapeutics committee that define promotional practices within the institution. These policies should be designed so that the pharmaceutical representatives' practices are not disruptive to the medical staff or contradictory to the policies and protocols approved by the therapeutics committee. Representatives can promote formulary drugs only according to the protocols or recommendations of the therapeutics committee.

We have a policy that states pharmaceutical representatives are not allowed to meet with physicians, nurses, or pharmacists in patient care areas, and can only meet with them by a prearranged appointment in a non–patient care area. Once business has been completed, the representative must proceed directly to a public hospital area (e.g., main lobby). In addition, in-servicing of nonformulary drugs on the hospital campus is prohibited.

To further control and monitor pharmaceutical representatives' activities, we have created a special committee composed of a hospital pharmacist and pharmaceutical representatives to investigate and punish those representatives who violate the policies mentioned above. In the case of a representative who is judged as having behavior inconsistent with these policies, the punishment usually involves banishment from the hospital facilities for 6 to 12 months. The members from industry on this committee are rotated on an annual basis.

Direct-to-consumer advertising policy by industry has also indirectly become a problem for therapeutics committees. These advertisements often encourage consumers to demand pricey drugs over cheaper ones that work just as well. The clinicians on the hospital staff then often make similar demands to the therapeutics committee to add the more expensive agents to the formulary. The percentage of industry spending on direct-to-consumer advertising has increased dramatically in the past 10 years. A review of this activity in 2002 by Competitive Media Reporting showed that about 60% of a company's spending on a drug may come from this form of advertising. The major classes of drugs that use this form of advertisement include, in decreasing order, anti-inflammatories, antihistamines, antihyperlipidemics, antiasthmatics, antiulcer drugs, antidepressants, erectile dysfunction drugs, weight loss drugs, oral contraceptives, genital herpes drugs, toenail fungus agents, and hormones. It is interesting that direct-to-consumer advertisement remains relatively low for antimicrobials.

IMPORTANCE OF THE COMPOSITION AND BACKGROUND OF THERAPEUTICS COMMITTEE MEMBERS

The chairperson of the therapeutics committee should be a physician who is economically independent of referrals from other physicians; hence, that person usually is a full-time hospital salaried employee. Unfortunately, chairpersons of many therapeutics committees, especially in small hospitals, often come from private practice, where they earn much, if not their entire income from referrals. This creates a practical dilemma for the chairperson, who is often reluctant to deny a request for a formulary addition, particularly from a colleague who is a major source of referrals.

The membership on the committee should be very broad based and should have representation from all areas of the hospital that have any involvement with drug usage, distribution, or purchase. For instance, at our hospital, we have representation from all medical and surgical departments and their divisions, nursing, nutritional services, pharmacy, research, risk management, emergency department, outpatient department, house staff, administration, drug informational services, clinical pharmacists, and even individuals from outside HMOs. It is unusual to have representatives from HMOs, but we have found that their presence on the committee often influences their formulary choices, resulting in a greater chance for similar formularies. This similarity usually creates more "seamless" care for the patient leaving the hospital for the community setting.

All members should sign a letter indicating whether they have any conflicts of interest, such as financial involvement with a pharmaceutical company as a paid consultant, major stockholder, recipient of large research grants, or member of speakers' bureaus. If a member has a conflict of interest of this type, that person should not be allowed to vote on the approval or disapproval of any of those companies' products. If a member is commonly absent for the meetings, that person should be replaced.

Except for unusual circumstances, the person requesting the addition of a drug to the formulary should not be present at the therapeutics committee meeting, especially if that person is highly influential. This person's presence may indirectly sway decisions owing to a tendency for members not to anger this person. On rare occasions, having such a person attend makes sense, but no vote should be made in his/her presence.

ESTABLISHMENT OF PRIORITIES BY THE THERAPEUTICS COMMITTEE

A common mistake of therapeutics committees is to spend an inordinate amount of time on drugs that are relatively inexpensive or nontoxic and devote minimal effort in controlling the expensive or toxic agents. Considerable attention should be directed at agents that create a major impact on the pharmacy budget. What is considered "major" will vary with the size of the hospital and the complexity of its services. At our tertiary hospital, any drug that requires more than $100,000 in expenditures is deemed worthy of special attention, to limit its inappropriate use. Special attention usually means the creation of a protocol for its usage along with a drug utilization review, which will be discussed later. Often drugs of this type may be given in an appropriate clinical situation but at the wrong dose, dosing interval, or mode of administration.

At our hospital, where many total knee and hip replacements are performed, about $200,000 was being spent annually on the use of tobramycin powder as a prophylactic agent impregnated in the bone cement. There were two reasons for this large expenditure: one was the large acquisition cost for aminoglycoside powder now that gentamicin powder is no longer available; the other was its use in primary implant procedures in which there were no evidence-based data for its use in this situation. After an extensive review of the literature and discussions with other large academic orthopedic departments, it became apparent that the use of tobramycin powder was inappropriate in primary joint replacements. The only possible acceptable situation for the use of the powder was in secondary or revision procedures. Through meeting with our orthopedic department, we were able to convince them to adhere to these restrictions. Because only 8% of the orthopedic joint replacement at our hospital was for revisions, we immediately recognized $160,000 in savings.

It is important in deciding on the merits of a drug to avoid nonpharmacological issues that do not pertain to the responsibilities of the therapeutics committee. These could include items such as decisions made on the agent from nearby competitive hospitals' therapeutics committees, effects on referral patterns, and nursing time. These are issues that should be addressed by other committees in the hospital. It is crucial that therapeutics committees stay within their "therapeutic box." For instance, if the nursing department is displeased with the addition of a drug to the formulary because it creates more labor time for them, then that issue should be discussed by the nursing department with their administrator and the medical executive committee of the hospital. To maintain an efficient therapeutics committee, issues that cannot be resolved there should not be addressed there.

In highly controversial decisions made by the therapeutics committee, it often makes sense for the chairperson, as well as the director of pharmacy services, to attend the medical executive committee meeting to defend the decision and to respond to any questions or comments.

Because the medical executive committee of the staff must approve all decisions made by the therapeutics committee, this final approval may often be delayed for an excessive time period, resulting in prolonged delays before the actual implementation of an important cost-containing recommendation. To resolve this problem, we have developed a "fast-track" system whereby selective decisions of our therapeutics committee that may translate into major economic savings or the avoidance of serious adverse reactions are given priority at the next meeting of the executive committee.

Another important approach to maintain a well-managed and efficient therapeutics committee is not to review again a drug that was rejected for formulary addition unless acquisition cost has significantly decreased or some very unusual new favorable findings were published pertaining to this agent.

The creation of extremely expensive drugs from new technology has resulted in a huge increase in acquisition costs for pharmacies. Classic examples of this situation are drugs such as drotrecogin alfa (Xigris) and liposomal formulations. For these types of agents, it is crucial to establish a protocol that has to be followed by all physicians and can be monitored with respect to physician compliance to the protocol. Restricting the ordering of these drugs to a selected specialist(s) has been used by many hospitals; however, this policy may not only be ineffective, it also may worsen the economic situation, particularly if the designated specialist(s) uses this power to indirectly increase his/her consultation services. The answer to controlling the expenses of these extremely pricey drugs is to create protocols accompanied by drug utilization evaluations, which will be discussed later.

THE ROLE OF THE DRUG INFORMATION PHARMACISTS IN THE REVIEW OF DRUGS FOR THE HOSPITAL FORMULARY

The primary objective for the drug information pharmacist is to review drugs for formulary addition or deletion based on safety, efficacy, and cost that makes scientific sense. Information about an agent for possible addition to or deletion from the formulary should be compared with existing agents in the same drug class. The data for this review should come as much as possible from literature published in peer review journals. Moreover, the data are best when they are quantifiable and subject to statistical analysis. In some instances, further evaluation may require consultation with outside agencies (e.g., FDA) and recognized authorities from other medical institutions pertaining to the agent in question. In drug class reviews, we routinely obtain input and consensus from the appropriate medical or surgical department prior to presentation to the therapeutics committee.

The efficacy data are based almost exclusively on the drug's pharmacokinetic, pharmacodynamic, and safety properties, as well as on clinical outcomes. In comparing two closely similar agents for addition to the formulary, one should avoid making a choice exclusively on acquisition costs, often referred to as a *minimalization analysis*. To do this, both agents should be "mirror images" of each other.

After safety and efficacy are determined, it is important for the pharmacist to provide a comparative financial analysis that is reflective of the institution's cost and reimbursement policies in order to properly integrate cost with the safety and efficacy data in the final evaluation for presentation to the therapeutics committee. Many times, pharmaceutical companies will provide elaborate cost comparative analysis, but in most instances, the data are not reflective of your institution. The drug information pharmacist should seek the assistance of the finance department in analyzing complex reimbursement issues.

Sometimes expensive drugs that have excellent reimbursement by insurance companies or the government may actually create a net profit for the hospital because the reimbursement for the drug may exceed the acquisition cost. This has been a common observation with a number of drugs to treat AIDS and patients on hemodialysis. To determine the economic impact on a hospital's overall budget of bringing a drug onto the formulary, one must always compare revenue versus acquisition cost whenever possible.

It has been our policy that the drug information pharmacist must first evaluate all drugs submitted for formulary addition for a minimum of two weeks before its placement on the agenda of the therapeutics committee. If this review suggests that an agent should not be added to the hospital drug formulary, it has been our practice to have either the drug information pharmacist or the chairman of the therapeutics committee contact the requesting physician before the meeting as to the reasons for the negative review. This approach has been beneficial in our relationship with physicians because it allows them the opportunity to respond before the meeting. The physician is often unaware of the drawbacks to the requested drug and often will withdraw his/her request upon hearing this information. Occasionally the physician will provide us with very important information that we failed to uncover in our review.

After completion of all drug reviews for the agenda, it is very important for the drug information pharmacist to present the results of the reviews to the chairman of the therapeutics committee before the actual meeting so he/she will be prepared to explain the basis for the recommendations from the drug information pharmacist. In brief, the drug information pharmacist behaves as a consultant to the therapeutics committee and especially to its chairperson. As any other good consultant, it is always best to be "on tap," but not "on top."

THE IMPORTANCE OF DRUG USE EVALUATIONS AND PROTOCOLS IN CONTROLLING THE USE OF EXPENSIVE AND/ OR POTENTIALLY TOXIC AGENTS

Protocols provide for rational care and result in the best clinical outcomes, lower toxicity, and lower costs. Moreover, they often protect the prescribing physician from malpractice suits because the drug is being used according to acceptable standards. Protocols also create a measurable way to check on physician adherence to the appropriate use of drugs. Because of the importance of the information given in protocols, they should be developed by persons most knowledgeable with the use of the drug and, if possible, should coincide with recommendations given by nationally recognized academic groups (e.g., Infectious Disease Society, Centers for Disease Control, American Thoracic Society).

Enforcement of protocols is essential. Protocols that are not part of a drug use evaluation (DUE) are more prone to noncompliance, especially when there are staffing deficiencies within the clinical section of the department of pharmacy services. Although a protocol drug should not be dispensed by the pharmacy until all protocol criteria have been met, it is often difficult to enforce when clinical pharmacists are not available and/or not assigned to monitor compliance to the protocol.

The establishment of a DUE protocol is preferable to the establishment of a non-DUE protocol because the criteria in a DUE protocol are usually tracked on a prospective or concurrent basis. At our hospital, noncompliant physicians who arbitrarily and consistently ignore DUE protocol criteria are reported to the therapeutics committee on a monthly basis. The chairperson of the therapeutics committee then sends a formal letter to that physician's department chief requesting him/her to take action on the noncompliance of the prescriber and to report back to the chairperson that appropriate action has been taken. This action is also documented with a letter placed into the physician's file. If the physician continues to be noncompliant, he/she is requested to explain his/her activities to the medical executive committee of the staff and faces potential loss of staff privileges. This quality assurance process for DUEs provides for enhanced compliance to therapeutics committee–approved protocols. In addition, the performing of DUEs meets a requirement of the Joint Commission on the Accreditation of Healthcare Organizations (JCAHO).

In a closely similar fashion, by the use of a "one-time-use" form, we maintain a tightly controlled formulary and do not allow physicians to carelessly use nonformulary drugs when there are appropriate and less expensive alternatives. At our hospital, the physician must complete this one-time-use form describing the reasons for requesting a nonformulary drug. The pharmacists must document that formulary alternatives were suggested to the physician and make a clinical decision as to whether there is agreement or disagreement with the physician's request. Although we do not hold up medical therapy, if there is disagreement between the physician and the pharmacist, our drug information services and the therapeutics committee, on a monthly basis, review all the one-time-use requests for appropriateness. If the therapeutics committee deems the nonformulary request to be inappropriate, a formal letter is sent from the chairperson of the therapeutics committee to the prescribing physician and copied to his/her department chief indicating the therapeutics committee's reasons for this view and stressing that this practice should not occur again. This practice at our hospital has significantly curtailed the inappropriate use of nonformulary agents.

It must be stressed that protocols are not guidelines. Unfortunately, guidelines, as the word implies, are only suggestions as to how a drug should be used, resulting in too many arbitrary choices by clinicians and the false sense that the hospital is actually controlling drug usage.

THE PHARMACY DEPARTMENT'S ROLE IN THE CREATION OF A THERAPEUTICS COMMITTEE THAT IS SCIENTIFICALLY AND ECONOMICALLY SOUND

Pharmacy services should be integrated in a major way with the activities of the therapeutics committee and the hospital's responsibility to patient care and safety. In addition to the role of the drug information pharmacist discussed above, the following constitutes some of the other major responsibilities of other members of the pharmacy department in ensuring proper drug usage:

- Chair DUE subcommittee of the therapeutics committee and ensure development and implementation of DUE programs.
- Correct improper dosing before the patient actually receives the agent.

- Be allowed to automatically replace intravenous antibiotics with oral agents that have high bioavailability (e.g., greater than 90%) in a clinically stable patient who can ingest and digest a medication. These interchanges are ones that have been approved by the therapeutics committee and the medical executive committee of the staff.
- Alert clinicians to possible adverse reactions and interactions of prescribed drugs.
- Ensure that the physician for nonformulary medications properly completes one-time-use request forms.
- Replace expensive drugs with less expensive, therapeutically equivalent agents that have been established by the therapeutics committee.
- Monitor compliance with protocols for selective drugs and report to the therapeutics committee clinicians who consistently ignore them.
- Make rounds with house staff, particularly in intensive care units, serving as a consultant on drug dosing and interactions.
- Distribute monthly information, usually in the form of a newsletter to all members of the staff, on drugs that have been added or withdrawn from the formulary.

Of all the activities mentioned above, the most effective ones have been those that have involved automatic conversions, particularly the replacement of intravenous with oral agents or so-called transitional or switch therapy (6, 7). Unfortunately, often clinicians feel threatened by empowering pharmacists to change their orders, usually from a concern that the pharmacist is usurping the role of the physician. This is obviously not the case, because it is the clinician who initially establishes the choice of therapy; all the pharmacist is doing is customizing therapy according to appropriate pharmacokinetic and pharmacoeconomic reasons. If transition programs are left entirely up to physicians, they rarely occur at all or occur too late to reap the economic gains (less drug acquisition and supply costs, less nursing and pharmacy labor costs) or the avoidance of intravenous line sepsis, the leading cause of nosocomial bacteremia or fungemia.

Physicians are often reluctant to change to an oral drug for two major reasons. The first one is that they view "injectables" as more "potent" than oral therapy. It is true that the modest bioavailability, i.e., less than 50%, of some oral antibiotics may be a legitimate reason not to use such agents; however, for drugs with 90% or greater bioavailability, this concern makes little, if any, sense. In fact, we now have a number of antimicrobial agents that meet this criterion, including levofloxacin, gatifloxacin, moxifloxacin, doxycycline, minocycline, trimethoprim/sulfamethoxazole, clindamycin, cephalexin, cefadroxil, cefprozil, ceftibuten, linezolid, rifampin, fluconazole, metronidazole, and voriconazole. It may sound cynical, but we like to remind clinicians that organisms have no idea whether the drug was given intravenously, intramuscularly, or orally, or whether it was given within or outside a hospital!

The second major reason for the poor acceptance of transitional therapy by clinicians relates to the pressures placed on them by some utilization review committees and insurance companies to discharge their patient once the patient has been changed to an oral antibiotic. Pressuring physicians to discharge patients once they are on oral therapy should no longer be done, for often there are many other reasons a particular patient should remain hospitalized. This behavior of utilization review committees and insurance companies has really backfired because the clinicians' response has been merely to leave the intravenous line in place, resulting in a marked increase in the chances for line sepsis, which in turn, causes an appreciable increase in cost, morbidity, and mortality. It is well known that the likelihood of line sepsis increases precipitously in patients in whom the line has stayed in place beyond 4 days. Because of these confounding problems, we have used our pharmacist as a major way to develop a highly effective proactive transitional program, with most conversions to oral therapy occurring within 2 to 3 days.

Successful transitional antibiotic programs require physician acceptance. Indeed, all clinicians within an institution must trust that transition programs will not only be safe and effective for patients but also provide benefits for the institution. One way to enhance acceptance is to make it clear that even though transitional therapy is appropriate in most cases, it is not expected to be used in all patients. In other words, transition therapy program changes are not intended to supersede clinical judgment.

Some practical steps that we have found to optimize cooperation and support from clinicians include the following:

- Review and present literature demonstrating the benefit of transition therapy.
- Conduct educational sessions to review the goals of the program and practical issues in implementation. Stress that the program addresses not only the financial concerns of the hospital but also the health of the patient, offering the possibility of earlier discharge and a reduced potential for hospitalization-related complications, such as line sepsis.
- Create user-friendly tools to assist in clinical decision making; these may include computer programs for screening and monitoring or simple algorithms with criteria for transition therapy and/or discharge.
- Create an infrastructure for implementing the program with components that include a system for tracking both clinical and economic outcomes.
- Strive to communicate successful results among clinical colleagues and enhance overall confidence in the process through newsletters and in-services.
- Allocate a budget for staffing and support. Consider that the overall savings will be greater than additional costs for support services and staff.
- Empower pharmacy to make automatic conversions based on criteria established by the therapeutics committee and approved by the medical executive committee of the staff.

CONCLUSIONS

Owing to the many confounding problems facing therapeutics committees, it has become extremely difficult to develop a committee that is both economically and scientifically sound. Most of these confounding problems come from the pressures of non-scientific, immeasurable variables, such as anecdotal observations, testimonials, and unreliable and unpublished data from meetings, abstracts, and non–peer reviewed journals. Quantifiable data are always the best because they are subject to statistical analysis. In fact, many curmudgeons feel if you cannot measure it, it is not worth addressing and until data are published in highly peer-reviewed scientific journals, there are no data! Strong integration of the activities of the therapeutics committee with pharmacy services has become crucial for the creation of a therapeutics committee that is both economically and scientifically sound and is the reason the term *therapeutics committee* is often replaced in hospitals by the name *pharmacy and therapeutics committee*.

REFERENCES

1. Richerson MA, Ambrose PG, Bui KQ, Grant E. Pharmacokinetic and economic evaluation of piperacillin/tazobactam administered as either continuous or intermittent infusion with once-daily gentamicin Infect Dis Clin Pract 1999; 8:195–200.

2. Nicolau DP, Freeman CD, Belliveau PP, Nightingale CH, Ross JW, Quintiliani R. Experience with a once-daily aminoglycoside program administered to 2,184 adult patients Antimicrob Agents Chemother 1995; 39:650–655.

3. Quintiliani R. Strategies for the Cost-Effective Use of Antibiotics. In: Gorbach SL,, Blacklow NR, Eds Infectious Diseases, Part IV. Treatment of Infectious Disease. Philadelphia: W.B. Saunders, 1998.

4. McNabb JC, Quintiliani R, Nicolau DP. Cost Effectiveness in the Use of Antibiotics In: Current Topics in Infectious Diseases, 2000:24–42.

5. Craig WA. Pharmacokinetic/pharmacodynamic parameters: rationale for antibacterial dosing of mice and men Clin Infect Dis 1998; 26:1–12.

6. Milkovich G. Intravenous-to-oral transition therapy in community-acquired pneumonia: the INOVA Health System experience Pharmacotherapy 2001; 21(7 Pt 2):83S–88S.

7. Kuti JL, Thuy NL, Nightingale CH, Nicolau DP, Quintiliani R. Pharmacoeconomics of a pharmacist-managed program for automatically converting levofloxacin route from i.v. to oral Am J Health Syst Pharm 2002; 59:2209–2215.

2

The *Public Health Action Plan to Combat Antimicrobial Resistance* and the Prevention of Antimicrobial Resistance in Health Care Settings

J. TODD WEBER

National Center for Infectious Diseases,
Centers for Disease Control and Prevention
Atlanta, Georgia, U.S.A.

THE *PUBLIC HEALTH ACTION PLAN TO COMBAT ANTIMICROBIAL RESISTANCE*

Antimicrobial resistance (AR) will always be with us. The challenge before us is to transform this increasingly urgent threat into a manageable problem. Over the past 10 years, the Institute of Medicine (1,2), the American Society for Microbiology (3), the World Health Organization (4,5), the Congressional

Office of Technology Assessment (6), the General Accounting Office (7,8), and other panels of distinguished experts have provided recommendations and options for government action to address the dangers posed by AR. The experts agree that we need to improve surveillance for emerging AR problems, to prolong the useful life of antimicrobial drugs, to develop new drugs, and to improve vaccine, diagnostic, and infection control measures to prevent and control AR.

Despite the urgency of the problem, the achievement of these goals has not been simple or straightforward, and accomplishments to date have been modest. Monitoring, preventing, and controlling AR requires sustained effort, commitment, and collaboration among many groups in the public and private sectors, and the involvement of the general public. Support and leadership are required from the federal government, combined with a willingness to address complex and sometimes controversial scientific, medical, and economic issues.

To provide a blueprint for federal actions to address the emerging threat of AR, the *Public Health Action Plan to Combat Antimicrobial Resistance* was developed by the Federal Interagency Task Force on AR and released in January 2001 (http://www.cdc.gov/drugresistance/actionplan/index.htm) (9). The task force was formed in 1999 because federal government experts in infectious diseases and AR understood that to adequately address the multifaceted problem of AR, cooperative action by multiple agencies and departments would be required. Co-chaired by the Centers for Disease Control and Prevention (CDC), the Food and Drug Administration (FDA), and the National Institutes of Health (NIH), the task force also includes the Agency for Healthcare Research and Quality (AHRQ), the Centers for Medicare and Medicaid Services (CMS), the Health Resources and Services Administration (HRSA), the Department of Agriculture (USDA), the Department of Defense (DOD), the Department of Veterans Affairs (VA), the Environmental Protection Agency (EPA), and, since 2001, the U.S. Agency for International Development (USAID). Encouraging the creation of the task force were a forum and a hearing on AR that were held by the U.S. Senate committees in 1999 and 2000, respectively, chaired by Senators Bill Frist (R-Tenn.) and Edward Kennedy (D-Mass.).

The plan was developed based on input from consultants from state and local health agencies, universities, professional societies, pharmaceutical companies, health care delivery organizations, agricultural producers, consumer groups, and other members of the public. The plan has been and will continue to be implemented incrementally, in collaboration with these and other partners, as resources become available. The plan has four focus areas: surveillance, prevention and control, research, and product development. Of eighty-four action items, thirteen are designated top priority (Box 1). Activities have been launched or completed for the thirteen top priority items as well as most of the other action items. The task force continues to meet to monitor implementation of the plan, releases annual progress reports, and seeks comment at public meetings (http://www.cdc.gov/drugresistance/actionplan/2003report/index.htm). This chapter focuses on issues and activities that are relevant to surveillance and prevention and control of AR in the community and health care settings.

Surveillance

In the United States, disease reporting is under state jurisdiction, but most states do not require reporting of drug susceptibility information, and the completeness of reporting varies. In collaboration with state health departments and other partners, CDC monitors resistance for several pathogens of public health importance and collects limited data on antimicrobial drug prescribing. For example, resistance in invasive *Streptococcus pneumoniae* infections is monitored on a population basis in nine states or portions thereof (with two additional states planning similar surveillance) through the Emerging Infections Program (EIP); similarly, health care–associated infections (e.g., *Staphylococcus aureus*, enterococci, gram-negative bacteria) are monitored in approximately 300 hospitals, and food-borne pathogens such as *Salmonella* are monitored in fifty states in a joint project that also involves FDA and USDA. In this project, resistance in food-borne pathogens

Box 1   Top Priority Action Items to Combat Antimicrobial
Resistance   (All thirteen items have top priority, regardless of
their order in the list)

Surveillance

With partners, design and implement a national antimicrobial resistance
  (AR) surveillance plan that defines national, regional, state, and local
  surveillance activities and the roles of clinical, reference, public health,
  and veterinary laboratories. The plan should be consistent with local and
  national surveillance methodology and infrastructure that currently exist
  or are being developed. (Action Item #2)
Develop and implement procedures for monitoring patterns of antimicrobial
  drug use in human medicine, agriculture, veterinary medicine, and consumer products. (Action Item #5)

Prevention and control

Conduct a public health education campaign to promote appropriate antimicrobial use as a national health priority. (Action Item #25)
In collaboration with many partners, develop and facilitate the implementation of educational and behavioral interventions that will assist clinicians in appropriate antimicrobial prescribing. (Action Item #26)
Evaluate the effectiveness (including cost-effectiveness) of current and
  novel infection-control practices for health care and extended care settings and in the community. Promote adherence to practices proven to be
  effective. (Action Item #39)
In consultation with stakeholders, refine and implement the proposed FDA
  framework for approving new antimicrobial drugs for use in food-animal
  production and, when appropriate, for re-evaluating currently approved
  veterinary antimicrobial drugs. (Action Item #58)
Support demonstration projects to evaluate comprehensive strategies that
  use multiple interventions to promote appropriate drug use and reduce
  infection rates, in order to assess how interventions found effective in research studies can be applied routinely and most cost-effectively on a
  large scale. (Action Item #63)

Research

Provide the research community genomics and other powerful technologies
  to identify targets in critical areas for the development of new rapid diagnostics methodologies, novel therapeutics, and interventions to prevent
  the emergence and spread of resistant pathogens. (Action Item #70)

Box 1 *Continued*

Research (*Con't*)

In consultation with academia and the private sector, identify and conduct human clinical studies addressing AR issues of public health significance that are unlikely to be studied in the private sector (e.g., novel therapies, new treatment regimens, and other products and practices). (Action Item #75)

Identify, develop, test, and evaluate new rapid diagnostic methods for human and veterinary uses with partners, including academia and the private sector. Such methods should be accurate, affordable, and easily implemented in routine clinical settings (e.g., tests for resistance genes, point-of-care diagnostics for patients with respiratory infections and syndromes, and diagnostics for drug resistance in microbial pathogens, including in nonculture specimens). (Action Item #76)

Encourage basic and clinical research in support of the development and appropriate use of vaccines in human and veterinary medicine in partnership with academia and the private sector. (Action Item #77)

Product development

Create an Interagency AR Product Development Working Group to identify and publicize priority public health needs in human and animal medicine for new AR products (e.g., innovative drugs, targeted spectrum antibiotics, point-of-care diagnostics, vaccines and other biologics, anti-infective medical devices, and disinfectants). (Action Item #79)

Identify ways (e.g., financial and/or other incentives or investments) to promote the development and/or appropriate use of priority AR products, such as novel compounds and approaches, for human and veterinary medicine for which market incentives are inadequate. (Action Item #80)

---

and commensal organisms is also monitored in animals (and, beginning in 2001, in retail meat products). For the past 10 years, the United States has had a national tuberculosis (TB) surveillance system that includes susceptibility data. The TB surveillance system collects information on drug susceptibility testing (initial and final results), initial drug regimen, and date therapy started and date therapy stopped for culture-positive patients. This information allows monitoring of the epidemiology of drug resistance so that appropriate interventions can be implemented. For example, information on the initial drug regimen prescribed coupled with information on initial drug susceptibility results allows a judgment about the adequacy of therapy and corrective action on individual cases by public health officials and health care providers if the regimen is judged to be inadequate or suboptimal.

For most other infections in most communities, a similar system that provides patient specific data is not needed to help develop and evaluate national prevention and control strategies. However, awareness of the extent to which resistance is present locally is important to guide treatment decisions and to generate support for local public health interventions such as appropriate drug use and vaccine campaigns. To implement the action plan, CDC seeks to support coordinated national surveillance of drug resistance and use at two levels. One involves surveillance that can be done by most states, communities, and health care systems to meet their local needs; the second consists of more specialized projects to monitor emerging problems and addresses in more detail specific national needs.

At a meeting held at CDC among state health department personnel and other experts in surveillance, there was consensus that statistically sound methods of data collection that capture valid, meaningful, and useful data must also meet the financial restrictions of state budgets (10). Active, population-based surveillance for collecting relevant isolates is considered the gold standard. Unfortunately, this type of surveillance is labor intensive and costly, making it an impractical choice for many states. The challenges of isolate collection, packaging and transport, data collection, and analysis may place an unacceptable workload on laboratory and epidemiology personnel.

Several state health departments have elected to implement enhanced antimicrobial drug-resistance surveillance programs using alternative surveillance methods. Two methods frequently used by states are sentinel (i.e., survey of subset of laboratories) and antibiogram (i.e., cumulative susceptibility data) surveillance. Common difficulties have been identified with implementing sentinel systems. Those difficulties include logistical obstacles with isolate or data processing and communication breakdowns between laboratory, epidemiology, and hospital infection control personnel. Care must be taken in selecting the numbers and types of laboratories to participate in a sentinel network. States collecting antibiograms from hospitals and state laboratories may also face challenges, including incompatible formatting of drug-testing panels, the inconsistent inclusion of duplicate or repeat isolates, and inconsistent reporting of denominator data. Solutions to these problems commonly involve improving communication between clinical microbiology laboratories and state health departments, including laboratory input in decision making and providing feedback of data from the system to participants. Guidance for aggregating cumulative susceptibility data (i.e., antibiograms) has been published and may serve as a guide for states and clinical microbiology laboratories in conducting surveillance (11). Another aspect of surveillance focuses on detecting rare events. Such events may include new changes in susceptibility, new mechanisms of resistance, susceptibility of unusual pathogens, and unexpected sources of resistant organisms. Establishing good communication among personnel in health departments and clinical laboratories is important for improving detection and reporting of such events. Allocating resources for improved surveillance is a practical and responsive step for states interested in tracking local resistant trends. Local data are important for raising public awareness, establishing resources and prevention activities, developing and informing treatment guidelines, monitoring trends, and motivating behavior change among clinicians.

At nine CDC EIP sites, surveillance is conducted for invasive bacterial diseases due to pathogens of public health importance through a project called Active Bacterial Core Surveillance (ABCs). For each case of invasive disease in the study population, a case report with basic demographic information is filed and, in most cases, the isolates (which have been cultured from a sample obtained from a normally sterile site such as blood or cerebral spinal fluid) from patients are sent to CDC for laboratory study. For *S. pneumoniae*, objectives are to track AR in pneumococcal isolates, to evaluate the impact of new pneumococcal conjugate vaccines for infants on disease burden, and to evaluate prevention among the elderly through pneumococcal polysaccharide vaccine use. Other infections under surveillance in this system include group A streptococcus, group B streptococcus, *Haemophilus influenzae*, and *Neisseria meningitidis*. Case finding is active and laboratory based. Because isolation of one of these organisms from a normally sterile site is essential to the case definition, the microbiology laboratories in acute care hospitals and appropriate reference laboratories processing sterile site specimens for residents of the surveillance area are the sources for case identification. Data that are essential for describing the population-based epidemiology of these diseases (e.g., age, residence within the surveillance area, outcome) are not available in many microbiology laboratories. Therefore, the case identification is complemented by additional data collection to complete a standard case report form. ABCs can be utilized to conduct surveillance for emerging infections, as is the case with community-associated methicillin-resistant *S. aureus* (CA-MRSA). Population-based surveillance for MRSA will be conducted in eight ABCs sites starting in 2004. Cases in these areas, with MRSA isolated from a normally sterile site, will be followed up by the health department or its public health partners, to measure the incidence and prevalence of MRSA in the population, characterize risk factors for infection, and describe the molecular epidemiologic patterns and microbiologic characteristics of health care–associated or CA-MRSA. Other population-based data on drug resistance include MRSA carriage in the community through the National Nutrition and Health Examination Survey (NHANES; http://www.cdc.gov/nchs/nhanes.htm) conducted by the National Center for Health Statistics. In NHANES, beginning in 2001, all participants 1 year of age or older were examined for nasal carriage of *S. aureus* and isolates underwent antibiotic susceptibility testing (AST). In addition, demographic and epidemiologic data were collected from participants and a selection of their households.

CDC is developing The National Healthcare Safety Network (NHSN), an Internet-based nationwide network that will monitor trends in adverse events associated with invasive devices, procedures, and medications used in the delivery of health care. Existing surveillance systems, including the National Nosocomial Infections System, the Dialysis Surveillance Network, and the National Surveillance System for Healthcare Workers will be a part of NHSN. In addition, under the NHSN's medication-associated Adverse Event Module, initial focus will be on use of and resistance to antimicrobial agents and on establishing electronic reporting of antimicrobial use and resistance data to increase efficiency, timeliness, and accuracy of the monitoring effort. When implemented, the NHSN will significantly enhance the ability to monitor and track trends of usage and resistance of microbes to antimicrobial agents in a variety of health care delivery settings. These data can then be used to enhance patient safety by enabling health care workers to develop and deploy strategies to prevent overuse and inappropriate use of these agents, as well as strategies to prevent other pathogens from becoming resistant.

CDC-supported projects monitor drug resistance for several other pathogens or infections, e.g., gonorrhea, influenza, *Helicobacter pylori*, HIV, and malaria.

Reliable surveillance information, as well as patient care and safety, depends on the accurate detection of drug resistance by clinical laboratories. New antimicrobial agents and new resistance patterns pose a challenge to clinical laboratories because testing methods vary with organism/antimicrobial agent combinations. NCCLS standards outline recommended procedures for AST but are difficult for some laboratories to interpret. To improve AST in clinical laboratories, CDC is working with partners such as the Association of Public Health Laboratories and the American Society for Microbiology to develop training and proficiency testing programs. In 2001, the Multilevel Antimicrobial Susceptibility Testing Educational Resource (MASTER) program was introduced on a website that includes discussions of difficult cases in diagnostic microbiology, recommendations and references, and opportunities to question CDC microbiologists (www.phppo.cdc.gov/dls/master/default.asp). In its first year of operation, this site received approximately 33,000 hits from twenty countries. The need for constant updating of clinical laboratory proficiency offers an opportunity for state public health laboratories to provide important leadership and strengthen their linkages with clinical laboratories. Through the National Laboratory Training Network and other programs, CDC's goal is to work with partners to ensure training and proficiency in drug resistance testing and reporting for clinical laboratories in all states and territories. In 2002, CDC produced a CD-ROM that assists laboratories in applying NCCLS standards, demonstrates the modes of action of each group of antimicrobial agents and the mechanisms organisms develop to resist the agents, describes quality control procedures needed to verify accuracy of testing results, and demonstrates specific procedures laboratories must use to detect resistance in different organisms. The CD may be requested at http://www.aphl.org/ast.cfm. More than 8,000 copies of the CD have been distributed throughout the United States and internationally.

Prevention and Control

Prevention and control of drug resistance primarily involves promoting appropriate use of antimicrobial drugs to extend their useful life and preventing infection transmission (e.g., through appropriate infection control and vaccine use). Appropriate antimicrobial drug use is defined as use that maximizes therapeutic impact while minimizing toxicity and the development of resistance. In practice, this means prescribing antimicrobial therapy when, and only when, beneficial to a patient; targeting therapy to the desired pathogens; and using the appropriate drug, dose, and duration. Prevention and control programs do not obviate the need for a constantly flowing "pipeline" of new drugs, as current drugs will inevitably become less effective with time because of resistance. CDC has been working with a variety of partners to promote appropriate antimicrobial use in the community (outpatient prescribing), in health care settings, and in agriculture (12).

For acute infections in outpatients, a major objective is to reduce antimicrobial drug prescribing for illnesses (e.g., viral respiratory infections) for which these drugs offer no benefit.

In 1995, CDC launched a National Campaign for Appropriate Antibiotic Use that involves partnerships with state and local health departments, health care delivery organizations, health care purchasers and insurers, professional societies, consumer groups, and others. Often working through state-based coalitions, these partners implement coordinated educational and behavioral interventions directed to patients and clinicians, including public education programs, prescribing principles, clinical training materials, and aids (e.g., "viral prescription pads") to help clinicians avoid prescribing an antibiotic when not indicated. Data from controlled trials indicate that these interventions may be effective in reducing inappropriate antibiotic prescribing for respiratory infections in the United States, as has been reported in other countries— although resistance rates of respiratory pathogens, having reached a certain level, may not necessarily decline thereafter (13–16). Encouraging data from the National Ambulatory Medical Care Survey indicate that antibiotic prescribing rates for children seen in physician offices declined in the 1990s, after having increased in the late 1980s (17). Initially focused primarily on pediatrics, the campaign was expanded in 2001 to target prescribing for adults (18) and to develop a model medical curriculum and Health Plan Employer Data and Information Set (HEDIS) Performance Measures (benchmarks for health plans) for appropriate prescribing. In 2003, the campaign was renamed Get Smart: Know When Antibiotics Work, concurrent with the launching of a media campaign targeting parents of young children.

Promoting appropriate antimicrobial drug use in agriculture and veterinary medicine has been complicated by long-standing disagreement between public health and agricultural communities regarding the benefits and risks of these uses, which may have economic implications for major industries. The American Veterinary Medical Association has developed principles for judicious therapeutic use of antimicrobials in veterinary medicine with input from CDC and FDA. CDC has also awarded cooperative agreements to four schools of veterinary medicine to assess the impact of antibiotic use in swine and dairy cattle, develop alternatives to the use of antimicrobials as growth promotants, and evaluate new practices to reduce resistant bacteria in food animals. The FDA issued a guidance document titled *Guidance for Industry: Evaluating the Safety of Antimicrobial New Animal Drugs with Regard to Their Microbiological Effects on Bacteria of Human Health Concern* in 2003. This guidance document discusses a recommended approach for assessing the safety of antimicrobial new animal drugs with regard to their microbiologic effects on bacteria of human health concern. The guidance document provides an approach drug sponsors can use before seeking approval to estimate the likelihood of risk to humans if a particular antimicrobial product was used to treat food-producing animals. The estimation is made up of three parts: (i) release assessment—determines the probability that bacteria resistant to an antimicrobial would be present in an animal treated with the antimicrobial; (ii) exposure estimate—estimates the probability that humans would ingest the resistant bacteria; and (iii) consequence assessment—assesses the likelihood that human exposure to the resistant bacteria would result in a human health consequence. A human health consequence is defined as a situation in which a physician would have difficulty treating a person with an antimicrobial drug because the bacteria infecting the human had acquired resistance to the drug and that resistance came from use of the drug in animals (19). The FDA's Center for Veterinary Medicine (CVM) has proposed withdrawing approval for use of the fluoroquinolones in poultry. This action was based on CVM's determinations that the use of fluoroquinolones in poultry causes the development of fluoroquinolone-resistant *Campylobacter*, a pathogen to humans, in poultry; that fluoroquinolone-resistant *Campylobacter* is transferred to humans and is a significant cause of the development of fluoroquinolone-resistant *Campylobacter* infections in humans; and that fluoroquinolone-resistant *Campylobacter* infections are a hazard to human health.

Preventing transmission of infections (e.g., through appropriate use of vaccines, infection control in health care, food safety) reduces disease incidence and drug prescribing (20–22). CDC has supported projects to evaluate the impact of pneumococcal conjugate vaccine in reducing infections with drug-resistant pneumococci, demonstration programs evaluating comprehensive approaches to infection control in health care settings in Chicago and Pittsburgh, and infection prevention and control research and evaluation programs at seven university-based Centers of Excellence in Healthcare Epidemiology. Regional approaches are important, as illustrated by the early recognition and successful control of the spread of vancomycin-resistant enterococci (VRE) in acute and long-term care facilities in the tristate area surrounding Sioux City, Iowa. With leadership from the Sioux City health department and support from the Iowa, South Dakota, and Nebraska state health departments and CDC, health care institutions rigorously implemented surveillance, prevention and control guidelines, and communicated openly with each other. As a result, they were able to eliminate VRE from hospitals and drastically reduce VRE rates in long-term care facilities, an unprecedented success (23).

CAMPAIGN TO PREVENT ANTIMICROBIAL RESISTANCE IN HEALTH CARE SETTINGS

In health care settings, where infection with multidrug-resistant organisms is a major patient safety issue, promoting appropriate antimicrobial drug prescribing is complicated by the higher stakes involved in treating sicker patients and the need to develop partnerships with a greater number of medical and surgical specialties involved in their care, as well as with other clinical staff and administrators. The CDC's Campaign to Prevent Antimicrobial Resistance in Healthcare Settings aims to prevent AR in health care settings by improving clinician practices. The campaign's programs are created in close partnership with professional societies and key opinion leaders in relevant specialties. The program translates published (i.e., peer-reviewed journals) scientific evidence and guidelines into action steps designed to optimize the care of individual patients in the era of widespread AR. The campaign centers on four main strategies: prevent infection, diagnose and treat infection, use antimicrobials wisely, and prevent transmission. Within the context of these strategies, multiple twelve-step programs are being developed targeting clinicians who treat specialty-specific, high-risk patient populations, including hospitalized adults (Box 2), dialysis patients, surgical patients, hospitalized children, and long-term care patients. Educational tools and materials are being developed for each patient population. The communication strategy includes the goals of informing clinicians, patients, and other stakeholders, raising awareness about the escalating problem of AR in health care settings, and motivating interest in and acceptance of interventional programs to prevent resistance. The campaign targets practicing clinicians, patient care partners, health care organizations, purchasers, patients, and the general public. Educational tools are being developed, including web-based didactic learning modules, pocket cards, and slide presentations. CDC is working with many public, professional, and private sector partners to market the twelve steps for each target group and promote their implementation. Educational tools are available with other supporting material on the Internet at http://www.cdc.gov/drugresistance/healthcare.htm.

Papers have been published discussing the principles of the campaign tailored to dialysis and surgical patients (24,25). For the strategy of "Prevent Infection," recommendations for dialysis patients include use of influenza and pneumococcal vaccines, reducing hemodialysis catheter use, using the lowest risk vascular access (i.e., arteriovenous [AV] fistulae in preference to grafts and minimizing use of hemodialysis catheters), and reducing hemodialysis and peritoneal access–related infections through various means, including consistent use of sterile technique, proper catheter procedures, appropriate dressings, and aseptic techniques, all by trained personnel. Among surgical patients, key principles in the strategy include minimizing the use of invasive devices and vaccinating at-risk surgical patients and staff. Guidelines are provided for prevention of catheter-associated urinary tract infections and prevention of health care–associated pneumonia.

For the strategy of "Diagnose and Treat Infection Effectively," physicians taking care of dialysis patients are in-

Box 2 Twelve Steps to Prevent Antimicrobial Resistance Among Hospitalized Adults

Strategy: Prevent Infection

Step 1. Vaccinate
–Give influenza/pneumococcal vaccine to at-risk patients before discharge.
–Get influenza vaccine annually.

Step 2. Get the catheters out
–Use catheters only when essential.
–Use the correct catheter.
–Use proper insertion and catheter-care protocols.
–Remove catheters when no longer essential.

Strategy: Diagnose and Treat Infection Effectively

Step 3. Target the pathogen
–Culture the patient.
–Target empiric therapy to likely pathogens and local antibiogram.
–Target definitive therapy to known pathogens and antimicrobial suscepti- bility test results.

Step 4. Access the experts
–Consult infectious disease experts for patients with serious infections.

Strategy: Use Antimicrobials Wisely

Step 5. Practice antimicrobial control
–Engage in local antimicrobial control efforts.

Step 6. Use local data
–Know your antibiogram.
–Know your patient population.

Step 7. Treat infection, not contamination
–Use proper antisepsis for blood and other cultures.
–Culture the blood, not the skin or catheter hub.
–Use proper methods to obtain and process all cultures.

Step 8. Treat infection, not colonization
–Treat pneumonia, not the tracheal aspirate.
–Treat bacteremia, not the catheter tip or hub.
–Treat urinary tract infection, not the indwelling catheter.

Step 9. Know when to say no to vanco
–Treat infection, not contaminants or colonization.
–Fever in a patient with an intravenous catheter is not a routine indication for vancomycin.

Box 2 *Continued*

Strategy: Use Antimicrobials Wisely *(Con't)*

Step 10. Stop antimicrobial treatment
–When infection is cured.
–When cultures are negative and infection is unlikely
–When infection is not diagnosed.

Strategy: Prevent transmission

Step 11. Isolate the pathogen
–Use standard infection control precautions.
–Contain infectious body fluids (use approved airborne/droplet/contact isolation precautions).
–When in doubt, consult infection control experts.

Step 12. Break the chain of contagion
–Stay home when you are sick.
–Keep your hands clean.
–Set an example.

structed in the proper collection and interpretation of blood, peritoneal dialysis exit site, tunnel, and dialysate cultures. Among surgical patients, key principles include targeting likely pathogens, using microbiologic data to tailor antimicrobial therapy, accessing the experts (guidance with difficult issues), and provision of surgical representation on committees that determine hospital formularies, guidelines, and other matters related to health care epidemiology and infection control. Most surgeons cannot remain current on all infectious disease issues; therefore, the identification of a medical or surgical colleague for guidance who is an expert in this area is helpful.

"Use Antimicrobials Wisely" is a strategy among dialysis patients that includes general principles of antimicrobial use defined as "the ideal is to have all patients treated with the most effective, least toxic, and least costly antibiotic for the precise duration of time needed to cure or prevent an infection" (26). Recommendations include proper use of vancomycin and alternatives to vancomycin; reducing use in situations in which it is inappropriate or for which there are alternatives, such as routine surgical prophylaxis; and continued empiric use when there are negative beta-lactam-resistant organisms. For example, antimicrobial prophylaxis should not routinely include vancomycin for placement of AV grafts or fistulae in the absence of serious beta-lactam allergy. Among patients on dialysis, there are issues of dosing and drug choice that must be considered, including inconvenience and expense of alternatives to vancomycin and lack of supporting pharmacokinetic data for some drugs. Among surgical patients, key principles include practice of thoughtful antimicrobial control, using local data on common pathogens and resistance patterns to guide empiric therapy, limiting treatment of contamination, and treating infection aggressively but not colonization.

Actions that comprise the "Prevent Transmission" strategy among dialysis patients include careful infection control with hand hygiene—the single most important infection-control measure—using soap and water or waterless alcohol-based gels or foams. Additional infection-control precautions should be considered for treatment of patients who might be at increased risk for transmitting pathogenic bacteria. Among surgical patients, hand hygiene is also paramount.

In summary, U.S. federal agencies now have a strategy and an action plan to address AR domestically. Progress to date is encouraging, indicating that additional investments can be expected to pay dividends in converting AR from an urgent to a manageable problem that does not compromise the availability of safe and effective therapy for patients today and in future generations.

REFERENCES

1. National Academy of Sciences, Institute of Medicine., Forum on Emerging Infections, Antimicrobial Resistance: Issues and Options [Workshop Report], 1998, Washington, DC.

2. National Academy of Sciences, Institute of Medicine., Forum on Emerging Infections, the Resistance Phenomenon in Microbes and Infectious Disease Vectors: Implications for Human

Health and Strategies for Containment [Workshop Summary], 2003, Washington, DC.

3. American Society for Microbiology., Report of the ASM Task Force on Antibiotic Resistance, 1995, Washington, DC.

4. World Health Organization., World Health Organization Report on Infectious Diseases 2000; Overcoming Antimicrobial Resistance. WHO/CDS/2000.2, 2000.

5. World Health Organization., WHO Global Strategy for Containment of Antimicrobial Resistance. WHO/CDS/CSR/DRS/ 2001.2. Geneva, 2001.

6. U.S. Congress, Office of Technology Assessment., Impact of Antibiotic-Resistant Bacteria, OTA-H-629, U.S. Government Printing Office, September 1995.

7. General Accounting Office, Antimicrobial Resistance., Data to assess public health threat from resistant bacteria are limited [GAO/HEHS/NSIAD/RCED-99-132], April 1999.

8. General Accounting Office, Food Safety., The agricultural use of antibiotics and its implications for human health [GAO/ RCED-99-74], April 1999.

9. Bell D. Development of the *Public Health Action Plan to Combat Antimicrobial Resistance.* In: Knobler SL, Lemon SM, Najafi M, Burroughs T, Eds The Resistance Phenomenon in Microbes and Infectious Disease Vectors: Implications for Human Health and Strategies for Containment—Workshop Summary.. Washington, DC: Forum on Emerging Infections, National Academy Press, 2003.

10. Hawley LA, Fridkin SK, Whitney CG. Drug-resistant *Streptococcus pneumoniae* and methicillin-resistant *Staphylococcus aureus* surveillance. Emerg Infect Dis [serial online]. October 2003. Available from: http://www.cdc.gov/ncidod/EID/vol9no10/ 03-03-0454.htm.

11. NCCLS (National Committee for Clinical Laboratory Standards)., Analysis and Presentation of Cumulative Antimicrobial Susceptibility Test Data; Approved Guideline., 2002.

12. Bell DM. Promoting appropriate antimicrobial drug use: perspective from the Centers for Disease Control and Prevention. Clin Infect Dis 2001; 33(Suppl 3):S245–S250.

13. Gonzales R, Steiner JF, Lum A, Barrett PH. Decreasing antibiotic use in ambulatory practice: impact of a multidimensional intervention on the treatment of uncomplicated acute bronchitis in adults. JAMA 1999; 281:1512–1519.

14. Finkelstein JA, Davis RL, Dowell SF, Metlay JP, Soumerai SB, Rifas-Shiman SL, Higham M, Miller Z, Miroshnik I, Pedan A, Platt R. Reducing antibiotic use in children: a randomized trial in 12 practices. Pediatrics 2001; 108:1–7.

15. Belongia EA, Sullivan BJ, Chyou PH, Madagame E, Reed KD, Schwartz B. A community intervention trial to promote judicious antibiotic use and reduce penicillin-resistant *Streptococcus pneumoniae* carriage in children. Pediatrics 2001; 108: 575–583.

16. Hennessy TW, Petersen KM, Bruden D, Parkinson AJ, Hurlburt D, Getty M, Schwartz B, Butler JC. Changes in antibiotic-prescribing practices and carriage of penicillin-resistant *Streptococcus pneumoniae*: A controlled intervention trial in rural Alaska. Clin Infect Dis 2002; 34:1543–1550.

17. McCaig LF, Besser RE, Hughes JM. Trends in antimicrobial prescribing rates for children and adolescents. JAMA 2002; 287: 3096–3102.

18. Gonzales R, Bartlett JG, Besser RE, Cooper RJ, Hickner JM, Hoffman JR, Sande MA. Principles of appropriate antibiotic use for treatment of acute respiratory infections in adults: Background, specific aims, and methods. Ann Intern Med 2001; 134: 479–486.

19. Food and Drug Administration., Guidance for Industry 152—Evaluating the Safety of Antimicrobial New Animal Drugs With Regard to Their Microbiological Effects on Bacteria of Human Health Concern.. Available at: http://www.fda.gov/cvm/guidance/fguide152.pdf. Accessed October 23, 2003.

20. Whitney CG, Farley MM, Hadler J, Harrison LH, Bennett NM, Lynfield R, Reingold A, Cieslak PR, Pilishvili T, Jackson D, Facklam RR, Jorgensen JH, Schuchat A. Active Bacterial Core Surveillance of the Emerging Infections Program Network. Decline in invasive pneumococcal disease after the introduction of protein-polysaccharide conjugate vaccine. N Engl J Med 2003; 348:1737–1746.

21. Neuzil KM, Mellen BG, Wright PF, Mitchel EF, Griffin MR. The effect of influenza on hospitalizations, outpatient visits, and courses of antibiotics in children. N Engl J Med 2000; 342: 225–231.

22. Fridkin SK, Edwards JR, Pichette SC, Pryor ER, McGowan JE, Tenover FC, Culver DH, Gaynes RP. Determinants of vancomycin use in adult intensive care units in 41 United States hospitals. Clin Infect Dis 1999; 28:1119–1125.

23. Ostrowsky BE, Trick WE, Sohn AH, Quirk SB, Holt S, Carson LA, Hill BC, Arduino MJ, Kuehnert MJ, Jarvis WR. Control of vancomycin-resistant enterococcus in health care facilities in a region. N Engl J Med 2001; 344:1427–1433.

24. Berns JS, Tokars JI. Preventing bacterial infections and antimicrobial resistance in dialysis patients Am J Kidney Dis 2002; 40:886–898.

25. Raymond DP, Kuehnert MJ, Sawyer RG. Preventing antimicrobial-resistant bacterial infections in surgical patients. Surg Infect 2002; 3:375–385.

26. Shlaes DM, Gerding DN, John JF, Craig WA, Bornstein DL, Duncan RA, Eckman MR, Farrer WE, Greene WH, Lorian V, Levy S, McGowan JE, Paul SM, Ruskin J, Tenover FC, Watanakunakorn C. Society for Healthcare Epidemiology of America and Infectious Diseases Society of America Joint Committee on the Prevention Antimicrobial Resistance: guidelines for the prevention of antimicrobial resistance in hospitals. Clin Infect Dis 1997; 25:584–599.

3

Why Appropriate Antimicrobial Selection Is Important: Focus on Outcomes

MARIN H. KOLLEF

Washington University School of Medicine and
Barnes-Jewish Hospital
St. Louis, Missouri, U.S.A.

INTRODUCTION

There is a general consensus that antimicrobial resistance in the hospital setting has emerged as an important variable that influences patient outcomes and overall resource utilization (1–3). Hospitals worldwide are faced with increasingly rapid emergence and spread of antibiotic-resistant bacteria. Both antibiotic-resistant gram-negative bacilli and gram-positive bacteria are reported as important causes of hospital-acquired infections (4,5). In many cases, few antimicrobial agents remain for effective treatment, particularly with methicillin-resistant and vancomycin-resistant *Staphylococcus aureus* (MRSA, VRSA) and gram-negative bacteria producing extended-spectrum beta-lactamases with resistance to many other antibiotics (6–8).

The increasing presence of antibiotic-resistant bacterial infections among hospitalized patients is likely related to numerous pressures promoting resistance as well as the administration of inappropriate antimicrobial therapy. These pressures include the frequent use of broad-spectrum antibiotics; prolonged use of antibiotics; crowding of patients with high levels of disease acuity within relatively small specialized areas of the hospital; reductions in nursing and ancillary support staff due to economic pressures, which increase the likelihood of person-to-person transmission of antibiotic-resistant bacteria; and presence of more chronically and acutely ill patients who require prolonged hospitalizations and often harbor antibiotic-resistant bacteria (9–11). This review focuses on antimicrobial resistance and the importance of administering initial appropriate antimicrobial treatment for serious infections as it applies to hospital-acquired infections, especially hospital-acquired pneumonia (HAP).

IMPORTANCE OF APPROPRIATE INITIAL ANTIMICROBIAL THERAPY

One of the consequences of greater antimicrobial resistance is an increased recognition of inappropriate antimicrobial treatment of infections (12). Inappropriate antimicrobial treatment of serious infections in the hospital setting has been demonstrated to be an important determinant of hospital mortality (Fig. 1) (13–15). Inappropriate antimicrobial treatment represents the use of antibiotics with poor or no *in vitro* activity against the identified microorganisms causing infection at the tissue site of infection. Examples of inappropriate treatment include the absence of antimicrobial agents directed at a specific class of microorganisms (e.g., absence of therapy for fungemia due to *Candida* species) and the administration of

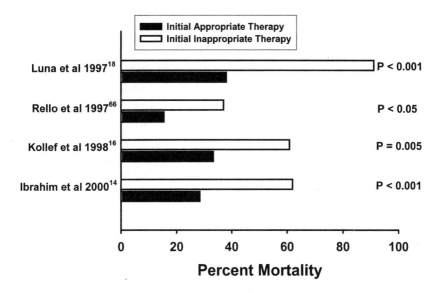

Figure 1 Crude hospital mortality from four clinical studies for patients receiving either appropriate or inappropriate initial antimicrobial therapy for hospital-acquired infections in the intensive care unit setting.

antimicrobial agents to which the microorganism responsible for the infection is resistant (e.g., empiric treatment with nafcillin for pneumonia subsequently attributed to MRSA). Changing antimicrobial therapy based on the subsequent available culture results and antibacterial susceptibilities may not reduce the excess risk of hospital mortality associated with inappropriate initial antibiotic treatment (16,17). Therefore, selection of initial appropriate therapy (i.e., getting antibiotic treatment right the first time) is an important aspect of care for hospitalized patients with serious infections.

Most inappropriate antimicrobial treatment of hospital-acquired infections appears to be the result of bacteria resistant to the prescribed antimicrobial agents (12–18). Although inappropriate antibiotic treatment may explain, in part, the greater mortality rates associated with antibiotic-resistant bacterial infections, other factors may also contribute to this excess mortality. Antibiotic-resistant gram-positive bacteria such as MRSA express a number of virulence factors potentially contributing to their higher rates of associated mortality (19,20). However, not all investigators have demonstrated greater mortality rates with infections due to MRSA compared with methicillin-susceptible *S. aureus* (21). Similarly, some antibiotic-resistant gram-negative bacteria (e.g., *Pseudomonas aeruginosa*) are associated with increased virulence factors as compared with antibiotic-susceptible pathogens (22,23). This may explain the excess attributable mortality observed with infections due to these pathogens as well.

Hospital-acquired bloodstream infections are among the most serious infections acquired by patients in the intensive care unit (ICU). Antibiotic resistance appears to have contributed to increasing administration of inappropriate antimicrobial therapy for hospital-acquired bloodstream infections that are associated with greater hospital mortality rates (13,14,24,25). The problem of antibiotic-resistant bacteremia also appears to be increasing in the hospital setting as well as in the community (26). Given the current trend of greater severity of illness for critically ill patients, it can be expected that infections due to antibiotic-resistant bacterial strains will be associated with greater morbidity and mortality, particularly when inappropriate empiric antimicrobial therapy is administered (12). Along with greater patient mortality rates, antibiotic-resistant bacterial infections and inappropriate antimicrobial treatment are associated with prolonged hospitalization and increased health care costs relative to antibiotic-sensitive bacterial infections (15,27,28). The overall national costs of antimicrobial resistance have been estimated to be between $100 million and $30 billion annually for the control and treatment of infections caused by antibiotic-resistant bacteria (29).

In addition to selecting the most appropriate antimicrobial agents for the treatment of serious infections, clinicians must insure that antibiotic administration follows certain minimal requirements. These minimal requirements include proper dosing, interval administration, optimal duration of treatment, monitoring of drug levels when appropriate, and avoidance of unwanted drug interactions (30). Lack of adherence to these minimal requirements may result in unforeseen administration of suboptimal or excessive antibiotic tissue concentrations, which increases the likelihood for antibiotic-resistance, patient toxicity, and lack of effectiveness, despite selecting an appropriate antimicrobial regimen (31).

THE TARGETED APPROACH TO ANTIBIOTIC UTILIZATION

Ideally, clinicians should prescribe antimicrobial therapy with the goals of providing appropriate initial therapy to hospitalized patients with serious infections and minimizing the emergence of bacterial resistance. Various strategies for the prevention of antibiotic resistance have been proposed in terms of improving overall antibiotic utilization (32,33). Table 1 highlights several of these strategies aimed at either limiting the unnecessary use of antibiotics or optimizing their effectiveness when prescribed to hospitalized patients. The targeted approach to empiric antimicrobial therapy is one approach to antibiotic utilization attempting to balance the need to provide appropriate initial treatment while limiting the emergence of antimicrobial resistance (Fig. 2).

An effective approach to targeted antimicrobial therapy necessitates that clinicians be aware of the microorganisms that are most likely to be associated with infection and inappropriate antimicrobial treatment in their practice setting. This requires that hospitals have updated and accurate antibiograms reflecting the bacterial pathogens and their antimicrobial susceptibility encountered at the local level. Variability in the microorganisms associated with hospital-acquired infections among hospitals, as well as within the wards of large hospitals, has been demonstrated to occur (34,35). Additionally, changing temporal patterns of nosocomial pathogens and antimicrobial susceptibility have been described (36). This suggests that hospitals may need to develop systems for updating local antibiograms on a regular basis because of the potential existence of intrahospital and temporal variations. Utiliz-

Table 1   Goals of Targeted Antibiotic Therapy in the
Hospital Setting

I. Optimize antimicrobial effectiveness

1. Prescribe initial appropriate empiric treatment based on local pathogen
   prevalence and antibiotic susceptibility.
2. Use combination antimicrobial treatment to cover the most common
   bacterial pathogens.
3. Provide education and professional detailing to clinicians on appropriate
   antibiotic therapy.
4. Use locally developed antibiotic management guidelines.
5. Consult with local infectious disease specialists.
6. Use antibiotic cycling and scheduled antibiotic changes according to
   changing patterns of pathogens and antimicrobial susceptibility.
7. Consider the use of area-specific empiric antimicrobial regimens in
   larger hospitals because of area-specific variability in pathogens and
   their susceptibility patterns.

II. Limit unnecessary antimicrobial utilization

1. De-escalation approach to therapy
   a. Use narrow-spectrum or older antibiotics based on patient risk profile
      and culture results.
   b. Use shortest course of antibiotic therapy that is clinically indicated.
2. Avoid prolonged use of prophylactic antibiotics.
3. Apply selective formulary control or restriction of specific "problem"
   antimicrobial agents or drug classes.
4. Develop/apply local guidelines or protocols detailing optimal indications
   for and durations of antimicrobial treatment.
5. Use quantitative cultures, when appropriate, to establish diagnostic
   thresholds for treating specific infections

ing such data can improve the efficacy of antimicrobial therapy
by increasing the likelihood that appropriate initial antibiotic
treatment will be prescribed to infected patients (36,37).

In order to appropriately target the initial empiric antimicrobial regimen, clinicians must be able to obtain culture specimens prior to starting antimicrobial therapy. However, it is
understood that prolonged delays in the administration of appropriate antibiotic treatment should not occur in seriously ill
patients while waiting for specific cultures to be obtained (e.g.,
bronchoalveolar lavage, cerebrospinal fluid). The most com-

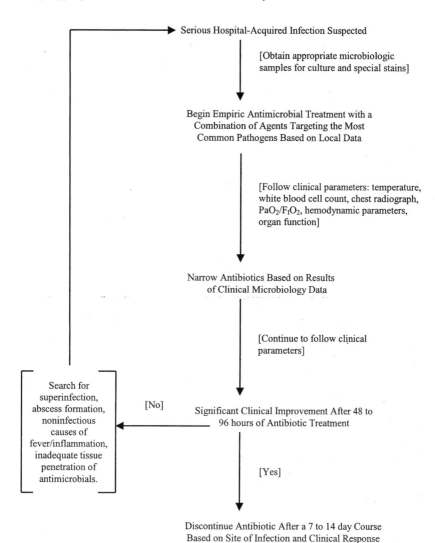

Figure 2 A flow diagram illustrating the targeted approach to antibiotic treatment for hospital-acquired infections.

mon pathogens associated with the administration of inappropriate antimicrobial treatment for hospital–acquired infections include potentially antibiotic-resistant gram-negative bacteria (*P. aeruginosa, Acinetobacter* species, *Klebsiella pneumoniae*, and *Enterobacter* species) and *S. aureus*, especially the strains with methicillin resistance (12–18). Therefore, clinicians should consider initial empiric therapy for these pathogens, especially in patients at high-risk for antibiotic-resistant infections.

Clinicians should also be aware that health care–acquired infections are similar to hospital-acquired infections in terms of the pathogens responsible for infection (38–41). Health care–acquired infections are defined by a positive culture obtained within 48 hours of hospital admission and one of the following criteria: (i) received intravenous therapy at home; received wound care or specialized nursing care through a health care agency, family, or friends; or had self-administered intravenous medical therapy in the 30 days before the infection; (ii) attended a hospital or hemodialysis clinic or received intravenous chemotherapy in the 30 days before the infection; (iii) was hospitalized in an acute care hospital for 2 or more days in the 90 days before the infection; (iv) resided in a nursing home or long-term care facility (38). Physicians should be aware of the factors that identify patients as having health care–acquired infections in order to avoid the prescription of inappropriate antibiotic treatment.

EXAMPLES OF THE TARGETED APPROACH TO EMPIRIC ANTIMICROBIAL THERAPY

Trouillet et al. (9) identified risk factors for ventilator-associated pneumonia (VAP) caused by potentially drug-resistant bacteria such as methicillin-resistant *S. aureus, P. aeruginosa, Acinetobacter baumannii*, and/or *Stenotrophomonas maltophilia* in 135 consecutive episodes of VAP observed in a single ICU over a 25-month period. Seventy-seven (57.0%) episodes of VAP were caused by "potentially resistant" bacteria and fifty-eight (43.0%) episodes were caused by "other" nonresistant organisms. According to logistic regression analysis, three variables were predictors for VAP due to potentially drug-resistant bacteria: duration of mechanical ventilation greater than or equal to 7 days (odds ratio [OR] = 6.0), prior antibiotic use (OR = 13.5), and prior use of broad-spectrum drugs (third-generation cephalosporin, fluoroquinolone, and/or a carbapenem) (OR = 4.1). Differences in the potential efficacies (ranging from 100% to 11%) against microorganisms for fifteen different antimicrobial regimens were studied to determine their overall level of activity for the pathogens associated with VAP. These investigators observed that the combination of a carbapenem plus amikacin and vancomycin provided the broadest *in vitro* coverage against the spectrum of gram-negative and gram-positive bacteria that were found in their ICU. Although clinical outcomes were not assessed, this study suggests that location-specific empiric antibiotic regimens, tailored to the susceptibility patterns of the local flora, are most likely to be effective. Additionally, this study demonstrates that patients at high-risk for infection with antibiotic-resistant bacteria can be identified based on risk factors that promote colonization with such pathogens (e.g., prior antibiotic therapy, exposure to high-risk environments including hospitals and long-term care facilities).

Ibrahim et al. (37) evaluated fifty consecutive patients in the ICU setting receiving antimicrobial therapy for VAP. They subsequently examined fifty-two consecutive patients with VAP whose antimicrobial treatment was administered according to a unit-specific antimicrobial guideline. The main goal of the guideline was to provide initial administration of appropriate antimicrobial treatment while avoiding the emergence of antimicrobial resistance. This meant providing initial coverage for *P. aeruginosa* and methicillin-resistant *S. aureus*, the two most common pathogens causing VAP in that specific ICU. This was accomplished by providing initial intravenous combination antimicrobial treatment with vancomycin, a carbapenem, and a fluoroquinolone. This combination was selected because it provided *in vitro* coverage for greater than 90% of all the bacterial isolates identified based on a unit-specific antibiogram. The guideline also required that antibiotic treatment be modified after 48 hours based on the available culture results and the clinical course of the patient. In fact, 61.5% of patients had two antibiotics discontinued within 48 hours of beginning therapy, based on special stains and culture data.

The second specified goal of the guideline developed by Ibrahim et al. was to reduce potentially unnecessary antimicrobial administration. This was accomplished by recommending a 7-day course of appropriate antimicrobial treatment for patients with VAP. Continued administration of antimicrobials beyond day 7 was only encouraged for patients with persistent signs and symptoms consistent with active infection (e.g., fever greater than 38.3°C, circulating leukocyte count greater than 10,000 mm^{-3}, lack of improvement on the chest radiograph, continued purulent sputum). Use of the guideline was associated with a statistically significant increase in the administration of appropriate antimicrobial treatment, a decrease in the development of secondary episodes of antibiotic-resistant VAP, and a reduction in the total duration of antimicrobial treatment.

The studies of Trouillet et al. and Ibrahim et al. employed local bacterial susceptibility data in order to develop recommendations for empiric therapy within their respective ICUs. The use of local data should always be taken into consideration when developing empiric regimens for treatment. The American Thoracic Society (ATS) released a consensus statement in 1996 on the diagnosis, assessment, treatment, and prevention of HAP that supported the de-escalation approach to antimicrobial treatment (42). This document identifies those microorganisms commonly implicated in HAP and provides antibiotic recommendations based on the infecting pathogens. According to the consensus statement, the management of HAP should be based on the following factors: severity of illness (i.e., mild to moderate vs. severe as defined in the ATS statement); presence of risk factors suggesting infection with specific microorganisms (to include the use of local data on pathogens and susceptibility patterns); and the time of pneumonia onset (i.e., less than 5 days after hospital admission vs. 5 days or more after admission).

The ATS guideline notes that patients with mild-to-moderate disease presenting less than 5 days after hospitalization generally are infected with *Haemophilus influenzae, Streptococcus pneumoniae*, methicillin-susceptible *S. aureus* (MSSA), or other "core microorganisms" (i.e., antibiotic-susceptible bacteria). However, the presence of risk factors (e.g., recent abdominal surgery, diabetes mellitus, head trauma, history of high-dose corticosteroids) or local patterns of pathogen prevalence and antimicrobial susceptibility can alter the type of predominant infecting microorganism needing coverage. The duration of hospitalization prior to the onset of pneumonia is one of the most important determinants for potential infecting pathogens. The risk of infection with MRSA, *P. aeruginosa*, and *Acinetobacter* species is increased if nosocomial pneumonia presents after the patient has been hospitalized for more than 5 days (43). In patients with specific risk factors, prolonged hospitalization, or severe disease, combination antimicrobial therapy should initially target this broader spectrum of likely infecting bacteria. In addition, combination therapy is required in suspected infections due to *P. aeruginosa* to improve survival rates and reduce the development of antibiotic resistance (42). Monotherapy may be adequate in some cases of severe nonpseudomonal infection, but few studies have evaluated the efficacy of single agents in severe disease (44–48).

TIMING OF ANTIMICROBIAL TREATMENT

A number of investigators have found that delays in the administration of appropriate antimicrobial treatment are associated with excess hospital mortality. Alvarez-Lerma (17) showed that among 490 episodes of pneumonia acquired in the ICU setting, 214 episodes (43.7%) required modification of the initial antibiotic regimen because of either isolation of a resistant microorganism (62.1%) or lack of clinical response to therapy (36.0%). Attributable mortality from VAP was significantly lower among patients receiving initial appropriate antibiotic treatment compared with patients receiving inappropriate treatment requiring a treatment change (16.2% vs. 24.7%; $p = 0.034$).

Iregui et al. (49) examined the influence of initially delayed appropriate antimicrobial treatment on the outcomes of 107 patients with VAP. All 107 patients eventually received treatment with an antibiotic regimen that was shown *in vitro* to be active against the bacterial pathogens isolated from their respiratory secretions. Thirty-three (30.8%) patients received appropriate antibiotic treatment that was delayed for 24 hours or more after patients initially met diagnostic criteria for VAP. The most common reason for the administration of delayed treatment was a delay in physicians recognizing the presence of VAP and writing the orders for antimicrobial treatment (n = 25; 75.8%). Patients receiving delayed antimicrobial treatment have a statistically greater hospital mortality compared with patients without the delay (69.7% vs. 28.4%); $p < 0.001$.

The studies of Alvarez-Lerma and Iregui et al. suggest that delaying the administration of appropriate antibiotic treatment is an important factor contributing to the excess hospital mortality of patients with serious infections. Delays in the administration of appropriate antibiotic treatment recently have also been associated with greater mortality for patients with severe sepsis (50,51; and H. Levy, personal communication, 2002). These studies demonstrate that initial selection of the "wrong" antibiotic regimen, because of a lack of efficacy for the identified microorganism(s) associated with infection, will delay appropriate antibiotic delivery to the tissue site of infection and result in worse clinical outcomes (12).

TARGETED ANTIMICROBIAL THERAPY AND RESISTANCE

The second goal of targeted antimicrobial therapy is to avoid the administration of unnecessary antibiotic treatment. This first requires narrowing the antimicrobial coverage after identification of the pathogen to which the infection is attributed and the microorganism's antimicrobial susceptibility profile.

Second, the duration of antimicrobial treatment should be limited to the shortest effective course of therapy. The following approaches are ways in which unnecessary antimicrobial therapy can be avoided in a de-escalation strategy.

Protocols/Guidelines

Antibiotic practice guidelines or protocols have emerged as a potentially effective means of both avoiding unnecessary antibiotic administration and increasing the therapeutic effectiveness of these agents. The potential benefits of antibiotic use guidelines in the hospital setting have been well demonstrated by the experience at LDS Hospital in Salt Lake City, Utah, which employs a computerized system guiding antibiotic use. This system has been successfully employed to reduce inappropriate empiric antibiotic administration as compared with individual physician prescribing practices (52). This automated guideline has also been shown to significantly reduce orders for drugs to which patients are allergic, overall adverse events caused by antibiotics, and the total number of anti-infective doses prescribed, as well as the medical costs associated with antimicrobial agents (53).

Nonautomated or partially automated protocols, usually driven by hospital-based quality improvement teams, have demonstrated results similar to those observed with the fully automated antibiotic utilization systems. Bailey et al. (54) randomized patients to have their physicians contacted by pharmacists with consensus recommendations to discontinue intravenous antibiotics versus no intervention in two teaching hospitals. The intervention significantly reduced antibiotic doses administered and mean antibiotic costs but was associated with increased labor costs. Similarly, Leibovici et al. (55) developed a problem-oriented data-base decision support system that significantly reduced the unnecessary use of antibiotics and decreased inadequate antibiotic administration, particularly to patients infected with multiresistant gram-negative isolates, enterococci, and *S. aureus*. With the advent of newly available technologies, to include handheld computers and portable communication devices, the ability to extend the influence of treatment protocols to the bedside is becoming increasingly possible.

Shorter Courses of Antimicrobial Therapy

Recently, several groups of investigators have demonstrated that shorter courses of therapy for VAP can be efficacious while reducing the emergence of antimicrobial resistance. Singh et al. (56) used a scoring system to identify patients with suspected VAP who could be treated with 3 days of antibiotics as opposed to the conventional practice of 10 to 21 days of antibiotic therapy. Patients receiving the shorter course of antibiotic therapy had clinical outcomes similar to the patients receiving longer therapy but with fewer subsequent superinfections attributed to antibiotic-resistant pathogens. Similarly, Ibrahim et al. (37) employed a pharmacist-directed protocol in the ICU setting to reduce the empiric administration of antibiotics for suspected VAP to 8.1 $\pm$ 5.1 days from 14.8 $\pm$ 8.1 days ($p < 0.001$).

Although recommended durations of antimicrobial therapy for VAP have generally ranged from 14 to 21 days in the past, these were not based on prospective studies. Dennesen et al. (57) evaluated twenty-seven patients with VAP to determine their resolution of signs and symptoms. All patients received appropriate antibiotic therapy, and the highest temperatures, leukocyte counts, P_aO_2/F_IO_2 ratios, and semiquantitative cultures of endotracheal aspirates were recorded from start of therapy until day 14. VAP was caused by Enterobacteriaceae (n = 14), *P. aeruginosa* (n = 7), *S. aureus* (n = 6), *H. influenzae* (n = 3), and *S. pneumoniae* (n = 1). *H. influenzae* and *S. pneumoniae* were eradicated from tracheal aspirates, whereas Enterobacteriaceae, *S. aureus*, and *P. aeruginosa* persisted despite *in vitro* susceptibility to antibiotics administered. Significant improvements were observed for all clinical parameters, most apparently within the first 6 days after start of antibiotics. Newly acquired colonization, especially with *P. aeruginosa* and Enterobacteriaceae, occurred in the second week of therapy. These data support the premise that most patients with VAP receiving appropriate antimicrobial therapy respond to treatment within the first 6 days and acquire colonization with antibiotic-resistant bacteria usually during the second week of therapy that frequently precedes a recurrent episode of VAP.

The available medical literature suggests that shorter courses of appropriate antimicrobial treatment for VAP should be employed because of their equivalent efficacy compared with longer courses of therapy and because of their reduced propensity for the emergence of bacterial resistance. The results of a European multicenter randomized trial of 8 days versus 15 days of antibiotic treatment for VAP were presented at the American Thoracic Society meeting in May 2003 and demonstrated equivalent clinical outcomes for both study groups (58). However, patients randomized to the shorter course of therapy had more antibiotic-free days and the emergence of fewer subsequent infections due to multiresistant gram-negative bacteria. This represents the first large (n = 401) randomized clinical trial to provide grade IA evidence in support of a shorter duration of therapy for VAP.

Scheduled Antibiotic Changes/Antibiotic Cycling/Antibiotic Rotation

Rahal et al. (59) introduced a new antibiotic guideline into their hospital that significantly restricted the use of the cephalosporin class. This was done to combat an outbreak of extended-spectrum beta-lactamase (ESBL)-producing *Klebsiella* infection. The restriction of cephalosporins was successful, with an 80% reduction in their hospital-wide use that was accompanied by a 44% reduction in infection and colonization with the ESBL-producing *Klebsiella*. However, the use of imipenem increased by 140% during the intervention year and was associated with a 69% increase in the incidence of imipenem-resistant *P. aeruginosa* throughout the medical center. Therefore, this represented a change or switch from one predominant antibiotic class to another. Although the number of multiresistant pathogens decreased with this formulary restriction, its overall effectiveness can be questioned.

Kollef et al. (60) examined the influence of a scheduled antibiotic change on the incidence of nosocomial infections among patients undergoing cardiac surgery. A 6-month before-period, during which the traditional practice of prescribing a third-generation cephalosporin (ceftazidime) for the empiric treatment of gram-negative bacterial infections, was followed by a 6-month after-period during which a fluoroquinolone (ciprofloxacin) was employed. Unexpectedly, the overall incidence of VAP was significantly reduced in the after-period compared with the before-period. This was primarily the result of a significant reduction in the incidence of VAP attributed to antibiotic-resistant gram-negative bacteria. Similarly, a lower incidence of antibiotic-resistant gram-negative bacteremia was observed in the after-period. This experience was followed by a series of scheduled antibiotic changes for the treatment of suspected gram-negative bacterial infections among patients admitted to the medical and surgical ICUs (61). Overall prescription of appropriate antimicrobial therapy was statistically increased for gram-negative bacterial infections during this experience.

The concept of antibiotic class cycling or rotation has been advocated as a potential strategy for reducing the emergence of antimicrobial resistance (62). In theory, a class of antibiotics or a specific antibiotic drug is withdrawn from use for a defined time period and reintroduced at a later point in time in an attempt to limit bacterial resistance to the cycled antimicrobial agents. Gerding et al. (63) evaluated cycling of aminoglycosides over 10 years at the Minneapolis Veterans Affairs Medical Center, cycling amikacin and gentamicin. Resistance to gentamicin had emerged as a clinical problem, limiting the use of that specific aminoglycoside at this hospital. Using cycle times of 12 to 51 months, the investigators found significantly reduced resistance to gentamicin when amikacin was used, but return of resistance with the rapid reintroduction of gentamicin, followed by more gradual reintroduction of gentamicin a second time without increased levels of resistance recurring. This experience suggested that the cycling of antibiotics within the same drug class, in some circumstances, could be an effective strategy for curbing antimicrobial resistance.

Gruson et al. (36) observed a reduction in the incidence of VAP after introducing an antimicrobial program that consisted of supervised rotation and restricted use of ceftazidime and ciprofloxacin, which were widely prescribed before institution of the antibiotic program. The antibiotic selection was based on monthly reviews of the pathogens isolated from the ICU and their antibiotic susceptibility patterns. Therefore, these clinicians were rotating antimicrobial agents based on "real-time" information, which allowed potentially more effective antibiotics to be prescribed to their patients. They observed a decrease in the incidence of VAP, which was primarily the result of a reduction in the number of episodes attributed to potentially antibiotic-resistant gram-negative bacteria, including *P. aeruginosa*, *Burkholderia cepacia*, *Stenotrophomonas maltophilia*, and *A. baumannii*. These same investigators have now demonstrated that their initial results could be sustained over a 5-year time period (64).

CONCLUSIONS

Clinicians caring for patients in the hospital setting must champion and employ strategies for more effective antimicrobial utilization. The most successful strategies will be multidisciplinary, involving cooperation from the pharmacy, nursing staff, treating physicians, and infectious disease consultants. Antimicrobial utilization programs should also be linked to infection control practices in order to minimize the future emergence and spread of antibiotic-resistant microorganisms. The targeted approach to antibiotic therapy is a method of providing appropriate initial treatment to patients with serious bacterial infections ("getting it right the first time") while avoiding the unnecessary use of antibiotics in order to prevent the emergence of resistance.

REFERENCES

1. Goldmann DA, Weinstein RA, Wenzel RP, Tablan OC, Duma RJ, Gaynes RP, Schlosser J, Martone WJ. Strategies to prevent and control the emergence and spread of antimicrobial-resis-

tant microorganisms in hospitals. A challenge to hospital leadership. JAMA; 1996; 275:234–240.

2. Gold HS, Moellering RC. Antimicrobial-drug resistance. N Engl J Med; 1996; 335:1445–1453.

3. Shlaes DM, Gerding DN, John JF Jr, Craig WA, Bornstein DL, Duncan RA, Eckman MR, Farrer WE, Greene WH, Lorian V, Levy S, McGowan JE Jr, Paul SM, Ruskin J, Tenover FC, Watanakunakorn C. Society for Healthcare Epidemiology of America and Infectious Diseases Society of America Joint Committee on the Prevention of Antimicrobial Resistance: guidelines for the prevention of antimicrobial resistance in hospitals. Clin Infect Dis; 1997; 25:584–599.

4. Vincent JL, Bihari DJ, Suter PM, Bruining HA, White J, Nicolas-Chanoin MH, Wolff M, Spencer RC, Hemmer M. The prevalence of nosocomial infection in intensive care units in Europe: results of the European Prevalence of Infection in Intensive Care (EPIC) Study. EPIC International Advisory Committee. JAMA; 1995; 274:639–644.

5. Richards MJ, Edwards JR, Culver DH, Gaynes RP. Nosocomial infections in medical intensive care units in the United States. National Nosocomial Infections Surveillance System. Crit Care Med; 1999; 27:887–892.

6. Quinn JP. Clinical problems posed by multiresistant nonfermenting gram-negative pathogens. Clin Infect Dis; 1998; 27(Suppl):S117–S124.

7. Smith TL, Pearson ML, Wilcox KR, Cruz C, Lancaster MV, Robinson-Dunn B, Tenover FC, Zervos MJ, Band JD, White E, Jarvis WR. Emergence of vancomycin resistance in *Staphylococcus aureus*. N Engl J Med; 1999; 349:493–501.

8. Jarvis WR. *Staphylococcus aureus* resistant to vancomycin—United States, 2002. MMWR Morb Mortal Wkly Rep; 2002; 51:565–566.

9. Trouillet JL, Chastre J, Vuagnat A, Joly-Guillou ML, Combaux D, Dombret MC, Gibert C. Ventilator-associated pneumonia caused by potentially drug-resistant bacteria. Am J Respir Crit Care Med; 1998; 157:531–539.

10. Fridkin SK, Pear SM, Williamson TH, Galgiani JN, Jarvis WR. The role of understaffing in central venous catheter-associated

bloodstream infections. Infect Control Hosp Epidemiol; 1996; 17:150–158.

11. Hardbarth S, Sudre P, Dharan S, Cadenas M, Pittet D. Outbreak of *Enterobacter cloacae* related to understaffing, overcrowding, and poor hygiene practices. Infect Control Hosp Epidemiol; 1999; 20:598–603.

12. Kollef MH. Inadequate antimicrobial treatment: an important determinant of outcome for hospitalized patients. Clin Infect Dis; 2000; 31(Suppl):S131–S138.

13. Kollef MH, Sherman G, Ward S, Fraser VJ. Inadequate antimicrobial treatment of infections. A risk factor for hospital mortality among critically ill patients. Chest; 1999; 115:462–474.

14. Ibrahim EH, Sherman G, Ward S, Fraser VJ, Kollef MH. The influence of inadequate antimicrobial treatment of bloodstream infections on patient outcomes in the ICU setting. Chest; 2000; 118:146–155.

15. Cosgrove SE, Kaye KS, Eliopoulous GM, Carmeli Y. Health and economic outcomes of the emergence of third-generation cephalosporin resistance in *Enterobacter* species. Arch Intern Med; 2002; 162:185–190.

16. Kollef MH, Ward S. The influence of mini-BAL cultures on patient outcomes: implications for the antibiotic management of ventilator-associated pneumonia. Chest; 1998; 113:412–420.

17. Alvarez-Lerma F. Modification of empiric antibiotic treatment in patients with pneumonia acquired in the intensive care unit. ICU-Acquired Pneumonia Study Group. Intensive Care Med; 1996; 22:387–394.

18. Luna CM, Vujacich P, Niederman MS, Vay C, Gherardi C, Matera J, Jolly EC. Impact of BAL data on the therapy and outcome of ventilator-associated pneumonia. Chest; 1997; 111: 676–685.

19. Winzer K, Williams P. Quorum sensing and the regulation of virulence gene expression in pathogenic bacteria. Int J Med Microbiol; 2001; 291:131–143.

20. Dufour P, Gillet Y, Bes M, Lina G, Vandenesch F, Floret D, Etienne J, Richet H. Community-acquired methicillin-resistant *Staphylococcus aureus* infections in France: emergence of a sin-

gle clone that produces Panton-Valentine leukocidin. Clin Infect Dis; 2002; 35:819–824.

21. Selvey LA, Whitby M, Johnson B. Nosocomial methicillin-resistant *Staphylococcus aureus* bacteremia: is it any worse than nosocomial methicillin-sensitive *Staphylococcus aureus* bacteremia? Infect Control Hosp Epidemiol; 2000; 21:645–648.

22. Hauser AR, Cobb E, Bodi M, Mariscal D, Valles J, Engel JN, Rello J. Type III protein secretion is associated with poor clinical outcomes in patients with ventilator-associated pneumonia caused by *Pseudomonas aeruginosa*. Crit Care Med; 2002; 30: 521–528.

23. Roy-Burman A, Savel RH, Racine S, Swanson BL, Revadigar NS, Fujimoto J, Sawa T, Frank DW, Wiener-Kronish JP. Type III protein secretion is associated with death in lower respiratory and systemic *Pseudomonas aeruginosa* infections. J Infect Dis; 2001; 183:1767–1774.

24. Leibovici L, Shraga I, Drucker M, Konigsberger H, Samra Z, Pitlik SD. The benefit of appropriate empirical antibiotic treatment in patients with bloodstream infection. J Intern Med; 1998; 244:379–386.

25. Chow JW, Fine MJ, Shlaes DM, Quinn JP, Hooper DC, Johnson MP, Ramphal R, Wagener MM, Miyashiro DK, Yu VL. *Enterobacter* bacteremia: clinical features and emergence of antibiotic resistance during therapy. Ann Intern Med; 1991; 115:585–590.

26. Morin CA, Hadler JL. Population-based incidence and characteristics of community-onset *Staphylococcus aureus* infections with bacteremia in 4 metropolitan Connecticut areas, 1998. J Infect Dis; 2001; 184:1029–1034.

27. Carmeli Y, Troillet N, Karchmer AW, Samore MH. Health and economic outcomes of antibiotic resistance in *Pseudomonas aeruginosa*. Arch Intern Med; 1999; 159:1127–1132.

28. Webb M, Riley LW, Roberts RB. Cost of hospitalization for and risk factors associated with vancomycin-resistant *Enterococcus faecium* infection and colonization. Clin Infect Dis; 2001; 33: 445–452.

29. Howard D, Cordell R, McGowan JE Jr, Packard RM, Scott RD 2nd, Solomon SL. Workshop Group. Measuring the economic

costs of antimicrobial resistance in hospital settings: summary of the Centers for Disease Control and Prevention–Emory Workshop. Clin Infect Dis; 2001; 33:1573–1578.

30. Niederman MS. Appropriate use of antimicrobial agents: challenges and strategies for improvement. Crit Care Med; 2003; 31:608–616.

31. Kollef MH, Fraser VJ. Antibiotic resistance in the intensive care unit. Ann Intern Med; 2001; 134:298–314.

32. Hoffken G, Neiderman MS. Nosocomial pneumonia: The importance of a de-escalation strategy for antibiotic treatment of pneumonia in the ICU. Chest; 2002; 122:2183–2196.

33. Kollef MH. Hospital-acquired pneumonia and de-escalation of antimicrobial treatment. Crit Care Med; 2001; 29:1473–1475.

34. Rello J, Sa-Borges M, Correa H, Leal SR, Baraibar J. Variations in etiology of ventilator-associated pneumonia across four treatment sites. Am J Respir Crit Care Med; 1999; 160:608–613.

35. Namias N, Samiian L, Nino D, Shirazi E, O'Neill K, Kett DH, Ginzburg E, McKenney MG, Sleeman D, Cohn SM. Incidence and susceptibility of pathogenic bacteria vary between intensive care units within a single hospital: implications for empiric antibiotic strategies. J Trauma; 2000; 49:638–645.

36. Gruson D, Hilbert G, Vargas F, Valentino R, Bebear C, Allery A, Bebear C, Gbikpi-Benissan G, Cardinaud JP. Rotation and restricted use of antibiotics in a medical intensive care unit: impact on the incidence of ventilator-associated pneumonia caused by antibiotic-resistant gram-negative bacteria. Am J Respir Crit Care Med; 2000; 162:837–843.

37. Ibrahim EH, Ward S, Sherman G, Schaiff R, Fraser VJ, Kollef MH. Experience with a clinical guideline for the treatment of ventilator-associated pneumonia. Crit Care Med; 2001; 29: 1109–1115.

38. Friedman ND, Kaye KS, Stout JE, McGarry SA, Trivette SL, Briggs JP, Lamm W, Clark C, MacFarquhar J, Walton AL, Reller LB, Sexton DJ. Health-care associated bloodstream infection in adults: a reason to change the accepted definition of community-acquired infections. Ann Intern Med; 2002; 137: 791–797.

39. Gaynes R. Health-care associated bloodstream infections: a change in thinking. Ann Intern Med; 2002; 137:850–851.

40. Mylotte JM. Nursing home-acquired pneumonia. Clin Infect Dis; 2002; 35:1205–1211.

41. Hutt E, Kramer AM. Evidence-based guidelines for management of nursing home–acquired pneumonia. J Fam Pract; 2002; 51:709–716.

42. Kramer AM. Hospital-acquired pneumonia: diagnosis, assessment of severity, initial antimicrobial therapy, and preventive strategies; a consensus statement, American Thoracic Society, November 1995. Am J Respir Crit Care Med; 1996; 153: 1711–1725.

43. Rello J, Ollendorf DA, Oster DA, Vera-Llonch M, Bellm L, Redman R, Kollef MH. VAP Outcomes Scientific Advisory Group. Epidemiology and outcomes of ventilator-associated pneumonia in a large US database. Chest; 2002; 122:2115–2121.

44. Siegman-Igra Y, Ravona R, Primerman H, Giladi M. *Pseudomonas aeruginosa* bacteremia: an analysis of 123 episodes, with particular emphasis on the effect of antibiotic therapy. Int J Infect Dis; 1998; 2:211–215.

45. Leibovici L, Paul M, Poznanski O, Drucker M, Samra Z, Konigsberger H, Pitlik SD. Monotherapy versus beta-lactam-aminoglycoside combination treatment for gram-negative bacteremia: a prospective, observational study. Antimicrob Agents Chemother; 1997; 41:1127–1133.

46. Fink MP, Snydman DR, Niederman MS, Leeper KV Jr, Johnson RH, Heard SO, Wunderink RG, Caldwell JW, Schentag JJ, Siami GA. Treatment of severe pneumonia in hospitalized patients: results of a multicenter, randomized, double-blind trial comparing intravenous ciprofloxacin with imipenem-cilastin: the Severe Pneumonia Study Group. Antimicrob Agents Chemother; 1994; 38:547–557.

47. Cometta A, Baumgartner JD, Lew D, Zimmerli W, Pittet D, Chopart P, Schaad U, Herter C, Eggimann P, Huber O. Prospective randomized comparison of imipenem monotherapy with imipenem plus netilmicin for treatment of severe infections in nonneutropenic patients. Antimicrob Agents Chemother; 1994; 38:1309–1313.

48. Sieger B, Berman SJ, Geckler RW, Farkas SA. Empiric treatment of hospital-acquired lower respiratory tract infections with meropenem or ceftazidime with tobramycin: a randomized study. Crit Care Med; 1997; 25:1663–1670.

49. Iregui M, Ward S, Sherman G, Fraser VJ, Kollef MH. Clinical importance of delays in the initiation of appropriate antibiotic treatment for ventilator-associated pneumonia. Chest; 2002; 122:262–268.

50. Garnacho-Montero J, Garcia-Garmendia JL, Barrero-Almodovar AE. Impact of the outcome of adequate empirical antibiotherapy in patients admitted to the ICU for sepsis. Crit Care Med. In press.

51. Leone M, Bourgoin A, Cambon S, Dubuc M, Albanese J, Martin C. Empirical antimicrobial therapy of septic shock patients: adequacy and impact on outcome. Crit Care Med; 2003; 31: 462–467.

52. Evans RS, Classen DC, Pestotnik SL, Lundsgaarde HP, Burke JP. Improving empiric antibiotic selection using computer decision support. Arch Intern Med; 1994; 154:878–884.

53. Evans RS, Pestotnik SL, Classen DC, Clemmer TP, Weaver LK, Orme JF Jr, Lloyd JF, Burke JP. A computer-assisted management program for antibiotics and other antiinfective agents. N Engl J Med; 1998; 338:232–238.

54. Bailey TC, Ritchie DJ, McMullin ST, Kahn M, Reichley RM, Casabar E, Shannon W, Dunagan WC. A randomized, prospective evaluation of an interventional program to discontinue intravenous antibiotics at two tertiary care teaching institutions. Pharmacotherapy; 1997; 17:277–281.

55. Leibovici L, Gitelman V, Yehezkelli Y, Poznanski O, Milo G, Paul M, Ein-Dor P. Improving empirical antibiotic treatment: prospective, nonintervention testing of a decision support system. J Intern Med; 1997; 242:395–400.

56. Singh N, Rogers P, Atwood CW, Wagener MM, Yu VL. Short-course empiric antibiotic therapy for patients with pulmonary infiltrates in the intensive care unit. A proposed solution for indiscriminate antibiotic prescription. Am J Respir Crit Care Med; 2000; 162:505–511.

57. Dennesen PJ, van der Ven AJ, Kessels AG, Ramsay G, Bonten MJ. Resolution of infectious parameters after antimicrobial therapy in patients with ventilator-associated pneumonia. Am J Respir Crit Care Med; 2001; 163:1371–1375.

58. Chastre J, Wolff M, Fagon JY,. Comparison of two durations of antibiotic therapy to treat ventilator-associated pneumonia (VAP). Am J Respir Crit Care Med; 2003.

59. Rahal JJ, Urban C, Horn D, Freeman K, Segal-Maurer S, Maurer J, Mariano N, Marks S, Burns JM, Dominick D, Lim M. Class restriction of cephalosporin use to control total cephalosporin resistance in nosocomial *Klebsiella*. JAMA; 1998; 280: 1233–1237.

60. Kollef MH, Vlasnik J, Sharpless L, Pasque C, Murphy D, Fraser V. Scheduled change of antibiotic classes: a strategy to decrease the incidence of ventilator-associated pneumonia. Am J Respir Crit Care Med; 1997; 156:1040–1048.

61. Kollef MH, Ward S, Sherman G, Prentice D, Schaiff R, Huey W, Fraser VJ. Inadequate treatment of nosocomial infections is associated with certain antibiotic choices. Crit Care Med; 2000; 28:3456–3464.

62. Kollef MH. Is there a role for antibiotic cycling in the intensive care unit? Crit Care Med; 2001; 29(Suppl):N135–N142.

63. Gerding DN, Larson TA, Hughes RA, Weiler M, Shanholtzer C, Peterson LR. Aminoglycoside resistance and aminoglycoside usage: ten years of experience in one hospital. Antimicrob Agents Chemother; 1991:1284–1290.

64. Gruson D, Hilbert G, Vargas F, Valentino R, Bui N, Pereyre S, Bebear C, Bebear CM, Gbikpi-Benissan G. Strategy of antibiotic rotation: long term effect on the incidence and the susceptibilities of gram-negative bacilli responsible for ventilator-associated pneumonia. Crit Care Med; 2003:1908–1914.

65. Rello J, Gallego M, Mariscal D, Sonora R, Valles J. The value of routine microbial investigation in ventilator-associated pneumonia. Am J Respir Crit Care Med; 1997:196–200.

4

Understanding Pharmacokinetics and Pharmacodynamics: Application to the Antimicrobial Formulary Decision Process

DAVID ANDES and WILLIAM A. CRAIG

Department of Medicine, Section of Infectious
Diseases, University of Wisconsin
Madison, Wisconsin, U.S.A.

INTRODUCTION

The formulary decision process is complex and includes consideration of a variety of preclinical and clinical efficacy and toxicity data as well as economic factors. The field of pharmacokinetics and pharmacodynamics (PK-PD) allows one to integrate the information available from these preclinical and clinical studies and accurately compare various antibiotic drugs.

For any individual infectious process, there are often several drug classes and drugs within a class that may have acquired a Food and Drug Administration (FDA)-approved indication. However, not all drugs with a similar indication are equivalent in terms of their likelihood of effecting a cure or causing toxicity, patient compliance, and cost. There are numerous reasons why drugs with comparable indications may not be expected to perform similarly, including inherent potency, pharmacokinetic differences, and toxicity. Pharmacodynamics provides a means to consider these variables by critically examining the relationship between drug potency against a microorganism, serum and infection site pharmacokinetics, and treatment outcome. Regulatory agencies, including the FDA and National Committee for Clinical Laboratory Standards (NCCLS) have recently recognized the importance of PK-PD analyses and have adopted this area of study to the drug development process. Pharmacodynamic considerations have also played an increasingly important role in the development of a number of antimicrobial treatment guidelines.

The goal of this chapter is to summarize current knowledge of pharmacokinetics and pharmacodynamics of antibiotics and describe how these considerations may be used in the antimicrobial formulary decision process.

TRADITIONAL PREDICTORS OF ANTIMICROBIAL EFFICACY

Among the factors important for choice of an antibiotic is the strength or potency of a drug against the targeted microbial pathogen. Laboratory-based susceptibility testing provides reports of the minimum inhibitory concentration (MIC) that are used to predict the activity of an antibiotic against a microorganism. Although these observations can accurately describe the potency of the drug–organism interaction in this *in vitro* test system, they do not necessarily predict relative treatment efficacy. It is important to understand the usefulness and limitations of these tests. For example, simply because drug A has a lower MIC value than drug B against a pathogen of interest does not necessarily mean that drug A would be more effective than drug B.

The MIC measurement describes antibiotic effect at a fixed concentration at a single point in time. These measurements do not account for the pharmacokinetic properties of antimicrobial agents; therefore, their ability to predict therapeutic efficacy is limited. Specifically, the MIC test does not allow determination of the impact of varying drug concentrations on the rate or extent of bacterial killing. In addition, this test method does not establish whether there are enduring or persistent inhibitory effects following exposure to an antibiotic. Consideration of the effects of changing antibiotic concentrations over time provides a more accurate understanding of the effects of drugs in patients at the site of infection, where drug concentrations increase and decrease following drug administration. The field of pharmacodynamics specifically examines the impact of drug concentration over time on organism killing and growth at the site of infection (1).

PHARMACOKINETICS AND PHARMACODYNAMICS

Pharmacokinetics describes the absorption, distribution, metabolism, and elimination of drugs in serum and at sites of infection. *Pharmacodynamics* relates the time course of drug levels or pharmacokinetics to the therapeutic action and pharmacologic toxicity of the drug (1–3). For an antibiotic, it describes the relationship that exists between the drug concentration to which the bacteria is exposed at various sites of infection and bacterial killing. The integral of these pharmacokinetic parameters (drug concentration and time of drug exposure) in serum throughout the dosing interval is expressed as the area under the concentration-time curve (AUC). Outcome of infection in animal models and human studies has been shown to correlate with one of three pharmacodynamic parameters: (i) ratio of peak serum concentration of the antimicrobial agent in relation to the MIC of the agent against the pathogen (peak/MIC ratio), (ii) ratio of the AUC in relation to the MIC of the agent against the pathogen (AUC/MIC ratio), and (iii) time (T) of exposure of a microorganism to concentrations of the antibiotic exceeding the MIC of the agent against the pathogen (T>MIC) (Fig. 1)(1,4,5). Antimicrobial agents can be classified based on the pharmacodynamic parameter that best describes their *in vivo* pattern of bactericidal activity (Table 1).

The evolution of the science of pharmacodynamics has augmented the body of knowledge about how antimicrobials are best used to treat infections. In addition, pharmacodynamics can be utilized to determine the impact of antimicrobial resistance (6–11). Consideration of pharmacodynamics can help define the MIC limit at which the pharmacokinetics of a specific antimicrobial drug would not be expected to result in

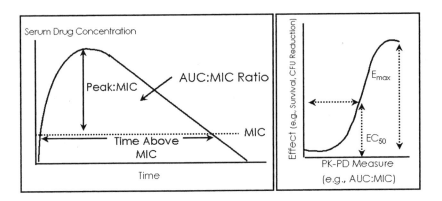

Figure 1 Three pharmacodynamic-pharmacokinetic (PK-PD) measures have been correlated with efficacy (**left**): (i) time (T) of exposure of the pathogen to concentrations exceeding the minimum inhibitory concentration (MIC) of the agent against the pathogen (T>MIC) (ii) ratio of the peak concentration of the agent to the MIC of pathogen (peak:MIC ratio), and (iii) ratio of the 24-hour area under the concentration-time curve (AUC) of the agent to the MIC of the pathogen (AUC:MIC ratio). The response *in vivo* to major classes of antibacterial agents can be mapped to a relationship between pharmacokinetics and the MIC (**right**). CFU, colony-forming unit; EC_{50}, median effective concentration; E_{max}, maximum effect. (Courtesy of MN Dudley.)

Table 1 Antimicrobial Pharmacodynamic Characteristics

Drug class	Pattern of activity	PK-PD parameter	PK-PD target*
Beta-lactams PCNs Cephalosporins Carbapenems	Time-dependent killing and minimal persistent effects	T>MIC	40%–50% T>MIC
Aminoglycosides	Concentration-dependent killing and prolonged persistent effects	Peak/MIC	Peak/MIC 10
Amphotericin B Echinocandins	Concentration-dependent killing and prolonged persistent effects	Peak/MIC	Peak/MIC 10
Fluoroquinolones	Concentration-dependent killing and prolonged persistent effects	24 h AUC/MIC	24 h AUC/MIC 25 for pneumococci 24 h AUC/MIC 100 for gram-negative bacilli
Macrolides Clindamycin Tetracycline Ketolides	Time-dependent killing and prolonged persistent effects	24 h AUC/MIC	24 h AUC/MIC 25
Triazoles	Time-dependent killing and prolonged persistent effects	24 h AUC/MIC	24 h AUC/MIC 25
Linezolid	Time-dependent killing and prolonged persistent effects	24 h AUC/MIC	24 h AUC/MIC 50–100

* Free or unbound drug levels.
24 h AUC/MIC, 24-hour area under the serum concentration curve in relation to the MIC; MIC, minimum inhibitory concentration; peak/MIC, ratio of peak serum concentration of the antimicrobial agent in relation to the MIC of the agent against the pathogen; PCN, penicillin; PK-PD, pharmacokinetic-pharmacodynamic; T.MIC, time above MIC.

treatment success. Pharmacodynamics has also established rational scientific principles that provide the basis for developing dosing strategies that optimize clinical outcomes (12–16).

PK-PD PATTERNS OF ACTIVITY AND PHARMACODYNAMIC MEASURES

There are two qualities of antimicrobial activity that determine the time course of antimicrobial effect. The first characteristic important for determination of the pharmacodynamic pattern of activity is whether drug killing of microorganisms is dependent on the drug concentration or on the duration of exposure (Fig. 2) (1,4,17). In other words, is antimicrobial kill-

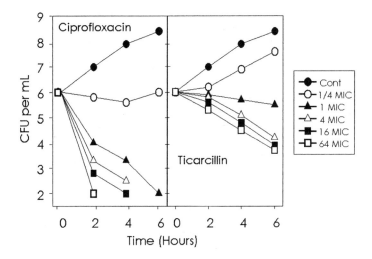

Figure 2 Time-kill curves of *Pseudomonas aeruginosa* ATCC 27853 with exposure to ciprofloxacin and ticarcillin at concentrations from one-fourth to sixty-four times the minimum inhibitory concentration (MIC). CFU, colony-forming units. (Adapted from: Craig WA. Pharmacodynamics of antimicrobials: general concepts and application. In: Nightingale CH, Murakawa T, Ambrose PG, eds. Antimicrobial Pharmacodynamics in Theory and Clinical Practice. New York: Marcel-Dekker, 2002:1–21.)

ing enhanced by increasing drug concentration or is killing optimized by extending bacterial exposure to the antibiotic for a prolonged period of time? The second quality important in pharmacodynamic description is whether a drug produces persistent effects that last after antimicrobial exposure (3,18). These persistent effects are termed *postantibiotic effects* and include persistent suppression of organism growth or regrowth following antibiotic exposure. These persistent effects have been described using *in vitro* test systems that identify the extent and/or duration of growth retardation that occurs when drug levels are suddenly eliminated. The persistent effects have also been described *in vivo* where drug is gradually eliminated over time and describes antimicrobial effects after drug concentrations fall below the MIC or at sub-MIC concentrations.

In examination of these two time course activity characteristics, three patterns of bactericidal have been identified. The first group includes antimicrobials that induce concentration-dependent killing and produce moderate to prolonged persistent effects. Antimicrobial drug classes exhibiting this pharmacodynamic pattern include several antibacterial classes—aminoglycosides, fluoroquinolones, metronidazole, and ketolides—and the antifungal drug classes polyenes and echinocandins (1,8,17,19–26). The goal of a dosing regimen with a drug exhibiting these pharmacodynamic characteristics would be to maximize concentrations with large doses. In addition, widely spaced dosing intervals are often feasible because of the persistence of antimicrobial activity or postantibiotic effects after drug is eliminated from the body and levels fall below the MIC of the infecting pathogen. The pharmacodynamic parameters that are associated with this pattern of activity include the peak serum drug level in relation to the MIC (peak/MIC) and the 24-hour area under the serum concentration curve in relation to the MIC (24 h AUC/MIC).

The second group of agents, including penicillins, cephalosporins, and carbapenems, exhibit minimal concentration-dependent killing and produce minimal persistent effects (14,24,25,27). High drug concentrations do not offer an advantage, and organisms begin to recover or regrow soon after drug is eliminated from the body. For these antibiotics, maximal bacterial killing is observed when serum levels exceed the MIC of the infecting bacteria by only fourfold. The goal of dosing of these antibiotics is to maximize the duration of time that drug concentrations remain above the MIC of the infecting pathogen. With these drugs, the frequency of administration and the dose are both important determinants of their antimicrobial activity. The percent of the dosing interval that serum levels exceed the MIC (%T>MIC) is the pharmacodynamic parameter representative of this pattern of activity.

The final pattern of bactericidal activity is also characterized by a lack of concentration-dependent killing, but differs from the second group in that there are more prolonged postantibiotic periods of growth suppression. With drugs from the tetracycline, glycopeptide, streptogramin, macrolide, lincomycin, and triazole drug classes, it is the total amount of drug administered that is the important determinant of activity (1,8,20,28–30). The dosing frequency is usually not a major factor in the efficacy of these drugs. The 24 h AUC/MIC ratio is the most important determinant of efficacy of these drugs.

PK-PD CHARACTERISTICS—MAGNITUDE OF MEASURE PREDICTIVE OF ACTIVITY

Knowing which pharmacodynamic measure is representative of the antimicrobial activity of a drug allows an optimal dosing strategy to be devised. For example, because the peak/MIC ratio best describes activity of drugs from the aminoglycoside class, large, infrequent, even once-daily administrations can be adopted. On the other hand, with beta-lactam antibiotics, the goal of dosing would be to optimize duration of drug exposure; more frequent administration or even continuous drug infusion strategies may be implemented (19,26,31).

Pharmacodynamic study analyses, however, have also been useful for determining the amount of drug necessary for efficacy in treatment against a number of microbial species, including drug-resistant strains. Both nonclinical (*in vitro* and animal infection models) and clinical trials have allowed the identification of a pharmacodynamic magnitude or target required for efficacy (4,9,12,17,32–37). For example, a study in an animal model with the penicillin derivative amoxicillin observed bacteriologic efficacy when dosing regimens produced a %T>MIC of 40 to 50 in treatment against a large number of *Streptococcus. pneumoniae* isolates (4,6,38). This T>MIC target was similar regardless of the MIC of the organism. So, for example, against an organism with a MIC of 1 µg/mL, serum levels of amoxicillin had to remain above a concentration of 1 µg/mL for at least 2.5 hours of the 6-hour dosing interval, or 40% of the dosing interval. For most drug–pathogen combinations, the magnitude of the parameter required for treatment success is most often similar among different microbiologic species (1,4,24,25,27). For example, studies with numerous beta-lactam antibiotics in a murine infection model against a variety of gram-positive and gram-negative bacteria produced maximal bacterial killing when the free-drug T>MIC exceeded 50% of the dosing interval (24,25). These studies included both susceptible and resistant strains. A large number of similar studies have also shown that the pharmacodynamic target or magnitude predictive of efficacy is similar for drugs within the same class (1,4,8,22,27). So, for example, the T>MIC needed for efficacy of penicillin is relatively similar to the T>MIC necessary for efficacy of the cephalosporin ceftriaxone, as long as free drug concentrations are considered. Protein binding limits distribution of antibiotics to the site of infection and binding to microbial drug targets, thus only unbound or free concentrations are available for microbiologic activity at the site of infection (8,39,40). Thus, it is critical that protein binding be taken into consideration when comparing potency among drugs. This is particularly important for drugs with a high degree of binding (e.g., greater than 80%).

A variety of experiments have also demonstrated that the pharmacodynamic target is similar in treatment of infections at different sites of infection and for different infecting microbial species (1,4,6,24,25,38). For example, Leggett et al. (25) demonstrated that the 24 h AUC/MIC of the fluoroquinolone ciprofloxacin necessary for efficacy (1 to 2 log reduction in bacterial numbers) against a species of *Klebsiella pneumoniae* and

Pseudomonas aeruginosa, in both a thigh sepsis and pneumonia models was similar (approximately 24 h AUC/MIC 100). Most importantly, the pharmacodynamic target associated with outcome has been shown to be similar among different animal species, including humans. For example, study T>MIC needed for efficacy with amoxicillin against pneumococci has been shown to be 40% to 50% in mice, rats, children with otitis media, and adults with sinusitis (4,6,12,36–38). The concordance of this pharmacodynamic target among animal species is not surprising, as the receptor (e.g., penicillin-binding protein, ribosome, DNA gyrase) for the antimicrobial agent is associated with pathogen and not the host.

PK-PD CHARACTERISTICS—BETA-LACTAMS

Beta-lactams are agents that exhibit time-dependent killing. These agents do not kill more efficiently when the concentration exceeds a value that is two- to fourfold higher than the MIC (17). Increasing the drug concentration beyond this magnitude does not improve the rate or extent of bacterial killing. The best predictor of clinical outcome is the duration of time the concentration at the site of infection remains above the MIC (T>MIC). In simplistic terms, the antibiotic needs to be at a high enough concentration for a long enough period of time at the site of infection. Data from *in vitro* and animal infection models, and human clinical studies suggest that the T>MIC needed to achieve bacterial eradication should generally be greater than 40% to 50% of the dosing interval for time-dependent antibiotics (1,4,6,12,25,41).

For example, the relationship between the beta-lactam T>MIC and efficacy has been evaluated in patients with acute otitis media caused by *S. pneumoniae* and *Haemophilus influenzae* (12,35–37). Bacteriologic cure rates of 80% to 85% were observed when the T>MIC for various beta-lactams were greater than 40% to 50% of the dosing interval. Similarly, in hospitalized patients with community-acquired pneumonia, no differences in clinical outcome were observed between patients receiving the cephalosporin cefuroxime as a 1,500-mg per day continuous infusion (T>MIC = 100%) compared with 750 mg administered three times daily (estimated T>MIC = 50% to 60%), suggesting a T>MIC target of 50% is adequate (42).

MACROLIDES

Macrolides and azalides (e.g., azithromycin) exhibit time-dependent killing; however, they produce prolonged postantibiotic effects (1,20,43). The pharmacodynamic parameter for these agents that correlates with efficacy is the AUC/MIC ratio, rather than T>MIC. The AUC/MIC ratio of free drug that predicts efficacy with drugs from the macrolide and azalide class in animal infection models is approximately 25 (20). Because the AUC is the integral of concentration over time, this value of 25 is essentially like averaging a drug concentration at one times the MIC over a 24-hour period, or 1 X 24. Studies in otitis media examining bacteriologic outcomes of azithromycin against pneumococci with varying *in vitro* susceptibility observed treatment success against organisms with lower MIC when the AUC/MIC ratio would exceed a value of 25 (35). However, in treatment of infection due to less susceptible strains, the AUC/MIC value was far below this target value and frequent bacteriologic failures were described.

FLUOROQUINOLONES

Fluoroquinolones kill bacteria most efficiently when their concentrations are appreciably above the MIC of the pathogen (2,3,19,21,22). The AUC/MIC ratio and the peak/MIC ratio are the major parameters correlating with efficacy (1,21,33). In most fluoroquinolone dose-fractionation studies, the AUC/MIC ratio is better correlated with efficacy than peak-to-MIC ratio. Data obtained from several sources, including animal infection models of sepsis, *in vitro* pharmacodynamic experiments, and clinical outcome studies, have found a similar AUC/MIC magnitude predictive of outcomes (5,7,32,33,44). For example, examination of data from several quinolones in several animal infection models in therapy against gram-negative bacilli found an AUC/MIC value of 100 was associated with maximal survival (1,9). Similarly, Forrest et al. (32) demonstrated that an AUC-to-MIC ratio of 125 or greater was associated with the highest bacterial eradication rates in the treatment of infections caused by gram-negative enteric pathogens.

However, for gram-positive bacteria, it appears that effective AUC/MIC ratios can be appreciably lower (1,4,9). For instance, Lister and Sanders (33) reported that for levofloxacin and ciprofloxacin, an AUC/MIC ratio of 32 to 44 was associated with maximal eradication of *S. pneumoniae* in an *in vitro* model of infection. These observations are supported by data from non-neutropenic animal models of infection, in which maximal survival was associated with an AUC/MIC ratio of 25 to 30 against the pneumococcus (44–46). Moreover, these observations from *in vitro* and *in vivo* models of infection are supported by clinical data. The relationship between microbiologic response and the AUC/MIC ratio for gatifloxacin and levofloxacin was recently evaluated in patients with pneumococcal respiratory tract infections (7). AUC/MIC ratios greater than 33.7 were associated with 100% of patients having a positive microbiologic response to therapy, whereas those patients with AUC/MIC ratios less than 33.7 had only a 64% response to therapy.

AMINOGLYCOSIDES

Both *in vitro* and animal infection models have demonstrated that aminoglycoside antibiotics have a concentration-dependent pattern of bactericidal activity and produce prolonged postantibiotic effects (2,3,18,19,23,26). The PK-PD measure predictive of efficacy from extensive study *in vitro, in vivo*, and in clinical trials is the peak/MIC ratio. The optimal dosing strategy to maximize the peak level has led to once-daily dosing of these compounds (26,31,47). In addition, toxicology studies in animals and humans have demonstrated that end-organ aminoglycoside toxicity in the kidney and inner ear is also pharmacodynamically related (48,49). Toxicity at both sites is saturable; thus the very high drug levels provided by once-daily dosing result in fewer adverse events than if smaller doses were to be administered more frequently. The latter strategy results in prolonged drug concentrations at a level associated with toxicity.

OXAZOLIDINONES

Linezolid is the first approved drug of a new class of antibacterial known as oxazolidinones. The bacterial-killing characteristics of the drug shows minimal dependence on drug concentration and produces modest persistent effects. In animal infection model studies, the 24 h AUC/MIC ratio was the pharmacodynamic parameter that correlated best with efficacy (28). The magnitude of the mean AUC/MIC ratio necessary to produce a bacteriostatic effect in this *in vivo* model ranged from near 50 to 100. These values are equivalent to averaging two and four times the MIC of a day of therapy. Supporting clinical pharmacodynamic data are not available.

KETOLIDES

Studies in animal infection models suggest that the AUC/MIC ratio is the measure best correlating with drug activity. The AUC/MIC ratio that predicted efficacy against *S. pneumoniae* for most ketolides is 25 to 100 (11,20,43).

ANTIFUNGALS

Similar pharmacodynamic analyses have been undertaken with drugs from several antifungal drug classes. The concepts developed with antibacterials appear to also be important for these compounds. Each of the three pharmacodynamic measures (peak/MIC ratio, AUC/MIC ratio, and T>MIC) are represented. Drugs from the polyene class, such as amphotericin B, and from the new echinocandin class demonstrate concentration-dependent killing and prolonged persistent effects (8). The peak/MIC ratio is the critical PK-PD determinant of activity. However, for the pyrimidine analogue flucytosine, high drug concentrations do not induce extensive killing and only minimal post-antifungal effects are observed. T>MIC is the important PK-PD measure. For the many drugs from the triazole class, there is a lack of concentration-dependent antifungal activity; however, prolonged post-antifungal effects have been described in animal models. The 24 h AUC/MIC ratio has been found important in predicting efficacy in a variety of animal models. The target AUC/MIC value in treatment of *Candida* infections in animals and in clinical trials is near 25 (8,50). In the largest analysis of the relationship between *Candida* spp MIC and efficacy, the fluconazole dosing regimen producing efficacy against organisms labeled susceptible supports the AUC/MIC target of 25. In studies of several drugs from the triazole antifungal class, free drug levels were demonstrated to be important.

CLINICAL USE OF PHARMACOKINETICS AND PHARMACODYNAMICS

Knowledge of pharmacodynamics has had a remarkable impact on the clinical use and regulatory development of antimicrobials. For example, the ability to predict efficacy against both drug-susceptible and -resistant pathogens based on achieving a defined pharmacodynamic target has been useful in the design of treatment strategies in the face of emerging antimicrobial drug resistance. This impact has been most evident in prediction of treatment outcome against increasing multidrug-resistant *S. pneumoniae* (6,13,14,16,41,51). Although there are numerous beta-lactam antibiotics approved for the treatment of pneumococcal respiratory tract infections, in the face of resistant pneumococci, pharmacodynamic analysis would predict treatment failure for many of the antibiotics included in this group. The elevation in MIC reduces the %T>MIC for all available oral cephalosporins well below the 40% target, and treatment failure would be anticipated

(13,16,51). These predictions have been confirmed in studies of patients with both community-acquired pneumonia and upper respiratory tract infection (12,35–37,41). This type of pharmacodynamic knowledge has been used to develop treatment guidelines for otitis media, sinusitis, and community-acquired pneumonia, and these differences in pharmacodynamic potency are reflected in recent recommendations (13,14,16). In addition, these approaches to understanding antimicrobial efficacy have been used to determine the MIC levels for which organisms should be labeled susceptible or resistant, termed *susceptibility breakpoints* (10,52).

POPULATION PHARMACOKINETICS AND STOCHASTIC MODELING

As discussed above, an important factor influencing the effectiveness of a particular antibiotic regimen includes the drug exposure in the individual, which is reflected by the pharmacokinetics. However, because of natural variation in biological systems, pharmacokinetics distribute across a range of values (7,10). Some individuals absorb, metabolize, distribute and excrete a drug more rapidly than others and some more slowly, leading to considerable variations in pharmacokinetic parameters (53,54). As a result of these variations, antimicrobial agent efficacy *in vivo* may differ. To determine the true efficacy of an agent in every patient, the MIC of the causative organism against the agent used and the serum pharmacokinetics of the agent would need to be determined in each patient. This is, of course, physically impossible, and has only been performed on a small scale, for obvious reasons. Another source of variation in treatment of patients is that found in the infecting organism. There is considerable variation in the susceptibility of a specific pathogen to an antimicrobial agent.

Often the pharmacokinetic portion of pharmacodynamic predictions has been based on mean serum pharmacokinetic values from healthy patients. These values obviously do not reflect potential variation in pharmacokinetics from patient to patient, so that some patients will not achieve the target needed, whereas others will exceed the target (54). More recently, investigators have used population pharmacokinetic methods to better account for variation in drug levels among different patients and to identify factors that account for these variations (10,34).

Both the pharmacokinetic variability and the entire distribution can be taken into account by more sophisticated statistical modeling. The term *Monte Carlo simulation* refers to the method that is used to extend the variation in pharmacokinetics in a small population to one as large as 5,000 to 10,000 patients. One then determines what percentage of this large population attains the PK-PD target required for efficacy with the drug being studied (10,55). The performance of such analyses provides the likelihood that a particular dosing regimen will result in drug levels that will achieve the defined pharmacodynamic target or magnitude of exposure associated with efficacy. For example, the approach can quantify the probability that a twice-daily administration of the beta-lactam antibiotic X will result in a T>MIC of 40% to 50% in the treatment of pneumococcal infections expected to be encountered in one's community. This type of data modeling has been shown to be quite powerful and is being used by the pharmaceutical industry in selection of dosing regimens for clinical trials and by regulatory agencies such as the NCCLS and the FDA to aid in development of susceptibility breakpoints for various drug–organism combinations (51,56).

PK-PD AND HOSPITAL TREATMENT GUIDELINES/ALGORITHMS

Pharmacokinetic and pharmacodynamic principles play an important role in the evaluation and selection of antimicrobial therapy for treatment guidelines (13,14,16). PK-PD analyses have been particularly useful for the development of guidelines for the treatment of infections for which antimicrobial resistance has recently emerged. Recent guidelines for antibacterial therapy for the respiratory tract have relied heavily on PK-PD concepts.

Similar to the modeling process described above, first the PK-PD measure that best predicts antimicrobial activity *in vivo* for the drug classes under consideration is identified. Next, the magnitude of the PK-PD parameter required for efficacy is determined (i.e., PK-PD target) for each drug–organism combination, and resistance may be defined for situations in which the PK-PD goal cannot be achieved. Subsequently, data from population pharmacokinetics and large *in vitro* susceptibility surveillance projects may be considered in the context of the PK-PD target. Finally, the likelihood of treatment success in the empiric therapy of the infection for each of the drugs can be determined. The most detailed prediction analysis has been undertaken by the Sinus and Allergy Health Partnership (16) for the development of appropriate antibacterial therapies for bacterial sinusitis and otitis media.

DEFINING APPROPRIATE *IN VITRO* SUSCEPTIBILITY BREAKPOINTS

These concepts likewise have been used as a tool for defining susceptibility breakpoints for antibiotics. Therapeutic decisions for treatment of infections in patients are frequently guided by the definition of the implicated pathogen as susceptible or resistant. Thus, the MIC above which organisms are termed resistant is quite important. The criteria used to categorize organisms as susceptible or resistant have traditionally been based on the distribution of organism MIC values. Many times, the distribution of organisms is distinct and far below clinical drug levels, making this decision straightforward. However, most recently, the use of pharmacodynamics has provided a means to examine the relationship among the MIC, serum drug concentrations, and effect. Using PK-PD to aid in defining susceptibility breakpoints for antimicrobial agents does not require special data sets or extensive *in vitro* or clinical studies. First, the PK-PD target is defined in animal infection or *in vitro* infection models. With this target in mind, one can then use Monte Carlo simulation to consider variation in drug levels using population pharmacokinetics to define the

MIC for which a certain drug and dosing regimen would be anticipated to achieve the PK-PD target for the majority of patients (e.g., 90% to 95% target attainment) (10). Resistance can then be defined as MIC values above the PK-PD breakpoint MIC.

For example, the PK-PD breakpoint MIC for beta-lactam antibiotics can be determined by using Monte Carlo simulation of population pharmacokinetics to define the drug concentration that corresponds with 40% to 50% of the dosing interval. This drug concentration would then be defined as the PK-PD susceptibility limit or breakpoint. In the treatment of organisms with MIC values at or below this concentration, one would anticipate therapeutic success. Additionally, the proportion of bacteria that are therefore susceptible can be defined from large surveillance studies based on the proportion of isolates with MIC values at or below these susceptibility limits or breakpoints.

APPLICATION TO ANTIBIOTIC FORMULARY DECISIONS

With emerging resistance, not all drugs within a drug class or from different classes would be expected to perform similarly. Utilization of PK-PD analyses by pharmacy and therapeutic committees and antibiotic subcommittees as decision support tools when comparing competing alternatives will likely result in optimizing clinical outcomes and decreasing the probability of selecting for resistance.

REFERENCES

1. Craig WA. Pharmacokinetic/pharmacodynamic parameters: rationale for antibacterial dosing of mice and men. Clin Infect Dis 1998; 26:1–12.

2. Vogelman B, Gudmundsson S, Leggett J, Turnidge J, Ebert S, Craig WA. Correlation of antimicrobial pharmacokinetic parameters with therapeutic efficacy in an animal model. J Infect Dis. 1988; 158:831–847.

3. Vogelman B, Gudmundsson S, Turnidge J, Leggett J, Craig WA. *In vivo* postantibiotic effect in a thigh infection in neutropenic mice. J Infect Dis 1988; 157:287–298.

4. Andes D, Craig WA. Animal model pharmacokinetics and pharmacodynamics: a critical review. Int J Antimicrob Agents 2002; 19:261–268.

5. Preston SL, Drusano GL, Berman AL, Fowler CL, Chow AT, Dornseif B, Reichl V, Natarajan J, Corrado M. Pharmacodynamics of levofloxacin: a new paradigm for early clinical trials. JAMA 1998; 279:125–129.

6. Andes D, Craig WA. *In vivo* activities of amoxicillin and amoxicillin-clavulanate against *Streptococcus pneumoniae*: application to breakpoint determination. Antimicrob Agents Chemother 1998; 42:2375–2379.

7. Ambrose PG, Grasela DM, Grasela TH, Passarell J, Mayer HB, Pierce PF. Pharmacodynamics of fluoroquinolones against *Streptococcus pneumoniae* in patients with community-acquired respiratory tract infections. Antimicrob Agents Chemother 2001; 45:2793–2797.

8. Andes D. *In vivo* pharmacodynamics of antifungal drugs in the treatment of candidiasis. Antimicrob Agents Chemother 2003; 47:1179–1186.

9. Craig WA. Does the dose matter? Clin Infect Dis 2001; 33(Suppl 3):S233–S237.

10. Dudley MN, Ambrose PG. Pharmacodynamics in the study of drug resistance and establishing *in vitro* susceptibility breakpoints: ready for prime time. Curr Opin Microbiol 2000; 3: 515–521.

11. Vesga O, Craig WA. Impact of macrolide resistance on the *in vivo* activity of a new ketolide, HMR 3647, against *S. pneumoniae* and *S. aureus* [abstr F259], 37th Interscience Conference on Antimicrobial Agents and Chemotherapy, Toronto, Sept 28–Oct 1, 1997.

12. Craig WA, Andes D. Pharmacokinetics and pharmacodynamics of antibiotics in otitis media. Pediatr Infect Dis J 1996; 15: 255–259.

13. Dowell SF, Butler JC, Giebink GS, Jacobs MR, Jernigan D, Musher DM, Rakowsky A, Schwartz B. Acute otitis media: man-

agement and surveillance in an era of pneumococcal resistance—report from the Drug-Resistant Streptococcus Pneumoniae Therapeutic Working Group. Pediatr Infect Dis J 1999; 18:1–9.

14. Heffelfinger JD, Dowell SF, Jorgensen JH, Klugman KP, Mabry LR, Musher DM, Plouffe JF, Rakowsky A, Schuchat A, Whitney CG. Management of community-acquired pneumonia in the era of pneumococcal resistance: a report from the drug-resistant *Streptococcus pneumoniae* therapeutic working group. Arch Intern Med 2000; 160:1399–1408.

16. Whitney CG. Antimicrobial treatment guidelines for acute bacterial rhinosinusitis. Otolaryngol Head Neck Surg 2000; 123: 1–32.

17. Craig WA, Ebert SC. Killing and regrowth of bacteria *in vitro*: a review. Scand J Infect Dis 1991; 74(Suppl):63–70.

18. Craig WA, Gudmundsson S. Postantibiotic Effect. In: Lorian V,, Ed Antibiotics in Laboratory Medicine.. 4th ed.. Baltimore: Williams & Wilkins, 1996:296–329.

19. Blaser J, Stone BB, Groner MC, Zinner SH. Comparative study with enoxacin and netilmicin in a pharmacodynamic model to determine importance of ratio of antibiotic peak concentration to MIC for bactericidal activity and emergence of resistance. Antimicrob Agents Chemother 1987; 31:1054–1060.

20. Craig WA, Kiem S, Andes DR. Free drug 24-hr AUC/MIC is the PK/PD target that correlates with *in vivo* efficacy of macrolides, azalides, ketolides, and clindamycin [abstr A-1264], 42nd Interscience Conference on Antimicrobial Agents and Chemotherapy, San Diego, CA, Sept 27–30, 2002.

21. Drusano GL, Johnson DE, Rosen M, Standiford HC. Pharmacodynamics of a fluoroquinolone antimicrobial agent in a neutropenic rat model of *Pseudomonas* sepsis. Antimicrob Agents Chemother 1993; 37:483–490.

22. Lacy MK, Lu W, Xu X, Tessier PR, Nicolau DP, Quintiliani R, Nightingale CH. Pharmacodynamic comparisons of levofloxacin, ciprofloxacin, and ampicillin against *Streptococcus pneumoniae* in an *in vitro* model of infection. Antimicrob Agents Chemother 1999; 43:672–677.

23. Lacy MK, Nicolau DP, Nightengale CH, Quintiliani R. The pharmacodynamics of aminoglycosides. Clin Infect Dis 1998; 27: 23–27.

24. Leggett JE, Fantin B, Ebert S, Totsuka K, Vogelman B, Calame W, Mattie H, Craig WA. Comparative dose-effect relationships at several dosing intervals in murine pneumonitis and thigh-infection models. J Infect Dis 1989; 159:281–292.

25. Leggett JE, Ebert S, Fantin B, Craig WA. Comparative dose-effect relations at several dosing intervals for beta-lactam, aminoglycoside and quinolone antibiotics against gram-negative bacilli in murine thigh-infection and pneumonitis models. Scand J Infect Dis 1990; 74:179–184.

26. Moore RD, Lietman PS, Smith CR. Clinical response to aminoglycoside therapy: importance of the ratio of peak concentration to minimal inhibitory concentration. J Infect Dis 1987; 155: 93–99.

27. Craig WA. Interrelationships between pharmacokinetics and pharmacodynamics in determining dosage regimens for broad-spectrum cephalosporins. Drug Microbiol Infect Dis 1995; 22: 89–93.

28. Andes D, Peng J, Craig WA. *In vivo* characterization of the pharmacodynamics of a new oxazolidinone (linezolid). Antimicrob Agents Chemother 2002; 46:3484–3489.

29. Christianson J, Andes D, Craig W. Characterization of the pharmacodynamics of clindamycin against Streptococcus pneumoniae in a murine thigh infection model [abstr], 41st Interscience Conference on Antimicrobial Agents and Chemotherapy, Chicago, Dec 16–19, 2001.

30. Christianson J, Andes D, Craig W. Magnitude of the 24h AUC/ MIC required for doxycycline against *Streptococcus pneumoniae* in a murine thigh infection model [abstr], 41st Interscience Conference on Antimicrobial Agents and Chemotherapy, Chicago, Dec 16–19, 2001.

31. Bailey TC, Little JR, Littenberg B, Reichley RM, Dunagan WC. A meta-analysis of extended-interval dosing versus multiple daily dosing of aminoglycosides. Clin Infect Dis 1997; 24: 786–795.

32. Forrest A, Nix DE, Ballow CH, Goss TF, Birmingham MC, Schentag JJ. Pharmacodynamics of intravenous ciprofloxacin in seriously ill patients. Antimicrob Agents Chemother 1993; 37:1073–1081.

33. Lister PD, Sanders CC. Pharmacodynamics of levofloxacin and ciprofloxacin against *Streptococcus pneumoniae*. J Antimicrob Chemother 1999; 43:79–86.

34. Preston SL, Drusano GL, Berman AL. Levofloxacin population pharmacokinetic and creation of a demographic model for prediction of individual drug clearance in patients with serious community-acquired infection. Antimicrob Agents Chemother; 1998:1098–1104.

35. Dagan R, Leibovitz E, Fliss DM, Leiberman A, Jacobs MR, Craig W, Yagupsky P. Bacteriologic efficacies of oral azithromycin and oral cefaclor in treatment of acute otitis media in infants and young children. Antimicrob Agents Chemother 2000; 44:43–50.

36. Dagan R, Johnson CE, McLinn S, Abughali N, Feris J, Leibovitz E, Burch DJ, Jacobs MR. Bacteriologic and clinical efficacy of amoxicillin/clavulanate vs. azithromycin in acute otitis media. Pediatr Infect Dis J 2000; 19:95–104.

37. Dagan R, Hoberman A, Johnson C, Leibovitz EL, Arguedas A, Rose FV, Wynne BR, Jacobs MR. Bacteriologic and clinical efficacy of high dose amoxicillin/clavulanate in children with acute otitis media. Pediatr Infect Dis J 2001; 20:829–837.

38. Woodnut G, Berry V. Two pharmacodynamic models for assessing the efficacy of amoxicillin-clavulante against experimental respiratory tract infections caused by strains of *Streptococcus pneumoniae*. Antimicrob Agents Chemother 1999; 43:29–34.

39. Craig WA, Suh B. Protein Binding. In: Lorian V, Ed Antibiotics in Laboratory Medicine.. 3d ed.. Baltimore: Williams & Wilkins, 1991:367–402.

40. Kunin CM, Craig WA, Kornguth M, Monson R. Influence of binding to the pharmacologic activity of antibiotics. Ann NY Acad Sci 1973; 226:214–224.

41. File TM Jr, Jacobs MR, Poole MD, Wynne B. Outcome of treatment of respiratory tract infections due to *Streptococcus pneu-*

moniae, including drug-resistant strains, with pharmacokinetically enhanced amoxicillin/clavulanate. Int J Antimicrob Agents 2002; 20:235–247.

42. Ambrose PG, Quintiliani R, Nightingale CH. Continuous vs intermittent infusion of cefuroxime for the treatment of community-acquired pneumonia. Infect Dis Clin Prac 1997; 7:463–470.

43. Vesga O, Andes D, Craig WA. Comparative *in vivo* activity of HMR 3647, azithromycin, clarithromycin, and roxithromycin against *S. pneumoniae* and *S. aureus* [abstr F258], 37th Interscience Conference on Antimicrobial Agents and Chemotherapy, Toronto, Sept 28–Oct 1, 1997.

44. Andes D, Craig WA. Pharmacokinetics of fluoroquinolones in experimental endocarditis. Clin Infect Dis 1998; 27:47–50.

45. Andes D, Craig WA. Characterization of the pharmacodynamics of the new fluoroquinolone, gatifloxaxin, in murine thigh and lung infection models. Antimicrob Agents Chemother 2002; 46:1665–1670.

46. Nicolau DP, Mattoes HM, Banevicius M, Xuan D, Nightingale CH. Pharmacodynamics of a novel des-F(6)-quinolone, BMS-284756, against *Streptococcus pneumoniae* in the thigh infection model. Antimicrob Agents Chemother 2003; 47:1630–1635.

47. Kashuba ADM, Nafziger AN, Drusano GL, Bertino JS. Optimizing aminoglycoside therapy for nosocomial pneumonia caused by gram-negative bacteria. Antimicrob Agents Chemother 1999; 43:623–629.

48. Rybak MJ, Abate BJ, Kang SL, Ruffing ML, Lerner SA, Drusano GL. Prospective evaluation of the effect of an aminoglycoside dosing regimen on rates of observed nephrotoxicity and ototoxicity. Antimicrob Agents Chemother 1999; 43:1549–1555.

49. Verpooten GA, Biulinao RA, Verbist L, Eestermans G, De Broe ME. Once-daily dosing decreases renal accumulation of gentamicin and netilmicin. Clin Pharmacol Ther 1989; 45:22–27.

50. Rex JH, Pfaller MA, Galgiani JN, Bartlett MS, Espinel-Ingroff A, Ghannoum MA, Lancaster M, Odds FC, Rinaldi MG, Walsh TJ, Barry AL, for the NCCLS Subcommittee on Antifungal Susceptibility Testing. Development of interpretive breakpoints for antifungal susceptibility testing: conceptual framework and

analysis of *in vitro* and *in vivo* correlation data for fluconazole, itraconazole, and *Candida* infections. Clin Infect Dis 1997; 24: 235–247.

51. Ambrose PG, Garsela DM. The use of Monte Carlo simulation to examine pharmacodynamic variance of drugs: fluoroquinolone pharmacodynamics against *Streptococcus pneumoniae*. Diagn Microbiol Infect Dis 2000; 38:151–157.

52. Garsela DM. NCCLS Document M100-S11: Performance Standards for Antimicrobial Susceptibility Testing; Eleventh Informational Supplement.. Philadelphia: NCCL, 2001.

53. Ambrose PG, Bhavnani SM, Cirincione BB, Piedmonte M, Grasela TH. Gatifloxacin and the elderly: pharmacokinetic-pharmacodynamic rationale for a potential age-related dose reduction. J Antimicrob Chemother 2003; 52:435–440.

54. Ambrose PG, Quintiliani R. Limitations of single point pharmacodynamic analysis. Pediatr Infect Dis J 2000; 19:769.

55. Bonate PL. A brief introduction to Monte Carlo simulation. Clin Pharmacokinet 2001; 40:15–22.

56. http://FDA.gov/cder/guidance/2580dft.pdf.

5

Optimization of Antibacterial Therapy to Minimize Costs, Medication Errors, and Adverse Outcomes

DAVID E. NIX and BRIAN L. ERSTAD

University of Arizona College of Pharmacy
Tucson, Arizona, U.S.A.

As noted in the widely publicized Institute of Medicine report, medical errors are a major cause of mortality, morbidity, and excess health care costs (1). A substantial portion of these medical errors are medication errors that lead to preventable adverse drug events (ADEs). In the United States, the estimated cost of a preventable ADE ranges from $2,600 to $6,800 (based on year 2000 values) in hospitalized patients and from $700 to $2,200 in outpatients requiring emergency department evaluation or hospital admission. When extrapolated to a nationwide basis, the combined annual cost is in the range of $2 billion to $3 billion (2). Antibacterial agents represent the class of drugs most cited as the subject of ADEs (3,4). Furthermore, the adverse effects attributable to antibacterial agents are not limited to minor reactions. This class has been found to be a major cause of fatal ADEs (5).

Although antibacterial agents may be costly and associated with ADEs, the consequences and costs associated with infection are also substantial. Approximately 2 million patients develop nosocomial infections each year in U.S. acute care facilities, with associated costs exceeding $4 billion (6). When nosocomial infection occurs, the clinician must select among available agents based on effectiveness, safety, and cost. This chapter reviews medication errors and associated ADEs involving antibacterial drugs, including errors related to inappropriate and suboptimal use. The discussion includes antibacterial strategies that may prevent these events, as well as issues to consider when making formulary and economic decisions concerning antibacterial agents.

DIAGNOSIS

An accurate diagnosis is the first step in deciding whether an antibacterial drug is needed and selecting the particular drug(s). Antibacterial drugs are frequently prescribed for unexplained fever or vague complaints without a specific diagnosis having been made. Elderly patients, for example, may present only with nonspecific signs of infection, such as fever, fatigue, decreased appetite, mental confusion, or trauma due to a fall. Some patients may benefit from antibacterial therapy, whereas others may receive antibacterial drugs needlessly and risk suffering an ADE. A study of the diagnosis of Lyme disease in children revealed a correct diagnosis in only 51% of 146 patients. Thirty-eight percent were overdiagnosed, whereas a smaller percentage was underdiagnosed for Lyme disease (7). In the southwestern United States, many patients receive antibacterial drugs for treatment of pulmonary coccidioidomycosis. If the correct diagnosis were made, antibacterial therapy could be avoided, and only patients with complications of the primary pulmonary infection would require antifungal treatment (8). Appropriate therapy requires a thorough evaluation of the disease process and knowledge of the clinical entity.

Most of the literature has focused on overuse of antibacterial agents in situations where antibacterial treatment may not provide benefit. Examples of these situations include upper respiratory infection syndromes, acute non–β-hemolytic streptococcal pharyngitis, and acute bronchitis. Data from the 1996 National Ambulatory Medical Care Survey revealed that 61% to 72% of patients diagnosed with a cold, upper respiratory infection, or acute bronchitis were prescribed an antibacterial drug. Such prescriptions accounted for 15% of the total prescriptions for antibacterial drugs (9). Colds, upper respiratory infection syndromes, and acute bronchitis (in adults) are almost always caused by viral infection, and antibacterial therapy does not improve the outcome (10). Although acute sinusitis is frequently managed with antibacterial drugs, most patients have spontaneous resolution of symptoms. A recent placebo-controlled trial of amoxicillin treatment of acute sinusitis did not show a statistically significant improvement with amoxicillin compared with placebo (11). Serious complications associated with acute sinusitis occur primarily in patients who have underlying chronic sinusitis or who are immunocompromised. Antibiotics have only modest benefits in children with acute otitis media or otitis media with effusion. As with acute sinusitis, the spontaneous resolution rate is high. Current recommendations involve waiting 3 to 6 months before considering a trial of antibiotics for otitis media with effusion (12). For acute otitis media in children at least 2 years of age, waiting up to 3 days before initiating antibiotic therapy is a valid treatment option (13,14). Acute otitis media will spontaneously improve in the majority of children, resulting in substantially fewer antibacterial prescriptions. Acute bronchitis is almost always caused by a viral pathogen and is self-limiting without specific therapy. There is no benefit from antibacterial therapy. In contrast to these common respiratory infections, community-acquired pneumonia should be treated with antibacterial agents unless bacterial infection is excluded (15). Influenza is another disease in which antibacterial therapy would be inappropriate. Signs, symptoms, and history of influenza vaccination are not reliable to differentiate influenza from other infectious diseases. The availability of a rapid influenza antigen detection test along with white blood cell count has been shown to improve clinical decisions (16). However, the possibility of secondary bacterial pneumonia must be considered in a patient with influenza. When and when not to treat patients for acute exacerbation of chronic bronchitis is less clear than with pneumonia; however, the need for treatment is based on the stage of chronic bronchitis, severity of symptoms, and other risk factors (17).

ETIOLOGY

After the diagnosis is made and the clinician determines that antibacterial treatment is warranted, the infectious etiology needs further consideration. The etiology for some infections may be established on the basis of clinical presentation, whereas further diagnostic testing is needed in other cases. In considering the need for etiologic diagnosis, clinicians must consider the difficulty of obtaining an appropriate specimen, laboratory costs, the likelihood of finding the etiology, the likelihood of serious outcome or complication with inappropriate therapy, and often, knowing how the etiology will alter treatment. For example, culture and pathogen identification is generally not needed for acute otitis media, acute rhinosinusitis, or uncomplicated urinary tract infections. In cases of simple cellulitis, the difficulty of obtaining uncontaminated specimens and low yield precludes routine culturing. The role of sputum cultures with community-acquired pneumonia is controversial for the same reasons. Although blood cultures are quite specific, sensitivity is low. The value of culture to determine specific etiology is quite clear for some infections, such as blood cultures in suspected sepsis or endocarditis, cerebrospinal fluid cultures in suspected meningitis, or bone biopsy in osteomyelitis. Defining exactly when culture is required and when susceptibility testing should be performed is beyond the scope of this chapter. However, a potential pathogen in situations of clinically apparent infection may not be cultured despite appropriate culturing methods. In the case of community-acquired pneumonia, sputum and blood cultures identify a specific etiology in less than half the cases (18). When cultures are negative, empiric therapy may be appropriate, depending on the clinical entity and likelihood of a bacterial pathogen. Susceptibility testing should clearly be performed for invasive infections and for clinical isolates in which resistance has been documented with relative frequency. Given modern resistance problems, susceptibility testing is usually indicated any time a culture is taken and a probable pathogen is isolated. The susceptibility results may not always influence therapy in the individual patient, but the results are also important for local susceptibility surveillance.

DRUG SELECTION AND DOSING

If a specific etiology is not or cannot be determined, treatment must be determined on the basis of clinical trials (proof of efficacy) and knowledge of usual etiologies. Clinical trials of antibacterial agents do not typically address optimal therapy for a particular infection. Given design constraints of including only patients who are likely to respond (i.e., have susceptible organism and no conditions that complicate response) and study goals of demonstrating equivalence between treatments, few treatments are demonstrated to be superior (19). Clinical trials are focused on a specific disease, such as community-acquired pneumonia or intra-abdominal infection. Consideration of etiology is usually a secondary concern unless *in vitro* resistance is documented at protocol entry. Antibacterial drugs are labeled for indications that include specific pathogens based on an adequate number of cases entered into phase III clinical trials. However, such label information does not ensure that the antibacterial agent is the best available drug. In many cases, the science available may support nonlabeled uses for the agent. A pharmacodynamic (PD) approach considers the etiology (pathogen susceptibility) and antibacterial exposure (pharmacokinetics [PK]) as most important. Excluding specialized infection sites such as the cerebrospinal space, middle ear space, or urine, serum concentrations may be used as a surrogate for concentrations at the site of infection. For agents that have significant protein binding (particularly agents that are 85% or more bound), the free concentration represents the bioactive concentration and should be used for defining exposure (20). Special considerations are needed for bacteria that survive and multiply within cells, such as *Chlamydia* spp. and *Legionella* spp (21). Likewise, PK/PD relationships may differ substantially among agents. Free serum concentrations of a beta-lactam agent may predict response to infections caused by extracellular pathogens, for example. However, agents that have high tissue affinity (e.g., azithromycin) may have greater efficacy than would be predicted based on serum concentrations (22). Optimally, one would have PK/PD studies performed for each type of infection and groups of antibacterial drugs and would understand the relationships among dose, biophase exposure, antibacterial activity, and clinical efficacy. Whether antibacterial activity is predictable on the basis of antibacterial exposure and pathogen susceptibility would be established. Common organisms that behave differently than predicted would also be identified. Our knowledge of PK/PD is clearly lacking for many infections; however, the information available does provide a framework for designing optimal therapy. Prevention of medication errors and adverse events involving antibacterial drugs requires a broad-based, integrated effort. Potential adverse effects would be avoided in patients who do not receive antibacterial therapy when such therapy is not indicated. These adverse effects include not only adverse effects in the individual patient, but also adverse effects to society, such as increasing bacterial resistance and increased health care costs. However, the risk of overtreatment should be balanced with the risk of undertreatment. Failure to administer an antibacterial agent to patients who have an active infection and could benefit from antibacterial therapy could lead to more serious illness and long-term and/or permanent complications. Thus, the first principle is to use antibacterial drugs in appropriate circumstances. The second principle is to administer the right drug in appropriate clinical situations. Achieving this second principle is less defined. Is the right drug one that is Food and Drug Administration (FDA) approved for the specific indication, generally accepted as effective for the specific indication, the drug of choice for the specific indication, or the best drug for the individual patient? Clinical trials, as currently performed, are not designed to provide the information needed to promote optimal use of antibacterial drugs in individual patients. Obstacles to individualized antibacterial selection and dosing include failure to identify a specific pathogen(s), uncertainty of etiology, semiquantitative susceptibility testing, lack of predictive pharmacokinetic models or analytical capabilities, and uncertainties as to whether more scientifically based antibacterial prescribing will enhance outcomes. The application of PK/PD strategies has not been demonstrated to be cost-effective. In the end, the desire to have simplified marketing and dosing is a major obstacle to using a PK/PD approach.

Pharmacodynamic principles allow for individualization of drug selection. Clinicians will need to be familiar with pharmacokinetics as they relate to drug exposure at different sites of infection, *in vitro* susceptibility, and pharmacodynamic goals as they relate to different classes of antibacterial drugs. Exposure parameters such as maximum drug concentration/minimum inhibitory concentration (C_{max}/MIC) ratio are useful for many drugs, including aminoglycosides and fluoroquinolones. Here, the population C_{max} may be used with the MIC_{90} (MIC for 90%) of the species or with the individualized pathogen MIC. In the original description, the agent with the highest C_{max}/MIC would be selected (23). In reality, there may be several agents that have C_{max}/MIC ratios that are sufficient for optimal response, and other factors (cost, dosing convenience, safety) can be used to select between the agents. For aminoglycosides and fluoroquinolones, C_{max}/MIC ratios of 8 to 10 or greater are considered optimal for most infections (24,25). Generally the serum C_{max} can be used except when the site of infection involves a barrier to drug penetration. For example, cerebrospinal fluid (CSF) concentration should be used with meningeal infection and middle ear fluid concentrations for the treatment of otitis media (26). The area under the plasma concentration-time curve divided by MIC (AUC/ MIC) is also useful for optimal use of fluoroquinolones. In fact, this parameter predicts outcome slightly better than C_{max}/ MIC. The goal for AUC/MIC may vary depending on the specific fluoroquinolone and specific infection; however, in general, the AUC/MIC should optimally exceed 100 to 125 for gram-negative infections (25).

Antimicrobial activity is best explained by the free drug concentration and exposure parameters based on free drug concentrations. However, many of the clinical PK/PD study reports provide conclusions based on total drug exposure rather than free (unbound) drug exposure. A better understanding of PK/PD targets is needed before extrapolating a study involving one drug to other drugs in the same class. Differences in penetration to the site of infection, protein binding, and other undetermined factors may affect the exposure parameter target values.

After the correct drug is selected, dosing needs to be optimized using the same pharmacodynamic principles. The susceptibility breakpoints for gentamicin are 4 μg/mL or greater for susceptible pathogens and 8 μg/mL for intermediate pathogens (27). Current recommendations for high-dose extended-interval dosing target maximum concentrations of 14 to 20 μg/ mL. A pathogen could be reported susceptible to gentamicin, whereas maximum doses would achieve a C_{max}/MIC ratio of only 3.5 to 5 and AUC/MIC of 13 to 19. Optimal pharmacodynamics is believed to be associated with a C_{max}/MIC ratio of 10 or greater and AUC/MIC of 70 or greater (24,28). Use of gentamicin in this setting would be acceptable only in combination with a primary antibacterial agent that would achieve more optimal pharmacodynamic end points. Although a drug-free period is generally desirable with aminoglycosides, this is difficult to achieve among patients with markedly impaired renal function. One also must guard against having too long a drug-free interval, although *too long* is not currently defined. Examples of "medication errors" could include the use of aminoglycoside in a patient with renal impairment when other, less toxic drugs are considered equally effective, or the use of high-dose, once-daily gentamicin without extending the dosing interval.

For other drugs, such as beta-lactams and vancomycin, the percent of time above the MIC (%T>MIC) should be optimized (29). In some infections, %T>MIC of at least 40 may be just as effective as %T>MIC of 100 (30). The optimal %T>MIC has been defined only in limited circumstances, and more research is needed. If the pathogen is *Streptococcus pneumoniae*, %T>MIC of 40 or greater may be adequate, whereas %T>MIC of 60 to 70 or greater may be needed for gram-negative pathogens (30–32). Protein binding may also play a role in response because the observed activity in serum containing media is reduced for highly protein-bound (greater than 85%) drugs. Some investigators have suggested that activity is best characterized using free drug concentrations and exposure parameters instead of total serum concentrations (33). This principle seems more important for gram-positive organisms (e.g., *Staphylococcus aureus*) than for gram-negative pathogens (e.g., *Pseudomonas aeruginosa* and Enterobacteriaceae) (34,35). As with aminoglycosides and fluoroquinolones, doses need to be based on pharmacodynamic principles, although the principles are different. On the basis of CSF concentrations, the MIC breakpoint for penicillin susceptibility is less than 0.1 µg/mL and intermediate susceptibility is defined by a MIC of 0.1 to 1 µg/mL (27). However, patients with pneumonia due to *S. pneumoniae* with an MIC of 2 or 4 µg/mL may well respond to standard doses of penicillin G. The administration of 500,000 units of penicillin G per hour by continuous infusion can be expected to provide steady-state serum concentrations of about 14 µg/mL (36). Concentrations would also be expected to exceed 2 µg/mL more than 50% of a dosing interval if 2 million units were administered every 4 hours or if 3 million units were administered every 6 hours. Discussion of methods for calculating %T>MIC is beyond the scope of this chapter. Ideally, population-based pharmacokinetic parameters should be available for antibacterial drugs, and these should be determined from infected patients (target population). The parameters should be individualized based on patient specific characteristics (e.g., weight, creatinine clearance). %T>MIC can then be determined using pharmacokinetic simulation and a designated MIC value. For time-dependent antibacterial drugs, continuous infusion is the most efficient means to deliver the drug. Although there is increasing interest in continuous infusion of beta-lactam drugs and vancomycin, many situations favor the use of intermittent dosing for practical reasons (37,38). As an example, one could deliver cefepime as a continuous infusion, 125 mg/hour, or as 1 g every 8 hours, 1.5 g every 12 hours, or 3 g every 24 hours. Based on a two-compartment model and typical pharmacokinetic parameters (CL_T = 7.07 L/h; V_1 = 14.3 L; (8_1 = 0.988 h^{-1}; and (8_2 = 0.233 h^{-1}), steady-state concentrations would remain above 8 g/mL for 100%, 68%, 55%, and 38% of the time, respectively. Achieving %T>MIC of 100 (8 g/mL) would require almost 6 g/day for every-8-hour dosing and 11 g/day for every-12-hour dosing, compared with 1.5 g/day for continuous infusion.

MEDICATION ERRORS AND ADVERSE DRUG EVENTS

Medication errors are errors that result in preventable (actual or potential) ADEs. These errors are usually considered by the stage during which they occurred: prescription, transcription, dispensation, or administration. Examples of prescription medication errors leading to an adverse event would include using an aminoglycoside in a patient with moderate renal impairment or other concomitant nephrotoxic drugs leading to worsening renal failure. The "error" component would enter the situation if gentamicin therapy could not be justified. Another example involves administration of a penicillin derivative to a patient with a known history of immediate hypersensitivity reaction. A medication error includes use of a drug without considering a contraindication or special risk applicable to an individual case. If the clinician is aware of the contraindication or special risk and makes a decision to use the drug by weighing the potential benefits and risks, this is not a medication error.

Transcription medication errors are usually due to the result of illegible or inaccurate orders in systems that do not have computerized order entry. Transcription errors may also occur in systems that require rewriting or re-entering (in the case of computers) of an appropriate order other than by the prescriber. The latter type of error could occur in hospitals that have computerized order entry but have a different software program in the pharmacy that requires pharmacy personnel to enter the order into their system. A variety of ADEs could result from transcription errors, depending on whether the error involved the wrong patient, wrong medication, wrong time, wrong dose, or wrong route.

Dispensing errors usually occur in the pharmacy, although they may occur in any setting where dispensing takes place (e.g., emergency department, operating room). As with transcription errors, a variety of ADEs may result from errors in the dispensing process.

The last stage of medication error, and administration errors, is least likely to be prevented because there is usually no redundancy in the system. The administration phase of the medication use process is the final event in which the medication is given to the patient. Except in rare instances, such as nurse-check-nurse, such errors are unlikely to be intercepted. An ADE may be the first suspicion that such an error has occurred. Table 1 lists common causes of medication errors and ways to prevent their occurrence.

Adverse drug events could include failure to respond to therapy or inadequate response to therapy. One must evaluate individual cases to determine whether (i) the appropriate antibacterial drug(s) was used, (ii) the dose selected was appropriate considering PK/PD principles, (iii) the duration of therapy was adequate, and (iv) the patient received adequate supportive and surgical care. One of the more common examples of inadequate duration of therapy involves *S. aureus* bacteremia with evidence of metastatic lesions. In such cases, at least 4 weeks of treatment are warranted; however, patients managed with only 10 to 14 days of therapy continue to present with recurrent bacteremia and endocarditis following the initial treatment.

Table 1 Examples of Potentially Serious Medication Errors and Possible Prevention Strategies

Stage of medication error	Problem	Prevention strategy*
Prescription	Allergy	Accurate assessment and recording of allergies
	Underdose/overdose	Literature-based dosing that takes into account patient-specific factors such as age, height/weight, and clinical condition (e.g., renal dysfunction); computerized order entry may prevent some of these errors by limiting possibility of inappropriate dosing options
	Wrong drug	Limited use of phone orders; appropriate use of consulting services and clinical pharmacy personnel; utilization of updated antibiograms; use of narrow spectrum antimicrobial agents once susceptibility data are available
	Drug–drug or drug–nutrient interactions	Computerized order entry systems that detect and notify prescriber of significant interactions
Transcription	Illegible/inaccurate orders	Computerized order entry systems that avoid illegible handwriting errors and errors related to decimal points, abbreviations, and units of measurement; systems that avoid the need to rewrite/re-enter the original order (presuming no errors in the original order are found during the order verification process)

| Dispensing and delivery | Wrong drug, dose, time, or patient; lack of sterility | Appropriate use of supportive personnel and technology (e.g., bar coding, drug interactions software, alerts for high-risk problems); as much consistency as possible in dosage formulations (e.g., standard concentrations for IV solutions); appropriate labeling and packaging, particularly for medications compounded or packaged in-house; use of special labeling/packaging for high-risk antimicrobial agents; procedures in place to minimize medication turn-around time, particularly for first doses of antimicrobials; limiting of compounding, particularly of sterile products, to pharmacy |
| Administration | Wrong drug, dose, time, or patient | Appropriate use of supportive personnel and technology (e.g., avoid unnecessary use of automated dispensing machines that preclude possibility of system redundancy); nurse-check-nurse for high-risk prescriptions (e.g. penicillin G in neonates); appropriate storage prior to use (e.g., refrigeration if needed); avoidance of point-of-care mixing of sterile fluids; discussion of medication with patient prior to administration (when possible); prompt identification and reporting of possible antimicrobial-related adverse drug events (multidisciplinary effort); no reuse of IV single-dose products or products without preservatives |

* All prevention strategies should have system redundancy (e.g., allergies checked by physician, pharmacist, and nurse), ongoing system analysis for possible improvements and evaluation of system failures, ongoing educational efforts/materials (including ease of access to medication information), and fostering of interdisciplinary communication.

FORMULARY AND ECONOMIC CONSIDERATIONS

The high cost of new antibacterial therapies has forced institutions to develop strategies for limiting inappropriate prescribing. For institutions that have well-controlled formularies, the pharmacy and therapeutics (P&T) committee is often the gatekeeper when it comes to evaluating new products for formulary admission and creating restrictions for product use. When making such decisions, it is important that the P&T committee take into account the consequences and costs of untreated or inappropriately treated infections in addition to the safety profiles and costs of competing antibacterial agents. The consequences of infection, whether treated appropriately or not, are enormous, considering that 5% to 10% of patients admitted to acute care facilities develop at least one nosocomial infection and 90,000 of these patients die each year as a result of infectious complications (6). The cost to treat these infections is approximately $5 billion per year (6), and this figure is likely an underestimate, considering the indirect costs associated with nosocomial infections such as surgical site infections that frequently occur after discharge and are treated in outpatient settings (39). Recently, the Joint Commission on Accreditation of Hospitals included death due to nosocomial infection as a sentinel event requiring reporting and root cause investigation.

A basic understanding of outcomes research and particularly pharmacoeconomics is necessary when evaluating new antibacterials for formulary admission. This evaluation should go beyond simple cost comparisons. The need for this understanding has been recognized by P&T committee members as evidenced by a survey of pharmacy directors in acute care facilities in which more than 90% of respondents indicated that pharmacoeconomic information was used in formulary development (40). Despite the increased use of outcomes research in the decision-making process, some clinicians are skeptical of the value of health economics in evaluating new therapies. The skepticism will likely diminish as increased standardization occurs relative to the methodology and reporting of outcomes research. The U.S. Public Health Service has published a series of articles pertaining to this issue (41–43), and other specialty organizations, such as the American Thoracic Society, have developed recommendations for their respective areas (44).

There are four general types of pharmacoeconomic analyses that are used to help determine the possible value of any given therapy. The first type, cost minimization analysis, is the most common type reported in the medical literature. This analysis is used to compare the costs associated with competing therapies and does not consider outcomes or benefits. In fact, it usually presumes that outcomes are equivalent. For example, antibacterial X costs $1,000 for a course of therapy compared with $500 for therapy Y, so therapy Y is the preferred approach because it is less costly. What if therapy X decreased the length of hospital stay or time on mechanical ventilation compared with therapy Y in patients with ventilator-associated pneumonia? In this case, the savings associated with therapy X could be large, considering that the development of ventilator-associated pneumonia has been shown to increase mean hospital charges per patient by more than $40,000 (45). What if therapy Y causes thrombocytopenia in 10% of patients receiving a course of therapy? These benefits and risks have associated costs that could easily offset the extra $500 cost of therapy X. The required presumption of therapeutic equivalence limits the usefulness of cost-minimization data.

Cost–benefit analysis is another type of pharmacoeconomic assessment that can be used to compare competing therapeutic strategies. In cost–benefit analysis, both the numerator (i.e., the benefit) and the denominator (i.e., the cost) are expressed in dollars. The advantage of this form of analysis is that it allows for comparisons of totally different treatment modalities. For example, the cost of infectious complications associated with the use of antibacterial-impregnated catheters could be compared to the cost of treating such complications with systemic antibacterial agents once infection occurs. In this example, the hypothesized benefit might be reduced cost of infectious complications associated with the catheters. If the benefit was clearly in favor of the catheters, the use of the catheters might be justified even if the relative costs associated with product acquisition (the denominator) were the same with both approaches. The major limitation of cost–benefit analysis is that it requires conversion of all benefits into a dollar figure, which may be very difficult with certain study end points (e.g., cost of death). Therefore, cost–benefit analysis tends to be used more for programmatic analyses than for therapeutic comparisons.

The last two types of pharmacoeconomic analysis are similar and are generally viewed as the preferred approaches when outcomes are not, or cannot be assumed to be, similar. In cost-effectiveness analysis the numerator (i.e., cost) is expressed as dollars but the denominator is expressed as an effectiveness measure, such as the number of infections cured. As in the cost–benefit calculation, the cost-effectiveness ratio must take into account all substantial cost differences associated with competing therapies, including the costs of adverse drug effects and hospitalization. Assigning these costs may be difficult, and there is debate among experts as to which form of medical resources evaluation (e.g., costs vs. charges) is preferred (46). Once calculated, the cost-effectiveness ratios of competing strategies are easy to compare. The situation becomes more complicated when there is no directly competing therapy, as occurred when drotrecogin alfa was marketed. Because drotrecogin alfa decreased mortality in a large, well-controlled trial, a cost-effectiveness calculation would require that a value judgment be made concerning the appropriate cost per year of life gained (47).

A variant of cost-effectiveness analysis is cost utility analysis, in which the denominator is expressed as a utility, most commonly, quality-adjusted life years (QALYs). The QALY is a unit of measurement on a numeric scale of 0 (usually representing death) to 1 (perfect health) and is determined using a variety of techniques, most notably, surveys. Although some authorities consider cost utility analysis to be the optimal economic analysis, utility data are rarely available for recently released medications. On the other hand, cost-effectiveness analyses are being increasingly performed with new medications. In the absence of published cost-effectiveness analyses, it is often possible for P&T committee members to perform rudimentary analyses based on published clinical studies. As with cost–benefit analysis, both forms of cost-effectiveness analysis measure consequences as well as costs.

Figure 1 is a decision tree that models a hypothetical scenario in which three antibacterial agents are being compared for the treatment of pneumonia. A cost-effectiveness analysis is being used in which the numerator (i.e., cost) of each of the

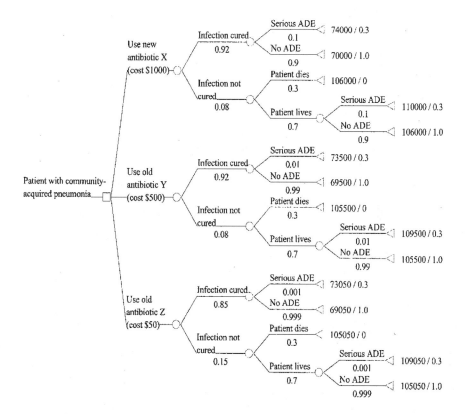

Figure 1 Decision tree for cost utility comparison of three hypothetical antibacterial drugs for the treatment of community-acquired pneumonia. Numbers below each branch represent event probabilities. The event cost and quality-of-life adjustment ($/QALY) is provided for each terminal branch. ADE, adverse drug event.

antibacterial pathways is the total cost of therapy associated with hospitalization, including costs for the antibacterial agent and its ADEs. It was assumed that the baseline cost of successful treatment was $69,000, whereas the cost associated with unsuccessful treatment was $105,000 (45). The cost of death was assumed to cost the hospital $105,000; note that this assumption demonstrates the importance of the perspective of the economic analysis, which in this case, is the institution. In addition to the antibacterial cost that is shown in the tree, the cost of a serious ADE was assumed to cost an additional $4,000 (2). The denominator (i.e., effectiveness) is based on hypothetical QALYs. Figure 1 provides the probabilities that specific events will occur. As an example, cost utility calculations are shown in Table 2 for drug X. The cure rates were based on two recent clinical trials in which antibacterial agents were compared for the treatment of community-acquired pneumonia (48,49). The decision tree demonstrates the problem with simply looking at medication cost to determine the best treatment scenario. In this example, the most cost-effective option (i.e., antibiotic Y) exhibited the lowest cost per treatment, considering overall cost of treatment. However, antibiotic Y was ten times more expensive than antibiotic Z. A simple cost assessment resulted in the following order of preference: antibiotic Y = $72,419/patient > antibiotic X = $73,270/patient > antibiotic Z = $74,454/patient. After ad-

Table 2 Example Cost Utility Calculation for Treatment X Based on the Hypothetical Decision Tree (Fig. 1)*

Cost per typical patient	Quality-of-life adjustment
$0.92 \times 0.1 \times \$74,000 = \$6,808$	$0.92 \times 0.1 \times 0.3 = 0.0276$
$0.92 \times 0.9 \times \$70,000 = \$57,960$	$0.92 \times 0.9 \times 1 = 0.828$
$0.08 \times 0.3 \times \$106,000 = \$2,544$	$0.08 \times 0.3 \times 0 = 0$
$0.08 \times 0.7 \times 0.1 \times \$110,000 = \$616$	$0.08 \times 0.7 \times 0.1 \times 0.3 = 0.00168$
$0.08 \times 0.7 \times 0.9 \times \$106,000 = \$5,342$	$0.08 \times 0.7 \times 0.9 \times 1 = 0.0504$
Sum of event costs = $73,270	QALYs (sum) 5 0.90768

* The cost utility value, defined as the cost divided by the quality-adjusted life year (QALY) adjustment, is $80,723/QALY.

justment for quality of life, the order of preference for antibiotics X and Z was different. The resulting preference order was antibiotic Y = \$74,723/QALY > antibiotic Z = \$78,017/QALY > antibiotic X/QALY = \$80,723. When looking at the decision tree and calculating results, it becomes obvious that pharmacoeconomic calculations may become complex depending on the assumptions of the modeling process.

A number of approaches have been used to control the high costs of antibacterial agents and their associated adverse events, beginning with formulary evaluation and continuing with a variety of medication and disease management programs. Examples include therapeutic interchange strategies for antibacterial agents deemed to have equivalent efficacy and adverse effect profiles, intravenous to oral substitution, dosing regimen optimization programs, clinical pathways or protocols, and therapeutic guidelines (50). Some of these strategies, such as initiation of antibacterial agents within 4 to 8 hours of hospital admission for patients with pneumonia, are relatively easy to implement and have been shown to reduce length of stay and mortality (51–53). Other strategies that focus on alterations in prescribing (e.g., broad-spectrum antibacterials initially, with rapid streamlining based on microbiologic results) are usually more difficult to implement but may yield rewards in terms of reduced antibacterial consumption, decreased resistance, and possibly decreased mortality (54,55).

Guidelines for many infectious diseases have been published, and many of the evidence-based versions can be found on the National Guideline Clearinghouse website (56). Although these guidelines are based on evidence from clinical trials, opinions of the contributors enter into the guidelines when published studies do not allow evidence-based conclusions. Despite any shortcomings, consensus guidelines provide an important framework for clinical decisions. However, they should not be applied without careful evaluation of individual situations.

Some of the more controversial approaches used primarily to prevent resistance (but that have economic implications) involve infection control measures such as antibacterial agent cycling or other attempts to restrict prescribing (57,58). These types of mandated control measures are the focus of much debate, given the disagreement among experts regarding treatment options, as exemplified by an international conference that attempted to derive consensus on the diagnosis and treatment of ventilator-associated pneumonia (59). The participants reached consensus on issues such as the importance of local surveillance programs, but there was little agreement on the appropriate choice of antibacterial agents other than the need to customize empiric therapy.

Most of the approaches used to control costs or prevent resistance have not been evaluated by formal economic analyses, and the evidence of their resource savings is usually based on cost minimization. As noted in one review of these strategies, no savings are likely to occur if a strategy is developed but never directly applied to patient care (60). Ways to insure that the strategies are utilized include their development and implementation using a multidisciplinary, systems-based approach that takes into account institution-specific issues (61).

SUMMARY

The majority of infectious diseases, particularly bacterial infections, may be managed using several alternative treatment regimens. Clinicians need to select the most appropriate therapy based on individual case circumstances and information available on efficacy, PK/PD, potential adverse effects, and patient-specific risk factors for adverse effects. All drugs have potential adverse effects, whether predictable or idiosyncratic. The most effective way to prevent ADEs is to use antibacterial drugs only when appropriate and, when appropriate, to select the best drug for the individual patient. A thorough medical history including any drug allergies can identify patient-specific risk factors that may help narrow the list of alternative regimens. Once the treatment regimen is selected, optimal dosing should be attempted based on PK/PD principles. Programs aimed at preventing medication errors are essential, given the health and economic implications. Such programs should focus on process evaluation and continuous improvement rather than punitive reactions. Applications of pharmacoeconomic data can provide further discrimination between regimens that are perceived as therapeutically equivalent. This chapter expands the definition of medication errors to include any inappropriate or suboptimal uses of antibacterial drugs. PK/PD principles may be applied in infectious disease practice to ensure more optimal selection and dosing of antibacterial drugs. Further consideration of error prevention and pharmacoeconomics is also necessary. Application and integration of these aspects will undoubtedly contribute to a reduction in inappropriate use, medication errors, and ADEs involving antibacterial drugs.

REFERENCES

1. Errors in health care: a leading cause of death and injury. In: Kohn LT, Corrigan JM, Donaldson MS, Eds To Err Is Human: Building a Safer Health System. Institute of Medicine Report. Washington, DC: National Academy Press, 1999:22–41.

2. Rodriguez-Monguio R, Otero MJ, Rovira J. Assessing the economic impact of adverse drug events. Pharmacoeconomics 2003; 21:623–650.

3. Cullen DJ, Sweitzer BJ, Bates DW, Burdick E, Edmondson A, Leape LL. Preventable adverse drug events in hospitalized patients: a comparative study of intensive care and general care units. Crit Care Med 1997; 25:1289–1297.

4. Suh D-C, Wsoodall BS, Shin S-K, Hermes-De Santis ER. Clinical and economic impact of adverse drug reactions in hospitalized patients. Ann Pharmacother 2000; 34:1373–1379.

5. Kelly W. Potential risks and prevention, part 1: fatal adverse drug events. Am J Health Syst Pharm 2001; 58:1317–1324.

6. Burke JP. Infection control—a problem for patient safety. N Engl J Med 2003; 348:651–656.

7. Feder HM Jr, Hunt MS. Pitfalls in the diagnosis and treatment of Lyme disease in children. JAMA 1995; 274:66–68.

8. Galgiani JN, Ampel NM, Catanzaro A, Johnson RH, Stevens DA, Williams PL. Practice guidelines for the treatment of coccidioidomycosis. Clin Infect Dis 2000; 30:658–661.

9. Cantrell R, Young AF, Martin BC. Antibiotic prescribing in ambulatory care settings for adults with colds, upper respiratory tract infections, and bronchitis. Clin Ther 2002; 24:170–182.

10. Gonzales R, Bartlett JG, Besser RE, Cooper RJ, Hickner JM, Hoffman JR, Sande MA. Centers for Disease Control and Prevention. Principles of appropriate antibiotic use for treatment of uncomplicated acute bronchitis: background. Ann Emerg Med 2001; 37:720–727.

11. van Buchem FL, Knottnerus JA, Schrijnemaekers VJ, Peeters MF. Primary-care-based randomised placebo-controlled trial of antibiotic treatment in acute maxillary sinusitis. Lancet 1997; 349:683–687.

12. Poehlman GS. Chronic otitis media with effusion. Prim Care 1996; 23:687–699.

13. Little P, Gould C, Williamson I, Moore M, Warner G, Dunleavy J. Pragmatic randomized controlled trial of two prescribing strategies for childhood acute otitis media. Br Med J 2001; 322: 336–342.

14. Rosenfeld RM. Observation option toolkit for acute otitis media. Int J Pediatr Otorhinolaryngol 2001; 58:1–8.

15. Ortquist A. Treatment of community-acquired lower respiratory tract infection in adults. Eur Respir J 2002; 36(suppl): 40S–53S.

16. Hulson TD, Mold JW, Scheid D, Aaron M, Aspy CB, Ballard NL, Boren N, Gregory ME, Truong TC. Diagnosing influenza: the value of clinical clues and laboratory tests. J Fam Pract 2001; 50:1051–1056.

17. Niederman MS. Antibiotic therapy of exacerbations of chronic bronchitis. Sem Resp Infect 2000; 15:59–70.

18. Bartlett JG, Dowell SF, Mandell LA, File TM Jr, Musher DM, Fine MJ. Practice guidelines for the management of community-acquired pneumonia in adults. Clin Infect Dis 2000; 31: 347–382.

19. Polk RE, Hepler CD. Controversies in antimicrobial therapy: critical analysis of clinical trials. Am J Hosp Pharm 1986; 43: 630–640.

20. Nicolau DP, Mattoes HM, Banevicius M, Xuan D, Nightingale CH. Pharmacodynamics of a novel des-F(6)-quinolone, BMS-284756, against *Streptococcus pneumoniae* in the thigh infection model. Antimicrob Agents Chemother 2003; 47:1630–1635.

21. Nix DE, Goodwin SD, Peloquin CA, Rotella DL, Schentag JJ. Antibiotic tissue penetration and its relevance: impact of tissue penetration on infection response. Antimicrob Agents Chemother 1991; 35:1953–1959.

22. Retsema JA, Bergeron JM, Girard D, Milisen WB, Girard AE. Preferential concentration of azithromycin in an infected mouse thigh model. J Antimicrob Chemother 1993; 31(suppl E):5–16.

23. Ellner PD, Neu HC. The inhibitory quotient. A method for interpreting minimum inhibitory concentration data. JAMA 1981; 246:1575–1578.

24. Craig WA. Once-daily versus multiple-daily dosing of aminoglycosides. J Chemother 1995; 7(suppl 2):47–52.

25. Wright DH, Brown GH, Peterson ML, Rotschafer JC. Application of fluoroquinolone pharmacodynamics. J Antimicrob Chemother 2000; 46:669–683.

26. Craig WA. Choosing an antibiotic on the basis of pharmacodynamics. Ear Nose Throat J 1998; 77(suppl 6):7–11.

27. Craig WA. Performance Standards for Antimicrobial Susceptibility Testing. NCCLS Document M100-S12. Wayne. PA: National Committee for Clinical Laboratory Standards, 2002.

28. Barclay ML, Duffull SB, Begg EJ, Buttimore RC. Experience of once-daily aminoglycoside dosing using a target area under the concentration-time curve. Aust N Z J Med 1995; 25: 230–235.

29. Levison ME. Pharmacodynamics of antibacterial drugs. Infect Dis Clin N Am 2000; 14:281–291.

30. Craig WA. Interrelationship between pharmacokinetics and pharmacodynamics in determining dosage regimens for broad-

spectrum cephalosporins. Diag Microbiol Infect Dis 1995; 22: 89–96.

31. Goldstein FW. Choice of an oral beta-lactam antibiotic for infections due to penicillin-resistant *Streptococcus pneumoniae*. Scand J Infect Dis 1997; 29:255–257.

32. Drusano GL, Craig WA. Relevance of pharmacokinetics and pharmacodynamics in the selection of antibiotics for respiratory tract infections. J Chemother 1997; 9(suppl 3):38–44.

33. Redington J, Ebert SC, Craig WA. Role of antimicrobial pharmacokinetics and pharmacodynamics in surgical prophylaxis. Rev Infect Dis 1991; 13(suppl 10):S790–S799.

34. Barry AL, Jones RN, Packer RR. Antistaphylococcal activity of ceforanide and cefonicid in the presence of human serum. Antimicrob Agents Chemother 1986; 29:147–149.

35. Perl TM, Pfaller MA, Houston A, Wenzel RP. Effect of serum on the *in vitro* activities of 11 broad-spectrum antibiotics. Antimicrob Agents Chemother 1990; 34:2234–2239.

36. Visser LG, Arnouts P, van Furth R, Mattie H, van den Broek PJ. Clinical pharmacokinetics of continuous intravenous administration of penicillins. Clin Infect Dis 1993; 17:491–495.

37. Wysocki M, Delatour F, Faurisson F, Rauss A, Pean Y, Misset B, Thomas F, Timsit JF, Similowski T, Mentec H, Mier L, Dreyfuss D. Continuous versus intermittent infusion of vancomycin in severe staphylococcal infections: prospective multicenter randomized study. Antimicrob Agents Chemother 2001; 45: 2460–2467.

38. Grant EM, Kuti JL, Nicolau DP, Nightingale C, Quintiliani R. Clinical efficacy and pharmacoeconomics of a continuous-infusion piperacillin-tazobactam program in a large community teaching hospital. Pharmacother 2002; 22:471–483.

39. Perencevich EN, Sands KE, Cosgrove SE, Guadagnoli E, Meara E, Platt R. Health and economic impact of surgical site infections diagnosed after hospital discharge. Emerg Infect Dis 2003; 9:196–203.

40. Ringold DJ, Santell JP, Schneider PJ, Arenberg S. ASHP national survey of pharmacy practice in acute care settings: Pre-

scribing and transcribing—1998. Am J Health Syst Pharm 199; 56:142–157.

41. Russell LB, Gold MR, Siegel JE, Daniels N, Weinstein MC. The role of cost-effectiveness analysis in health and medicine. JAMA 1996; 276:1172–1177.

42. Weinstein MC, Siegel JE, Gold MR, Kamlet MS, Russell LB. Recommendations of the panel on cost-effectiveness in health and medicine. JAMA 1996; 276:1253–1258.

43. Russell JE, Weinstein MC, Russell LB, Gold MR. Recommendations for reporting cost-effectiveness analyses. JAMA 1996; 276:1339–1341.

44. Gold MR. Report from the Second American Thoracic Society Workshop on Outcomes Research. Understanding costs and cost-effectiveness in critical care. Am J Respir Crit Care Med 2002; 165:540–550.

45. Rello J, Ollendorf DA, Oster G, Vera-Llonch M, Bellm L, Redman R, Kollef MH;. VAP Outcomes Scientific Advisory Group. Epidemiology and outcomes of ventilator-associated pneumonia in a large US database. Chest 2002; 122:2115–2121.

46. Copley-Merriman C, Lair TJ. Valuation of medical resource units collected in health economic studies. Clin Ther 1994; 16: 553–568.

47. Couglin MT, Angus DC. Economic evaluation of new therapies in critical illness. Crit Care Med 2003; 31(suppl):S7–S16.

48. Ortiz-Ruiz G, Caballaro-Lopez J, Friedland IR, Woods GL, Carides A. A study evaluating the efficacy, safety, and tolerability of ertapenem versus ceftriaxone for the treatment of community-acquired pneumonia. Clin Infect Dis 2002; 34:1076–1083.

49. Finch R, Schurmann D, Collins O, Kubin R, McGivern J, Bobbaers H, Izquierdo JL, Nikolaides P, Ogundare F, Raz R, Zuck P, Hoeffken G. Randomized controlled trial of sequential intravenous (i.v.) and oral moxifloxacin compared with sequential i.v. and oral co-amoxiclav with or without clarithromycin in patients community-acquired pneumonia requiring initial parenteral treatment. Antimicrob Agents Chemother 2002; 46: 1746–1754.

50. Weber RJ, Kane SL, Oriolo VA, Saul M, Skledar SJ, Dasta JF. Impact of intensive care unit (ICU) drug use on hospital costs:

a descriptive analysis, with recommendations for optimizing ICU pharmacotherapy. Crit Care Med 2003; 31(suppl): S17–S24.

51. Meehan TP, Fine MJ, Krumholz HM, Scinto JD, Galusha DH, Mockalis JT, Weber GF, Petrillo MK, Houck PM, Fine JM. Quality of care, process, and outcomes in elderly patients with pneumonia. JAMA 1997; 278:2080–2084.

52. Battleman DS, Callahan M, Thaler HT. Rapid antibiotic delivery and appropriate antibiotic selection reduce length of hospital stay of patients with community-acquired pneumonia. Arch Inter Med 2002; 162:682–688.

53. Mandell LA, Bartlett, Dowell SF, File TM, Jr., Musher DM, Whilney C. Update of practice guideline for the management of community-acquired pneumonia in inmunocompetent adults. Clin Infect Dis. 2003; 37:1404–1433.

54. Harbarth S, Garbino J, Pugin J, Romand JA, Lew D, Pittet D. Inappropriate initial antimicrobial therapy and its effect on survival in a clinical trial of immunomodulating therapy for severe sepsis. Am J Med 2003; 115:529–535.

55. Hoffken G, Niederman MS. Nosocomial pneumonia: The importance of a de-escalating strategy for antibiotic treatment of pneumonia in the ICU. Chest 2002; 122:2183–2196.

56. National Guideline Clearinghouse. About NGC. http://www.guidelines.gov/about/about.aspx (accessed 2003 Nov 10).

57. Fridkin SK. Routine cycling of antimicrobial agents as an infection-control measure. Clin Infect Dis 2003; 36:1438–1444.

58. Paterson DL. Restrictive antibiotic policies are appropriate in intensive care units. Crit Care Med 2003; 31(suppl):S25–S28.

59. Rello J, Paiva JA, Baraibar J, Barcenilla F, Bodi M, Castander D, Correa H, Diaz E, Garnacho J, Llorio M, Rios M, Rodriguez A, Sole-Violan J. International Conference for the Development of Consensus on the Diagnosis and Treatment of Ventilator-Associated Pneumonia. Chest 2001; 120:955–970.

60. Kuti JL, Capitano B, Nicolau DP. Cost-effective approaches to the treatment of community-acquired pneumonia in the era of resistance. Pharmacoeconomics 2002; 20:513–528.

61. Niederman MS. Appropriate use of antimicrobial agents: challenges and strategies for improvement. Crit Care Med 2003; 31:608–616.

6

Basic Pharmacoeconomics for the Hospital Decision-Maker

MARIANNE MCCOLLUM

School of Pharmacy, University of Colorado
Health Sciences Center
Denver, Colorado, U.S.A.

Arguably, the most important challenge in health care today is cost. National health expenditures have increased dramatically over the last 20 years, and will continue to do so, according to the Centers for Medicare and Medicaid Services (CMS) (1). Expenditures for health care increased fourfold between 1980 and 2000, and are projected by CMS to reach $3 trillion annually by 2012. Pharmaceuticals comprise a growing component of health spending, with expenditures increasing tenfold between 1980 and 2000 and CMS projections exceeding $445 billion by 2012.

Increases in prescription drug spending can be attributed to several factors. First, the population is aging. Between 1990 and 2000, the proportion of the population aged 45 to 54 years increased by 49%, whereas the population of those 85 years and older increased by 39% (2). Second, use of new pharmaceuticals continues to be subsidized by expanding insurance coverage (3). According to a survey conducted by *The News Hour with Jim Lehrer*, the Kaiser Family Foundation, and the Harvard School of Public Health (4), three out of four Americans have prescription drug coverage. Third, new drug development by the pharmaceutical industry has yielded effective new treatments for a wide range of diseases. These factors support the CMS spending projections and point to the enormous impact pharmaceutical expenditures will have on total health care costs in the coming decades.

Given the forces driving the increased use of pharmaceuticals, finding ways to control spending on prescription drugs will be difficult. Population demographics cannot be altered, and the extent of prescription drug coverage is increasing (e.g., through changes to Medicare benefits). Budget constraints make it essential that pharmaceuticals be used effectively in order to achieve maximum benefit from the associated expenditures. Therefore, the key to controlling expenditures on prescription drugs may be found in the field generally referred to as *technology assessment*: determining the costs and outcomes associated with the use of effective, yet expensive, pharmaceuticals (5).

The need to control expenditures on health care in general and pharmaceuticals in particular arises from the basic economic concept of scarcity; we have limited resources and unlimited wants and needs. As a society, we will never have enough resources to meet our needs. The response by health care systems to the concept of scarcity of resources typically includes the use of a formulary to manage medication costs (6). This chapter addresses the methods available to pharmacy and therapeutics (P&T) committees to assess the costs and effectiveness of pharmaceuticals in order to inform the formulary decision-making process, including outcomes research and prospective modeling. Methods for retrospective formulary decision assessment, examining the impact of decisions after they are implemented, are also described.

OUTCOMES RESEARCH

The outcomes associated with health care interventions are often classified according to the ECHO model, describing *economic*, *clinical*, and *humanistic* outcomes of health care interventions (7). Economic outcomes are the direct, indirect, and intangible costs associated with medical treatment. Clinical outcomes are the medical or health-related outcomes of treatment. Humanistic outcomes are the patient-focused consequences of treatment. Outcomes research focusing on the economic, clinical, and humanistic consequences pharmaceutical-based interventions is often referred to as *pharmacoeconomics*. This field encompasses a number of analytic tools that assess costs and consequences of treatment, including cost, benefit, cost-effectiveness, and cost-utility analyses. Other pharmacoeconomic evaluation methods assess only costs of treatment, such as simple cost analyses and cost-of-illness analyses. The methods included within the framework of the field of pharmacoeconomics are presented in Table 1.

Cost Analyses

Cost analyses consider the costs associated with treatment, without assessing the impact on outcomes. Two types of cost analyses are generally used: cost-of-care and cost-of-illness. Each method considers only costs of treatment, exclusive of outcomes.

Table 1 Commonly Used Pharmacoeconomic Methodologies

Method	Cost measurement	Outcome measurement
Cost analyses		
Cost-of-care	Dollars	Not assessed
Cost-of-illness	Dollars	Not assessed
Cost-outcomes analyses		
Cost-benefit	Dollars	Dollars
Cost-effectiveness	Dollars	Natural health units
Cost-minimization	Dollars	Natural health units
Cost-utility	Dollars	Quality-adjusted life years

Cost-of-Care

Cost-of-care analysis includes total costs of the resources consumed with the use of a pharmaceutical intervention. The patient population and time period are specified. Costs for all resources (e.g., drugs, hospitalizations, physician's services) would be included.

Cost-of-Illness

Cost-of-illness analyses go beyond cost of care analyses in that they include estimates of the cost impact of a disease on society. Overall costs of treatment are included as in a cost-of-care analysis. Unlike cost-of-care analyses, societal costs such as lost productivity due to morbidity and mortality are also included.

Cost-Outcomes Analyses

Cost-outcomes analyses take into account both the costs and the outcomes associated with an intervention, with the results expressed in terms of a cost:outcomes ratio. Cost:outcomes ratios compare the costs and outcomes of one intervention with the costs and outcomes of an alternative intervention. In all cost-outcomes methods, costs are measured in monetary units (e.g., U.S. dollars). The methods differ in how the outcomes are expressed, as detailed in the overview presented here. For a more comprehensive discussion of the methods, the reader is referred to Drummond et al. (8) or Gold et al. (9).

Cost-Benefit Analysis

Cost-benefit analysis compares the costs of alternative treatments with the dollar value of the outcome associated with those treatments. Results are expressed as a ratio of cost($)-outcome($). For example, an intervention with a cost-benefit ratio of 1:5 yields benefits valued at $5 for every $1 in costs. The expression of all outcomes in the same units allows comparison of interventions with disparate benefits, such as a vaccination program and an intervention that treats infections.

When conducting cost-benefit analyses, the outcomes, or benefits, are expressed in terms of their value in monetary units. Health care interventions which lead to increased survival might be expressed as a ratio of the dollar value of the cost of the intervention to the dollar value of life years gained as a result of the intervention. Three common methods used to convert life years to a dollar equivalent are human capital, willingness-to-pay, and revealed preferences.

The human capital approach equates a year of life with the market value of wages earned during that year. The benefits of an intervention are valued in terms of the present value of future wage earnings gained as a result of that intervention.

Willingness-to-pay methods use survey techniques to determine what people are willing to pay to attain the benefits from a health care intervention. Consider the addition of a new trauma center which will decrease the probability of death from major trauma for those living nearby. Respondents would be asked what they are willing to pay for this treatment center, keeping in mind what they can afford. The amount they are willing to pay is equated to the number of lives saved by the timely availability of treatment at the center. In this way, respondents implicitly state the value they place on life, in the same way the maximum price consumers are willing to pay for a good or service is an implicit measure of the value of that good or service.

Revealed preferences is a method that is based on consumer behavior, primarily in wage markets. A value is placed on human life based on the increased wages paid to workers employed in occupations with an increased probability of death.

It is important to note that in the willingness-to-pay and revealed preferences methods, the lives in question are statistical lives, representing lower probability of death in a population. Society typically places a much higher value on an identified life, as evidenced by the extreme and costly efforts undertaken to rescue people lost or trapped.

Cost-effectiveness Analysis

Cost-effectiveness analysis compares the costs of alternative treatments with the benefits of those treatments expressed in terms of natural health units. Avoiding the process of assigning a dollar value to the benefits of an intervention is a major advantage of cost-effectiveness analysis. For that reason, the majority of the cost-outcomes research conducted is in the form of cost-effectiveness analyses (10,11). Although the valuation of benefits in natural health units is appealing in terms of conducting a cost-outcomes study, comparing the results of interventions with benefits of varying types is difficult. The costs and outcomes of the vaccination program and the antibiotic treatment which were easily compared using cost-benefit analysis are not easily compared using cost-effectiveness analysis.

Cost-Minimization Analysis

Cost-minimization analysis considers both costs and outcomes of alternative treatments, but involves a situation in which the outcomes have been assessed and shown to be equivalent between the alternative treatments. In this case, costs are compared to determine the treatment with the lowest cost. It is important in these studies that equivalency of outcomes be documented explicitly and not assumed.

Cost-Utility Analysis

Cost-utility analysis compares the costs and benefits of alternative treatments, with the outcomes adjusted for quality-of-life and expressed in terms of quality-adjusted life years, or QALYs. By expressing all outcomes in terms of QALYs, costs and benefits of programs with varying outcomes can be compared, similar to cost-benefit analysis. Cost-utility analysis has been described as a distinct cost-outcomes method (8) or as a form of cost-effectiveness analysis in which the outcome is expressed as QALYs (9).

To convert the outcomes to QALYs, the final outcomes or benefits of a program (e.g., morbidity and/or mortality) are expressed as life years gained, lives saved, or functional days gained. These outcomes are then adjusted by multiplying them by a score that approximates the preference for that outcome, measured on a scale from 0 to 1.0 corresponding to death and perfect health, respectively. Consider two treatments for cancer. Costs and outcomes associated with each are assessed, with the outcomes measured in terms of life years gained. The outcomes, life years gained, are converted to QALYs by multiplying the quantity of life years gained by the preference score. If the preference for the first treatment is 0.6 (as a result of toxicities of treatment, for example), each life year gained is adjusted to 0.6 QALYs. If the preference for the second treatment is 0.8 (as a result of fewer associated toxicities), each life year gained with that treatment is adjusted to 0.8 QALYs. Using cost-utility analysis allows the comparison of both the magnitude of the outcome (e.g., life years gained) and the quality of those years.

Evaluating Cost-Outcomes Studies

Rubrics for evaluating published cost-outcomes studies can be helpful in understanding the methods and components of the analyses. Presented here is an overview of the ten-step assessment process proposed by Drummond et al. (8).

1. Was the Question Well Defined?

One of the key components of a cost-outcomes analysis is that both costs and outcomes are considered. Care should be taken with studies making claims about cost-effective treatment to ensure that the study did indeed address both costs and outcomes. Alternative therapies should be compared with any type of cost-outcomes research, and each alternative should be described thoroughly.

The perspective of the study should be explicitly stated. From whose viewpoint is the analysis being conducted? Relevancy of costs to be included will be based on the perspective taken in the analysis.

2. Were the Alternative Therapies Described?

The therapies being compared should be important in terms of clinical practice. Therapies should be described completely, even if the relevant alternative is doing nothing.

3. Were the Interventions Effective?

The effectiveness of the interventions being compared should be well established. Cost-outcomes methodologies are concerned with demonstrating ways of delivering effective care, not just economically efficient ways of delivering ineffective care. Documentation of the effectiveness of the treatments (e.g., clinical trials, population-based studies) should be included, along with possible biases that may be introduced as a result of the methods used to demonstrate effectiveness.

4. Did the Analysis Include All Relevant Costs?

Costs may be relevant for a variety of different participants in the delivery of the intervention, including the health care system, the payer, the patient, and society. The costs to be included in an analysis depend on the perspective of the study. For example, analyses done from the perspective of society will include costs due to lost productivity, whereas analyses done from the perspective of a third-party payer will not include these costs.

5. Were Costs Measured Appropriately?

Costs included in the analysis should be measured in terms that are appropriate for each type of cost. For example, the societal costs might be the value of lost productivity when work days are lost. Physician and nursing time might be measured in terms of wages; procedure or laboratory costs in terms of labor and materials. Shared costs, such as overhead costs, might be measured in terms of the portion of those costs associated with the interventions being analyzed, with a clear description of how they were derived. Capital costs should also be included.

Regardless of the types of costs included in the analysis, the study should clearly state if the costs are actual costs or if they are charges to patients and/or payers (12). Actual costs may be available to the investigators but may be proprietary and, therefore, not publishable. In that case, the authors should clearly state that charges were used to estimate costs, and should discuss potential biases that may result.

6. Were Costs and Outcomes Valued Credibly?

Costs incurred over multiple years should be expressed in terms of their current value. Low prices resulting from subsidies or rebates should be adjusted, and significant contributions from volunteers should be valued in terms of the wages avoided.

Preference scores may vary widely based on whose preference is being measured and how. Cost-utility studies should describe the method used and population surveyed to determine the preference score—doctors, patients with the disease being treated, family members or caregivers, the general population? Similarly, cost-benefit analyses valuing life years based on willingness-to-pay surveys should describe the population surveyed.

7. Was Discounting Employed?

Discounting is one of the more difficult concepts in conducting cost-outcomes analyses. The issue here is that, in general, we value what we have now more than what we will have in the future. We value $100 in cash in hand today more than we would in the future, as evidenced by the interest banks must offer in order to entice us to deposit those funds in a savings account for future use. For this reason, the value of both costs and benefits must be reduced or discounted to their present value, and the discount rate should be specified.

8. Was an Incremental Analysis Performed?

Cost-outcomes analysis generates a cost-outcomes ratio for two alternative therapies. It may be tempting to decide which intervention to use based on a simple comparison of these two ratios. However, it is necessary to examine and compare the difference in costs between the two treatments with the difference in outcomes or benefits between the treatments. This approach is referred to as an *incremental analysis*, and estimates how much more (or less) it will cost to achieve how much more (or less) in benefits with a new treatment compared with the existing one. Table 2 describes the costs and benefits of two treatments, A and B, along with an incremental analysis. The costs and benefits of a new intervention are compared with the costs and benefits of an existing one.

As stated above, a simple comparison of the cost-effectiveness ratios of treatment A versus treatment B would seem to

Table 2   Incremental Analysis of Treatment A Compared with Treatment B*

	Treatment A	Treatment B	Incremental value
Cost	$50,000	$120,000	$70,000
Benefit (life years gained)	10	15	5
Cost-effectiveness ratio	$5,000 per life year gained	$8,000 per life year gained	$14,000 per additional life year gained

* The incremental cost-effectiveness ratio indicates that implementing treatment B will cost an additional $14,000 for each additional life year gained.

indicate that treatment B incurs a cost of only $8,000 per life year gained. However, the incremental cost-effectiveness ratio correctly estimates that use of treatment B in place of treatment A will cost an *additional* $14,000 for each *additional* year of life gained when compared with the existing treatment (treatment A).

9. Was a Sensitivity Analysis Performed?

Estimates of costs and benefits are often just that—estimates. As such, they involve some level of uncertainty that may or may not have an impact on the outcome of the study. Sensitivity analyses—varying the values for cost inputs and outcomes—should be conducted to determine the impact, if any, on the results.

10. Was the Discussion of Results Comprehensive?

The presentation of the results of a cost-outcomes analysis should include comparisons with other studies, along with discussions of generalizing the results and the feasibility of implementing the interventions.

Limitations of Cost-Outcomes Research

There are a number of methodologic and practical application issues that limit the usefulness of cost-outcomes analyses in making formulary decisions. The first and perhaps the most important issue to consider is the quality of the study. Each study should be evaluated for sound methodology using a rubric such as the one developed by Drummond et al. (8) and described here. One review of the literature indicated that as many as two-thirds of pharmacoeconomic studies had significant problems (13).

Economic analyses are often performed in conjunction with clinical trials, leading to potential problems with the results (14). Strict inclusion/exclusion criteria in well-controlled trials allow inferences about the efficacy of drugs being tested, but limit the extrapolation of the results beyond the study population. Costs assigned to treatments based on study protocols may overestimate costs as a result of protocol-driven care. Study patients may receive more laboratory tests and procedures as a result of the study protocol. Patients treated outside the trial environment may be more likely to receive less intensive and, therefore, less expensive care. Medication compliance rates are also likely to be higher in clinical trials than in general practice, a factor that may have an impact on success of treatment and the occurrence of adverse events.

Conducting a cost-benefit analysis requires valuing benefits in dollars—a difficult task at best. The human capital approach may be the easiest because of the availability of wage data, but these data may lead to undervaluation of the old and young, and disparities between wages earned by sex and race/ethnicity may also lead to undervaluing women and minorities. The willingness-to-pay method, using surveys to determine what people are willing to pay for specified benefits, may yield varying results depending on the demographics of those surveyed. Revealed preferences, using implied values for life based on hazard pay, do not take into account the degree of risk aversion among workers selecting those occupations.

Cost-effectiveness methods avoid having to place a value on benefits, but are also limiting. Intermediate outcomes, such as degree of lowering of diastolic blood pressure or low-density-lipoprotein cholesterol, are often the outcomes measured. Although technically sound, these analyses are difficult to incorporate into decision making. In addition, two interventions, such as two pharmaceutical agents, are compared with each other, whereas in a health system, not all patients being treated for a particular disease are clinically eligible to receive each drug. Users of cost-effectiveness studies must take into account the possible extent to which each treatment could be used in their own institution. Implementing a treatment with a favorable incremental cost-effectiveness ratio may have limited impact on total costs if it can be used only to treat a small portion of the relevant patient population.

Appropriate interpretation of the results of a cost-effectiveness analysis requires a solid understanding of the methodology. Cost-effectiveness studies, even when technically well-done, do not include a determination about whether an intervention is "cost-effective" or not. Common misperceptions about the cost-effectiveness of interventions include the belief that cost-effectiveness means cost saving, whereas the appropriate determination of cost-effectiveness takes into account incremental cost-effectiveness estimates, judgments about the value of the outcomes, and budgetary limitations of the health system that might influence willingness to pay for additional benefits (15).

The limitations of cost-utility analyses are both methodologic and practical. Estimates of preferences for different health states vary based on the population surveyed, leading to significant uncertainty in quality-of-life adjustments. Outcomes are adjusted to QALYs through use of preference scores of 0 (death) or 1.0 (perfect health). Problems arise when preference scores are measured using bounds that are defined differently, such as equating a score of 1.0 to a symptom-free state, not perfect health (16). Sensitivity analyses may be performed to estimate the impact of uncertainty inputs but do not address the bigger question: To what extent do decision-makers and third-party payers consider quality of life when making decisions about implementing health care interventions?

Limitations of cost-outcomes analysis, especially those that are related to the application of literature-based results to a specific health care system, can be overcome by conducting institution-specific studies. In that way, costs and outcomes specific to the potential treating population can be used to estimate the incremental cost-outcomes ratios necessary to inform formulary decisions. Although this approach theoretically would overcome some of the limitations presented here, the feasibility of the approach is not clear. P&T committees do not always have personnel or staff trained in pharmacoeconomics and with adequate time at their disposal to conduct these analyses on a routine basis, ultimately limiting the use of this methodology to aid in the formulary decision process.

PROSPECTIVE MODELING

Much effort is expended by P&T committees in deliberating formulary decisions. Nevertheless, recent surveys indicate that P&T committees consider pharmacoeconomic data only after considering drug efficacy, toxicity, side effects, and acquisition costs (6,17). Increasing the use of pharmacoeconomic data in making and assessing formulary decisions is essential in improving the quality of those decisions.

Despite their widespread acceptance, the risk remains that formularies will be used more for cost control than to improve the quality of care. In its *Principles of a Sound Formulary System* (18), The Academy of Managed Care Pharmacy (AMCP) proposes that a well-designed formulary system can "promote rational, clinically appropriate, safe, and cost-effective drug therapy...that can best serve the health interests of a given patient population." To that end, extensive guidelines developed to improve the quality of information considered by P&T committees in making formulary decisions recommend that drugs be evaluated in light of their impact on total health care costs and clinical outcomes (19). These guidelines, the *Format for Formulary Submissions* (AMCP *Format*), recommend that formulary submissions include clinical drug data along with a description of the drug's place in therapy and an evaluation of relevant published economic studies.

Economic models can facilitate formulary decision making by estimating the system-wide cost consequences of therapies. That said, the use of economic models in health care is still met with some skepticism. Models created by pharmaceutical firms with "hidden" formulas are often seen as marketing tools rather than providing valid information to aid in decision making.

Alternatively, Weinstein et al. (20) propose that economic modeling can be appropriately used to inform formulary decision making, provided they meet the following evaluation criteria:

  a. Transparency: model assumptions, input values, and methods of using each in computing outputs should be clearly stated.
  b. Verification: the model should be debugged and outputs should be consistent with observed data.
  c. Corroboration: outputs from varying models using the same assumptions and inputs should be consistent.
  d. Face validity: model results should make sense intuitively.
  e. Accreditation: models should be peer reviewed.

Support for the use of prospective economic modeling is evidenced by the recommendation of the AMCP *Format* that formulary submissions include economic models which allow incorporation of institution-specific data. Economic modeling may still be a black box to many, but there is clearly a growing trend toward use of the methodology as an aid in making formulary decisions.

A major advantage of the use of prospective modeling to inform formulary decision making is that the process occurs before the decision is made. The prospective nature of the process allows refinement of the decision based on the model outputs *prior to* implementation, avoiding the need to modify or reverse it later. Unlike a retrospective analysis conducted after a formulary decision is made, not all institution-specific data on costs, utilization patterns, and clinical and patient outcomes may be available at the time the model is created—an issue that is explored later in this discussion.

Two general approaches to prospective modeling are presented. The first involves a more formal, and perhaps more familiar, decision analytic framework. This type of model can be constructed using commercially available software. The second approach uses a simplified spreadsheet approach to demonstrate a specific point concerning feasibility. As mentioned earlier, hospital P&T committees do not always have personnel available who are trained in more sophisticated modeling techniques. The use of readily available and commonly used software to model the potential impact of a formulary decision may be the most reasonable approach to take, considering the real-world demands on the members of a hospital P&T committee. Well-constructed spreadsheet models can meet the evaluation criteria described earlier, and would be a better choice than not including modeling data because of lack of expertise in conducting a formal decision analysis. Regardless of the specific method used, the health care system should undertake a retrospective analysis of the decision at an appropriate time following implementation using site-specific data for treatment costs and outcomes. The issue of formulary decision assessment is discussed in more detail later in this chapter.

Modeling cost and outcome estimates to aid a health system's P& T committee in making a formulary decision requires the use of input data with minimum uncertainty. Therefore, data that are both as accurate as possible and relevant to the health care system should be used whenever possible. Data elements such as number of patients, input costs for specific resources utilized in treatment, drug costs, medication compliance rates, and so on, should be obtained from internal health care system records whenever possible. Literature-based estimates of data inputs may be used when site-specific data are not available. Specific issues to consider when constructing any type of model include:

Perspective—The goal of a model should take the perspective of the payer. In the case of a model constructed for a hospital P&T committee, the perspective should be that of the hospital.

Time horizon—The choice of time horizon, the duration of time covered by the model, should be based on the needs of the institution. Modeling the costs and outcomes over 1 year would provide information on the impact of the formulary decision over that year. Caution should be used extending the estimation of costs and outcomes beyond that time frame. Rapidly changing clinical guidelines and emergence of new treatment options may make a 1-year time frame reasonable. If the model is extended beyond 1 year, discounting should be employed.

Cohort size—The number of patients to be treated in the model could reflect the number of patients typically treated in the specific health care system, or could be based on a hypothetical cohort if actual patient numbers are not known. Use of actual patient numbers would facilitate estimation of the total budget impact of a decision. Use of a hypothetical cohort would provide information on a per-patient basis. Keep in mind the formulary decision should be made with budget constraints in mind. The decision may be different if the medication will affect treatment of a small versus large number of patients.

Compliance rates—Estimates for medication compliance for the relevant patient population can be obtained from pharmacy refill records (21) or from literature estimates. Use of drug acquisition cost per day multiplied by number of days treated may lead to an overestimation of drug cost by not accounting for noncompliance. This issue plays a larger role in modeling costs for treatment of chronic diseases, and less of a role in modeling costs for acute conditions. Compliance rates may, however, be an important factor in clinical outcomes such as treatment success rates achieved with use of antibiotics.

Drug acquisition costs—In most institutions, drug acquisition cost data are readily available. Costs of additional medications used along with the drug under consideration, such as those needed to treat side effects, should be included. Not all patients take these additional drugs, so total additional drug costs can be averaged over the total treatment cohort.

Additional health care costs—Costs associated with utilization of resources other than drugs should be included in the model. Total treatment costs for drugs that must be administered in the hospital should reflect the cost of inpatient care. Costs for placement and monitoring of intravenous catheters should be included for intravenous drugs, along with an estimate of the costs of catheter-related adverse events. Laboratory costs should be included for drugs that require monitoring of levels or clinical parameters such as renal function.

Sensitivity analysis—The impact of data inputs that are estimated should be evaluated using a sensitivity analysis. The model should be run using varying parameters for which estimates are uncertain to determine potential impact on the model outputs.

Decision Analytic Models

Decision analysis provides a tool for systematic evaluation of the relative value of competing health care interventions. As with any type of modeling, the first step is to identify the problem, such as a comparison of a new drug or the existing formulary alternative. The choices in this example are to treat patients with either the new or the existing drug. Use of each drug is associated with a probability of a defined outcome, either success or failure. The possibility of treatment side effects may also be included, and may occur in the case of treatment success or failure.

Once the issue is identified, a "decision tree" is built that represents all of the possible choices and outcomes. Graphically, decision points, or nodes, are represented by squares, circles represent chance nodes, and outcomes are represented by triangles. At chance nodes, probabilities are assigned to each possible outcome (Fig. 1). Costs for each treatment would be estimated, based on the number of patients, drug costs, other treatment costs, duration of treatment, adverse event rates, and costs.

After assigning probabilities to each of the identified outcomes, the decision tree is analyzed by multiplying the individual probabilities along each branch. For example, for each case in which the new drug is administered, the probability of suc-

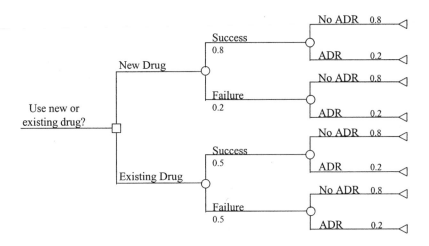

Figure 1 Decision tree for the use of two drugs, each with the probability of success or failure. Further, each success or failure is associated with the probability of adverse drug reactions (ADR) or no ADR.

cessful treatment without adverse drug reactions is $0.8 \times 0.8 = 0.64$. Costs may also be assigned to each branch of the tree, with total costs for each drug calculated by multiplying the cost of each outcome (i.e., branch) by the probability of the outcome, then adding it to the weighted cost of all other outcomes for that drug. For a more detailed discussion of decision analytic modeling, the reader is referred to Barr and Schumacher (22) or Weinstein and Fineberg (23). Decision analysis models can be constructed and run using commercially available software such as DATA (TreeAge Software, Williamstown, MA)™ and Precision Tree (Palisade Corporation, Newfield, NY)™.

Decision analysis would be an appropriate method to use when multiple outcomes are possible. One advantage of the methodology is that it breaks down complex medical treatments into components. The timeline aspect of the decision tree facilitates sequencing of events in a logical way. Treatments are selected followed by probabilities of success or failure. Estimates of outcome probabilities from the literature or from expert opinion may be used, allowing the investigator to construct and analyze a decision tree before making a decision for a particular patient population. The use of uncertain estimates for data inputs increases the importance of conducting sensitivity analyses to test their impact.

The "linearity" of decision analysis also constitutes one of the method's disadvantages. Recurrent events, repeating over time, may result in a decision tree that has become an unwieldy "bush." Under those circumstances, alternate techniques, such as Markov modeling, may be more appropriate (24).

Spreadsheet Models

The same treatment decision (new drug vs. existing drug) used in the decision analytic model can be evaluated using a spreadsheet model. This approach can provide a simplified, straightforward method for incorporating pharmacoeconomic data into the decision-making process that might otherwise be prohibited by staffing and expertise limitations. Cohort sizes, treatment duration, and costs of care used in the spreadsheet model are the same as those that would be used to model the same decision using decision analytic software. To illustrate the use of a spreadsheet model to inform the formulary decision-making process, consider the following case.

Intervention

Linezolid, a novel agent in the oxazolidinone class of antimicrobials, has clinical efficacy profiles and toxicity rates similar to vancomycin for methicillin-resistant *Staphylococcus* species (MRSS) and demonstrates virtually 100% bioavailability (25). The primary choice for treatment of MRSS infections has been intravenous (IV) vancomycin, but emerging vancomycin resistance in clinical staphylococcal isolates poses a threat to the efficacy of this agent in MRSS infections (26–28). The decision to be modeled is therefore the use of linezolid versus vancomycin for the treatment of MRSS infections in hospitalized patients.

Perspective

The perspective of this analysis becomes the payer, the entity liable for covering the cost of care for the patient with an MRSS infection. Because of high drug acquisition costs and the high bioavailability of the oral formulation of linezolid, the P&T committee in this case is considering use of the drug in patients who could be discharged home if they were being treated with an oral antibiotic.

Time Horizon and Cohort Size

The model will consider the impact on patients with MRSS infections treated during the next year, and a hypothetical cohort of 100 patients will be treated.

Clinical Outcomes

A published retrospective chart review indicates that patients receiving vancomycin for the treatment of suspected or confirmed MRSS infections meet eligibility criteria for switching to oral linezolid and discharge home an average of 3.3 ($\pm$ 2.9) days prior to actual discharge (29).

Resource Utilization

For this model, we will assume that the treatment decision point occurs when patients meet oral therapy and discharge criteria. From that point, treatment with vancomycin or linezolid will continue for 3.3 ($\pm$ 2.9) days. Continued use of vancomycin will incur costs for inpatient care and medication. Switching to linezolid will allow the patient to be discharged, so only drug acquisition costs will be included in the model ($18 per day for vancomycin, $125 per day for linezolid). As stated earlier, efficacy and toxicity rates of linezolid and vancomycin are equal (25), so costs for treatment failures and adverse drug reactions will not be included. Several resource cost assumptions can be made based on the short duration of treatment remaining. First, no costs will be included for monitoring vancomycin levels. Second, the model will assume that peripheral venous catheters will be used to administer vancomycin in the hospital, with no significant side effects related to catheter use. Third, because patients are eligible for discharge, hospitalization costs associated with continued vancomycin will reflect costs for an inpatient general medicine (i.e., non-intensive care) ward ($1,600 per day). All costs used in this example are hypothetical.

The treatment options are shown in the spreadsheet model in Figure 2, developed using Excel 2000 (Microsoft Corporation)™. Although not relevant when treatment outcomes are similar, as they are here, costs associated with adverse events and treatment failures could be included in this type of model. To do so, the probability of events (adverse drug reactions or treatment failures) would be multiplied by the number of patients in the cohort and the costs associated with each event. These costs would then be added to the costs for each treatment arm. As with other modeling software programs, spreadsheets allow model inputs to be varied easily. Use of spreadsheets provides an added advantage in that users can view the formulas used in obtaining outputs. This feature can be helpful in overcoming modeling's "black box" image.

FORMULARY DECISION ASSESSMENT

Once a formulary decision has been made, assessment of the decision does not always occur. A retrospective review evaluating the impact of a formulary decision after implementation is a method of evaluating the appropriateness of a formulary decision and identifying the need to modify or reverse the decision based on postimplementation data. The retrospective review process has the advantage of allowing a health care system to use internal data to conduct the analyses. The use of fewer estimated data inputs should provide a more precise estimate of the total cost and outcomes associated with the decision. An obvious drawback to a retrospective review is that the decision has already been made and revisions or rescissions may be difficult to implement.

An important methodologic issue in a retrospective evaluation of a formulary decision is whether or not to include all costs and outcomes for all patients with a specific diagnosis, regardless of whether they were eligible for treatment with the drug in question. The alternative would be to include in the analysis only those patients eligible to receive the treatment. The approach to take will depend on the goal of the analysis. One goal might be to evaluate the impact of adding

Comparison of Inpatient IV Vancomycin with Outpatient Oral Linezoid

Input Data	Range of Estimates		
	Low	**Base**	**High**
Number of cases	100	100	100
Vancomycin ($ per day)	15	18	20
Linezolid ($ per day)	85	125	150
Hospitalization ($ per day)	1250	1600	1850
Days of treatment	0.4	3.3	6.2

Resource Utilization [Using base cost inputs as entered]

A. Inpatient vancomycin	Per day ($)	Per case ($)	Cohort ($)
Hospitalization	1,600	5,280	528,000
Drug acquisition cost	18	59	5,940
Totals	**$1,618**	**$5,339**	**$533,940**

B. Outpatient linezolid	Per day ($)	Per case ($)	Cohort ($)
Drug acquisition cost	125	413	41,250
Totals	**$125**	**$413**	**$41,250**

Sensitivity Analysis	Total Cohort Costs		
	Low	**Base**	**High**
A. Inpatient vancomycin	$50,600	$533,940	$1,159,400
B. Outpatient linezolid	$3,400	$41,250	$93,000
Cost Differences	-$47,200	-$492,690	-$1,066,400

Summary

Using the base estimates for costs, compared with continued inpatient treatment with vancomycin, discharge of patient followed by treatment with linezolid results in a cost estimated to be

− $492,690

Based on the sensitivity analysis, the range of the difference is between:

− $47,200   and   − $1,066,400

Figure 2 Spreadsheet model comparing inpatient treatment with intravenous (IV) vancomycin with outpatient treatment with oral linezolid.

the drug to the formulary on total costs of care for the relevant patient population, such as all patients with heart failure. In that case, limiting the analysis to only those patients eligible to receive the drug would not take into account the impact of the proportion of patients ineligible to receive the drug. A subgroup analysis using only drug-eligible patients would be appropriate to inform the question of the impact of using the drug on costs and outcomes for that population only. It would not inform the question of how system-wide costs and clinical outcomes would be affected by the formulary decision. In other words, it is less likely that using that treatment will have a substantial impact on total population care costs. The design of the study will depend on the question being asked.

Another methodologic issue is the need to control for, or at least be aware of, systemic trends within the health system (trends that are occurring in the health system regardless of the use of the drug in question). Are there other factors, such as new treatment guidelines, that may have an impact on the costs and outcomes being studied?

The time frame of the study is also an issue that depends on the drug in question. Data should be collected representing a clinically relevant period of time. The observation time should be sufficient to allow events of interest to occur, but also to allow inclusion of an appropriate number of patients. Differences between the drug in question and the comparator drug may be seen in 6 months. On the other hand, it may be that only a few patients were treated with the new drug during the 6 months after the formulary decision was implemented. Patient availability and clinical issues should be considered when determining when a retrospective formulary decision should be conducted.

CONCLUSIONS

When conducted in accordance with the recommendations presented in this chapter, prospective modeling can be a useful tool to aid in formulary decision-making. Sophisticated computer programs need not be used in order to incorporate pharmacoeconomic data into the formulary decision process. In all cases, however, the model should be verified retrospectively to identify the need for revisions in the formulary decision, and to improve the ability to construct models initially.

REFERENCES

1. Centers for Medicare and Medicaid Services. National health expenditures. Available at: http://www.cms.hhs.gov/statistics/nhe/projections-2003/t2.asp.

2. U.S. Census Bureau. Age: 2000. Census 2000 brief. Available at: http://www.census.gov/prod/2001pubs/c2kbr01-12.pdf.

3. Weisbrod BA. The health care quadrilemma: an essay on technological change, insurance, quality of care, and cost containment. J Econ Lit 1991; 29:523–552.

4. The NewsHour with Jim Lehrer, Kaiser Family Foundation, Harvard School of Public Health. National Survey on Prescription Drugs. 2000. Available at: http://www.pbs.org/newshour/health/prescriptions/summaryandchartpack.pdf.

5. Garber AM. Can technology assessment control health spending? Health Aff 1994:116–126.

6. Pedersen CA, Schneider PJ, Santell JP. ASHP national survey of pharmacy practice in hospital settings: prescribing and transcribing—2001. Am J Health Syst Pharm 2001; 58:2251–2266.

7. Kozma CM, Reeder CE, Schulz RM. Economic, clinical, and humanistic outcomes: a planning model for pharmacoeconomic research. Clin Ther 1993; 15:1121–1132.

8. Drummond MF, Torrance G, O'Brien B, Stoddart G. Methods for the Economic Evaluation of Health Care Programmes. 2d ed. New York: Oxford University Press, 1997.

9. Gold MR, Siegel JE, Russell LB, Weinstein MC, EdsCost-Effectiveness in Health and Medicine.. New York: Oxford University Press, 1996.

10. Elixhauser A, Luce BR, Taylor WR, Reblando J. Health care CBA/CEA: an update on the growth and composition of the literature. Med Care 1993; 31(suppl 7):JS18–JS149.

11. Elixhauser A, Halpern M, Schmier J, Luce BR. Health care CBA and CEA from 1991 to 1996: an updated bibliography. Med Care 1998; 36:MS1–MS9.

12. Finkler SA. The distinction between costs and charges. Ann Intern Med 1982; 96:102–109.

13. Hill SR, Mitchell AS, Henry DA. Problems with the interpretation of pharmacoeconomic analyses. JAMA 2000; 283: 2116–2121.

14. O'Brien B. Economic evaluation of pharmaceuticals: Frankenstein's monster or vampire of trials? Med Care 1996; 34: DS99–DS108.

15. Doubilet P, Weinstein MC, McNeil BJ. Use and misuse of the term "cost effective" in medicine. N Engl J Med 1986; 314: 253–255.

16. O'Brien B. Health state utility anchors: being clear on what "1" means. Med Decis Making 1997; 17:352–353.

17. Odedina FT, Sullivan J, Nash R, Clemmons CD. Use of pharmacoeconomic data in making formulary decisions. Am J Health Syst Pharm 2002; 59:1441–1444.

18. Academy of Managed Care Pharmacy. Formulary Principles Coalition: Principles of a Sound Formulary System. October 2000. Available at: http://www.amcp.org/publications/drugformulary.pdf.

19. Academy of Managed Care Pharmacy. Format for Formulary Submissions, Version 2.0. October 2002. Available at: http://www.fmcpnet.org/data/resource/formatv20.pdf.

20. Weinstein MD, Toy EL, Sandberg EA, Neumann PJ, Evans JS, Kuntz KM, Graham JD, Hammitt JK. Modeling for health care and other policy decisions: uses, roles, and validity. Value Health 2001; 4:348–361.

21. Steiner JF, Koepsell TD, Fihn SD, Inui TS. A general method of compliance assessment using centralized pharmacy records. Description and validation. Med Care 1988; 26:814–823.

22. Barr JT, Schumacher GE. Decision analysis and pharmacoeconomic evaluations. In: Bootman JL, Townsend RJ, McGhan

WF, Eds Principles of Pharmacoeconomics.. Cincinnati, OH: Harvey Whitney Books Company, 1991.

23. Weinstein MC, Fineberg FV. Clinical Decision Analysis.. Philadelphia: WB Saunders, 1980.

24. Tom E, Schulman KA. Mathematical models in decision making. Infect Control Hosp Epidemiol 1997; 18:65–73.

25. Stevens DL, Herr D, Lampiris H, Hunt JL, Batts DH, Hafkin B, and the Linezolid MRSA Study Group. Linezolid versus vancomycin for the treatment of methicillin-resistant *Staphylococcus aureus* infections. Clin Infect Dis 2002; 34:1481–1490.

26. Hiramatsu K, Aritaka N, Hanaki H, Kawasaki S, Hosoda Y, Hori S, Fukuchi Y, Kobayashi I. Dissemination in Japanese hospitals of strains of *Staphylococcus aureus* heterogeneously resistant to vancomycin. Lancet 1997; 350:1670–1673.

27. Smith TL, Pearson ML, Wilcox KR, Cruz C, Lancaster MV, Robinson-Dunn B, Tenover FC, Zervos MJ, Band JD, White E, Jarvis WR. Emergence of vancomycin resistance in *Staphylococcus aureus*. Glycopeptide-Intermediate *Staphylococcus aureus* Working Group. N Engl J Med 1999; 340:493–501.

28. Sieradzki K, Roberts RB, Haber SW, Tomasz A. The development of vancomycin resistance in a patient with methicillin-resistant *Staphylococcus aureus* infection. N Engl J Med 1999; 340:517–523.

29. Parodi S, Rhew DC, Goetz MB. Early switch and early discharge opportunities in intravenous vancomycin treatment of suspected methicillin-resistant staphylococcal species infections. J Managed Care Pharm 2003; 9:317–326.

7

Measuring the Attributable Costs of Resistant Infections in Hospital Settings

R. DOUGLAS SCOTT II and STEVE L. SOLOMON

Centers for Disease Control and Prevention,
National Center for Infectious Diseases, Division
of Healthcare Quality Promotion
Atlanta, Georgia, U.S.A.

RALPH CORDELL

Centers for Disease Control and Prevention,
National Center for Chronic Disease Prevention
and Health Promotion, Division of Adolescent
and School Health
Atlanta, Georgia, U.S.A.

REBECCA R. ROBERTS

Department of Emergency Medicine, John H.
Stroger Jr. Hospital of Cook County
Chicago, Illinois, U.S.A.

DAVID HOWARD

Rollins School of Public Health,
Emory University
Atlanta, Georgia, U.S.A.

JOHN E. MCGOWAN, JR.

School of Medicine, Emory University
Atlanta, Georgia, U.S.A.

Infections with microorganisms resistant to conventional anti-microbial drug therapy (resistance resulting from microorganisms evolving to decrease their susceptibility to antimicrobial drugs) present difficult problems for hospital management and administration. Such infections complicate patient treatment, often requiring the use of broader spectrum (and usually more expensive) drugs (1). Just as important, many resistant infections are acquired within hospitals and other health care settings and thus are an important patient safety issue (2). Estimating the economic costs to hospitals and society has proven challenging because of difficulties both in understanding the epidemiology of drug resistance and in developing economic estimates that accurately reflect the additional costs attributable to resistant infections. Various published estimates of the aggregate economic cost of antimicrobial resistance in the United States range from $4 million to $5 million to $100 million to $30 billion (3,4). The wide disparity in estimates illustrates how differing assumptions and the varying perspectives of an analytic framework can influence the results of an analysis.

This chapter focuses on methods of measuring the attributable cost of resistant infections from the perspective of the hospital. As many resistant infections are nosocomial, hospitals absorb much of the direct medical cost of their treatment. Although the direct excess medical cost due to resistant infections comprises only a small portion of the potential costs to society, economic analysis conducted within the perspective of hospital administrators is most likely to encourage hospitals to make the financial investment in improved infection control programs and interventions. To prepare the reader, the chapter begins with an explanation of the theory of perfectly competitive markets and the related concepts of opportunity cost and relative price ratios. The second section discusses the divergence of perspectives on costs in health care resulting from the imperfect nature of markets for health care and how perspectives on cost vary when considering antimicrobial resistance. The third section focuses on the epidemiologic models used to measure the attributable costs to hospitals of resistant nosocomial infections, and considers both the choice of surrogates used to represent costs and the use of severity-of-illness indexes to control for confounding. Finally, the chapter concludes with some recommendations to improve the quality of the economic information that can be provided by hospital-based observational studies.

OVERVIEW OF ECONOMIC THEORY

Economic analysis of antimicrobial resistance and the infection control interventions needed to minimize its impact involves the use of concepts that are viewed with some skepticism by the public health community. Many clinicians and public health practitioners are troubled by the use of money to value health outcomes without addressing issues of equity (5,6). Confusion also results from the evaluation of this problem from the different perspectives of clinical medicine, with its focus on individual outcomes, and of economics, with its focus on allocating resources (within a given system of property rights) to achieve the highest (most efficient) level of output for the overall benefit of society.

It is important, therefore, to emphasize the role of resource allocation in assessing economic impact, for this distinguishes economics from accounting. Economics is essentially a behavioral science that is concerned with determining the best allocation of limited resources among competing unlimited demands. Accounting practices are concerned with financial cost—the actual monetary payments made for resources that are used. Measuring cost in economics involves much more than financial cost in that it embodies opportunity cost—the value of a resource when it is employed in its next best alternative use. Opportunity cost indicates whether an employed resource is being utilized to its full productive potential. Because hospital and health care resources are limited, it is socially desirable to get the most output from these limited resources.

A key function of economic theory is the design of resource allocation mechanisms (or markets) that can allocate scarce resources among unlimited demands. The fundamental underlying economic assumption about human behavior is that individuals will strive to maximize their own welfare (happiness). With this in mind, there are three main issues to consider when designing a resource allocation mechanism. First, suppliers will desire an allocation mechanism that promotes efficiency—getting the greatest output of goods and services from the inputs (resources) used in production. Second, consumers desire an allocation mechanism that will provide the goods and services they demand. And finally, the mechanism must be able to efficiently distribute the products among those who wish to consume them.

The Perfectly Competitive Market Model

In economics, the idealized form or "gold standard" of resource allocation mechanisms is the perfectly competitive market (the model that is presented in introductory courses on economics) (7). Characteristics of a perfectly competitive market include (i) many buyers and sellers where no single individual consumer or supplier can influence the exchange of goods among market participants, (ii) a homogeneous or standardized product (i.e., goods that individual producers cannot alter or differentiate to collect a higher price), (iii) no barriers to the movement of firms in or out of the market, (iv) perfect information about market conditions that is available to all market participants, and (v) a fully defined system of property rights in which ownership of all products and productive resources is assigned (8).

This allocation mechanism provides a social environment in which producers and consumers can freely interact. Consumer preferences about a particular product are revealed where greater quantities of product are purchased as price declines (labeled *demand curve* in Fig. 1); producer preferences become apparent where greater quantities of product are supplied as product price increases (labeled *supply curve* in Fig. 1). As market participants interact, an equilibrium price level will emerge so that the quantity demanded at price P_E by consumers is equal to the quantity that producers will supply (Q_E) at price P_E. P_E is the price that "clears the market"

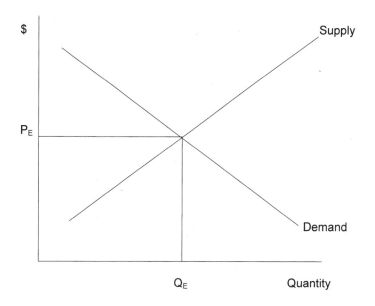

Figure 1   Supply and demand curves. The x axis represents a quantity of goods purchased for demand curve and quantity of goods supplied for supply curve. The y axis represents the price of goods in dollars. P_E and Q_E are defined in the text. (Adapted from Scott RD, Solomon SL, McGowan JE. Applying economic principles to health care. Emerg Infect Dis 2001; 7:282–285.)

because at no other price level does the quantity demanded by consumers equal the quantity supplied by producers. Prices greater than this level will result in excess supply (buildup of inventories), whereas prices below this level will result in excess demand (pressing prices to increase).

An advantage of a perfectly competitive market is that the prices observed in the marketplace capture the full opportunity costs associated with each resource, service, or output traded in the market. Prices act as a feedback mechanism to all market participants, reflecting the value to suppliers (or the opportunity cost) of resources used in production and the value to consumers of the final goods and services produced.

Within a perfectly competitive market, the perspectives of consumers, producers, and society as a whole converge. This resource allocation mechanism provides incentives for individual economic agents to produce the greatest possible output from the scarce resources available. In order to make a reasonable profit, producers must be efficient with their resources or be forced to leave the market. Across the various markets, consumer demands are met as consumers select the goods and services in the quantities they prefer to consume, producers are providing the most output possible (thereby maximizing profits), and society gets the most output from the scarce resources available.

Determining the opportunity cost of resources utilized in health care is difficult because of the organizational structure of health care markets and characteristics of health care as a good or service (7). Health care markets are considered imperfect markets, as many of the market attributes needed for the functioning of a perfectly competitive market do not exist for health care services. Problems are encountered in evaluating this market in the United States because (i) health care is a heterogeneous product in which patients may experience a range of different health outcomes, (ii) full information on market characteristics and conditions are not available to market participants, (iii) many health care consumers are insured by third-party payers who are responsible for direct medical expenses, and (iv) a market price (or feedback mechanism) that reflects the full opportunity costs of the resources used by health care providers does not exist.

The prices observed in imperfect markets, such as health care markets, will not embody the full opportunity costs of resources employed in production. In the United States, hospital services are not like other typical commodities that are traded in markets. With the advent of the prospective payment system, hospitals face fixed reimbursement schedules for patients covered by third-party payers, notably Medicare and Medicaid. Also, health outcomes cannot be guaranteed, even with the best treatment. Relief from the pain and suffering from illness and its impact on individuals is not readily translated into prices that can be reflected in a market. Without market-generated prices to observe, surrogate measures must be found to represent the opportunity costs of resources that are consumed due to resistant infections. Surrogates for opportunity costs can come from adjustments to observed charges or estimates that have been developed using analytical models.

The Role of Relative Prices

Opportunity costs are measured using relative prices (expressing the prices of a good or product in terms of another good) (8). An important implication of the role of prices in resource allocation is that prices relative to each other, and not the absolute level of nominal prices (the price of a good expressed in terms of money), are important when considering changes in the demand for goods and services (9). In the exchange of goods and services in a perfectly competitive market, consumers will base their purchases on product prices and their own tastes and preferences. As prices change in the market, goods that are less expensive may be substituted for other higher-priced goods. For example, if the price of pizza increases, consumers may switch to eating more of a less expensive item (e.g., hamburger) as opposed to paying more for pizza, because income is limited. With changes in product prices, the quantities of goods purchased will depend on whether they are substitutes, where one good can be consumed in place of another (e.g. switching from sodas to fruit juice), or complements, where consumption of one product will depend on the consumption of another (e.g. consumption of automobile tires and owning a car).

Relative prices are expressed as ratios that show how much of one good a consumer must give up in order to purchase an additional unit of another good (see discussion in Gould and Ferguson) (10). If one has two goods, X and Y, then the relative price of good X to good Y can be expressed as P_x/P_y (where P_x is the price of X and P_y is the price of Y). If the price ratio is 1.2, then 1.2 units of Y must be given up to get an additional unit of good X. In circumstances in which income remains constant and nominal prices change proportionately (e.g., all prices double), the relative price ratio stays the same (e.g., $2P_x/2P_y = P_x/P_y$). In this case, a proportional increase (decrease) in prices will produce the same results as when there is a decrease (increase) in income. The rate at which one trades good Y for good X stays the same, but the overall quantities purchased will decline.

This illustrates that prices and the value of products consumed provide *ordinal* measures (as opposed to *cardinal* measures) of economic well-being.[1] The dollar values associated with the various bundles of goods and services that consumers purchase are used to rank whether consumers are improving their own economic well-being with the choices made in the marketplace within their finite budgets.

This result has implications for studies on attributable costs of resistant infections because it is important to have all the necessary information to make cost comparisons among the three clinical situations ("states") related to resistance: noninfection, susceptible infection (infections due to organisms that can be treated by the usual antimicrobials), and resistant infection. The absolute difference in the attributable costs of these three various states has no real meaning without making comparisons to a reference state—in effect, constructing a relative price ratio. For example, if the attributable costs of an infection due to a specific resistant pathogen is estimated at $20,000, the magnitude of the attributable difference (when compared with the costs of treating noninfected patients) will

---

[1] In economic theory, the purchases that consumers make in the marketplace are observed and then evaluated to assess the economic well-being (defined in terms of the value of the purchases made) of consumers. The dollar values associated with various bundles of consumer goods are used to rank economic states, with higher-value bundles implying higher attainment of economic well-being (in most cases). In this sense, dollars are used as ordinal measures. The absolute difference in dollar values between states does not have any real meaning outside of this ranking. If the dollar values of economic bundles were cardinal measures, the absolute difference would have meaning. This would imply that the subjective taste and preferences of consumers are quantifiable and that consumers can always determine exactly how much their economic well-being changes with different levels of consumption. Because of the obstacles in finding a quantifiable way to measure tastes and preferences, economic theory has rested on the less-stringent behavioral assumption that consumers can at least ordinally rank various economic states according to their tastes and preferences.

vary depending on whether the reference group comprises less–resource-intensive patients (e.g., general medicine patients whose hospital costs average $10,000) or more–resource-intensive patients (e.g., patients in intensive care units [ICU] whose costs average $50,000). This information is vital in ranking the various economic states of well-being and estimating the opportunity costs associated with susceptible and resistant infections.

As an example of the importance of the relative ranking of economic states for antibacterial resistance, the U.S. Office of Technology Assessment (OTA) in 1995 determined that the national aggregated direct hospital cost of infections due to six different resistant pathogens (methicillin-resistant *Staphylococcus aureus* [MRSA], vancomycin-resistant enterococci [VRE], imipenem-resistant *Pseudomonas aeruginosa*, methicillin-resistant coagulase-negative staphylococci, ampicillin-resistant *Escherichia coli,* and resistant *Enterobacter*) for five different categories of infections (surgical site infection, pneumonia, bacteremia, urinary tract infection, and other miscellaneous infections) was approximately $1.3 billion (1992 U.S. dollars) annually (11). Because of the lack of specific studies on the economic impact of these resistant organisms, this figure was derived using an estimate (based on limited evidence) that the cost of infection when these organisms are antibiotic resistant is double the cost of infection when these nosocomial pathogens are antibiotic susceptible (12). However, there has been very little evidence published to verify the accuracy of this rough estimate of the relative ranking between the costs of susceptible and resistant infections (11). Such economic information is crucial in order to develop national aggregate estimates of the economic cost of the various aspects of antimicrobial resistance.

THE ANALYTIC PERSPECTIVES ON THE COSTS OF RESISTANT INFECTIONS

What are the implications for conducting cost studies of resistant infections in hospitals? There are three important decisions an analyst must make when beginning any economic evaluation: choosing an analytic perspective, determining the relevant costs, and deciding how to measure costs (13). Because of the heterogeneous nature of the health care market, the economic impact of changes in the allocation of resources will be viewed differently by the various market participants. The costs and benefits of an expensive new health care intervention to mitigate antimicrobial resistance may be perceived differently by physicians, patients, health care businesses, drug industry firms, and society. The perspective that is chosen for the study will determine which costs and benefits should be included in the analysis. For example, the analytic perspective chosen for the OTA study mentioned above was from the hospital administration's point of view, in which the primary economic impact stems from the direct medical costs of additional patient care resulting from infection. Alternatively, a broader societal perspective would consider other cost considerations, including pain and suffering and the loss of working productivity due to the infection. This section discusses the various cost perspectives related to antimicrobial resistance (Table 1) (14).

Physicians

Physicians' main concerns are with the individual patient and are motivated by a desire to eliminate disease in patients (Table 1). The economic consequences of resistant infections are related to ineffective treatment (consequences arising from the patient's continued illness or death). From the clinician's perspective, it becomes a concern if the available supply of antimicrobials becomes "ineffective." The economic impact of diminishing effectiveness of a given drug or group of drugs depends on the availability of other drugs which could be substituted to treat a given type of infection.

Patients

Infected patients have a perspective on cost similar to that of physicians, because the patient's focus is on successful treatment. Patients are motivated by their desire to obtain im-

Table 1 Different Perspectives of Economic Impact of Antimicrobial Resistance

	Medical	Patient	Health care business	Drug industry	Public ("society")
Focus	Individual	Individual	Care group	Potential clients	Population
Outcome	Absence of disease	Absence of disease	Reduced cost of care	Product sales	Maximization of health
Time frame	Short	Short	Short	Short, long	Long
Motivation	Professionalism	Personal well-being	Profit	Profit	Social good
Approach	Treatment	Treatment	Cost containment	Development of new drugs, maintaining life of old drugs	Reduction in forces leading to resistance

* From Cordell RE, Solomon SE, Scott RD, McGowan, unpublished data, 2000.

proved health. The costs of resistant infections to patients include the extra cost of drugs and of health services (resulting from the infection) which are paid either directly (out of pocket) or indirectly (through insurance premiums). From this perspective, costs of resistant infections should include not only the added costs of treatment but also the costs associated with morbidity or mortality, including pain and suffering, and other indirect costs, such as time lost from work.

Health Care Businesses

In the United States, a large share of the financial resources of the health system, and their allocation, are controlled by a myriad of hospital administrators, financial managers, insurance companies, and the government (local, state, and federal agencies), with less control by the health care providers. Here, the perspective on the costs of resistant infections and their economic impact comes from a focus of treating patients (i.e., customers) who are part of a well-defined population being served, but doing so to maximize financial returns (or minimize costs) to boards of directors or shareholders. Resistance becomes a problem when drug effectiveness becomes reduced and the corresponding patient-care costs rise as additional resources (alternative drugs, personnel time, supplies, space, and equipment) must be employed for patient care. To minimize this cost, health system administrators often attempt to monitor and/or control drug effectiveness through pharmacy and therapeutics committees, drug utilization reviews, and formularies.

From this perspective, a resistant infection in settings outside the population served by a particular health care organization becomes of interest only when it may affect its client population. Health care businesses (particularly hospitals) may provide the easiest setting for measuring the economic impact of resistant infections on their costs. The economic impact is limited to the costs of specific antimicrobial drugs and the extra costs of care to specific patient groups. These costs can be calculated for a specific health care organization and used to assess the cost-effectiveness of programs that preserve the effectiveness of available drugs.

Even among health care businesses, perspectives on costs may diverge. Health insurance businesses (and other third-party payers) are interested in having health care services delivered in a cost-effective manner to minimize reimbursements. Reimbursement policies that allow hospitals to pass along the added treatment expenses from resistant nosocomial infections could act as a financial disincentive to hospitals to invest in improved infection control programs, because the hospital does not absorb any of these costs.

Drug Industry Firms

Pharmaceutical firms operate similarly to health care businesses in that they seek to generate profits. They produce a variety of antimicrobial compounds and vaccines used to treat or prevent infectious diseases for potential users of their products (either direct users such as patient/clients or indirect users such as health care systems and government health agencies). Firms look to high product sales (usually in the short term) as the desired outcome. However, firms must also take a longer view and consider the impact of resistance as a potential for the introduction and sale of new products. This requires a two-pronged strategy. First, the firm wishes to extend the effective life of its current drug line against resistance. Second, the pattern of resistance may make competitors' products obsolete, thus providing the firm with a new marketing opportunity for an existing product of its own (that may have in the past been more expensive, less safe, or less effective than the now-obsolete drug) or producing a niche for a new antimicrobial agent that the firm can manufacture.

Public or Societal View

The societal perspective is concerned with the well-being of members of society, which may be expressed in terms of populations (of cities, states, countries, or even the entire world). The goal of this perspective is to maximize health for the entire defined population, usually over a long time horizon. For this reason, antimicrobials are a scarce resource that must be managed wisely to prevent and treat infectious diseases. Appropriate use of antimicrobial drugs for treatment and prevention of infection might lead to an eventual, but acceptable, decrease in antimicrobial effectiveness, whereas overuse or misuse of antimicrobial drugs would lead to an inappropriate (i.e., too rapid) decrease in effectiveness. If the treatment of one patient leads to decreased effectiveness in treating the next person using the same drug, society is affected adversely.

Antimicrobials possess characteristics that make it difficult to allocate their effectiveness between current and future consumers, within the perfectly competitive market model described earlier. An important attribute of antimicrobials is that over time, consumption (current use) decreases their effectiveness (future value) (15,16). On one hand, antimicrobials are given to promote an individual patient's health, but the decision to provide antimicrobial treatment to one patient can affect the future efficacy and quality of treatments to others (17). In the broader societal view, this feature of antimicrobial drug use places these agents within a class of economic goods called *common property resources*. The characteristic that distinguishes common property resources from other goods and services is that an individual's consumption of such a good can affect the consumption of the resource by others without their permission. In economics, this phenomenon is called an *externality* (18). A popular example of a common property resource in basic economics is a fishery (based on a frequently referenced paper published by Gordon) (19). Individual commercial fishermen seek to maximize their profit by attempting to catch as many fish as their boats will hold. However, the operation of one boat catching as many fish as possible causes an increase in the costs of fishing for every fisherman by reducing the fish stock—the externality being reflected in the increasing average unit cost for fish harvested. The result is overfishing, which in the long run could lead to the biologic collapse of the fish population, which ultimately is detrimental to all users of the fishery (although Gordon's model predicted most fishermen would be forced to quit fishing because of high harvest costs before this level of biologic collapse takes place).

The problem of externalities stems from violating the last condition for a perfectly competitive market: a fully defined system of property rights. Because the resource belongs to no one particular individual or group of individuals, the resource is held "in common." No user of the resource (in the example above, the fishermen who catch fish to bring to market) must pay anyone to get access to the fishery and harvest fish. Without prices to provide feedback concerning the long-term economic value of maintaining a sustainable fish population, the perfectly competitive market "fails." In cases of market failure such as this, the resource allocation mechanism designed for common property resources is usually a modified market mechanism with rights to use the resource held within a government agency or some collective organization made up of users. These bodies oversee the use of regulations, taxes, and subsidies to act as surrogates for market prices to reflect the value of a sustainable resource (e.g., the fishery); in effect, internalizing the externality.

For antimicrobial resistance, the externality stems from the decision of an individual clinician to administer antimicrobial treatment to an infected patient without consideration of the impact on future users of the drug. Such use for one patient may increase the costs of care for other patients without their permission. At present, there is no broadly applicable formal regulatory mechanism in place that attempts to "internalize" the externality (i.e., provide the feedback about the future effectiveness of antimicrobials based on current use). However, hospitals, government health agencies, and various organizations of health care professionals are developing and advocating appropriate-use guidelines and, in some cases, antimicrobial management programs (20). Time will tell if these types of institutional arrangements, based on voluntary associations or local controls, will be capable of responding to the challenges that the emerging pattern of resistance places on public health, globally as well as nationally.

The Appropriate Perspective?

The economic costs and benefits of programs to preserve antimicrobial effectiveness must be interpreted in the context of the differing points of view illustrated above. In any single study, it is essential to keep the same perspective consistently throughout. The business viewpoint might place a positive value on the loss of effectiveness of a competitor's cheap antimicrobial if it leads to use of the same manufacturer's more expensive agent in treatment. The physician's viewpoint might consider the loss of effectiveness of the cheaper drug of little consequence as long as other effective drugs are available and there is no clinical or economic impact (from the physician's perspective) to using a different drug.

Another example of varying perspectives is the use of policies and formularies to control the physician's choice of antimicrobial agents. This step may make great sense to hospital or other health care administrators when it is likely to produce more efficient use of resources. However, these measures might be seen as having no positive value to clinicians who are willing to use any and all resources to cure their patients.

Antimicrobial drugs could potentially be managed collectively with a market-based resource allocation mechanism which can distribute the current supply of antimicrobials between current and future users. However, the detrimental effect of current use on long-term effectiveness has not been quantifiably determined for most situations (21). This makes it difficult to design a resource allocation mechanism that can distribute antimicrobial effectiveness from a social perspective.

The net economic impact of resistant infections, from the hospital perspective, can be narrowly viewed as the attributable cost of medical treatment due to the presence of a resistant pathogen (these costs would be the benefits or the cost savings of avoiding additional treatment resulting from interventions to curb resistance) minus the cost of preventing such resistant infections. Cost analysis under a broader social perspective should include consideration of all resources affected by the illness or any interventions, including lost days of work and productivity, diminished quality of life, and the value of resources (such as volunteer labor), that have not been paid for (22). Table 2 illustrates the variety of cost factors that are important to the differing perspectives when conducting an economic analysis of antimicrobial resistance (14). When com-

Table 2 Elements of the Economic Impact of Antimicrobial Resistance, by Perspective Affected

Element	Measurement	Perspective affected
Mortality	Costs associated with treatment failure (R) (S)	Physician, patient, HCB
Morbidity	Costs associated with pain, suffering, inconvenience (R) (S)	Physician, patient
Care cost	Charges for care (R) (S)	Patient
Care time	Time devoted to care (R) (S)	Physician, HCB
	Length of process (R) (S)*	Patient, society
Diagnosis costs	Costs for diagnosis (R) (S)	HCB
Treatment costs	Costs for drugs, etc. (R) (S) (additional drugs and treatments, more expensive drugs, etc.)	HCB
Diminished marketability	Market for drug use (R) (S)	Drug industry
New markets	Market for new drug (S) (R) (replace current market leader; replace inexpensive drug with more expensive drug; provide new product)	Drug industry
Impact on nontreated	Increased resistance (R) (S)	Society

* Costs associated with lack of usual function during infection, including cost of patient's loss of work time, quality of life, etc. (note: includes both inpatient and outpatient components); for society, costs are associated with reduction of useful function in workforce.
HCB, health care business; (R), extent in patients infected with resistant organism; (S), extent in patients infected with susceptible organism

paring the costs of resistant infections to susceptible infections, the added cost for each factor is shown along with its impact on the various perspectives.

For example, in Table 2, the direct medical costs for diagnostic procedures (e.g., laboratory tests, radiology, bronchoscopy), the costs for additional or more expensive antimicrobial drugs and therapeutic agents, and the increased length of hospital stay are primarily of concern to health care institutions when these costs cannot be passed on to third-party payers or the patients. Patients also experience indirect costs due to losses in income from missed workdays, travel costs associated with increased hospital or doctor visits, and possible declines in quality of life whereas businesses in which the patients are employed experience a loss in productivity. The drug industry may also experience indirect costs due to the diminishing marketability of their drugs.

Studies of the economic impact of resistance have not included measurement of the full range of these variables. Most studies on nosocomial pathogens have conducted their economic analysis from the cost perspective of hospital administrators or third-party payers (usually using hospital charges for costs). From this perspective, the additional direct costs of diagnosis and treatment due to a resistant pathogen (i.e., direct medical care costs) are measured to determine the magnitude of the potential per-patient cost savings that could result from reducing the incidence of resistant infections. The Study on the Efficacy of Nosocomial Infection Control (SCENIC) project, conducted during the late 1970s to early 1980s, showed that hospitals employing infection control surveillance and other preventive interventions had lower rates of nosocomial infections (23). In order to further justify investment in surveillance programs, researchers conducted economic studies of the cost-effectiveness of infection control programs and the cost savings they could generate from the perspective of both the hospital and society at large. The analytic approaches used to examine the overall economic impact of nosocomial infections in hospital settings were later used to assess the economic impact of resistant infections. Because most of the work was done from the hospital perspective, the remainder of this discussion focuses specifically on the economic studies of resistant infections taken from that point of view.

EPIDEMIOLOGIC MODELS OF THE ATTRIBUTABLE COST OF RESISTANT INFECTIONS FROM THE HOSPITAL PERSPECTIVE

The most common analytic approach for measuring the attributable costs of resistant infections in hospitals has been to conduct an observational epidemiologic study (24). This approach was routinely used in studies of the attributable cost of susceptible nosocomial infections and was adopted by researchers to measure the attributable cost of resistant nosocomial infections when these became more prominent. Two groups of patients with similar characteristics but different exposure status (e.g., susceptible infection vs. resistant infection) are followed to see if the outcome variable (patient cost) differs between the groups. To better understand the epidemiologic studies used to analyze cost outcomes in hospitals, we need to address in particular the use of severity of illness (SOI) indexes to control for the confounding caused by the high cost of underlying disease severity, and the use of cost measures for hospital resources.

Focusing on susceptible nosocomial infections, Haley (25) provided a summary of the observational study designs and cost measurement issues that may be considered when estimating the cost savings to a hospital from infection control programs and interventions. Two study designs have been used to assess the cost savings achieved by infection control programs: the concurrent method and the comparative method. The concurrent method involves following each case of infection on a daily basis and itemizing all the resources consumed (e.g., labor, supplies, equipment) to treat the infection. Costs associated with each resource are then combined with the volume of resources used to estimate the total costs attributable to the infection. Such studies usually employ an appropriateness evaluation protocol, which serves as a guide in determining whether a particular service, procedure, or day in the hospital is attributable to the nosocomial infection (26).

Most comparative studies, although erroneously referred to as *case-control studies*, have used a cohort or case-cohort approach. Exposed subjects are defined as those with an identified nosocomial infection, whereas a comparison group is selected from patients who do not have a nosocomial infection. Common outcome variables include some measure of cost (often hospital charges), length of hospital stay, or mortality. A true case-control study would involve assigning subjects to groups on the basis of their having or not having a particular outcome variable—in this instance, a high cost of care—and then looking for risk factors, such as having a nosocomial infection (susceptible or resistant), that are positively associated with the outcome.

In studies of the overall excess cost of nosocomial infections, it was recognized that patients acquiring nosocomial infections might have a greater severity of underlying disease upon admission to the hospital than patients who did not become infected (25,27–29). This introduced an upward bias in cost estimates because the infected patient group, on the whole, already had patients more costly to treat than the corresponding control group. Investigators frequently match subjects with and without resistant infections on other factors, such as age, diagnosis, and/or severity of underlying illness, in an attempt to improve the comparability of the two groups.

For this reason, these same concerns and issues hold true for measuring the excess costs of resistant infections as well (30,14). Controlling for the confounding effects of severity of underlying disease both in patients with susceptible nosocomial infections and in those with resistant nosocomial infections has been a particularly difficult analytic issue to overcome in epidemiologic studies of antimicrobial resistance. A number of recommendations have been advanced on the best way to adjust for differences in patient characteristics and severity of disease in studies of nosocomial infections. Haley (25) recommended that researchers use multiple matching criteria, by selecting one or more control patients for every infected patient, in order to obtain control subjects that would have "the same expected length of hospital stay and hospital costs" as infected patients would have had if they had not developed an infection. He further suggested the use of diagnosis-related groups (DRGs) as the best measure to predict patient length of stay and total hospital costs. Alternatively, Gross et al. (31) advocated using the number of comorbidities as a measure to control for severity of disease. Harris et al. (32) suggested that using SOI indexes that possess standardized scores would promote the comparison of results from different studies. Standardized scores that have been used include the Acute Physiology and Chronic Health Evaluation (APACHE) system, the Charlson index, and the McCabe-Jackson scale (33–35).

The Measurement of Costs

Once the perspective of the analysis is determined, the types of benefits and costs that are consistent with the perspective can be measured. When taking the hospital perspective, studies of resistant infections must find an appropriate measure for the opportunity costs of resources used in a hospital. As stated earlier, market prices for hospital care do not exist, so surrogates for opportunity costs must be found. An obvious candidate for opportunity costs is the total patient charges at discharge from the hospital. An important consideration in the measurement of costs is making the distinction between costs (the expenditures the hospital makes for goods and services) and charges (what the hospital charges the patient) (36,37). However, the reimbursement system leads to distortions such as cost shifting, in which the hospital raises charges above those that would accurately reflect costs so that payers with more generous reimbursement schedules are, in effect, subsidizing less generous payers as well as patients whose care is uncompensated. Thus, hospital charges will probably overestimate the actual costs of resources consumed (38,39). Similarly, cost shifting may occur within the hospital when some services are reimbursed at a higher rate (percentage of time cost) than others.

Recognizing the limitations of using charges as a surrogate for costs, Haley (25) offered several methods to overcome the problem of this substitution. One approach involves adjusting charges by the overall hospital cost-to-charge ratio to get an improved surrogate measure for costs. A modification would be to determine the cost-to-charge ratio for each service department and then sum all subtotals for each department in which the patient received services. This eliminates the distortion in costs introduced by cost shifting between departments. Another approach would be to use micro-costing or cost accounting data, which are usually available from hospital expenditure reports or hospital accounting departments. These costs are the actual hospital expenditures on all resources hospitals consume in order to provide health services (e.g., see Stone et al. and Roberts et al.) (40,41). Of the various approaches, micro-costing provides the most accurate direct measure of costs and, although difficult to obtain, would most likely prove to be more credible to administrators interested in the study results (30).

When choosing between methods, it is important to consider the issue of statistical power. Medical cost data are highly skewed, and standard deviations are typically large relative to the mean. The implication is that studies with small- to medium-sized samples will be underpowered (i.e., they will fail to reject the null hypothesis that costs are equal between groups even when they are not). Indeed, most of the studies reviewed below lack statistical power, and thus findings of no difference in costs (in attributable cost studies of either susceptible infections or resistant infections) must be viewed with caution.

Micro-costing methods in which costs are imputed to units of service will tend to reduce the measured variance of costs. Although ordinarily this would be viewed as a drawback, sounder conclusions about the implications of resistance for resource use may be reached by counting intermediate measures of resource use, such as utilization or imputed costs, than by examining medical costs directly.

Overview of Studies on Economic Impact of Resistant Infections in Hospitals

The perspective having been determined, the key considerations from economic theory for conducting cost studies of resistant infections are that (i) prices are ordinal and are used to rank whether different states (or bundles of consumption) result in a higher level of economic well-being, (ii) measures of hospital costs should reflect the opportunity costs of resources used in hospital services, and (iii) noninfected patients selected to be controls must be as ill as infected patients in order to address the potential confounding of the severity of the underlying disease. Without comparable controls, the economic resources consumed will always be different between the two groups. Table 3 summarizes recent studies (papers and abstracts that report results in U.S. dollars) examining the hospital costs associated with resistant pathogens. The study results are evaluated for the cost comparisons between groups of patients (providing information to assess the opportunity costs of hospital resources across the various infection states of no infection, susceptible infection, and resistant infection), the variables used to control for the confounding associated with SOI, and the surrogates used to measure opportunity costs.

The evidence from the selected studies presents a varied picture as to the magnitude of the attributable cost of resistant nosocomial infections, the use of SOI measures, and the surrogates used for patient costs. With the exception of the studies by Rubin et al. (42) and Engemann et al. (43), most of the studies do not compare the costs across patients in the possible infection states: those without infection to those with a susceptible infection to those with a resistant infection. Rubin et al. (42) suggested that methicillin-sensitive *S. aureus* (MSSA) infection results in a 2.08-fold ($27,700), or a 108% increase, in the direct medical costs in nonobstetrical patients as compared with these costs in noninfected nonobstetrical patients. MRSA infection increased costs by 137% of the average cost for treating noninfected patients ($13,263). The increase in average costs when comparing MSSA-infected patients ($27,700) to MRSA-infected patients ($31,400) was approximately 13%. In the Engemann paper (43), separate cost comparisons were made of noninfected surgical patients with both surgical patients acquiring MSSA and surgical patients acquiring MRSA. Although relative costs were not reported in the paper, these can be calculated for both the mean and median cost estimates based on the data presented in the paper. The presence of MSSA resulted in a 79% increase over unadjusted median cost and a 113% increase over unadjusted mean cost of treating noninfected surgical patients. MRSA-infected patients had a 214% increase over median cost and a 244% increase over mean cost. MRSA surgical site infections were 75% greater in median costs and 62% greater in mean costs when compared

Table 3 Studies on the Direct Medical Costs of Resistant Nosocomial

Study (ref. no.)	Design (n)	Study setting	Type of (resistant) infection	Site of infection	Total noninfected patient costs	Measure of cost for sensitive infections
Rubin et al., 1999 (42)	Retrospective cohort and modeling (1,351,362, including 6,300 NIs)	All New York state nonobstetrical discharges	Noninfected vs. MSSA; noninfected vs. MRSA	Pneumonia, bacteremia, endocarditis, SSI, osteomyelitis, septic arthritis	$13,263 (mean)	$27,700 (mean total costs)
Chaix et al., 1999 (44)	Matched retrospective case-control; modeling† (54)	ICU in French hospital	MRSA	Bacteremia, catheter-related, lower respiratory tract, UTI	$20,950 (mean)	NA
Abramson and Sexton, 1999 (46)	Prospective nested case-control study† (38)	U.S. university tertiary-care hospital	MSSA vs. MRSA	Primary BSI	NR	$9,661 (median attributable cost)
Welch et al., 1999 (47)	Retrospective case-control; matched (296)	U.S.; multicenter hospitals	MSSA vs. MRSA	All patients with MRSA or MSSA bacteremia	NA	$19,487 (total MSSA patient cost)
Reed et al., 2003 (48)	Prospectively identified cohort (92)	U.S teaching tertiary-care hospital	MRSA vs. MSSA	Bacteremia in ESRD patients	NA	$13,706 (mean total cost)
Engemann et al., 2003 (43)	Prospective cohort; retrospective cost data, modeling (479)	U.S. teaching tertiary-care hospital	Noninfected vs. MSSA; noninfected vs. MRSA	SSIs	$29,455 (median) $34,395 (mean)	$23,336 (unadjusted median attributable cost)* $38,770 (unadjusted mean attributable cost)*
Carmeli et al., 1999 (52)	Modeling and matched cohort analysis (489)	U.S. teaching tertiary-care hospital	Resistant *P. aeruginosa*	BSI, respiratory tract, UTI, wound, soft tissue	NR	NA
McKinnon et al., 2000 (49)	Matched case-control (72)	U.S. hospital level-1 trauma center	VREF vs. VSEF	Urinary, skin, IV catheter, intra-abdominal	NA	$16,692 (mean total VSEF patient cost)
Linden et al., 1998 (50)	Case-control; matched (34)	U.S. teaching tertiary-care hospital	VREF vs. VSEF	Bacteremia in liver transplant patients	NA	$91,833 (mean total VSEF patient cost)
Roughmann et al., 2000 (45)	Retrospective cohort (190)	U.S. hospital adult ICU unit	MSSA vs. MRSA; VSE vs. VRE	BSIs	NA	$25,888 (mean total cost) $34,469 (mean total cost)
Song et al., 2003 (51)	Retrospective matched cohort (277)	U.S. teaching tertiary-care hospital	VRE	VRE bacteremia	$46,699 (mean)	NA
Cosgrove et al., 2002 (53)	Nested matched cohort (477)	U.S. teaching tertiary-care hospital	Sensitive vs. resistant cephalosporin *Enterobacter*	BSI, respiratory tract, UTI, wound, effusion	NA	$57,606 (mean total cost)

* Increases in relative costs are estimated when not directly reported. Relative costs are based on crude cost comparisons of infection states using the following formulas:
Increase in relative cost of patients with sensitive infection over costs for noninfected patients cost = total patient cost of sensitive infections/total cost of noninfected patients
Increase in relative cost of patients with resistant infection over costs for noninfected patients cost = total patient costs of resistant infection/total patient costs of noninfected patient
Increase in relative cost of patients with resistant infection over costs for patients with sensitive infection = total patient cost with resistant infections/total patient costs with sensitive infections
† Authors report as case-control studies when the design is actually a matched retrospective cohort study.
‡ Estimate was reported but was not found to be significant in statistical analysis.
APACHE II, Acute Physiology, Age, Chronic Health Evaluation; APR-DRG, All Patient Refined Diagnosis Related Group; BSI, bloodstream infection; DRG, Diagnosis Related Group;
ESRD, hemodialysis-dependent end-stage renal disease; ICD-9, International Classification of Disease, version 9; ICU, intensive care unit; IV, intravenous;
MRSA, methicillin-resistant *Staphylococcus aureus*; MSSA, methicillin-sensitive *S. aureus*; NA, not measured in study; NIs, nosocomial infections; NR, estimate measured but not reported;
SAPS II, Simplified Acute Physiology Score; SOI, severity of illness; SSI, surgical site infection; UTI, urinary tract infection; VRE, vancomycin-resistant enterococci;
VREF, vancomycin-resistant *Enterococcus faecium*; VSE, vancomycin-sensitive enterococci; VSEF, vancomycin-sensitive *Enterococcus faecium*.

Infections

Increase in relative cost of sensitive infections over noninfected patient costs	Measure of cost for resistant infections	Increase in relative cost of resistance over noninfected patient costs	Increase in relative cost of resistance over sensitive infection costs	Cost data	SOI controls
2.08*	$31,400 (mean total cost)	2.37*	1.13*	Hospital charges, Medicare physician fees, wholesale drug prices	None
NA	$9,275 (mean attributable cost)	1.44*	NA	Hospital costs	McCabe-Jackson, SAPS II
NR	$27,083 (median attributable cost)	NR	NR	Hospital costs	Comorbidities, primary and secondary diagnosis
NA	$23,075 (total MRSA patient cost)	NA	1.18*	Hospital charges adjusted to costs	DRG, ICD-9 codes
NA	$22,010 (mean total cost)	NA	1.61*	NR	APACHE II
1.79 (unadjusted median)* 2.13 (unadjusted mean)*	$62,908 (unadjusted median attributable cost)* $84,020 (unadjusted mean attributable cost)*	3.14 (unadjusted median)* 3.44 (unadjusted mean)*	1.75 (unadjusted median)* 1.62 (unadjusted mean)*	Hospital charges	Comorbidities, ICD-9 codes
NA	$7,340 (mean attributable cost)‡	NA	NA	Hospital charges	Charlson, comorbidities
NA	$38,226 (mean total VRE patient cost)	NA	2.29*	NR	APACHE II
NA	$190,728 (mean total VREF patient cost)	NA	2.08*	Hospital charges adjusted to costs	None
NA	$50,440 (mean total cost) $60,798 (mean total cost)	NA	1.95 (MSSA vs. MRSA) 1.76 (VSE vs. VRE)	NR	None
NA	$81,208 (risk-adjusted estimate for total cost)	1.74*	NA	Hospital charges	APR-DRG complexity index
NA	$29,379 (attributable cost above total charges for controls with sensitive infections)	NA	1.51	Hospital charges	McCabe-Jackson

with MSSA infections (adjusted mean costs were 19% greater for MSRA over MSSA).

The remaining papers compared two of the three states of infection using various estimators of attributable cost. Chaix et al. (44) compared ICU patients with MRSA infection to ICU patients with no nosocomial infection, but did not specifically look at patient costs of MSSA. They estimated the mean attributable cost due to resistance to be $9,275 (a 44% increase over costs for similar noninfected control cases). Comparing patients with MRSA bloodstream infections (BSIs) to patients with MSSA infection, Roughman et al. (45) reported an average attributable direct cost of $24,552 (a 95% cost increase) above costs of patients with MSSA infection; Abramson and Sexton (46) reported a median attributable cost of $27,083; Welch et al. (47) reported a mean total patient cost of $23,075 (an 18% increase over total costs for MSSA-infected patients); and Reed et al. (48) reported a mean attributable cost of $22,010 (a 61% increase) over costs for hemodialysis-dependent end-stage renal disease (ESRD) MSSA-infected patients.

Patients infected with vancomycin-resistant *Enterococcus faecium* (VREF) had a mean total patient cost of $38,226 (a 129% increase in cost over vancomycin-sensitive *E. faecium* [VSEF] patients); for liver transplant patients, total patient cost for those with VREF infection was $190,728 (a 108% increase over the cost of VSEF cases) (49,50). For studies examining VRE, Song et al. (51) found that the costs for patients with VRE bacteremia were 66% higher than those for noninfected patients, while Roughman et al. (45) found that VRE resulted in a 76% increase in costs over those for vancomycin-sensitive enterococci (VSE) (51,45). Finally, resistant *P. aeruginosa* infections caused $7,340 in attributable cost compared with noninfected patients, and cephalosporin-resistant *Enterobacter* caused an excess cost of $29,379 (a 51% increase) compared with costs for patients with susceptible infections (52,53).

As presented above, the published evidence in recent years has offered little improvement on the relative cost estimates developed by Holmberg et al. (12) and used by the OTA (11) for antimicrobial-susceptible versus resistant infections. Based on the studies reviewed, the relative direct medical cost (i) doubles (100% increase) between noninfected patients and MSSA-infected patients, (ii) increases by 16% between MSSA- and MRSA-infected patients (a much smaller impact than the 100% increase estimated by Holmberg et al.), and (iii) increases 44% to 140% between noninfected patients and patients infected with a resistant pathogen. With the exception of the study by Rubin et al. (42), these studies were conducted at a single center, so the results could be influenced by a variety of localized patient management practices, particularly the transfer of infected patients between acute care hospitals and long-term care facilities and empiric therapy regimens (14). In hospitals where drugs active against resistant strains are used as empiric therapy, the cost differential for treating patients infected with resistant strains compared with patients infected with susceptible strains may be less.

Making inferences at the regional or national level based on single-center institutions is probably inappropriate. Much larger regional studies are needed to control for differences in hospital practices. Single-center studies should provide detailed information on antibiotic regimens to facilitate comparisons.

As shown in Table 3, several different types of SOI measures have been used to control for confounding in economic studies of the cost of resistant infections. Among these measures are the APACHE II, Simplified Acute Physiology Score (SAPS) II, Charlson, and McCabe-Jackson scores and the All Patient Refined Diagnosis Related Group (APR-DRG), as well as simply counting the number of comorbidities listed as primary and secondary diagnoses (34,35,54–56). The APACHE II and SAPS II are primarily physiologic indexes that were designed to predict death upon admission to an ICU, whereas the Charlson index was developed to predict death in breast cancer patients over 1 year and is based on identifying various comorbidities present in the patient. The McCabe-Jackson score is a subjective measure of the likelihood of mortality, based on observations of an attending physician upon patient admission to the hospital. The APR-DRG complexity index is an extension to DRG codes to reflect patient SOI.

The diversity of measures used in various studies demonstrates there is no consensus regarding which SOI indexes are the most appropriate controls in observational comparison studies of resistant infections. SOI scoring indexes are not good predictors of nosocomial infections in ICU populations (57). As indicated above, many of the standardized SOI indexes (such as the Charlson, APACHE, or SAPS scores) were developed for other uses and have not been evaluated as control measures in studies of resistant infections (58). This is a fruitful area for future research.

There appears to be more agreement regarding the choice of surrogates for opportunity costs of hospital resources. A majority of the studies we reviewed used actual hospital costs or charges adjusted by cost-to-charge ratios, whereas others used unadjusted hospital charges (Table 3). As unadjusted hospital charges may overstate the actual costs of resistant infections, the upward bias in these estimates may be substantial. Published cost-to-charge ratios for the United States range from just over 50% to 80% (59). These ratios are readily available and when cost accounting is not possible, should be used to adjust hospital charges to more accurately reflect the opportunity costs of resistant infections.

Implications for Future Epidemiologic Studies on Attributable Cost of Resistant Infections

Measuring the absolute attributable cost is useful in determining the potential cost savings associated with interventions that reduce resistant infections within a given hospital (or other health care) setting. In addition, it is important to measure the relative costs of nosocomial infections, both susceptible and resistant infections, because they indicate the magnitude of the social costs (in terms of hospital resources) resulting from these infections. Comparison studies are needed to evaluate the cost differences between the three states of infection status for the specific study population. The attributable costs of the different infection states should be examined within the same research study, in which the matching criteria, control variables (such as SOI indexes), and cost measures are internally consistent. Within this framework, hypothesis tests on the significance of the attributable cost differences can be made, the existence of the attributable cost differences can be verified, and the relative costs of the infection states can be estimated. By estimating relative costs, the estimates that come from various single institution studies can be used to make inferences about the cost impact, both regionally and nationally, of resistant infections (such as updating the OTA estimate).

Similarly, the use of various SOI indexes should be evaluated to determine if attributable cost study results are sensitive to the severity measures used as either matching criteria or controls in multivariate models. As noted earlier, clinical SOI indexes have not been good predictors of nosocomial infection risk; a simple tally of the number of comorbidities present appears to be more reliably predictive (60). The lack of predictive value may undermine the use of SOI indexes in controlling for confounding in economic studies of resistant infections. However, a recent study has shown that the APACHE III index is correlated with cost (61). In models with patient cost as a dependent variable, this index was used to control for the increased costs associated with the baseline underlying disease, independent of the occurrence of infection. More studies are needed to understand how SOI indexes can be used in both cost and disease models so that they can be compared and examined for disparities (if any) they may have on cost study results.

The advent of electronic surveillance to help curb the incidence of resistant infection can potentially influence how comparison studies of resistant infections are done. As electronic medical records become more common, studies of resistant nosocomial infections will be much cheaper (in terms of research and data collection costs) to conduct. This will allow the use of larger data sets which could greatly increase the robustness of these analyses (over studies with smaller sample sizes, as noted earlier) and address the same variability in relative (and nominal) costs. SOI indexes which can more easily be constructed from electronic patient data may prove to be the best measures to use in future comparison studies.

Further Considerations

Can comparative studies be successfully expanded to make comparisons of results for the three infection states? There are other measurement issues to be addressed in comparison studies. A workshop held at Emory University on methodologic issues concerning cost measurement of resistant infections in hospitals (30) resulted in a number of recommendations for such studies, including:

1. Increase study populations by using multicenter studies, because the lack of statistical power in single-center studies with small sample sizes limits the use of statistical controls for SOI as well as the ability to make generalizations to larger populations.
2. Develop standardized definitions of resistance, because several microorganisms of clinical importance lack well-defined criteria to be categorized as resistant.
3. Assess costs of infection longitudinally, as attributable costs may still accrue after the patient is discharged.

Although comparison studies can measure the attributable costs of resistant infections, the reporting of results needs to be consistent and complete (filling in the missing economic information, as identified in Table 3). The difficulty in conducting these studies (and the associated research cost) increases when the three states of infection are to be compared and matched. Because many comparison studies employ the strategy of matching, many patients who do not fit the matching criteria are excluded from the study population. A matching strategy may be appropriate in developing measures of relative risk of infection; however, such a strategy may exclude patients who have excess costs that should be measured, particularly if an intervention is hospital-wide.

In order to develop cost estimates to be used to evaluate a hospital-wide intervention to reduce resistant infections, an alternative analytic approach to concurrent and comparison studies was employed by Roberts et al. [61]. This pilot study measured the attributable costs of nosocomial infections in a random sample of adult medical patients hospitalized in a large urban teaching hospital. The patients in this study were grouped into three categories: no infection (n = 139); confirmed infection (n = 17), based on the National Nosocomial Infection Surveillance (NNIS) definitions (modified for use to retrospectively identify infections); and suspected infection (n = 8), representing patients who met some but not all of the NNIS definitions. Confounding effects of underlying disease were controlled using APACHE III scores and ICU admission in a linear regression model. Estimates from the model showed that the attributable cost due to confirmed nosocomial infection was approximately $15,000 and the excess cost for suspected infection was approximately $6,800 (excess costs due to resistant infections could not be measured in this pilot study because of an inadequate number of patients with resistant infections). This strategy is currently being used in a larger study at the same hospital that will capture a sufficient number of patients to measure costs due to resistant infections.

Another area of future research is the measurement of costs related to the increasing use of alternative antimicrobials for empiric therapy (1,62,63). Patients will often be given empiric therapy before an infecting organism has been identified; as the prevalence of resistant infection increases in a given hospital or geographic area, physicians are more likely to use alternative drugs that are often more costly than those that would have been used if resistance were absent or less prevalent. These excess costs, which include any side effects or complications that may result from the alternative treatment, have rarely been measured but potentially could exceed the costs of treatment failure (1). Although these costs may not be relevant from the perspective of the hospital (although they are relevant from a third-party payer and social perspective), economic models of hospital costs can be more readily adapted (than can comparison studies) to measure this component of costs (if patients who were not in need of alternative therapy can be identified).

Another important measurement issue in attributable cost studies of resistant infections is the endogenous relationship between hospital length of stay and the risk of acquiring a nosocomial infection (64). Patients experiencing longer hospital stays (and thus patients with higher hospital costs) have a greater chance of acquiring a nosocomial infection; conversely, patients acquiring a nosocomial infection tend to have longer hospital stays (and therefore have higher hospital costs). This implies that an endogenous problem exists between costs and infection. A two-stage modeling process that includes a model of the probability of acquiring infection (stage 1) and a model of patient costs (stage 2) can test the statistical significance of this endogenous relationship and correct the model estimates to account for this bias.

CONCLUSIONS

Recent studies of the attributable cost of resistant nosocomial infections from the hospital perspective have indicated that hospitals can realize cost savings by reducing the incidence of resistant nosocomial infections. The attributable cost studies published in the medical literature are mostly comparative (i.e., cohort) observational studies in which cost (as opposed to disease) becomes the outcome variable. The economic evidence presented in these studies (Table 3) tends to ignore the relative costs of the various states of infection and to make comparisons of just two of the three possible states of infection (no infection vs. resistant infection, or susceptible vs. resistant infection), rarely comparing all three. The limited evidence indicates that MRSA infections tend to increase costs anywhere from 44% to 244%. The wide disparity in estimates may be partly the result of the differing research strategies regarding the use of SOI measures as controls, the type of information used to represent patient hospital costs, and the site of infection (e.g., surgical, bloodstream). Although reporting the absolute dollar costs associated with resistance is important for conducting a cost-effectiveness or cost–benefit analysis of a particular intervention, reporting the cost differences as relative proportions between different infections will provide the evidence that can be used to estimate the economic burden of disease from the hospital perspective.

Comparative studies face challenges in controlling the confounding influence of the severity of the underlying disease and finding appropriate measures to represent opportunity cost of resources. More research is needed to evaluate various SOI measures that have been used in studies as controls to see if attributable cost estimates are sensitive to the measures used. Opportunity costs of hospital resources are best reflected in the micro-costing data of hospital expenditures, but such data are difficult to collect. At a minimum, when hospital charges are used as surrogates for opportunity cost, they must be adjusted by cost-to-charge ratios to remove the upward bias present in charges that are the result of cost shifting. Implementing the above recommendations can improve the quality of economic information from comparative studies but places additional informational burdens on such studies in terms of study populations (three comparison groups as opposed to two), matching of various cohort participants, and study costs.

REFERENCES

1. Howard DH, Scott RD, Packard R, Jones D. The global impact of drug resistance Clin Infect Dis 2003; 36(Suppl 1):S4–S10.

2. Jones D. To Err Is Human: Building a Safer Health System. Washington, DC: National Academy Press, 2000.

3. Jones D. Antimicrobial Drug Resistance: Issues and Options. Workshop Report. Washington, DC: National Academy Press, 1998.

4. Phelps DE. Bug/drug resistance Med Care 1989; 27:194–203.

5. Nord E, Pinto JL, Richardson J, Menzel P, Ubel P. Incorporating societal concerns for fairness in numerical valuations of health programmes Health Econ 1999; 8:25–39.

6. Williams A. Intergenerational equity Health Econ 1997; 6: 117–132.

7. Scott RD, Solomon SL, McGowan JE. Applying economic principles to health care Emerg Infect Dis 2001; 7:282–285.

8. Mankiw NG. Principles of Economics. Orlando, FL: The Dryden Press, 1998.

9. Varian HR. Microeconomic Analysis. New York: WW Norton, 1984.

10. Gould JP, Ferguson CE. Microeconomic Theory. Homewood, IL: Richard D. Irwin, Inc., 1980.

11. Ferguson CE. Impacts of Antibiotic Resistant Bacteria. OTA-H-629. Washington, DC: U.S. Government Printing Office, 1995.

12. Holmberg SD, Solomon SL, Blake PA. Health and economic impacts of antimicrobial resistance Rev Infect Dis 1987; 9: 1065–1078.

13. Farnham PG, Haddix AC. Study design. In: Haddix AC, Teutsch SM, Shaffer PA, Dunet DO, Eds Prevention Effectiveness: A Guide to Decision Analysis and Economic Evaluation. 2d edition. New York: Oxford University Press, 2003; 11–27.

14. McGowan JE. Economic impact of antimicrobial resistance Emerg Infect Dis 2001; 7:286–292.

15. McGowan JE. Antimicrobial resistance in hospital organisms and its relation to antibiotic use Rev Infect Dis 1983; 5: 1033–1048.

16. Tisdell C. Exploitation of techniques that decline in effectiveness Public Finance 1982; 3:428–437.

17. Coast J, Smith RD, Millar MR. Superbugs: should antimicrobial resistance be included as a cost in economic evaluation? Health Econ 1996; 5:217–226.

18. Hardin G. The tragedy of the commons Science 1968; 162: 1243–1247.

19. Gordon HS. Economic theory of a common property resource: the fishery J Political Econ 1954; 62:124–142.

20. Shlaes DM, Gerding DN, John JF Jr, Craig WA, Bornstein DL, Duncan RA, Eckman MR, Farrer WE, Greene WH, Lorian V, Levy S, McGowan JE Jr, Paul SM, Ruskin J, Tenover FC, Watanakunakorn C. Society for Healthcare Epidemiology of America and Infectious Diseases Society of America Joint Committee on the Prevention of Antimicrobial Resistance: guidelines for the prevention of antimicrobial resistance in hospitals Clin Infect Dis 1997; 25:584–599.

21. Zanetti G, Platt R. Cost-effectiveness of vancomycin use versus cefazolin for perioperative antibiotic prophylaxis in coronary artery bypass graft surgery [abstr] Am J Infect Control; 2000; 28:79.

22. Gorsky RD, Haddix AC, Schaffer PA. Cost of an intervention. In: Haddix AC, Teutsch SM, Shaffer PA, Dunet DO, Eds Pre-

vention Effectiveness: A Guide to Decision Analysis and Economic Evaluation.. New York: Oxford University Press, 1996; 57–75.

23. Haley RW, Culver DH, White JW, Morgan WM, Emori TG, Munn VP, Hooton TM. The efficacy of infection surveillance and control programs in preventing nosocomial infections in US hospitals Am J Epidemiol 1985; 121:182–205.

24. Lilienfeld DE, Stolly PD. Foundations of Epidemiology. 3d ed. New York: Oxford University Press, 1994.

25. Haley RW. Measuring the costs of nosocomial infections; methods for estimating economic burden on the hospital Am J Med 1991; 91(suppl 3B):32S–38S.

26. Wakefield DS, Pfaller MA, Hammons GT, Massanari RM. Use of the appropriateness evaluation protocol for estimating the incremental cost associated with nosocomial infections Med Care 1987; 25:481–488.

27. Haley RW, Schaberg DR, Von Allmen SD, McGowan JE. Estimating the extra charges and prolongation of hospitalization due to nosocomial infections: a comparison of methods J Infect Dis 1980; 141:248–257.

28. Freeman J, McGowan JE Jr. Methological issues in hospital epidemiology: III. investigating the modifying effects of time and severity of underlying illness on estimates of cost of nosocomial infection Rev Infect Dis 1984; 6:285–300.

29. Rello J. Impact of nosocomial infections on outcomes: myths and evidence Infect Control Hosp Epidemiol 1999; 20:392–394.

30. Howard D, Cordell R, McGowan JE, Packard RM, Scott RD 2d, Solomon SL;, Solomon SL. Measuring the economics of antimicrobial resistance in hospital settings: summary of the Centers for Disease Control and Prevention–Emory Workshop Clin Infect Dis 2001; 33:1573–1578.

31. Gross PA, DeMauro PJ, Van Antwerpen C, Wallenstein S, Chiang S. Number of co-morbidities as a predictor of nosocomial infection acquisition Infect Control Hosp Epidemiol 1988; 9: 497–500.

32. Harris AD, Karchmer TB, Carmeli Y, Samore MH. Methodological principles of case-control studies that analyzed risk factors

for antibiotic resistance: a systematic review Clin Infect Dis 2001; 32:1055–1061.

33. Knaus WA, Wagner DP, Draper EA, Zimmerman JE, Bergner M, Bastos PG, Sirio CA, Murphy DJ, Lotring T, Damiano A. The APACHE III prognostic system: risk prediction of hospital mortality for critically ill hospitalized adults Chest 1991; 100: 1619–1636.

34. Charleson ME, Pompei P, Ales KL, MacKenzie CR. A new method of classifying prognostic comorbidity in longitudinal studies: development and validation J Chronic Dis 1987; 40: 373–383.

35. McCabe WR, Jackson GG. Gram-negative bacteremia. I. Etiology and ecology Arch Intern Med 1962; 110:847–853.

36. Finkler SA. The distinction between cost and charges Ann Intern Med 1982; 96:102–109.

37. Haddix AC, Schaffer PA. Cost-effectiveness analysis. In: Haddix AC, Teutsch SM, Shaffer PA, Dunet DO, Eds Prevention Effectiveness: A Guide to Decision Analysis and Economic Evaluation. New York: Oxford University Press, 1996; 103–129.

38. Dranove D. Pricing by non-profit institutions: the case of hospital cost shifting J Health Econ 1988; 7:47–57.

39. Dor A, Farley DE. Payment source and the cost of hospital care: evidence from a multiproduct cost function with multiple payers J Health Econ 1996; 15:1–21.

40. Stone PW, Gupta A, Loughrey M, Della-Latta P, Cimiotti J, Larson E, Rubenstein D, Saiman L. Attributable costs and length of stay of an extended-spectrum beta-lactamase-producing *Klebsiella pneumoniae* outbreak in a neonatal intensive care unit Infect Control Hosp Epidemiol 2003; 24:601–606.

41. Roberts RR, Frutos PW, Ciavarella GG, Gussow LM, Mensah EK, Kampe LM, Straus HE, Joseph G, Rydman RJ. Distribution of variable vs fixed costs of hospital care JAMA 1999; 281: 644–649.

42. Rubin RJ, Harrington CA, Poon A, Dietrich K, Greene JA, Moiduddin A. The economic impact of *Staphylococcus aureus* Infection in New York hospitals Emerg Infect Dis 1999; 5:9–17.

43. Engemann JJ, Carmeli Y, Cosgrove SE, Fowler VG, Bronstein MZ, Trivette SL, Briggs JP, Sexton DJ, Kaye KS. Adverse clinical and economic Outcomes attributable to methicillin resistance among patients with *Staphylococcus aureus* surgical site infection Clin Infect Dis 2003; 36:592–598.

44. Chaix C, Durand-Zaleski I, Alberti C, Brun-Buisson C. Control of endemic methicillin-resistant *Staphylococcus aureus*: a cost-benefit analysis in an intensive care unit JAMA 1999; 282: 1745–1751.

45. Roughmann M, Bradham D, South B, Fridkin S, Perl T. The clinical and economic impact of antimicrobial drug resistance on nosocomial bloodstream infections [abstr] Infect Control Hosp Epidemiol 2000; 21:97.

46. Abramson MA, Sexton JS. Nosocomial methicillin-resistant and methicillin-susceptible *Staphylococcus aureus* primary bacteremia: at what costs Infect Control Hosp Epidemiol 1999; 20:408–411.

47. Welch KE, Goff DA, Fish N, Sierawski SJ, Paladino JA. A multicenter economic analysis of bacteremia caused by methicillin-resistant *Staphylococcus aureus* [abstr], 39th International Conference of Antimicrobial Agents and Chemotherapy, San Francisco, Sept 26–29, 1999.

48. Reed SD, Szczech LA, Kaye KS, Friedman JY, Engeman JJ, Stryjewski ME, Griffiths RI, Reiler LB, Corey GR, Fowler VG. Methicillin-resistant *Staphylococcus aureus* leads to higher inpatient costs, longer hospital stays, and higher mortality in end–stage renal disease patients on hemodialysis [abstr], 43rd International Conference of Antimicrobial Agents and Chemotherapy, Chicago, Sept 14–17, 2003.

49. McKinnon PS, Tam VH, Kwa AL, Rybak MJ. An economic analysis of bacteremia caused by vancomycin resistant *Enterococcus* in patients admitted to a level-1 trauma center [abstr], 40th International Conference of Antimicrobial Agents and Chemotherapy, Chicago, Sept 17–20, 2000.

50. Linden P, Paladino J, Saul M, Stoffer D. The economic impact of bacteremia due to vancomycin-resistant *Enterococcus faecium*: a case control study [abstr], 38th International Conference of Antimicrobial Agents and Chemotherapy, San Diego, CA, Sept 24–27, 1998.

51. Song X, Srinivasan A, Perl T. Effect of nosocomial vancomycin-resistant enterococcal bacteremia on mortality, length of stay, and costs Infect Control Hosp Epidemiol 2003; 24:251–256.

52. Carmeli Y, Troillet N, Karchmer AW, Samore MH. Health and economic outcomes of antibiotic resistance in *Pseudomonas aeruginosa* Arch Intern Med 1999; 159:1127–1132.

53. Cosgrove SE, Kaye KS, Eliopoulous GM, Carmeli Y. Health and economic outcomes of the emergence of third-generation cephalosporin resistance in *Enterobacter* species Arch Intern Med 2002; 162:185–190.

54. Knaus WA, Draper EA, Wagner DP, Zimmerman JE. The APACHE II: a severity of disease classification system Crit Care Med 1985; 13:818–829.

55. Le Gall JR, Lemeshow S, Saulnier F. A new Simplified Acute Physiology Score (SAPS II) based on a European/North American multicenter study JAMA 1993; 270:2957–2963.

56. Saulnier F. All Patient Refined-Diagnosis Related Groups Definitions Manual. Version 15.0. St. Paul. MN: 3M Health Information Systems, 1998.

57. Keita-Perse O, Gaynes RP. Severity of illness scoring systems to adjust nosocomial infection rates: a review and commentary Am J Infect Control 1996; 24:429–434.

58. Harris AD, Karchmer TB, Carmeli Y, Samore MB. Methodological principles of case-control studies that analyze risk factors for antibiotic resistance: a systematic review Clin Inf Dis 2001; 32:1055–1061.

59. Haddix AC, Teutsch SM, Shaffer PA. Prevention Effectiveness: A Guide to Decision Analysis and Economic Evaluation. 2d ed. New York: Oxford University Press, 2003.

60. Gross PA, Stein MR, van Antwerpen C, DeMauro PJ, Boscamp JR, Hess W, Wallenstein S. Comparison of severity of illness indicators in an intensive care unit Arch Intern Med 1991; 151: 2201–2205.

61. Roberts RR, Scott RD, Cordell R, Solomon SL, Steele L, Kampe LM, Trick WE, Weinstein RA. The use of economic modeling to determine the hospital costs associated with nosocomial infections Clin Infect Dis 2003; 36:1424–1432.

62. Howard DH, Rask KJ. The impact of resistance on antibiotic demand in patients with ear infections. In: Laxminarayan R, Brown G, Eds Battling Resistance to Antibiotics and Pesticides: An Economic Approach. Washington. DC: Resources for the Future, 2003.

63. Phillips M, Phillips-Howard P. Economic implications of resistance to antimalaria drugs Pharmacoeconomics 1996; 10: 225–238.

64. Graves N, Weinhold D, Roberts JA. Correcting for bias when estimating the cost of hospital acquired infections; an analysis of lower respiratory tract infections in non-surgical patients. Unpublished paper, June 2002.

8

Optimizing Antimicrobial Use and Combating Bacterial Resistance: Benchmarking and Beyond

SUJATA M. BHAVNANI and PAUL G. AMBROSE
School of Pharmacy and Pharmaceutical
Sciences, University at Buffalo, and
Cognigen Corporation,
Buffalo, New York, U.S.A.

The term *benchmarking* refers to a continuous process of measuring the products, services, or practices of an institution against those of its peer groups or leaders in the field (external benchmarking), or against its own past performance (internal benchmarking). In a data-driven manner and through a recurring review process, target goals are established, periodically assessed, and, if necessary, modified. Benchmarking requires a commitment to the assiduous collection of data, the critical evaluation of past performance, and the use of such data to increasingly enhance performance.

The process of benchmarking, though a relatively recent innovation in the health care setting, originally stemmed from the principles cited by Deming (1) through his use of continuous quality improvement in the automobile manufacturing industry in Japan. Benchmarking was imported to the United States in the early 1980s by the Xerox Corporation to institute a process whereby best practices could be identified, adopted, and optimized to achieve the highest-quality product while expending the least possible resources.

Benchmarking in institutional settings such as hospitals, long-term care facilities, and even in the outpatient setting, has proven to be of value in identifying potential problem areas in health care delivery and in aiding the establishment of appropriate and attainable target goals (2–5). Increasingly, there are reports in the literature of institutions and groups using national data sources to compare standards of practice and patient outcomes, including the identification and monitoring of infection rates. For example, Woomer et al. (2), in an effort to compare rates of urinary tract infections in home care, described a collaborative approach in which six home care agencies developed standards to define and monitor urinary tract infections. Narong et al. (3), using data from the National Nosocomial Infection Surveillance (NNIS) System as a reference, benchmarked rates of surgical site infections in patients undergoing major operations in a university hospital setting.

Benchmarking has also been used to reveal the positive impact of a change in practice. For example, Bissell (6) described the experience of the Latter Day Saints Hospital in Salt Lake City. Through the use of internal and retrospective data, the beneficial impact on patient outcomes of computerized decision-support based on laboratory and clinical data was demonstrated. Similarly, after collecting and benchmarking data on vancomycin use and the prevalence of vancomycin-resistant enterococci (VRE) in 50 intensive care units (ICUs) among 20 U.S. NNIS hospitals participating in Project Intensive Care Antimicrobial Resistance Epidemiology (Project ICARE), Fridkin et al. (7) assessed whether such comparative information led to quality improvement. These authors reported that specific and targeted changes in practices were associated with both decreases in vancomycin use and prevalence of VRE in the ICU.

Benchmarking has the potential to be an invaluable means to pursue continuous quality improvement in the health care setting. In the last few years, the benefits of benchmarking have been increasingly recognized, and the practice of benchmarking has become important to the hospital accreditation process. This chapter serves as a general introduction to the concept of benchmarking, with a focus on the institutional benchmarking of antimicrobial use and bacterial resistance.

RATIONALE FOR BENCHMARKING ANTIMICROBIAL USE AND BACTERIAL RESISTANCE

The goal of benchmarking in the health care setting is simple: achieving the best health care delivery possible within the constraints of available resources. However, the task of effectively balancing health-based decisions with cost-driven considerations is challenging. For example, every year there is a constant onslaught of new and often costly advancements in technology, treatment modalities, and related health care delivery systems that promise improved patient care. Without a set of criteria by which both the health-related and economic impacts of new treatments and devices may be measured, institutions are ill-equipped to make informed decisions as to which technologies or treatment modalities should be incorporated into their patient care arsenal.

By participating in a benchmarking effort with a group of similar institutions, a hospital or nursing home can benefit from the experiences of other equivalent institutions, thereby avoiding the necessity to continually reinvent the wheel. Similar complex issues arise when making formulary decisions; for example, selecting the most cost-effective formulary does not merely equate to choosing the least expensive drugs. In the case of antibiotics and the treatment of bacterial infections, for example, the cost of the antimicrobial agents themselves must be weighed against a number of factors, including time to infection resolution, length of hospital stay, and rate of infection recurrence and the potential for resistance selection.

There are many compelling reasons to monitor and benchmark the use of antimicrobial agents. Institutional antimicrobial use typically represents 20% of all annual drug expenditures (8). Given this level of spending, even a modest improvement in prescribing has the potential to make a significant impact. However, though important, cost is not the only reason to control antimicrobial usage; the association between increased use of antimicrobial agents and decreased susceptibility of bacteria, which has been well documented in the literature, is increasingly even more alarming (9,10). Historically, however, such reports have typically described hospital formulary practices and associated microbiologic observations within single institutions (11,12). Reports of relationships between usage and susceptibility patterns across groups of institutions, which are more compelling, are less frequent (8,13–16). The association between increasing antimicrobial use and bacterial resistance has been more apparent for microorganisms for which selection is the mechanism of resistance, including *Enterobacter* spp, *Streptococcus pneumoniae*, *Pseudomonas aeruginosa*, and *Escherichia coli*. Stemming the development of resistance in these organisms through sound antimicrobial management is an important and realistic goal. Microorganisms such as methicillin-resistant *Staphylococcus aureus*, for which the current widespread and high rates of resistance are largely the result of clonal spread, fall more under the purview of infection control. Although infection control practices can be, and have been, effectively benchmarked, they are not our present focus.

As demonstrated in a number of reports, changes in antimicrobial management programs have been associated with restoration of bacterial susceptibilities for certain microorganisms. A study performed by Rice et al. (17) demonstrated that a decrease in ceftazidime use and concurrent increase in piperacillin/tazobactam use was associated with a decrease in ceftazidime-resistant *Klebsiella pneumoniae* but without a concurrent increase in piperacillin/tazobactam-resistant strains. A study conducted in a New York hospital also demonstrated a decrease in the prevalence of extended-spectrum beta-lactamase-producing *K. pneumoniae* following a shift in antibiotic use from cephalosporins to other agents. An 80% reduction in hospital-wide cephalosporin use correlated with a 44% reduction in ceftazidime-resistant *K. pneumoniae* infection and colonization throughout the hospital ($p < 0.01$), a 71% reduction in all ICUs ($p < 0.001$), and an 88% reduction in the surgical ICU ($p < 0.001$). However, the resulting increase in use of imipenem/cilastatin in this same institution was associated with an increased incidence of imipenem-resistant *P. aeruginosa* (18). Patterson et al. (19) also reported similar experiences with a decrease in multidrug-resistant *K. pneumoniae* at two university-affiliated hospitals in Texas after a decrease in ceftazidime use. Given the commonly observed association between antimicrobial use and bacterial resistance, programs designed to monitor patterns of use and susceptibility can be used to quickly identify, investigate, and potentially remedy prescribing practices associated with the development of resistance. However, as observed in one of the above examples (18), a simple shift in antimicrobial use may merely being trading one problem for another. Thus, judicious use of antimicrobial agents and adherence to infectious control procedures are as important as formulary choices.

Although it is relatively simple to quantify the cost of antimicrobials, it is more challenging to quantify the economic burden of bacterial resistance. The annual cost associated with antimicrobial resistance in the U.S. was estimated to range from $100 million to $30 billion per year (20). Holmberg et al. (21), after their extensive review of the literature describing the outcomes for both nosocomial and community-acquired bacteria with reduced antibiotic susceptibilities, concluded that infections caused by resistant organisms were associated with substantially worse economic and health outcomes than those caused by susceptible organisms. Thus, the relative economic burden of bacterial resistance is a third compelling reason to monitor and benchmark antimicrobial use and bacterial resistance.

Given that clinical pharmacy antimicrobial management programs have been associated with improvement in certain outcomes (22–24), benchmarking of antimicrobial use and bacterial resistance, as well as factors affecting either of these measures, may also help to quantify the impact of particular services and even staffing levels. Studies documenting this impact may be used to support clinical pharmacy antimicrobial management programs. By obtaining data from other institutions, benchmarking techniques can be used to demonstrate the impact of services not currently offered at an institution. Such data may even provide a sufficiently compelling argument to justify to administrators the need for enhanced support of such clinical programs.

MEASURES TO BENCHMARK

In an ideal situation, an individual wishing to assess the performance of an institution or department would have all relevant data readily available. In an era of continual cost cutting, however, one of the greatest challenges to the benchmarking process is the simple allocation of personnel to collect and collate the required data. Ironically, in order to justify hiring more staff, a department within an institution may need to present administrators with a considerable amount of data, the collection of which is made infeasible because of staff shortages. Therefore, it is important to determine exactly what needs to be optimized within a system, collect only the most salient data, and benchmark the most effective measures.

Drug utilization is a measure that can be easily collected and benchmarked, though there are a number of ways to represent antibiotic use. For analyses conducted in the community setting, the number of treatment courses or prescriptions is a common way to represent gross usage. For analyses in hospital settings, where the volume of antibiotic use is quite high, the defined daily dose (DDD) is a common measure, often advocated over other measures. This measure was developed more than two decades ago as a means to standardize drug utilization data (sales statistics or pharmacy inventory data) into medically meaningful units. As described by agencies such as the World Health Organization or the Centers for Disease

Control and Prevention (CDC) (25), the DDD is derived by dividing the number of grams of a particular agent by the average daily dose. For example, the DDD for cefazolin, which is usually administered 1 g every 8 hours, is 3 g. However, because the DDD for a specific agent represents an average daily maintenance dose for a given indication (26,27) and there are discrepancies between definitions of DDD, one must be cognizant of such variances when comparing results from different studies or collecting data from different institutions. In the United States, definitions of DDD generally follow the recommendations of the CDC.

The total number of grams dispensed over a period of time is another common way to represent antimicrobial use. One obvious advantage of using DDDs rather than total grams as a measure of use is that the DDD allows for a more meaningful comparison of use within and across classes of antibiotics that differ in potency. Another common measure of drug use in the hospital setting is expenditure data that represent dollars of drug purchased. This type of data is limited by the fact that it is really a surrogate for actual use data, does not usually account for wastage, and is dependent on institutional purchasing patterns and fluctuations in pricing structures and discounts. However, because the majority of hospital pharmacy computer systems do not allow for retrospective tracking of number of doses dispensed, annual expenditure data have historically represented the most robust measure of drug use available. In any case, as discussed below, all of the above-described measures of drug use are more similar than dissimilar.

Irrespective of the measure of drug use chosen, it is important to select a denominator by which drug use can be normalized in order to make comparisons across institutions. The denominator is typically a measure of patient density to represent the potential number of patients that could be exposed. A common denominator is "1,000 inpatient days." The total number of hospital beds is also a commonly used denominator, but given that occupancy rates may vary within an institution by year and across hospitals, calculating the total number of occupied beds (OB = total number of beds × average occupancy rate) is preferable. Also, when benchmarking individual hospital data to data from a peer group of hospitals for which the acuity of the patient population varies greatly (e.g., a group of hospitals that are similar in size but not type), adjusting the individual data by the case mix index (CMI) may be prudent. For example, equation 1 could be applied to expenditure data ($/OB) to adjust for CMI:

$$\$/OB/CMI = [(\$/OB)/(\text{individual hospital CMI})] \times \text{median CMI of peer group} \tag{1}$$

For analyses of drug use in a community setting, a measure of the population density (e.g., 100 or 1,000 inhabitants) is commonly used as a denominator.

Although DDD appears to be the most strongly advocated measure of use, the relative merit of one measure over another may be debated. Although some studies have reported discrepancies in correlations between various measures of drug usage and DDDs (28,29), other reports (with larger sample sizes and using data from multiple centers) demonstrate that these measures are more similar than dissimilar. When antimicrobial use data from a European study are examined, one can see a high correlation coefficient (0.81) between DDDs per 1,000 inhabitants and number of prescriptions per 1,000 inhabitants (30,31). Similarly, using data collected from U.S. hospitals, correlation coefficients between fluoroquinolone use expressed as dollars per OB and both grams per OB and DDDs per 1,000 patient days ranged from 0.79 to 0.92 (8).

In the context of the most meaningful measure of use, i.e., the actual exposure in an individual patient, all of the above-described measures of population-based drug use are gross measures and suffer from the same limitations. That is, these measures do not tell us anything about the dosing regimens, the duration of the regimens, and most important, the appropriateness of the regimens in individual patients. Thus, by negating these factors, analyses evaluating associations between such drug use measures and bacterial resistance rates assume that the impact of the unit of measure is the same across patients of all types, organisms of all susceptibilities, infections of all types, and regimens differing by duration. Even DDDs, which are constructed by normalizing total grams by a standard daily dose, negate the impact of variations in dosing regimens that may occur when treating populations that are renally compromised or that have serious infections and normal renal function. In this regard, perhaps too much time is spent debating the merits of the gross measure to use when in fact, as discussed later in the chapter, there are other ways we can optimize these analyses.

Although there are few choices when considering hospital susceptibility measures, nonetheless, they merit consideration. Typically, hospitals summarize, in the form of an antibiogram, hospital-wide and/or unit-specific data showing the number of bacterial isolates tested against various antimicrobial agents during a specific period. For a given group of bacterial isolates, the proportion that was susceptible for all agents tested is reported. Analyses of hospital data examining the relationship between antimicrobial use and bacterial susceptibility have commonly made use of antibiogram data collected from hospitals. Although institutions generally adhere to the same standards for testing and reporting susceptibility results, one needs to be aware of the limitations of pooling such data across hospitals. For example, a group of *E. coli* isolates may come from different infection sites, such as blood or urine. Some institutions may report susceptibility for isolates by specimen type, whereas others may combine the data and report pooled results. Another example might involve the hospital size or occupancy rates. If hospitals in a sample are smaller or have a lower occupancy rate, relatively few isolates may be collected compared with those from larger hospitals over a designated period. Establishing a minimal sample size of isolates for inclusion or weighting by sample size across all observations may be prudent in the effort to minimize the effect of small samples.

In addition to comparing drug use itself, the effectiveness of various activities aimed at reducing inappropriate antibiotic use can also be benchmarked. Such activities might include staffing levels (measured as full-time equivalents) of pharmacists, technicians, clinical pharmacists, and infection control staff; pharmacy department computing resources; programs for switching or intravenous-to-oral (IV-to-PO) streamlining of antimicrobials; how often such programs are instituted; various infection control practices; computer access to microbiology results; and the impact of formulary guidelines.

IDENTIFYING PEER GROUPS AND LEADERS

For the benchmarking process to be valid, a great deal of care is required in selecting appropriate peer groups and in developing criteria for the identification of industry leaders. Benchmarking apples with oranges is both misleading and counterproductive. As a rule, the more data included in the analysis, the more narrowly defined, and therefore meaningful, the peer group comparisons become.

Thus, the selection of hospitals to constitute a peer group depends on the amount and types of specific data collected from each institution. For example, hospitals may be grouped according to their number of beds (e.g. fewer than 400 beds vs. more than 400 beds), the type of institution (e.g. tertiary-care university hospital vs. nonteaching community hospital), geographic region (e.g. Northeast vs. Southwest), formulary practices (e.g. fewer vs. greater antimicrobial choices), or any number of other criteria. Therefore, the ideal benchmarking program would collect a wide variety of data from a large number of hospitals of all sizes, types, and geographic locations. In this way, for example, a nonteaching community hospital in the Northwest region of the country with fewer than 150 beds could compare itself to ten or more similarly categorized hospitals. Nevertheless, as long as the data are approached cautiously, benchmarking efforts may be of considerable value to even small groups of institutions.

In addition to comparisons with peer groups, the benchmarking process allows for identification of, and comparison to, institutions that have proved to be the best performers, or *benchmark institutions* (32). Identifying such benchmark institutions is not always straightforward, and many issues must be considered. As a general guideline, a benchmark institution might be one in which expenditures were within the lowest twenty-fifth to fiftieth percentile of its peer group while quality of patient care was in the upper twenty-fifth percentile.

However, one must not lose sight of the forest for the trees. Tabulating total costs for any particular procedure or treatment course is relatively easy, and thus it is not difficult to determine whether an institution is spending more or less than peer hospitals for a given treatment (e.g., total cost of antibiotics for treatment of community-acquired pneumonia). However, the cost of any single procedure may not be as relevant as the overall cost of patient treatment, which may include a whole host of other expenditures. Cost savings in one arena may be compensated or even exceeded by cost inflations elsewhere, and the possibility of such compensation should be actively investigated.

It is even more difficult to identify factors that clearly indicate quality of patient care. For example, gross measures such as the mortality rate of patients with community-acquired pneumonia can be benchmarked fairly easily. However, the measure of quality, in this case, the mortality rate, takes no account of the acuity of the patient population or the number and severity of their comorbidities; such considerations are surely relevant to treatment success rates. A higher mortality rate may merely indicate that a patient population is sicker, not that there is anything fundamentally lacking in an institution's procedures. In the latter case, normalizing data by CMI can help negate such differences in patient population, but not all institutional differences can be so easy normalized.

When the results of any benchmarking effort are viewed cautiously and in the context of the specific type of data analyzed, they can provide an institution with important insights that can be obtained in no other way.

ANALYSIS AND PRESENTATION OF DATA

Whether the number of institutions participating in the benchmarking effort is great or small, analysis and presentation of the data may proceed in a similar fashion. Optimally, the sample size of the peer group should be as robust as possible. At the end of the period of observation, after all data have been collected and stored in a database, analysis can be performed. As described earlier in this chapter, in order to make the data suitable for direct comparison, all relevant data should be normalized by measures such as the total number of occupied beds or patient days and, where appropriate, CMI.

	Individual Hospital		Peer Group (n = 15)			Benchmark Hospital
Column	1	2	3	4	5	6
General Hospital Data			25th	50th	75th	
Licensed Beds	350		250	333	420	322
Occupied Beds	220		149	201	268	207
Hospital Type	CT		CT	CT	CT	CT
Inpatient Days	70,105		40,569	62,116	76,643	50,615
% Antibiotic Expenditures						
Antibiotics/Pharmacy	8		10	12	16	15
Antibiotics/Drugs	10		15	18	22	18
Individual Antibiotics						
Ceftriaxone	30,874	140	39	100	697	135
Ampicillin/Sulbactam	20,543	93	161	290	404	174
Piperacillin/Tazobactam	65,583	298	59	171	212	40
Ciprofloxacin IV	40,787	185	89	189	257	219
Totals						
Beta-Lactamase Inhibitors Comb	89,947	409	366	468	639	147
3rd Generation Cephalosporins	75,876	345	347	550	1011	821
Flouroquinolones	92,233	419	343	412	723	751

Figure 1 Sample table comparing annual data for an individual hospital, peer group of hospitals, and benchmark hospital. Column 1 shows raw data for the individual hospital. Column 2 shows expenditure data normalized by the number of occupied beds. Columns 3, 4, and 5 show the twenty-fifth percentile, median, and seventy-fifth percentile for the peer group. Column 6 shows the data for the benchmark hospital. CT, community-teaching hospital.

Although an array of statistical procedures may be performed, a report showing the profile of an individual hospital compared with a peer group using simple summary statistics is often all that is required. Depending on the nature of the data reported, the most informative parameters for continuous variables such as DDD per 1,000 inpatient days or expenditures per OB are central measures of tendency and measures of dispersion. Measures of central tendency include the mean or median, and measures of dispersion include the standard deviation, percent coefficient of variation, interquartile range, and range. For samples limited in size and with extreme variation in observations, nonparametric measures such as the median and the interquartile range are recommended. For a larger sample of hospitals, presentation of a range of percentiles including the tenth, twenty-fifth, fiftieth, seventy-fifth, and nintieth has proved to be informative (25).

Although the goal of a report should be to contain valuable information, it is also important to present data in a manner that is easiest to interpret. Reports should always include as much raw data as possible, to allow individual institutions to investigate issues of particular interest. Figure 1 shows a sample table comparing annual data for an individual hospital, peer group of hospitals, and selected hospitals identified as leaders (benchmark hospitals). In addition to displaying data in tables, however, an effective report should also contain data represented graphically, in order to allow for quick and easy comparisons between an individual institution, its peer groups, and benchmark hospitals. Figure 2 demonstrates how comparisons of antibiotic expenditures for an individual hospital and a peer group of hospitals can be represented graphically. As shown in Figure 3, box plots may be used to compare parameters such as annual drug expenditures per OB (*panel A*) or rates of bacterial resistance (*panel B*) over time between the individual site and the peer group. The heterogeneity of a sample can be shown visually using pie charts or bar graphs. Other characteristics of interest among the whole sample that can be displayed graphically include mean antimicrobial usage, antimicrobial expenditures, and bacterial resistance

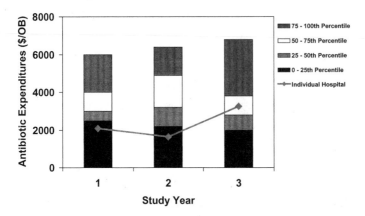

Figure 2 Comparison of antibiotic expenditures for an individual hospital and a peer group of hospitals. Percentiles of expenditures for the peer group are shown by contrast of shading. Expenditures for the individual hospital are shown by the diamond symbols.

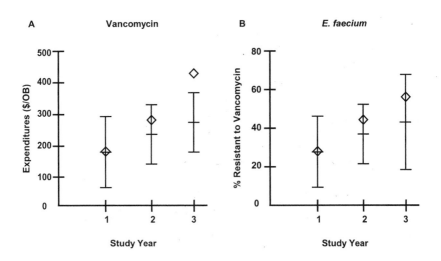

Figure 3 Interquartile-range plots demonstrating (**A**) expenditures per occupied bed and (**B**) percent of *Enterococcus faecium* isolates resistant to vancomycin by study year for the individual hospital (*diamonds*) compared with those of the peer group of hospitals (box plots showing twenty-fifth, fiftieth, and seventy-fifth percentiles).

patterns of interest, ranked by highest to lowest values. Box plots may be used to compare various parameters, such as measures of drug use across drug classes within a given period of time. Because the same data may be presented in a variety of ways, reports can be specifically tailored to their intended audience. For example, clinicians will be more interested in treatment-related comparisons, whereas administrators are also interested in the comparison of economic outcomes. With respect to measures of drug use, DDD per 1,000 inpatient days may be more informative for clinicians, whereas expenditures per OB may be preferred by administrators.

Once the peer group analysis is complete, the benchmark institution(s) may be identified. In the case of antimicrobial management, criteria for benchmark institutions might include having total antibiotic expenditures near or below the twenty-fifth percentile, total pharmacy expenditures and total drug expenditures near or below the median, performance of antibiotic management activities (e.g., aminoglycoside consults, IV-to-PO switch, streamlining of broad-spectrum IV antibiotics), and demonstrating efforts to reduce inappropriate vancomycin usage (32).

The presence or absence of various antibiotic management activities, such as switching and streamlining programs, may also be included in the reports, as may the rates at which these activities are performed (e.g., number of IV-to-PO switches per month). Insights may also be gained by benchmarking levels of clinical staffing. Such data may then be used to present strong arguments in favor of existing or even additional personnel to be dedicated to antimicrobial management programs. And finally, for those institutions that participate in a collaborative program annually, each new report affords an opportunity for internal benchmarking, which allows for the assessment of interventions or programs established in order to improve performance. Comparative data and internal trends can then be shared with all relevant departments in the institution for the purposes of discussing multidisciplinary approaches to optimizing processes and outcomes.

Having received a complete report, an individual institution can now readily see how its expenditures compare with peer groups and benchmark hospitals. At this point, the individual hospital may then choose to investigate why, or if, its own practice deviates from the middle of the peer group or from the benchmark hospitals. It is not necessarily the case that a higher expenditure for a particular agent should automatically be labeled inappropriate, but if a given expenditure seems unusually high in comparison with the peer groups, it would likely be an area meriting further examination. No health care staff has the time to continually investigate all of its practices, thus a benchmarking report can assist the staff in their selection of those areas most in need of scrutiny.

EXISTING BENCHMARKING PROGRAMS

Increasingly, national health care organizations such as the Infectious Diseases Society of America and the Society for Healthcare Epidemiology of America (IDSA/SHEA) and the Joint Commission on Accreditation of Healthcare Organizations (JCAHO) are promoting the use of microbiologic surveillance, benchmarking techniques, and multidisciplinary teams to monitor and control antimicrobial use and stem the development of bacterial resistance (33,34). There are several programs in the United States that monitor antimicrobial susceptibility of bacterial organisms, including the CDC's NNIS System, the SENTRY Antimicrobial Surveillance Program, and the TRUST Surveillance Program. However, because these programs do not collect antimicrobial usage data, they are unable to investigate the relationship, if any, between antimicrobial use and bacterial resistance.

Project ICARE, a collaborative effort between the CDC (using selected NNIS System hospitals from 1994 to 1999) and Emory University, has been one of the few large-scale programs to capture both antimicrobial use and bacterial susceptibility data within the hospital, though primarily the ICU, setting (35). Data from Project ICARE have been used to quantify the relationship between antimicrobial use and bacterial resistance for several organisms, characterize the epidemiology of vancomycin use, and develop rational and valid comparative data on antimicrobial use and resistance for intrahospital or interhospital comparison (7,36,37). Using such data, practice changes related to vancomycin use have been instituted, thereby lowering the amount of vancomycin used and the prevalence of VRE (7).

Although data collection for Project ICARE ended in 1999, the methodology from this program was adapted into the new Antimicrobial Use and Resistance (AUR) component of the NNIS system in a continuing effort to provide hospitals with a tool to combat bacterial resistance. The AUR has been designed to provide users with interhospital comparisons of aggregated data on drug use for select antimicrobial agents (represented as DDDs per 1,000 patient days) and resistance rates for certain antimicrobial-resistant pathogens. To be included in aggregate reports, hospitals submit at least 6 months of data in a given calendar year for a minimum of three hospital areas (at least one ICU, all inpatient areas combined, and all outpatient areas combined (25,36)).

Another program that has examined the relationship between antibiotic use and bacterial resistance is the SCOPE-MMIT (Surveillance and Control of Pathogens of Epidemiologic Importance—MediMedia Information Technology, North Wales, PA) Antimicrobial Network. In this collaborative program, MMIT extracts all antibiotic dispensing data from billing records at each hospital, based on electronic recognition of antibiotic codes using the Uniform System of Classification (IMS, Plymouth Meeting, PA) for antibacterial, antiviral, and antifungal drugs. Total grams of each agent dispensed to inpatients for all routes of administration are then provided to SCOPE investigators, along with total patient days for the period of interest (quarterly or annually). Using total grams and total patient days, the DDD per 1,000 patient days is calculated for each antibiotic at each hospital. These data are then compared with hospital bacterial susceptibility data (collected via hospital antibiograms), and changes in resistance rates from one period to the next are calculated (16,38).

Perhaps the longest-running program of this nature is the Benchmarking Program, coordinated by the Clinical Pharmacokinetics Laboratory in Buffalo, New York (32,39,40). Since 1993, the Benchmarking Program has been building a database that currently contains more than 450 hospital-years of antimicrobial use and bacterial susceptibility data from more than 200 U.S. hospitals. Participants complete an annual survey to report hospital demographic information such as number of beds, occupancy rates, number of inpatient days, and CMI. With respect to pharmacy data, annual inpatient expenditures for many individual antimicrobial agents are collected. Though there is some degree of error with such a measure, antimicrobial expenditures are collected because they are the most easily retrievable measure of usage for the vast majority of hospitals. To obtain microbiology data, hospital antibiograms are collected. In addition to these data, each participant provides information regarding the types of antibiotic management activities performed at the institution, including whether or not antibiotic formularies are enforced and, if so, how; what types and choices for therapeutic substitution are available; and whether programs such as streamlining broad-spectrum to narrow-spectrum antibiotics exist.

Like the results from Project ICARE/AUR, analyses of data from the Benchmarking Program database have also served to establish certain relationships. One analysis demonstrated that hospitals that encouraged an IV-to-PO switching program significantly reduced their antibiotic expenditures by an average of $320/occupied bed/year (32). More recently, the relationship between the intensity of use of various fluoroquinolone agents and the susceptibility of *P. aeruginosa* against ciprofloxacin was examined. It was discovered that the susceptibility of *P. aeruginosa* to ciprofloxacin significantly decreased as expenditures for both ofloxacin and levofloxacin increased (5.4% decrease in susceptibility for each increase of $300/occupied bed of ofloxacin or levofloxacin), but was unaffected by increasing expenditures of ciprofloxacin (8).

LIMITATIONS OF BENCHMARKING
ANTIMICROBIAL USE AND BACTERIAL
RESISTANCE

Benchmarking suffers from certain limitations that must not be overlooked. For example, in any but the largest benchmarking programs, the sample size of peer groups is likely to be a concern when evaluating for meaningful and statistically significant differences between institutions. One must always be on guard against attempting to make inferences from data that do not possess sufficient statistical power. Thus, when significant differences between institutions are not found, this does not necessarily imply that differences do not exist. Getting the right answer begins with asking the right question.

Although there have been numerous reports of an association between antibiotic use and bacterial resistance in the hospital setting (7,8,13–16), not all studies evaluating use and resistance have been able to demonstrate a statistically significant association (38). When no association is observed, it may be because of a genuine lack of association, though it may also be the result of small sample size, limited duration of observation, poor quality of data, limitations of study design, and/or the existence of interactions with other variables not captured. Antibiotic use is typically examined on an institutional level as a function of DDDs, annual tonnage, or annual expenditures normalized by the size of the inpatient population; it is rarely examined on a patient level. Thus, the nature of such institutional examinations, irrespective of the exact measure of drug utilization, does not permit an evaluation of the impact of actual drug exposure in individual patients (i.e., concentration and duration of dosing regimens) on the emergence of bacterial resistance. The fact that five similar hospitals, for example, all used the same total number of grams of a particular antimicrobial agent tells one nothing at all about the actual dosing regimens that clinicians chose for patients in different age ranges with varying levels of renal function, nor does it indicate anything about the duration of those regimens.

Over the last two decades, a wealth of knowledge regarding the relationship between drug concentrations and the pharmacologic or toxicologic effects of antimicrobial agents has been amassed. Using data from clinical and nonclinical models of infection, dosing regimens can be optimized to achieve pharmacokinetic-pharmacodynamic (PK-PD) target measures associated with efficacy. Thus, if an association between antimicrobial use and bacterial resistance is observed on an institutional level, poor dosing and the subsequent failure to achieve effective PK-PD targets in individual patients are likely contributory factors. Such ineffective dosing may be the result of insufficient care and consideration of the infection, though it may also simply be inherent in doses recommended in the product label.

Many epidemiologic studies conducted to date have demonstrated the multitude of risk factors associated with emergence of bacterial resistance (41–43). Examination of the impact of antimicrobial use alone on the percent of isolates that are resistant fails to account for other factors known to increase the likelihood of resistance. However, because risk factors reported have been predominantly patient related (e.g., comorbidities, prior length of stay, exposure to prior antimicrobials, presence of indwelling catheters), the institutional nature of the above-described studies evaluating the relationship between use and resistance limits the ability to assess these factors.

Perhaps the most important limitation of institutional-based analyses involving antimicrobial usage and bacterial resistance has been the qualitative nature of microbiologic data available. Microbiologic data are usually obtained from hospital antibiograms that show the proportion of isolates that were sensitive, intermediate, or resistant to a drug of interest over a given study period. Until recently, the more quantitative form of antimicrobial susceptibility data, i.e., the minimum inhibitory concentration (MIC), was not utilized. The problem with relying on qualitative susceptibility data is one of resolution. Only when a relatively large proportion of a bacterial population crosses the MIC breakpoint for resistance can one detect changes. Use of actual MIC values allows for detection of shifts in the MIC distribution much earlier; often allowing for an intervention before a clinical or epidemiologic crisis.

Analyses of antimicrobial use and bacterial resistance, which make use of quantitative MIC data, may help overcome such limitations. Although the data collected from individual hospitals are often qualitative, sources of quantitative susceptibility data from institutions are available. A number of large and long-standing surveillance systems, such as the SENTRY (44), TRUST (45), and MYSTIC (46) programs, have performed extensive MIC testing for isolates collected globally. Moreover, these surveillance systems frequently have more information about the patient and institution from which isolates were collected than is ever reported. Such data allow for multiple linear regression analyses evaluating the impact of various patient- and institution-specific variables on MIC data and thus represent a step forward in the effort to better understand the predictors of resistance (42,47,48).

Despite the above-described limitations, large multicenter benchmarking efforts are very important and serve a crucial role in monitoring trends and providing individual institutions with useful data to combat the growing problem of bacterial resistance. Without such efforts, there is a danger in failing to detect important changes in prescribing patterns and associated changes in bacterial susceptibility. Knowing how an individual institution's bacterial resistance rates compare to its peers also aids the institution in distinguishing between its own local resistance problems and problems of national significance.

CONCLUSIONS

Over the last few decades, benchmarking techniques have proved to be an enormously valuable aid in the institutional quest for continuous quality improvement and cost containment. Benchmarking antibiotic drug utilization in the institutional setting has been used to identify both the potential problem areas in pharmacy and prescribing practices as well as the successes of formulary guidelines and specific management and infection control practices. Furthermore, the ongoing process of benchmarking promotes a self-reflective atmosphere in which an institution comes to habitually track its own progress from year-to-year with respect to a wide array of specific and measurable parameters.

However, the optimal unit of study is often the patient rather than the institution. For example, in the early and mid-1990s, reports of an association between increasing vancomycin usage and VRE on an institutional level were generally absent from the literature, whereas both single- and multicenter case-control studies in patients consistently reported the finding that "prior vancomycin administration" was a risk factor for emergence of VRE (41). By using institutional benchmarking data in combination with data from patient outcome studies, an institution can most effectively evaluate the impact of new and existing therapeutic agents and programs, both from a clinical and pharmacoeconomic aspect. Furthermore, studies designed to identify factors associated with the development of bacterial resistance and using the best possible data sources (i.e., quantitative susceptibility data and patient-specific data) will provide us with greater insight into mechanisms of bacterial resistance. Bacterial resistance is a multifactorial problem, and combating its development and spread will require a multidisciplinary approach.

Finally, it is important to remember that benchmarking is not a one-time event, but rather a continuous process. The best practices of today will become the minimum standards of tomorrow. Just as bacteria are finding ever more novel mechanisms to survive exposure to antimicrobial agents, personnel in the arenas of drug development and drug utilization will need to continuously update their methods and practices. In order to meet the challenge, a continuous stream of new data will be required. It is to be expected that the introduction of widespread computer databasing in U.S. hospitals will greatly facilitate the collection and collation of such new data, and this task is one area in which pharmacy departments may be able to make an important contribution to improving the quality of health care.

REFERENCES

1. Deming WE. Out of the Crisis.. Cambridge: Massachusetts Institute of Technology Center for Advanced Engineering Study, 1986.

2. Woomer N, Long CO, Anderson C, Greenberg EA. Benchmarking in home health care: a collaborative approach. Caring 1999; 18:22–28.

3. Narong MN, Thongpiyapoom S, Thaikul N, Jamulitrat S, Kasatpibal N. Surgical site infections in patients undergoing major operations in a university hospital: using standardized infection ratio as a benchmarking tool. Am J Infect Control 2003; 31:274–279.

4. Stevenson KB. Regional data set of infection rates for long-term care facilities: description of a valuable benchmarking tool. Am J Infect Control 1999; 27:20–26.

5. Rudy EB, Lucke JF, Whitman GR, Davidson LJ. Benchmarking patient outcomes. J Nurs Scholarsh 2001; 33:185–189.

6. Bissell MG. The effect of benchmarking clinical practice with the clinical laboratory. Clin Lab Med 1999; 19:867–876.

7. Fridkin SK, Lawton R, Edwards JR, Tenover FC, McGowan JE, Gaynes RP. Intensive Care Antimicrobial Resistance Epidemiology Project. National Nosocomial Infections Surveillance Systems Hospitals. Monitoring antimicrobial use and resistance: comparison with a national benchmark on reducing vancomycin use and vancomycin-resistant enterococci. Emerg Infect Dis 2002; 8:702–707.

8. Bhavnani SM, Callen WA, Forrest A, Gilliland KK, Collins DA, Paladino JA, Schentag JJ. Effect of fluoroquinolone expenditures on susceptibility of *Pseudomonas aeruginosa* to ciprofloxacin in U.S. hospitals. Am J Health Syst Pharm 2003; 60: 1962–1970.

9. McGowan JE Jr. Antimicrobial resistance in hospital organisms and its relation to antibiotic use. Rev Infect Dis 1983; 5: 1033–1048.

10. McGowan JE Jr. Is antimicrobial resistance in hospital microorganisms related to antibiotic use? Bull NY Acad Med 1987; 63:253–268.

11. Quale J, Landman D, Saurina G, Atwood E, DiTore V, Patel K. Manipulation of a hospital antimicrobial formulary to control an outbreak of vancomycin-resistant enterococci. Clin Infect Dis 1996; 23:1020–1025.

12. Roberts NJ, Douglas RG. Gentimicin use and *Pseudomonas* and *Serratia* resistance: effect of a surgical prophylaxis regimen. Antimicrob Agents Chemother 1978; 13:214–220.

13. Ballow CH, Schentag JJ. Trends in antibiotic utilization and bacterial resistance. Diagn Microbiol Infect Dis 1992; 15(2 suppl):375–425.

14. Fridkin SK, Edwards JR, Courval JM, Hill H, Tenover FC, Lawton R, Gaynes RP, McGowan JE Jr. Intensive Care Antimicrobial Resistance Epidemiology (ICARE) Project and the National Nosocomial Infections Surveillance (NNIS) System Hospitals. The effect of vancomycin and third-generation cephalosporins on prevalence of vancomycin-resistant enterococci in 126 U.S. adult intensive care units. Ann Intern Med 2001; 135:175–183.

15. Lesch CA, Itokazu GS, Danziger LH, Weinstein RA. Multihospital analysis of antimicrobial usage and resistance trends. Diagn Microbiol Infect Dis 2001; 41:149–154.

16. Johnson CK, Polk R. Antimicrobial use in U.S hospitals and methicillin-resistant *Staphylococcus aureus* (MRSA) [abstr no. K-1399]., 43rd Interscience Conference on Antimicrobial Agents and Chemotherapy, Sept 16, 2003, Chicago.

17. Rice LB, Eckstein EC, DeVente J, Shlaes DM. Ceftazidime-resistant *Klebsiella pneumoniae* isolates recovered at the Cleveland Department of Veterans Affairs Medical Center. Clin Infect Dis 1996; 23:118–124.

18. Rahal JJ, Urban C, Horn D, Freeman K, Segal-Maurer S, Maurer J, Mariano N, Marks S, Burns JM, Dominick D, Lim M. Class restriction of cephalosporin use to control total cephalosporin resistance in nosocomial *Klebsiella*. JAMA 1998; 280: 1233–1237.

19. Patterson JE, Hardin TC, Kelly CA, Garcia RC, Jorgensen JH. Association of antibiotic utilization measures and control of multiple-drug resistance in *Klebsiella pneumoniae*. Infect Control Hosp Epidemiol 2000; 21:455–458.

20. Phelps CE. Bug/drug resistance: sometimes less is more. Med Care 1989; 27:194–203.

21. Holmberg SD, Solomon SL, Blake PA. Health and economic impacts of antimicrobial resistance. Rev Infect Dis 1987; 9: 1065–1078.

22. Himmelberg CJ, Pleasants RA, Weber DJ, Kessler JM, Samsa GP, Spivey JM, Morris TL. Use of antimicrobial drugs in adults before and after removal of a restriction policy. Am J of Hosp Pharm 1991; 48:1220–1227.

23. Briceland LL, Nightingale CH, Quintiliani R, Cooper BW, Smith KS. Antibiotic streamlining from combination therapy to monotherapy utilizing an interdisciplinary approach. Arch Intern Med 1988; 148:2019–2022.

24. Ramirez JA, Srinath L, Ahkee S, Huang A, Raff MJ. Early switch from intravenous to oral cephalosporins in the treatment of hospitalized patients with community-acquired pneumonia. Arch Intern Med 1995; 155:1273–1276.

25. National Nosocomial Infection Surveillance (NNIS) System Report, data summary from January 1992–June 2001, issued August 2001. Am J Infect Control 2001; 29:404–421.

26. Bergman U, Grimsson A, Wahba AHW, Westerholm B. Studies in Drug Utilization. European series, no. 8.. Copenhagen: WHO Regional Office for Europe, 1979.

27. Westerholm B. Consumption of Drugs: Report on a Symposium. Euro 3102. Copenhagen: WHO Regional Office for Europe, 1970.

28. Enzweiler K, Lorenz K, Bosso J, White R. Agreement among different markers of antibiotic use over an eight-year period., 41st Interscience Conference on Antimicrobial Agents and Chemotherapy, Dec 16–19, 2001, Chicago.

29. Bonapace CR, Lorenz KR, Bosso JA, White RL. Use of different measures of drug usage in assessing antibiotic use/susceptibility relationships., 40th Interscience Conference on Antimicrobial Agents and Chemotherapy, Sept 17–20, 2000, Toronto.

30. Cars O, Molstad S, Melander A. Variation in antibiotic use in European Union. Lancet 2001; 357:1851–1853.

31. Molstad S, Lundborg CS, Karlsson AK, Cars O. Antibiotic prescription rates vary markedly between 13 European countries. Scand J Infect Dis 2002; 34:366–371.

32. Bhavnani SM. Benchmarking in health-system pharmacy: current research and practical applications. Am J Health Syst Pharm 2000; 57(suppl 2):S13–S20.

33. Shlaes DM, Gerding DN, John JF Jr, Craig WA, Bornstein DL, Duncan RA, Eckman MR, Farrer WE, Greene WH, Lorian V, Levy S, McGowan JE Jr, Paul SM, Ruskin J, Tenover FC, Watanakunakorn C. Society for Healthcare Epidemiology of America and Infectious Diseases Society of America Joint Committee on the Prevention of Antimicrobial Resistance: guidelines for the prevention of antimicrobial resistance in hospitals. Infect Control Hosp Epidemiol 1997; 18:275–291.

34. Patton KA. Role of JCAHO standards and clinical practice guidelines in promoting appropriate antimicrobial use. Am J Health Syst Pharm 2002; 59(8 suppl 3):S16–S18.

35. Fridkin SK, Steward CD, Edwards JR, Pryor ER, McGowan JE, Archibald LK, Gaynes RP, Tenover FC. Surveillance of antimicrobial use and antimicrobial resistance in United States hospitals: project ICARE phase 2. Clin Infect Dis 1999; 29: 245–252.

36. Fridkin SK. The challanges and value of monitoring antimicrobial use and resistance [abstr no. K-1084]. 42nd Interscience Conference on Antimicrobial Agents and Chemotherapy, Sept 27–30, 2002, San Diego.

37. Hill HA, Haber MJ, McGowan JE Jr, Fridkin SK, Edwards JR, Tenover FC, Gaynes RP, Project ICARE Hospitals. A link between quinolone use and resistance in *P. aeruginosa* [abstr no. 495]. 39th Annual Meeting of the Infectious Diseases Society of America, Oct 25–28, 2001, San Francisco.

38. Johnson CK, Davis S, Polk R. No association between changes in hospital fluoroquinolone use and changes in rates of fluoroquinolone-resistant *P. aeruginosa* [abstr no. K-1427]. 43rd Interscience Conference on Antimicrobial Agents and Chemotherapy, Sept 14–17, 2003, Chicago.

39. Schentag JJ, Paladino JA, Birmingham MC, Zimmer G, Carr JR, Hanson SC. Use of benchmarking techniques to justify the evolution of antibiotic management programs in healthcare systems. J Pharm Tech 1995; 11:203–210.

40. Rifenburg RP, Paladino JA, Hanson SC, Tuttle JA, Schentag JJ. Benchmark analysis of strategies hospitals use to control antimicrobial expenditures. Am J Health Syst Pharm 1996; 53: 2054–2062.

41. Bhavnani SM, Drake JA, Forrest A, Deinhart JA, Jones RN, Biedenbach DJ, Ballow CH, and the National Nosocomial Re-

sistance Surveillance Group. A nationwide, multicenter, case-control study comparing risk factors, treatment, and outcome for vancomycin-resistant and -susceptible enterococcal bacteremia. Diagn Microbiol Infect Dis 2000; 36:145–158.

42. Bhavnani SM, Hammel JP, Forrest A, Jones RN, Ambrose PG. Relationships between patient- and institution-specific variables and decreased susceptibility of gram-negative pathogens. Clin Infect Dis 2003; 37:344–350.

43. Graffunder EM, Venezia RA. Risk factors associated with nosocomial methicillin-resistant *Staphylococcus aureus* (MRSA) infection including previous use of antimicrobials. J Antimicrob Chemother 2002; 49:999–1005.

44. Sader HS, Biedenbach DJ, Jones RN. Global patterns of susceptibility for 21 commonly utilized antimicrobial agents tested against 48,440 Enterobacteriaceae in the SENTRY Antimicrobial Surveillance Program (1997–2001). Diagn Microbiol Infect Dis 2003; 47:361–364.

45. Thornsberry C, Sahm DF, Kelly LJ, Critchley IA, Jones ME, Evangelista AT, Karlowsky JA. Regional trends in antimicrobial resistance among clinical isolates of *Streptococcus pneumoniae, Haemophilus influenzae*, and *Moraxella catarrhalis* in the United States: results from the TRUST Surveillance Program, 1999–2000. Clin Infect Dis 2002; 34:S4–S16.

46. Rhomberg PR, Jones RN. MYSTIC Program (USA) Study Group. Antimicrobial spectrum of activity for meropenom and nine broad spectrum antimicrobials: report from the MYSTIC Program (2002) in North America. Diagn Microbiol Infect Dis 2003; 47:365–372.

47. Hammel JP, Bhavnani SM, Ambrose PG, Jones RN, Forrest A, Piedmonte MR. Comparison of censored regression vs standard regression analyses for modeling relationships between minimum inhibitory concentrations and patient- and institution-specific variables., 104th American Society for Clinical Pharmacology and Therapeutics, April 2003, Washington, DC.

48. Bhavnani SM, Hammel JP, Jones RN, Ambrose PG. Relationship between increased levofloxacin use and decreased susceptibility of *Streptococcus pneumoniae*: report from the ARREST Program [abstr no. K-1397]., 43rd Interscience Conference on Antimicrobial Agents and Chemotherapy, Sept 14–17, 2003, Chicago.

9

The Role of Infection Control and Hospital Epidemiology in the Optimization of Antibiotic Use

AUGUST J. VALENTI

Director, Epidemiology and Infection
Prevention, Maine Medical Center
Portland, Maine, U.S.A.

No discussion of the optimization of antibiotic use in health care settings should take place without considering infection control. Infections drive antibiotic use, which contributes to the development of resistance, and resistance leads to increased utilization of antibiotics and resources. Interventions designed to interrupt or modify this use-resistance pathway are among the chief concerns of infection control programs. More than any interventional hospital program, infection control is founded on the traditions and proven methods of epidemiology.

209

The emphasis in infection control should really be on **prevention**: the primary prevention of infections, the prevention of transmission of infections, and the prevention of the development and spread of resistance. Identifying and understanding the processes that lead to health care-acquired infection, transmission, and resistance ideally progress to the development, implementation, and assessment of interventional strategies directed at correcting them.

Increasingly, hospital-acquired infections are framed within the context of adverse events affecting patient safety (1). This is not surprising given the attention patient safety has been receiving since the Institute of Medicine published its highly trumpeted report on errors in the health system (2). Nosocomial infections are the leading adverse events affecting patients in hospitals (1). Five percent to 10% of all patients admitted to acute care hospitals may be expected to develop one or more infections during their stay; approximately 2 million patients are affected annually (3). With nearly 90,000 deaths a year, at an annual cost in the billions of dollars, it is not difficult to understand why nosocomial infections are regarded as an important emerging infectious disease problem for the new millennium (4).

Yet, notwithstanding the fact that at least a third of hospital-acquired infections have been shown to be preventable through effective infection control programs (5), there is a growing tendency to view such programs as cost centers, and for hospitals to divert resources away from infection control. Indeed, a component distracting infection control professionals from their mission currently is making the case for its legitimate role in analyzing and reducing adverse outcomes, controlling costs, and improving patient satisfaction.

Emerging antibiotic resistance is a problem of particular concern for the hospital epidemiologist, and, depending on how a hospital's various quality programs are configured, hospital epidemiologists either administer or are closely allied with antibiotic stewardship programs at their institutions. Optimization of antibiotic use should be a priority for any good infection control program, and optimization of the infection control program should be a priority of every health care institution.

THE COMPONENTS OF A GOOD INFECTION CONTROL PROGRAM

In 1953, the Joint Commission on Accreditation of Healthcare Organizations (JCAHO) began promulgating infection control standards. Among other requirements, a hospital was expected to establish an infection control committee overseeing surveillance, have facilities for isolating infected patients, and have access to a competent microbiology laboratory (6). For more than 30 years, following outbreaks of staphylococcal infections in hospitals, the principles of hospital epidemiology based on case definition and classification, surveillance, reporting to responsible authorities, prevention, and control have been refined and integrated into health care.

In 1970, the Centers for Disease Control and Prevention (CDC) recommended that hospitals have an infection control nurse and a hospital epidemiologist (7). Subsequently, the Study on the Efficacy of Nosocomial Infection Control (SENIC) Project further invigorated the infection control movement by providing evidence that approximately one third of nosocomial infections could be prevented in hospitals that practiced good surveillance and control (5).

The body of literature supporting the efficacy of infection control methods continues to grow. Those responsible for infection control can look to a number of private and governmental agencies as well as professional societies for pertinent recommendations and guidelines; the Society for Healthcare Epidemiology of America (SHEA), the Association for Professionals in Infection Control and Epidemiology (APIC), the Surgical Infection Society, the Infectious Diseases Society of America (IDSA), the CDC—especially the Division of Healthcare Quality Promotion and the Healthcare Infection Control Practices Advisory Committee (HICPAC)—are among the most prominent.

In 1998, a SHEA consensus panel developed a position paper on the requirements for and the essential activities of infection control and hospital epidemiology (8). The overarching mission of an infection control program is to protect patients, hospital staff, health care providers, visitors, and others in the health care environment by providing cost-effective infection prevention and control. Among the considerations surrounding cost are the expense of diagnosing and treating infections, increased length of stay, delayed return to work, disability, legal issues, patient satisfaction, and adverse publicity (some hospital outbreaks have attracted significant media attention). In the context of affecting antibiotic use, effective infection control should decrease infections and the transmission of resistance, which reduces antibiotic use, mor-

---

Functions of Infection Control and Hospital Epidemiology

- Management of critical data and information, including **surveillance** of nosocomial infections and **reporting** of infection rates

- Setting and recommending policies and procedures to prevent adverse events

  - Assuring the appropriateness of policies and procedures

  - Compliance with regulations, guidelines, and accreditation requirements

  - Employee health, including post-exposure prophylaxis and vaccination

  - Other prevention strategies (e.g. surgical prophylaxis)

- The direct intervention to interrupt the transmission of infections (including the identification, investigation, and management of outbreaks)

- The education and training of healtcare personnel, patients, and family

---

Figure 1 Essential activities of an infection control department. (From Scheckler WE, Brimhall D, Buck AS, Farr BM, Friedman C. SHEA position paper: requirements for infrastructure and essential activities of infection control and epidemiology in hospitals: a consensus panel report. Infect Control Hosp Epidemiol 1998; 19:114–124.)

bidity, mortality, and costs. Currently, infection control departments have seen the scope of their activities increase to include quality assurance, facilities design, insuring compliance with Occupational Safety and Health Administration (OSHA) regulations, and preparing for biological terrorism; however, four core functions remain the essential components of an infection control program (Figure 1).

Management of Critical Data and Information

The most important activity of an infection control program is **surveillance**, the monitoring of definable events in a given population (8). A good surveillance program not only captures significant variations from expected infection rates ("clusters" and outbreaks), but collects, analyzes, interprets, and reports data on infection rates in a well-organized and timely fashion. Surveillance is the most labor-intensive and time-consuming activity of a department, but is the most important in preventing nosocomial infections(5). Therefore, surveillance should be simple, efficient, and able to meet the objectives set by the infection control committee, which ordinarily oversees the activities of the department.

The CDC recently updated its guidelines for evaluating public health surveillance systems (Figure 2) (9,10). A good system is not only simple, but is flexible, that is, responsive to new problems, case definitions, and technologic advances. Data should be complete and accurately collected and collated to minimize the inevitable challenges that come from recipients. Acceptance of data is sometimes the "rate-limiting step" in catalyzing change; therefore, it is important that data be valid, capturing cases that meet definitions and accurately excluding cases that do not. Timely identification of trends, clusters, and outbreaks is important. The sooner a surveillance system identifies a problem and gets the data into appropriate hands, the earlier the opportunity for intervention. Surveillance also helps measure the effects of interventions. Infection control departments should be given the appropriate resources and computer support to insure that surveillance systems provide data reliably with little "downtime" or delays.

8 Characteristics of Effective Surveillance Programs

Simplicity

Flexibility

High-quality data

Acceptability

Sensitivity and specificity

Timeliness

External validity

Reliability

Figure 2 The eight characteristics of an effective surveillance program. (From Centers for Disease Control and Prevention. Update guidelines for evaluating public health surveillance systems: recommendations from the guidelines working group. MMWR Morb Mortal Wkly Rep 2001; 50:13–24; and Edmond MB. National and international surveillance systems for nosocomial infections. In: Wenzel RP, ed. Prevention and Control of Nosocomial Infections. Philadelphia: Lippincott Williams & Wilkins, 2003:109–119.)

Although desirable, it is difficult and not always the best application of limited resources for most hospitals to identify every hospital-acquired infection in the institution ("total hospital surveillance"). An acceptable strategy is for surveillance to "target" specific units (especially intensive care units [ICUs]), procedures, or infections of particular concern or importance. The infection control committee should review the surveillance plan periodically (at least annually) and recommend areas to target. The most common nosocomial infections are urinary tract infections (UTIs), pneumonias, surgical site infections (SSIs), and bloodstream infections.

Using standard definitions of infections, such as those developed by the CDC (11), helps avert disputes that may arise when data are fed back to stakeholders. Standard definitions and appropriately **adjusted** rates are important for benchmarking purposes. Rates adjusted for factors such as severity of illness (**risk-indexed**), length of stay (**patient-days**), or exposure to devices (**device-days**) help correct for variations in the risk of infection among patient populations and allow for more meaningful comparisons of populations within a facility, over time or among hospitals (12,13). A rate for any nosocomial infection for a particular time period in a selected hospital population can be expressed in terms of patient-days; the denominator is the sum of the number of days each patient spent on the ward (multiplying the rate by 100 or 1,000 is a common convention). Infection rates associated with devices—central lines, urinary catheters, ventilators, or other devices—for a specified time period (e.g., 3 months), are frequently reported in terms of device-days, that is, the number of days each patient in a given population, during a particular time period has been exposed to the device (14). For example,

$$\frac{Number\ of\ urinary\ catheter\text{–}associated\ UTIs}{Number\ of\ catheter\text{-}days} \times 1{,}000\ \text{provides}$$

the number of urinary catheter-associated infections UTIs per 1,000 catheter-days. Similarly,

$$\frac{Number\ of\ ventilator\text{-}associated\ pneumonias}{Number\ of\ ventilator\text{-}days} \times 1{,}000\ \text{is com-}$$

monly used to derive a rate for ventilator-associated pneumonias in intensive care units. Surgical site infection (SSI) rates may be surgeon-specific, service-specific (e.g., cardiothoracic, neurosurgery, orthopedics), or procedure-specific. A surgeon-specific rate, represented as a percent, may be derived by using the following formula (15):

$$\frac{Number\ of\ SSIs\ in\ patients\ operated\ on\ by\ surgeon\ A}{Total\ number\ of\ patients\ operated\ on\ by\ surgeon\ A} \times 100$$

NNIS has developed a risk-index scoring system that is useful for comparisons (16). Patients are assigned a value based on the wound class of the procedure, the duration, the use of an endoscope, and the American Society of Anesthesiology (ASA) score assigned by the anesthesiologist.

Feedback to providers is an important tool in the reduction of health care-acquired infections. Figure 3 shows an example of a "dashboard" format used by some facilities. The calculation, adjustment, and display of rates are "bread-and-butter" issues for infection control professionals. For a more thorough treatment of this subject, the interested reader is referred to resources cited at the conclusion of this chapter.

Depending on the time and resources of the infection control department, it may be beneficial to belong to a surveillance

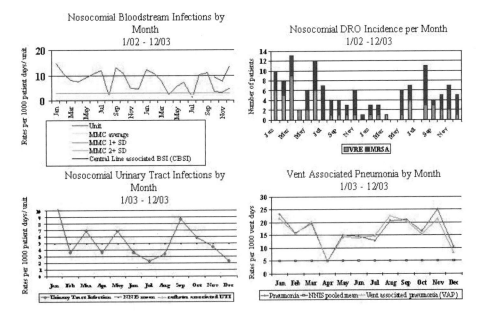

Figure 3 An example (fictitious) of how rates can be displayed for feedback to providers

network. A number of networks are active here and abroad (see Edmond) (10) and can help a hospital establish benchmarks for comparisons, which are increasingly requested by cost- and quality-conscious hospital administrators and insurers. Aggregate data from networks have shed light on important trends. In the United States, the oldest and best-known surveillance network is the National Nosocomial Infection Surveillance System. NNIS has significantly contributed to the understanding and control of hospital-acquired infections. Project ICARE (Intensive Care Antimicrobial Resistance Epidemiology), a joint venture of the CDC and Emory University, is providing information on antimicrobial use and the development of resistance.

Computer-enhanced surveillance is used in some hospitals but may be costly and limited in functionality. However, the merits of well-conceived medical information systems in infection control are apparent (1,17). One pertinent example is provided by a study in which computer-assisted surveillance helped identify and reduce inappropriate and redundant antibiotic usage (18). With increasing computational capabilities, automated surveillance systems, and data mining technology (see below), it is likely that hospitals will be able to broaden surveillance in the future, and we will witness an increase in interinstitutional surveillance networks (10).

The application of **data mining** technology to surveillance for hospital-acquired infections is a promising innovation. Data mining utilizes advances in machine learning (artificial intelligence), statistical analysis, and database technology to search for patterns in large amounts of data that are too subtle to be detected by traditional surveillance (19,20). Brossette et al. (21) developed a proprietary surveillance system that centers on a hospital's clinical microbiology database and the laboratory's information system to detect clusters, increases in colonization pressure, and changes in antibiotic resistance. Identifying trends and process breakdowns (sentinel events) in real time allows infection control personnel to investigate and correct the causes of these breakdowns more efficiently. Data mining could increase the sensitivity and specificity of surveillance, and there are indications that a broader application of this technology to health care is on the horizon (20–25).

Besides surveillance, computerized information systems can be used to store information on patients known to be infected or colonized with drug-resistant organisms so that appropriate precautions can be taken when they re-enter the facility. Admissions officers are alerted to the need for precautions before the patient is admitted to a unit, which saves time and decreases the risk of exposing other patients to resistant organisms.

Setting and Recommending Policies and Procedures to Prevent Infections

Hospital-wide policies and procedures pertaining to infection control should be based on the best available scientific evidence. Pertinent literature, including consensus statements and published guidelines, should be consulted. For convenience, Abrutyn et al. (26) brought many of these guidelines together in a single, very useful volume. Policies and procedures should be practical, enforceable, and cost-effective. To gain acceptance, key stakeholders should have a role in the process. Periodic reviews of compliance and efficacy in reducing adverse outcomes should be undertaken and are usually required for accreditation.

Strategies for Preventing the Transmission of Infection

The containment of pathogens through the **isolation** of patients and the use of barrier precautions (**hand hygiene, gloves, gowns, masks**, and **protective equipment**) has been traditionally associated with infection control. Over the past 30 years, significant revisions in isolation policies have been recommended by the CDC (27). Current precautions are more interaction driven than simply diagnosis driven, reflecting the experience and knowledge gained from managing the HIV epidemic.

Transmission of infection within a hospital requires a source, a susceptible population, and a means of transmission (contact, airborne, common source, droplet, or vector) (27). **Standard precautions** are applied to all hospitalized patients to reduce the spread of pathogenic organisms. **Transmission-based precautions** (airborne, droplet, contact) and the empiric use of transmission-based precautions supplement standard precautions in those situations in which patients are known or suspected to be colonized or infected with pathogens of epidemiologic significance. Because recommendations may not anticipate every contingency, it remains the prerogative of the hospital epidemiologist to modify precautions to fit the needs of an institution or a special situation.

Hand Hygiene

Although hand washing is nearly universally regarded as the single most important thing a health care worker can do to prevent the transmission of infection, studies have consistently demonstrated a significant lack of compliance (28). A host of reasons can be cited for this discordance and need to be considered in campaigns to increase compliance with hand hygiene policies (Fig. 4) (29).

Boyce and Pittet (29) prepared a comprehensive review of hand hygiene for HICPAC and the HICPAC/SHEA/APIC/IDSA Hand Hygiene Task Force. Based on studies of the efficacy of **alcohol-based hand rubs**, the task force strongly recommends the use of these products for routine decontamination of the hands, unless the hands are visibly soiled. Hand washing is recommended "when hands are visibly dirty or contaminated with proteinaceous material or are visibly soiled with blood or other body fluids." Alcohol-based hand rubs decrease the time needed for hand hygiene, are less irritating, and are better accepted by health care personnel (30). In addition, they can be conveniently placed in areas where it is difficult to provide sinks. The wearing of artificial fingernails for those whose responsibilities include direct contact with high-risk patients, such as those in surgery and ICUs, is discouraged. Adherence to hand hygiene should be monitored, and information regarding performance should be given to personnel.

Self-reported reasons for poor adherence to hand hygiene

- Irritation and dryness of the skin
- Inconveniently placed sinks or shortage of sinks
- Lack of soap or paper towels
- Too busy or insufficient time
- Understaffing or overcrowding
- Patient needs take priority
- Hand hygiene interferes with healthcare worker-patient relationship
- Low risk of acquiring infection from patient
- Wearing gloves or the belief that gloves obviate the need for hand hygiene
- Lack of knowledge of guidelines
- Forgetfulness or not thinking about it
- No role model from colleagues or superiors
- Doubts about the value of hand hygiene
- Disagreement with the recommendations
- Lack of scientific information on the impact of improved hand hygiene on healthcare associated infections

---

Figure 4 Reasons health care workers cite for poor adherence to hand hygiene. (From Boyce JM, Pittet D. Guidelines for hand hygiene in health-care settings: recommendations of the Healthcare Infection Control Practices Advisory Committee and the HICPAC HEA APIC IDSA Hand Hygiene Task Force. Am J of Infect Control 2002; 30:S1–S46)

Improved compliance with hand hygiene may easily reduce transmission in settings where the number of infected or colonized patients is low. In settings where the **average daily point prevalence** is high, that is, **colonization pressure** is increased, a few lapses in hand hygiene may be all that is needed to sustain cross-transmission (28,31). The efficacy of efforts to improve hand hygiene adherence requires further investigation, but institutions should make hand hygiene a priority.

Gloves

The hand hygiene guideline addresses glove use as well. Proper use of gloves requires that they be changed—not washed—after each patient or, if moving from a contaminated body site to a clean site, on the same patient. Glove use does not obviate the need for proper hand hygiene.

Universal gloving with disposable examination gloves during contact with high-risk patients or their environment has been proposed by Weinstein and Kabins (32) and others. It has been shown to reduce the spread of *Clostridium difficile*-associated diarrhea and transmission of vancomycin-resistant enterococci (VRE) (32–35). In a study by Tenorio et al. (36), gloving reduced the risk of acquisition of VRE on health care workers' hands by 71%. Hand hygiene remains important: Gloves are changed between patients, and hands are decontaminated by washing or applying alcohol-based rubs. The ease and convenience of this approach has a certain appeal over the gowning and gloving required by traditional contact precautions (37). In some studies, gowning offered no demonstrable advantage over universal gloving in the control of VRE, methicillin-resistant *Staphylococcus aureus* (MRSA), ceftazidime-resistant *Escherichia coli*, or *Klebsiella pneumoniae* (28,37,38). However, gowns have been shown to be of benefit in other studies (see the discussion later in this chapter on control of resistant organisms) and remain a recommendation for contact precautions.

Universal glove use is directed at the reservoir of colonized patients in hospitals who are unrecognized and have the potential to transmit pathogens. Some infection control experts advocate surveillance cultures on all patients or on those at high risk for colonization so that contact precautions (gloves and gowns) can be applied. In one institution where screening cultures and full contact precautions for infected or colonized patients were routinely practiced, universal gloving on high-risk units for patients whose colonization status was unknown was associated with significant reductions in the acquisition of VRE (39).

Compliance with Regulations and Accreditation Requirements

Infection control personnel need to be part of the compliance mechanisms of the institution. Collaboration with local, state, and federal health agencies is an important current and future role of infection control, especially in the management of emerging infections. Infection control professionals should offer support and guidance to public health officials and policy makers. Regulatory and accrediting bodies are increasing pressure on hospitals to identify, report, and reduce adverse events; infection control indicators are prominent in current efforts.

Employee Health

Employees play an undeniable role in introducing and spreading infections within a hospital. It is important for infection control to partner with the hospital's employee health unit or occupational health department to develop policies and procedures aimed at improving vaccination rates, compliance with tuberculosis screening, reasonable work restrictions for communicable infections, and prompt postexposure prophylaxis. Recognizing the less than desirable rates of immunization among employees and patients against influenza and pneumococcus—infections likely to increase antibiotic use—the CDC has made vaccination a priority in its twelve-step program to prevent antimicrobial resistance (40).

Other Prevention Strategies

Antibiotic Interventions

Application of intranasal mupirocin ointment may substantially reduce the prevalence of *S. aureus* nasal carriage, although the effect is often temporary (41,42). Decolonization strategies have been used to prevent surgical wound infections and infections in patients undergoing dialysis (43–45). Not surprisingly, resistance to mupirocin is increasing—a serious concern. However, Perl et al. (46) studied preoperative use of intranasal mupirocin ointment in 3,864 patients undergoing nonurgent, elective surgery in a university hospital system and concluded that a short, perioperative course of mupirocin did not contribute significantly to resistance and decreased the overall incidence of nosocomial *S. aureus* infections in colonized patients. They suggested that such an approach to nasal carriage before surgery may be cost-effective, but further study is needed before this practice can be recommended.

Antibiotic Stewardship

Inappropriate use of antibiotics when they are not indicated or improper selection, dosing, and duration contribute needlessly to the emergence and spread of resistant organisms. The CDC has made the appropriate use of antibiotics a key component in its twelve-step program for the management of antibiotic resistance (40). Choosing the appropriate agent, dose, and duration of therapy based on the proper collection and interpretation of cultures; improving laboratory performance; treating true infections as opposed to colonization; and limiting the use of certain antibiotics should be the goal of every clinician and hospital (40). This is part of an overall strategy to reduce resistance, and in many institutions, is within the purview of the infection control department, which should be closely allied with antibiotic management in any case.

IMPORTANT HOSPITAL-ACQUIRED INFECTIONS

Catheter-Associated Urinary Tract Infections

Urinary tract infections account for about 40% of all hospital-acquired infections (47). Instrumentation, particularly indwelling catheterization, is responsible for the majority of nosocomial UTIs (48). Therefore, using these catheters only when indicated, inserting and maintaining them properly, and removing them when they are no longer needed are important.

Urinary catheters are overused in many hospitals and are left in for longer than needed; catheters should never be used for convenience (49). Personnel who insert and maintain catheters should be trained in aseptic technique. Strict adherence to the **sterile continuously closed system** of urinary drainage is the standard and has been shown to be superior to open drainage (48). The use of prophylactic antibiotics in the prevention of catheter-related UTIs is not currently recommended and was shown to increase resistance in some studies (50,51). Studies of the efficacy of catheters coated with antibiotics or silver alloy in reducing bacteriuria and UTIs have had mixed results, but silver alloy/hydrogel-coated catheters have shown the most promise and may be cost-effective (52,53).

Nosocomial Pneumonia and Ventilator-Associated Pneumonia

The second most common nosocomial infection is pneumonia (54).The attributable mortality of nosocomial pneumonias is about 30%, and they are the leading cause of death from nosocomial infection in the United States (55). Mayhall (56) and Craven et al. (57) have published excellent scientific reviews of the concepts of diagnosis, management, and prophylaxis of nosocomial pneumonia. Guidelines published by the CDC present a comprehensive strategy for the prevention of this important hospital-acquired infection (54).

Pneumonia is the most common infection in medical-surgical intensive care units (58), and mechanical ventilation is the most significant risk factor for the development of pneumonia. This has been a widely studied area, with mostly disappointing results in terms of elucidating effective preventive measures. Reducing the number of ventilated patients and reducing the length of time on mechanical ventilation are obvious strategies. In this regard, studies of positive-pressure ventilation methods that do not require intubation are encouraging. Continuous suctioning of secretions that pool in the subglottic space over the tracheal cuff has been shown to be an effective strategy once patients are intubated and ventilated (59,60). Simply placing patients in a semirecumbent rather than supine position, aimed at reducing the aspiration of gastric contents, may be helpful (61).

The use of systemic or nonabsorbable antibiotics to selectively decontaminate the digestive tract (**selective digestive decontamination**) has been proposed, but is controversial, especially because increased antibiotic use could lead to the development of resistance. Although this strategy may decrease ventilator-associated pneumonias in select populations of ventilated patients, it has not been shown to significantly affect mortality (62).

Antibiotic cycling in the special care unit shows promise as an intervention in reducing ventilator-associated pneumonias. Antibiotic cycling is discussed in Chapter 17 of this book. Recent studies reported reductions in ventilator-associated pneumonias when antibiotics were rotated on a regular basis (63–65).

Bloodstream Infections

Health care-acquired bloodstream infections contribute significantly to increased costs, length of stay, mortality, and excess antibiotic use. The bulk of hospital-acquired bloodstream infections are related to intravascular catheterization. When the integrity of a vascular catheter system is broken for the purpose of introducing medications or fluids into a line or withdrawing blood from a line, bacteria may contaminate the lumen and enter the bloodstream. Bacteria also track along the outer surface of the catheter and penetrate the mechanical barrier to infection provided by the integument.

Mermel (66) published a concise overview of this area. Education of staff on proper insertion and care of catheters, the designation of special intravenous teams responsible for the insertion and maintenance of peripheral lines, and feedback of infection rates to personnel should be part of an overall strategy for the prevention of catheter-related infections. Institutional policies should focus on appropriate use of catheters, proper insertion and maintenance, minimizing interruptions in the integrity of intravascular access systems, and removing catheters when they are no longer necessary or when they become infected. Designating specially trained teams of personnel for the insertion and maintenance of vascular catheters appears to be an effective strategy (67). As with SSIs, the importance of infection control providing feedback to personnel may also be helpful in reducing bloodstream infections (68).

Insertion under sterile conditions using a full barrier technique including large drapes, sterile gowns, and surgical masks for all in attendance has been shown to be a highly cost-effective measure (69). Additional measures, such as tunneling catheters and avoiding the femoral area for intravenous catheterization, have also proven effective (70,71). Skin preparation with chlorhexidine has been shown to be superior to povidone-iodine; covering catheter insertion sites with chlorhexidine dressings may reduce line-associated bacteremias (66).

Technologic strategies have included the development of catheters impregnated with antiseptics or antibiotics, catheter hubs that contain antibiotics, and contamination shields on pulmonary artery catheters. Darouiche (72) outlined the characteristics of antimicrobial-coated vascular catheters that should enhance efficacy and guide product development and evaluations. The antimicrobial coating should have durable activity against most potential pathogens and be able to reach organisms on the external and internal catheter surface as well as those imbedded in the biofilm that surrounds the catheter. Properly conducted clinical trials on one or more units of the hospital with infection control comparing actual outcomes with expected outcomes and manufacturers' claims may help determine the acceptance and efficacy of such products in a particular setting.

Catheters treated with antiseptics and antibiotics have been associated with reductions in bloodstream infections in many studies, but they are costly. A recent review of eleven randomized, controlled trials of antimicrobial-impregnated central venous catheters pointed out methodologic and statistical flaws in these studies and concluded that no significant clinical advantage to antibiotic-impregnated central lines could be demonstrated (73).

Surgical Site Infections

Surgical site infections occur in up to 10% of operations in the United States (74), and approximately one-fourth of noso-comial infections are caused by SSIs (75). In 1999, HICPAC published guidelines that provide detailed information on the prevention of SSIs (76).

Although the most important factors in the prevention of SSIs are the skill of the surgeon, proper technique, and the health of the patient (77–79); infection control also has an important role in the reduction of SSIs. Surveillance of SSIs with feedback of surgeon-specific infection rates has been shown to be an effective intervention (80–82) and is strongly recommended by the CDC (76).

The practice of administering perioperative antibiotics for the prevention of surgical infections has evolved since Burke's landmark study in 1961 (83), which showed the relationship between the timing of antibiotic administration and efficacy in preventing experimental skin infection. Recommendations for antibiotic prophylaxis have emphasized that the appropri-ate antibiotic must have adequate levels in the target tissue before or at the time of expected contamination. Historically, many studies purporting to demonstrate the efficacy of antibi-otic prophylaxis in a host of procedures suffered from design flaws, but more recent work has made it possible to develop evidence-based recommendations (79).

An appropriate perioperative antibiotic should be chosen for procedures in which the evidence supports their use and given at a time that ensures bactericidal serum and tissue levels are present when the incision is made. It is not necessary to maintain therapeutic levels for more than a few hours after closure; therefore, additional doses should be given only when indicated in published guidelines (76). When antibiotics are not discontinued in a timely manner, cost and resistance are adversely affected.

Appropriate use and timing of preoperative antibiotics is emerging as an important quality indicator. Poor compliance with established guidelines is a problem for many hospitals. One technologic solution is to use a computer-based reminder system to prompt appropriate timing of antibiotics. Burke's group at LDS Hospital (84,85) improved the timing of preoperative antibiotic administration and observed a reduction in SSIs with a computerized reminder system.

Less certain than the efficacy of prophylactic antibiotics before surgery is the practice of elimination of intranasal carriage of *S. aureus* by the application of mupirocin to the nares. *S. aureus* is a common pathogen in wound infections and intranasal carriage is a risk factor for cardiovascular surgical infections (86). Decolonization requires further study, and, at present, this strategy cannot be routinely recommended for reducing SSIs.

DIRECT INTERVENTIONS FOR PREVENTING NOSOCOMIAL INFECTIONS

Investigation and control of outbreaks are best accomplished by personnel with training and experience in infection control and hospital epidemiology. Basic training in infection control and hospital epidemiology is offered to professionals by SHEA and CDC as well as APIC, and is highly recommended. Certification in infection control is a desirable qualification for infection control practitioners. Effective outbreak management requires the coordinated efforts of a good microbiology laboratory (access to molecular typing techniques such as pulsed-field gel electrophoresis); an effective antibiotic stewardship program; a compliant staff; and a responsive, supportive hospital administration. In significant outbreaks, infection control professionals should seek the help of their state health departments and/or the CDC. There may be a reluctance to go outside the institution for assistance in the investigation and control of an outbreak, but the help provided by public health professionals and epidemiologists may be extremely valuable and instructive, especially at institutions where resources are limited and experienced personnel are not available.

The Control of Antibiotic-Resistant Organisms

Hospitals, especially ICUs, are important epicenters for resistance. Unfortunately, some resistant organisms are endemic in many hospitals. Recent literature suggests that antibiotic-resistant organisms may be successfully managed by multidisciplinary efforts that include enhanced contact precautions, proper environmental cleaning, effective antibiotic stewardship, and a return to the basics of health care worker hand hygiene. Whether or not antibiotic-resistant organisms are endemic or epidemic at a hospital, policies aimed at reducing transmission of infectious agents still apply.

It is clear that resistance is related, in some way, to the intensity of antimicrobial use in a population (87). At least 70% of the bacteria responsible for nosocomial infections are resistant to at least one of the drugs most commonly selected to treat them (40). In the presence of resistant strains, treatment with an antibiotic to which the organisms are resistant provides selective pressure for the emergence of these strains (Table 1).

The rise of antibiotic resistance is a significant global health problem. The continuing spread of MRSA, VRE, and extended-spectrum beta-lactamase–producing organisms (ESBLs) and the recent appearance of vancomycin-resistant *S. aureus* (VRSA) are alarming. The CDC, U.S. Public Health Service, World Health Organization (WHO), and other agencies recognize infection control as a key component in curtailing the spread of resistance (40,88). Nicolle (88) reviewed the role of infection control programs in controlling antimicrobial resistance as a background document for WHO. More recently, Muto et al. (89) published an exhaustive review of interventions for controlling the transmission of MRSA and VRE and proposed evidence-based recommendations, which have been adopted as SHEA guidelines. There is debate in the literature over the strength of evidence for infection control measures in preventing the spread of resistant organisms, but the appearance of vancomycin-resistant strains of *S. aureus*—with some evidence that VRE isolates may transfer resistance to staphylococci—is viewed by some as a signal that more rigorous infection control measures are needed (90).

Table 1 Drug-Resistant Organisms of Epidemiologic Importance in Hospitals

Organism	Resistant to
Staphylococcus aureus	Methicillin (MRSA)
	Vancomycin (VISA, VRSA)
Staphylococcus epidermidis	Vancomycin
Enterococci	Ampicillin
	Vancomycin (VRE)
	Aminoglycosides
Streptococcus pneumoniae	Penicillin
	Cephalosporins
	Macrolides
	Fluoroquinolones
Enterobacteriaceae	Aminoglycosides
	Third-generation cephalosporins
	Monobactams
	Ceftazidime
Pseudomonas aeruginosa	Extended-spectrum penicillins
	Fluoroquinolones
	Ceftazidime
	Carbapenems
	Aminoglycosides
Acinetobacter spp	Aminoglycosides
	Ceftazidime
	Carbapenems
Mycobacterium tuberculosis	Isoniazid
	Rifampin
	Ethambutol
	Pyrazinamide
	Streptomycin
Candida spp	Amphotericin B
	Azoles
Herpes simplex	Acyclovir
Cytomegalovirus	Foscarnet

MRSA, methicillin-resistant *S. aureus*; VISA, vancomycin intermediate-susceptible *S. aureus*; VRE, vancomycin-resistant enterococci; VRSA, vancomycin-resistant *S. aureus*.
Modified from Nicolle L. Infection control programmes to contain antimicrobial resistance. Available at: http://www.who.int/csr/resources/publications/drugresist/WHO_CDS_CSR_DRS_2001_7/en/ (accessed on August 15, 2003).

Methicillin-Resistant *S. aureus*

The acquisition of the **staphylococcal cassette chromosome mec** by a sensitive strain confers resistance to methicillin (91; cited in 89). Epidemiologic evidence suggests that the spread of MRSA has been caused by a few clonal types, introduced into a population by infected or colonized patients, rather than the frequent de novo development of new MRSA clones (91–97; cited in 89). Interrupting transmission is an appropriate strategy in controlling this type of spread (89).

Muto et al. pointed out that countries in which transmission-based control policies (**surveillance cultures** to identify colonized patients and strict barrier precautions for patients infected or colonized) are in effect have seen substantial reductions in the prevalence of MRSA. The authors attributed sustained reductions in resistance in Denmark, Finland, and the Netherlands to national hospital infection control policies that include surveillance cultures to identify colonized patients and staff, cohort nursing, barrier precautions, and isolating patients from other countries until screening cultures indicate they are not colonized or infected with MRSA.

Methicillin-resistant *S. aureus* transmission occurs predominantly within health care settings, but community-acquired infection is well documented, and increasing spread in this venue could impede efforts to control hospital spread (98,99). There are selective advantages afforded MRSA strains by antibiotic use that favor person-to-person transmission, but antibiotic usage does not always correlate with MRSA prevalence (89). Therefore, infection control practices directed at interrupting transmission remain necessary for successful control of MRSA.

Vancomycin-Resistant Enterococci

The majority of vancomycin resistance in enterococci is the result of *van*A and *van*B gene clusters (100). Most, if not all, VRE infection and colonization are caused by the transmission of VRE or the transfer of these gene clusters; vancomycin resistance does not appear to arise spontaneously in patients exposed to vancomycin (101–103; cited in 89). VRE is almost always associated with health care in the United States, as opposed to Europe, where *van*A or *van*B VRE isolates have been found in healthy people, farm animals, and food products (89). In general, a single clonal strain is usually responsible for an initial outbreak of VRE in a health care setting. However, where the organism has persisted, multiple clones may be found—possibly because of the transfer of resistance genes to multiple strains of sensitive enterococci, the introduction of new strains, or both (89,104,105).

Antibiotics exert selective pressure that favors the growth of acquired VRE strains in the stool, making transmission more likely (106). The colonization pressure of VRE in a given unit is a strong predictor of VRE acquisition, and the effect of antibiotic pressure may be less of a factor when colonization pressure is high (31). Muto et al. (89) concluded that only modest reductions in VRE transmission can be achieved through antibiotic controls, and, as with MRSA, infection control interventions are more likely to be successful.

Interventions for the Control of Methicillin-Resistant *S. aureus* and Vancomycin-Resistant Enterococci

Hand Hygiene and Gloves

Both VRE and MRSA can survive on the hands of health care workers, and persistence on environmental surfaces may be a source of contamination of health care workers' hands and gloves (107–109). Proximity to patients with VRE, shared caregivers, and colonization pressure within a unit are predictors of VRE acquisition (31,110–112). One stochastic mathematical model predicted that even a moderate increase in hand hygiene during periods of understaffing or overcrowding—conditions that are likely to favor poor hand hygiene—in an ICU could decrease transmission as effectively as placing patients in cohorts (113). It can be inferred from these and other studies that improvement in hand hygiene should reduce the transmission of these organisms. Yet, compliance with hand hygiene guidelines has been distressingly poor, despite the acknowledged efficacy of this simple intervention. Therefore, hand hygiene should be a part of a broader set of interventions.

Gloves are known to reduce hand contamination and/or the transmission of pathogens in healthcare settings and, as previously noted, universal gloving has been associated with significant reductions in the transmission of VRE. Although studies support the role of gloves in reducing hand contamination, changing gloves between patients—VRE can be recovered from gloves following routine examination of a patient—and hand hygiene are still strongly advocated (107,109).

Gowns

Some transmission of drug-resistant organisms is probably the result of the contamination of health care workers' apparel. Although the role of gowns is not entirely clear, they have been shown to reduce transmission of VRE and MRSA, and most studies appear to support their utility (89). Although Slaughter et al. (38) could not demonstrate that gowns added additional benefit over gloving in their study, Puzniak et al. (112) demonstrated a beneficial effect of gowns in reducing VRE transmission in a medical ICU when colonization pressure was high.

Masks

The protective effect of masks is difficult to quantify. Because of potential airborne transmission of staphylococci, nasal colonization, and shedding of staphylococci by patients and health care workers, there is some theoretic rationale for the use of masks in contact precautions for MRSA, vancomycin intermediate-susceptible *S. aureus*, and VRSA (89).

Equipment and Environmental Disinfection

Portable equipment that is used on more than one patient—stethoscopes, for instance—can transport pathogens either directly or by contaminating hands and gloves (114–116). Using dedicated or disposable equipment and cleaning equipment between patients are recommended (89,117). The cleaning and disinfection of equipment and environmental surfaces to inactivate drug-resistant organisms, particularly in areas that come into frequent contact with the hands of health care workers, should be carried out as outlined in the current CDC guidelines for environmental infection control (117). Routine cultures of the environment add to the expense of controlling outbreaks and are *not* recommended, but they may be useful in verifying that adequate environmental cleaning is taking place, especially in settings where VRE transmission is continuing despite control measures (117).

Surveillance Cultures, Contact Isolation, and
Antibiotic Controls

In response to the rising incidence of VRE infections in the United States, HICPAC issued guidelines in 1994 that raised the possibility that periodic screening cultures of stool or rectal swabs might facilitate the control of VRE by identifying colonized patients, especially among high-risk populations. However, the incidence of vancomycin resistance among hospital isolates of enterococci continued to rise (118).

A number of studies have reported control of VRE when the CDC guidelines are rigorously applied, that is, when active surveillance cultures are part of control measures (119). An important investigation conducted by Ostrowsky et al. (120) in 32 health care facilities in the Siouxland region of South Dakota, Iowa, and Nebraska demonstrated that control of VRE could be accomplished in a health care system through surveillance cultures to detect colonization in high-risk patients, isolation of colonized patients, and the use of barrier precautions—without an active attempt to reduce antibiotic use. It also supported an approach that involves not only acute care facilities, but all facilities in a region—an approach that many experts feel is necessary for the control of emerging resistance.

Among the more controversial recommendations in the SHEA guideline is a call for broader application of active surveillance cultures to screen patients for colonization with MRSA or VRE. Yet, active surveillance cultures in conjunction with contact precautions for colonized or infected patients may be better than standard precautions alone and is associated with reductions in rates of colonization and infection with MRSA and VRE in many studies (89,121). Calfee et al. (119) reported sustained control of VRE at the University of Virginia Hospital over a 5-year period, which they largely attributed to the use of surveillance cultures to identify asymptomatic, colonized patients. As Harbarth and Pittet (122) pointed out, most published reports of successful control of these two organisms have included active surveillance cultures and contact precautions among their interventions.

Vriens et al. (123) reported a higher frequency of transmission of MRSA from unidentified carriers than from identified patients who were isolated in an ICU. In one epidemic, proximity to colonized, nonisolated patients with VRE was an important risk factor for acquisition of VRE; however, proximity to isolated patients who were VRE positive was not (111). Indeed, the proportion of colonized patients who are undetected in the absence of active surveillance cultures may be significant—86% in one study (119). The authors of the SHEA guideline found the correlation of these measures with control of MRSA and VRE in the many studies they analyzed compelling enough to strongly recommend instituting an active surveillance program for resistant pathogens (89).

The SHEA guideline also recommends surveillance cultures at the time of admission for patients at high-risk (or *all* patients if the facility has a high prevalence rate on initial screening) for carriage of MRSA and/or VRE, as well as periodic point-prevalence culture surveys in high-risk areas or throughout an institution, depending on prevalence (89).

However, a study by D'Agata et al. (124) raises concerns about the sensitivity of peri-rectal cultures for VRE colonization (only 58% in this study). Technologic innovations such as polymerase chain reaction assay for active surveillance may increase response times and reduce unnecessary isolation by identifying colonized patients more quickly than cultures (125).

Wider use of surveillance cultures as proposed in the SHEA guideline has already been challenged. Although some have argued that this is a cost-effective approach, the anticipated high cost of implementing these measures has generated concern, as the impact on health care resources could be considerable (126–128). Much of the evidence used to support these recommendations is derived from outbreak investigations in which multiple interventions are commonly instituted, making the contribution of individual interventions difficult to quantify. Our own experience in successfully achieving and sustaining reductions in the incidence of MRSA and VRE in a thirty-two bed ICU suggests the merits of a multifaceted approach, such as that advocated in the SHEA recommendations, but the difficulties of identifying the most effective interventions are apparent (129). In the future, mathematical models may lead to a better understanding of the proportional influence of particular interventions in multifaceted approaches and guide the development of rational strategies (130).

Extended-Spectrum and AmpC Beta-Lactamase–Producing Gram-Negative Bacteria

Extended-spectrum beta-lactamases were first recognized in 1983, shortly after the introduction of cefotaxime (131). Subsequently, AmpC beta-lactamases, which had been investigated since the late 1970s, were detected on bacterial plasmids and transferred to organisms that did not usually elaborate these enzymes (132). ESBL-producing gram-negative bacteria were initially detected in Europe, but outbreaks in the United States followed. Efforts to control these organisms are hampered by a lack of awareness of their clinical significance, largely because of under-reporting by hospital microbiology laboratories.

Most ESBLs are mutants of the older, broad-spectrum beta-lactamases: TEM-1, TEM-2, and SHV-1. These enzymes hydrolyze all cephalosporins, penicillins, and aztreonam; cephamycins and carbapenems are not affected. They are found most often in *Klebsiella* and *E.coli*, but they have been detected in other Enterobacteriaceae, *Pseudomonas aeruginosa*, *Burkholderia cepacia*, and *Capnocytophaga ochracea*. Plasmid-mediated AmpC beta-lactamases occur in *E. coli*,

Klebsiella pneumoniae, Salmonella, Citrobacter freundii, Enterobacter aerogenes, and *Proteus mirabilis* (131).

The National Committee for Clinical Laboratory Standards (NCCLS) guideline was issued in 1999 to help laboratories screen for and confirm ESBL production in *K. pneumonia, Klebsiella oxytoca,* and *E.coli.* (133) Potential producers are detected by the zone of inhibition (disk diffusion method) around disks containing cefpodoxime (22 mm or less), ceftazidime (22 mm or less), aztreonam (27 mm or less), cefotaxime (27 mm or less), or ceftriaxone (25 mm or less); or the minimum inhibitory concentration of these agents (2 µg/mL or greater) in the broth dilution method. Phenotypic confirmation requires further testing of the suspected isolate against ceftazidime and ceftazidime-clavulanate or cefotaxime and cefotaxime-clavulanate. The methods are relatively easy and should be available to most microbiology laboratories, but require extra labor and expense. Unfortunately, the test has a number of limitations: It does not detect ESBL-producing strains outside of *Klebsiella* and *E.coli,* it identifies the phenotype rather than genotype, and organisms that contain AmpC or other beta-lactamases can mask ESBL production, resulting in false-negative results (118,131).

Surveys done to determine the ability of laboratories to detect ESBLs have been disappointing. ICARE reported that 58% of laboratories were unable to detect them (134). A survey by Tenover et al. (135) of thirty-eight clinical laboratories reported that only seven correctly categorized and reported ESBLs and AmpC strains sent to them. Although underdetection is a problem, incorrect identification of a strain as an ESBL producer may also lead to improper antibiotic selection.

Rationale for Interventions in the Control of Extended-Spectrum Beta-Lactamase–Producing Organisms

As with other nosocomial gram-negative infections, risk factors for acquiring ESBLs include indwelling catheter, increased severity of illness, emergency abdominal surgery, ventilator use, and prolonged hospital stay, among others.

Lautenbach et al. (136) at the University of Pennsylvania Medical Center analyzed risk factors for infection with ESBL-producing *Klebsiella* and *E. coli* versus non–ESBL-producing *E. coli* and *Klebsiella* isolates and found that ESBL-infected patients had a greater cumulative antibiotic exposure than did controls. Total antibiotic exposure was the only independent predictor of infections with these organisms in their study. Certain antibiotics were associated with infection—extended-spectrum cephalosporins, cotrimoxazole, and aminoglycosides—suggesting that spread of ESBLs may be aided by the selective effect of other antibiotics with resistance factors on the same plasmid. Therefore, curbing inappropriate use of all classes may be important. The investigators concluded that control measures must focus on limiting contact transmission of resistant isolates as well as controlling antibiotic use (136). Here again, there may be a role for the kinds of interventions described for MRSA and VRE in controlling multidrug-resistant gram-negative bacteria (137).

These organisms are likely to have a significant impact in the future. Lautenbach et al. (136) found that infection with ESBL-producing *Klebsiella* and *E. coli* was associated with significantly longer durations of hospital stay and increased hospital charges than were infections due to susceptible organisms. Also, appropriate treatment of ESBLs may also lead to resistance; therefore, containing these organisms should be a priority (Fig. 5).

Before effective control of ESBLs can be accomplished, more education about these organisms is needed. Clinical microbiology laboratories should be encouraged to look for these organisms and be given adequate resources for appropriate screening and confirmation. As with MRSA and VRE, early detection of ESBLs should lead to earlier treatment of infected patients and enable infection control departments to muster appropriate interventions, such as periodic screening, the use of cohorts, and contact precautions for infected or colonized patients (138,139).

Multidrug-Resistant Tuberculosis

Multidrug-resistant tuberculosis is a globally important problem and a major concern of infection control. Known or sus-

---

- Laboratories should follow NCCLS guidelines for detecting ESBLs among **all** isolates of *Klebsiella pneumoniae* and *Escherichia coli* and should report these to clinicians and infection control.
- Proper hand hygiene, gloves, and gowns should be used when caring for infected orcolonized patients.
- Educate clinical and laboratory staff, visitors, and patients about these organisms.
- Affected patients should be grouped in cohorts, and staffing assignments should minimize the potential for cross-transmission.
- Periodic rectal swabs and urine cultures of patients in ICUs to identify carriers.
- Antibiotic controls, especially of extended-spectrum cephalosporins, should be instituted.
- Inform receiving units or other facilities of infected or colonized patients.
- Since carriage can persist for months, previously colonized or infected patients should be regarded as colonized until proven otherwise, and medical records should be flagged so that status is known at readmission.
- Colonized or infected patients may be admitted to nursing homes, where they should be placed in single rooms with private bathrooms. The use of common areas by these patients should be considered on an individual basis.

Figure 5 Suggested interventions for the control of extended-spectrum beta-lactamase (ESBL)-producing organisms in outbreaks. ICU, intensive care unit; NCCLS, National Committee for Clinical Laboratory Standards. (Adapted from Paterson DL, Yu VL. Editorial response: extended-spectrum β-lactamases: a call for improved detection and control. Clin Infect Dis 1999; 29:1419–1422.)

pected cases should be managed using airborne precautions. Negative-pressure rooms and the use of N95 masks or powered air-purifying respirators (PAPRs) protect other patients and employees. High-risk patients (those with HIV, immunocompromised patients) with pneumonias of unknown etiology should be placed on precautions until *Mycobacterium tuberculosis* is ruled out (140).

MANAGING THE ENVIRONMENT

A clean patient care environment and proper disinfection of reusable equipment should be part of an overall program to reduce the transmission of susceptible and resistant microbes. Outbreaks associated with equipment and environmental reservoirs are described. The exact contribution of the environment in hospital-acquired infections is difficult to prove in all cases, but the elimination, disinfection, or sterilization of environmental sources can contribute to control (88). Infection control personnel should review and contribute to all policies related to air handling, clinical waste disposal, laundry, and cleaning and disinfecting of the environment of care.

Nosocomial infections due to fungi, molds, and bacteria have been linked to hospital construction (141). Proper preparation before construction reduces the incidence of *Aspergillus* infections, which are costly to treat and often lethal (142). Therefore, it is important that infection control personnel be consulted in the planning, design, renovation, and construction of any new clinical facilities. Infection control professionals should work to ensure that designs incorporate the appropriate number and proper location of sinks, isolation rooms, clean and dirty utility rooms, storage areas, and so on. Several useful publications in this area can be retrieved or purchased online, including the CDC's *Guideline for Environmental Infection Control in Health-Care* (www.cdc.gov), the American Institute of Architecture's *Guidelines for Design and Construction of Hospital and Health Care Facilities* (www.aia.org), and APIC's *Construction and Renovation Toolkit* (www.apic.org) (117,143).

RESOURCES FOR INFECTION CONTROL

Information Resources

There are many resources available to the infection control-professional. Search engines and online journals have substantially improved access to information. The CDC (www.cdc.gov), SHEA (www.shea-online.org), IDSA (www.idsociety.org), APIC (www.apic.org), Hospital Infection Society (www.his.org.uk), Infection Control Nurses Association (www.icna.co.uk), and other sources of high-quality information may be accessed on the Internet. These sites provide links to their journals and guidelines. Some offer links to discussion groups in which information is shared or advice is available. Several web-based alert services are available, such as the Emerging Infectious Disease list-serve from the CDC, ProMED-mail (www.promed-mail.org), and the National Center for Infectious Diseases/ Division of Healthcare Quality Promotion Rapid Notification e-mail system (www.cdc.gov/ncidod/hip).

It is still necessary to have a reference library. Some recommended texts include:

Mayhall CG, ed. Hospital Epidemiology and Infection Control. 2nd ed. Philadelphia: Lippincott Williams & Wilkins, 1999.

Wenzel RP, ed. Prevention and Control of Nosocomial Infections. 4th ed. Philadelphia: Lippincott Williams & Wilkins, 2003.

Abrutyn E, Goldmann DA, Scheckler WE, eds. Saunders Infection Control Reference Service: The Experts' Guide to the Guidelines. 2nd ed. Philadelphia: WB Saunders, 2001.

Herwaldt LA, Decker MA, eds. A Practical Handbook for Hospital Epidemiologists/The Society for Healthcare Epidemiology of America. Thorofare, NJ: Slack Incorporated, 1998. *This is a highly recommended resource for beginners in hospital epidemiology. An updated edition is in preparation.*

Mandel GL, Bennett JE, Dolin R, eds. Principles and Practice of Infectious Diseases. 5th ed. Philadelphia: Churchill Livingstone, 2000.

Pickering LK, ed. 2003 Red Book: Report of the Committee on Infectious Diseases. 26th ed. Elk Grove Village, IL: American Academy of Pediatrics, 2003.

Financial Resources: An Uncertain Future

Although there is abundant evidence supporting the effectiveness of good infection control in reducing nosocomial infections, infection control personnel and hospital epidemiologists face the problem of functioning effectively in a cost-conscious environment. The cost-sparing effect of prevention is not appreciated as readily as the benefit of programs that generate revenue for an institution. Moreover, infection control programs are finding themselves competing with other quality initiatives for funding. There may be considerable overlap and duplication of efforts to monitor adverse events and improve performance.

Infection control professionals do not operate in a vacuum nor should they be viewed as having sole responsibility for reducing nosocomial infections (144). Infection control departments must collaborate with other health care professionals in a team-oriented approach to develop interventions for reducing infections (144,145). Hospitals should be encouraged to standardize and coordinate efforts to measure and improve outcomes.

It is clear that the cost of nosocomial infections represents a substantial burden for the health care system: Increased length of stay, the price of medications, private rooms, precautions, and numerous other factors contribute to cost. However, cost–benefit analyses of infection control interventions are plagued by complexity, especially when multiple interventions are initiated at the same time—a common practice in managing clusters and outbreaks. There is a need for better analytic tools and data. Despite the complexity, there is increasing interest in developing sound assessment guidelines (146).

Antimicrobial resistance is an additional burden on the resources of a hospital, and understanding the impact of antimicrobial resistance on outcomes and costs is critical for those responsible for allocating resources for surveillance and control of resistant organisms (146). Resistance can alter microbial virulence, delay appropriate therapy, increase toxicity, prolong hospital stays, and increase mortality. Studies have shown MRSA to be more costly than methicillin-susceptible

S. aureus bloodstream infections (147). Not surprisingly, the same is true of VRE infections compared with vancomycin-sensitive enterococci (148). The appearance of VRSA is likely to represent an even greater cost in lives and dollars in the future.

Paradoxically, antimicrobial resistance can be seen as having some beneficial effects on infection control (88). Often the drug-resistant isolate draws attention to process break-downs that would otherwise go unnoticed. Efforts aimed at control are likely to reduce the transmission of other organisms, improve outcomes, and lead to better practices. On the other hand, some infection control practices, such as anti-microbial prophylaxis and efforts to decolonize health care personnel or patients, may contribute to the development of resistance.

CONCLUSION

If infection control professionals wish to preserve their leader-ship in the patient safety arena, they must be willing to edu-cate a wider audience than ever before on the importance of reducing hospital-acquired infections, because the responsibil-ity for reducing these infections rests on the shoulders of all who work in or utilize health care. Whereas those who manage the financial resources of a hospital should have an apprecia-tion for the evolution, methodology, and effectiveness of infec-tion control, infection control professionals have an equally important obligation to understand and be willing to discuss the impact of their interventions on the resources of their facil-ities. Of course, this is of even greater importance at the state and national levels. This will require some shift in the focus of health care epidemiology, but making the "business case" for infection control is necessary if it is to remain a prominent advocate for patient safety (144). Along with antibiotic stew-ardship, a vigorous and comprehensively applied infection con-trol program can reduce infections, antimicrobial use, and resistance; preserve health care resources; and improve the well-being of patients (149).

The author wishes to thank Sheridan Dirrigl, RN, CIC, and Gwen Rogers, RN, MS, CIC, for their review and suggestions.

REFERENCES

1. Burke JP. Infection control—a problem for patient safety N Engl J Med 2003; 348;7:651–656.

2. Kohn LT, Corrigan JM, Donaldson MS. To Err Is Human: Building a Safer Health System. Washington, DC: National Academy Press, 1999.

3. Public health focus: surveillance, prevention, and control of nosocomial infections MMWR Morb Mortal Wkly Rep 1992; 41:783–787.

4. Weinstein RA. Nosocomial infection update Emerg Infect Dis 1998; 4:416–420.

5. Haley RW, Culver DH, White JW, Morgan WM, Emori TG, Munn VP, Hooton TM. The efficacy of infection surveillance and control programs in preventing nosocomial infections in U.S. hospitals Am J Epidemiol 1985; 121:182–205.

6. Hooton TM. Standards: Infection Control. JCAHO Accreditation Manual for Hospitals. Chicago: Joint Commission on Accreditation of Hospitals, 1964.

7. Garner JS, Bennett JV, Scheckler WE, Maki DG, Brachman PS. Surveillance of nosocomial infections, in Centers for Disease Control. In: Proceedings of the International Conference on Nosocomial Infections. Atlanta: Centers for Disease Control, 1970:277–281.

8. Scheckler WE, Brimhall D, Buck AS, Farr BM, Friedman C. SHEA position paper: requirements for infrastructure and essential activities of infection control and epidemiology in hospitals: a consensus panel report Infect Control Hosp Epidemiol 1998; 19:114–124.

9. Friedman C. Update guidelines for evaluating public health surveillance systems: recommendations from the guidelines working group MMWR Morb Mortal Wkly Rep 2001; 50: 13–24.

10. Edmond MB. National and international surveillance systems for nosocomial infections. In: Wenzel RP, Ed Prevention and Control of Nosocomial Infections. Philadelphia: Lippincott Williams & Wilkins, 2003:109–119.

11. Horan TC, Emori TG. Definitions of nosocomial infections. In: Abrutyn E, Goldmann DA, Scheckler WE, Eds Saunders Infection Control Reference Service: The Experts' Guide to the Guidelines. 2nd ed. Philadelphia: WB Saunders, 2001:25–40.

12. Gaynes RP, Emori TG. Surveillance of nosocomial infections. In: Abrutyn E, Goldmann DA, Scheckler WE, Eds Saunders Infection Control Reference Service: The Experts' Guide to the Guidelines. 2nd ed. Philadelphia: WB Saunders, 2001:41–44.

13. Pottinger JM, Herwaldt LA, Perl TM. Basics of surveillance. In: Herwaldt LA, Decker MA, Eds A Practical Handbook for Hospital Epidemiologists/The Society for Healthcare Epidemiology of America. Thorofare, NJ: Slack Incorporated, 1998: 59–78.

14. Decker MA. National Nosocomial Infections Surveillance (NNIS) System Report, data summary from January 1992 to June 2002, issued August 2002 Am J Infect Control 2002; 30: 458–75.

15. Roy M, Perl TM. Basics of surgical site infection surveillance. In: Herwaldt LA, Decker MA, Eds. A Practical Handbook for Hospital Epidemiologists/The Society for Healthcare Epidemiology of America. Thorofare, NJ: Slack Incorporated, 1998: 59–78.

16. Culver DH, Horan TC, Gaynes RP, Martone WJ, Jarvis WR, Emori TG, Banerjee SN, Edwards JR, Tolson JS, Henderson TS. Surgical wound infection rates by wound class, operative procedure, and patient risk index Am J Med 1991; 91(suppl 3B):152S–157S.

17. Burke JP, Classen DC, Pestotnik SL, Evans RS, Stevens LE. The HELP system and its application to infection control J Hosp Infect 1991; 18:(suppl A):424–431.

18. Glowacki RC, Schwartz DN, Itokazu GS, Wisniewski MF, Kieszkowski P. Antibiotic combinations with redundant antimicrobial spectra: clinical epidemiology and pilot intervention

of computer-assisted surveillance Clin Infect Dis 2003; 37: 59–64.

19. Fayyad UM, Piatetsky-Shapiro B, Smyth P, Uthurusamy R. From data mining to knowledge discovery: an overview. In: Fayyad UM, Piatetsky-Shapiro B, Smyth P, Uthurusamy R, Eds Advances in Knowledge Discovery and Data Mining. Cambridge, MA: AAAI Press, 1996:1–34.

20. Peterson LR, Brossette SE. Hunting health care–associated infections from the clinical microbiology laboratory: passive, active, and virtual surveillance J Clin Microbiol 2002; 40:1–4.

21. Brossette SE, Sprague AP, Jones WT, Moser SA. A data mining system for infection control surveillance Methods Inf Med 2000; 39:303–310.

22. Hymel PA, Brossette SE. Data mining enhanced infection control surveillance—sensitivity and specificity [abstr], Society for Healthcare Epidemiology of America Annual Meeting, April 1–3, 2001, Toronto.

23. Brosette SE, Taylor BD, Warren B, Avent KC, Moser SA. Improving infection control surveillance using data mining technology [abstr #1215], 41st Interscience Conference on Antimicrobial Agents and Chemotherapy, Dec 16–19, 2001, Chicago.

24. Branca D, Gould MA. A reduction in bloodstream infections in an oncology unit following data mining surveillance and targeted interventions [abstr #108], 13th Annual Scientific Meeting of the Society for Healthcare Epidemiology of America, April 5–8, 2003, Arlington, VA.

25. Vason B, Gould MA. Cluster of community-acquired, respiratory infections of *Serratia marcescens* identified at a children's hospital employing data mining surveillance [abstr #118], 13th Annual Scientific Meeting of the Society for Healthcare Epidemiology of America, April 5–8, Arlington, VA.

26. Abrutyn E, Goldmann DA, Scheckler WE. Saunders Infection Control Reference Service: The Experts' Guide to the Guidelines. 2nd ed. Philadelphia: WB Saunders, 2001.

27. Garner JS,. the Hospital Infection Control Practices Advisory Committee: Guidelines for isolation precautions in hospitals Infect Control Hosp Epidemiol 1996; 17:53–80.

28. Weinstein RA. Controlling antimicrobial resistance in hospitals: infection control and use of antibiotics Emerg Infect Dis 2001; 7:188–192.

29. Boyce JM, Pittet D. Guidelines for hand hygiene in healthcare settings: recommendations of the Healthcare Infection Control Practices Advisory Committee and the HICPAC HEA APIC IDSA Hand Hygiene Task Force Am J of Infect Control; 2002; 30:S1–S46.

30. Boyce JM, Kelliher S, Valleande N, Korber S, Denicola G, Fedo J. Hand disinfection with an alcoholic gel causes less skin irritation and dryness of nurses' hands than soap and water handwashing. [abstr #78], 9th Annual Society for Healthcare Epidemiology of America Meeting, April 19–20, 1999, San Francisco.

31. Bonten JM, Slaughter S, Ambergen A, Hayden MK, van Voorhis J, Nathan C, Weinstein RA. The role of "colonization pressure" in the spread of vancomycin-resistant enterococci Arch Intern Med 1998; 158:1127–1132.

32. Weinstein RA, Kabins SA. Strategies for the prevention and control of multiple drug resistant nosocomial infections Am J Med 1981; 70:449–454.

33. Johnson S, Gerding DN, Olson MM, Weiler MD, Hughes RA, Clabots CR, Peterson LR. Prospective, controlled study of vinyl glove use to interrupt *Clostridium difficile* nosocomial transmission Am J Med 1990; 88:137–140.

34. Hartstein AI, Denny MA, Morthland VH, LeMonte AM, Pfaller MA. Control of methicillin-resistant *Staphylococcus aureus* in a hospital intensive care unit Infect Control Hosp Epidemiol 1995; 16:405–411.

35. Badri SM, Sahgal NB, Tenorio AR, Law K, Hota B, Matushek M. Effectiveness of gloves in preventing the transmission of vancomycin-resistant *Enterococcus* (VRE) during patient care activities. [abstr #599], 36th Annual Meeting of the Infectious Diseases Society of America, Nov 11–14, 1998, Denver, CO.

36. Tenorio AR, Badri SM, Sahgal NB, Hota B, Matushek M, Hayden MK, Trenholme GM, Weinstein RA. Effectiveness of gloves in the prevention of hand carriage of vancomycin-resis-

tant *Enterococcus* species by health-care workers after patient care Clin Infect Dis 2001; 32:826–829.

37. Trick WE, DeMarais PL, Jarvis WR, Tomaska W, Ohlrich S, Hagemean J. Comparison of universal gloving to contact isolation precautions to prevent transmission of multidrug-resistant bacteria in a long-term care facility, 4th Decennial International Conference, March 5–9, 2000, Atlanta.

38. Slaughter S, Hayden MK, Nathan C, Hu TC, Rice T, van Voorhis J, Matushek M, Franklin C, Weinstein RA. A comparison of the effect of universal gloves and gowns with that of glove use alone on acquisition of vancomycin-resistant enterococci in a medical intensive care unit Ann Intern Med 1996; 125:448–456.

39. Muto CA, Byers KE, Karchmer TB, Dill JB, Durbin LJ, Farr BM. Controlling vancomycin-resistant enterococcus (VRE) at a university hospital [abstr 52:28], 7th Annual Meeting of the Society for Healthcare Epidemiology of America, April 27–29, 2000, St. Louis, MO.

40. Centers for Disease Control and Prevention. Campaign to Prevent Antimicrobial Resistance in Healthcare Settings: Why a Campaign? Atlanta: Centers for Disease Control and Prevention, 2001. Available at: www.cdc.gov/drugresistance/health care/problem.htm.

41. Doebbeling BN, Breneman DL, Neu HC, Aly R, Yangco BG, Holley HP Jr, Marsh RJ, Pfaller MA, McGowan JE Jr, Scully BE. Elimination of *Staphylococcus aureus* nasal carriage in health care workers: analysis of six clinical trials with mupirocin calcium ointment. The Mupirocin Collaborative Study Group Clin Infect Dis 1993; 17:466–474.

42. Doebbeling BN, Regan DR, Pfaller MA, Houston AK, Hollis RJ, Wenzel RP. Long term efficacy of intranasal mupirocin ointment: a prospective cohort study of *Staphylococcus aureus* carriage Arch Intern Med 1994; 154:1505–1508.

43. Boelaert JR, Van Landuyt HW, Godard CA, Daneels RF, Schurgers ML, Matthys EG, De Baere YA, Gheyle DW, Gordts BZ, Herwaldt LA. Nasal mupirocin ointment decreases the incidence of *Staphylococcus aureus* bacteraemias in haemodialysis patients Nephrol Dial Transplant 1993; 8:235–239.

44. Herwaldt LA. Nasal mupirocin prevents *Staphylococcus aureus* exit site infection during peritoneal dialysis J Am Soc Nephrol 1996; 7:2403–2408.

45. Mehtar S. New strategies for the use of mupirocin for the prevention of serious infection J Hosp Infect 1998; 40(suppl B): S39–S44.

46. Perl TM, Cullen JJ, Wenzel RP, Zimmerman MB, Pfaller MA, Sheppard D, Twombley J, French PP, Herwaldt LA. Mupirocin and the Risk of *Staphylococcus aureus* Study Team. Intranasal mupirocin to prevent postoperative staphylococcus aureus infections N Engl J Med 2002; 346:1871–1877.

47. Centers for Disease Control. National Nosocomial Infections Study Report. Atlanta: Centers for Disease Control, Nov 1979: 2–14.

48. Wong ES, Hooton TM. Guideline for Prevention of Catheter-Associated Urinary Tract Infections. Atlanta: U.S. Department of Health and Human Services, US Department of Commerce, National Technical Information Service. 1982:1–5.

49. Jain P, Parada JP, David A, Smith LG. Overuse of the indwelling urinary tract catheter in hospitalized medical patients Arch Intern Med 1995; 155:1425–1429.

50. Gribble MJ, Puterman ML. Prophylaxis of urinary tract infection in persons with recent spinal cord injury: a prospective, randomized, double-blind, placebo-controlled study of trimethoprim-sulfamethoxazole Am J Med;; 1993:141–152.

51. Saint S, Lipsky BA. Preventing catheter-related bacteriuria: Can we? How? Arch Intern Med 1999; 159:800–808.

52. Salgado CD, Karchmer TB, Farr BM. Prevention of catheter-associated urinary tract infections. In: Wenzel RP, Ed Prevention and Control of Nosocomial Infections. Philadelphia: Lippincott Williams & Wilkins, 2003:297–311.

53. Karchmer TB, Giannetta ET, Muto CA, Strain BA, Farr BM. A randomized crossover study of silver-coated urinary catheters in hospitalized patients Arch Intern Med 2000; 160: 3294–3298.

54. Farr BM. Guidelines for the prevention of nosocomial pneumonia MMWR Morb Mortal Wkly Rep 1997; 46:1–79.

55. Steger KA, Tablan OC, Mir J, Craven DE. Preventing nosocomial pneumonia: guidelines for health care workers. In: Abrutyn E, Goldmann DA, Scheckler WE, Eds Saunders Infection Control Reference Service: The Experts' Guide to the Guidelines. 2nd ed. Philadelphia: WB Saunders, 2001:269–279.

56. Mayhall CG. Nosocomial pneumonia: diagnosis and prevention Infect Dis Clin North Am. 1997; 11:427–457.

57. Craven SE, De Rosa FG, Thornton D. Nosocomial pneumonia: emerging concepts in diagnosis, management, and prophylaxis Curr Opin Crit Care 2002; 8:421–429.

58. Richards MJ, Edwards JR, Culver DH, Gaynes RP. Nosocomial infections in combined medical-surgical intensive care units in the United States Infect Contol Hosp Epidemiol 2000; 21:510–515.

59. Vallès J, Artigas A, Rello J, Bonsoms N, Fontanals D, Blanch L, Fernandez R, Baigorri F, Mestre J. Continuous aspiration of subglottic secretions in preventing ventilator-associated pneumonia Ann Intern Med 1995; 122:179–186.

60. Kollef MH, Skubas NJ, Sundt TM. A randomized clinical trial of continuous aspiration of subglottic secretions in cardiac surgery patients Chest 1999; 116:1339–1346.

61. Torres A, Serra-Batlles J, Ros E, Piera C, Puig de la Bellacasa J, Cobos A, Lomena F, Rodriguez-Roisin R. Pulmonary aspiration of gastric contents in patients receiving mechanical ventilation: the effect of body position Ann Intern Med 1992; 116: 540–543.

62. Eggimann P, Pittet D. Infection control in the ICU Chest 2001; 120:2059–2093.

63. Kollef MH, Vlasnik J, Sharpless L, Pasque C, Murphy D, Fraser V. Scheduled change of antibiotic classes: a strategy to decrease the incidence of ventilator-associated pneumonia Am J Respir Crit Care Med 1997; 156:1040–1048.

64. Gruson D, Hilbert G, Vargas F, Valentino R, Bebear C, Allery A, Bebear C, Gbikpi-Benissan G, Cardinaud JP. Rotation and restricted use of antibiotics in a medical intensive care unit. Impact on the incidence of ventilator-associated pneumonia caused by antibiotic-resistant gram-negative bacteria Am J Respir Crit Care Med 2000; 162:837–843.

65. Gruson D, Hilbert G, Vargas F, Valentino R, Bui N, Pereyre S, Bebear C, Bebear CM, Gbikpi-Benissan G. Strategy of antibiotic rotation: long-term effect on incidence and susceptibilities of Gram-negative bacilli responsible for ventilator-associated pneumonia Crit Care Med 2003; 31:1908–1914.

66. Mermel LA. New technologies to prevent intravascular catheter-related bloodstream infections Emerg Inf Dis 2000; 7:197–199.

67. Soifer NE, Borzak S, Edlin BR, Weinstein RA. Prevention of peripheral venous catheter complications with an intravenous therapy team. A randomized controlled study Arch Int Med; 1998; 158:473–477.

68. Curran ET, Coia JE, Gilmour H, McNamee S, Hood J. Multicentre research surveillance project to reduce infections/phlebitis associated with peripheral vascular catheters J Hosp Infect 2000; 46:194–202.

69. Raad II, Hohn DC, Gilbreath J, Suleiman N, Hill LA, Bruso PA, Marts K, Mansfield PF, Bodey GP. Prevention of central venous catheter-related infections by using maximal sterile barrier precautions during insertion Infect Control Hosp Epidemiol 1994; 15:231–238.

70. Timsit JF, Bruneel F, Cheval C, Mamzer MF, Garrouste-Orgeas M, Wolff M, Misset B, Chevret S, Regnier B, Carlet J. Use of tunneled femoral catheters to prevent catheter-related infection. A randomized, controlled trial Ann Intern Med 1999; 130:729–735.

71. Merrer J, De Jonghe B, Golliot F, Lefrant JY, Raffy B, Barre E, Rigaud JP, Casciani D, Misset B, Bosquet C, Outin H, Brun-Buisson C, Nitenberg G. French Catheter Study Group in Intensive Care. Complications of femoral and subclavian venous catheterization in critically ill patients: a randomized controlled trial JAMA 2001; 286:700–707.

72. Darouiche RO. Nosocomial bloodstream infections and second-generation vascular catheters. In: Wenzel RP, Ed Prevention and Control of Nosocomial Infections. Philadelphia: Lippincott Williams & Wilkins, 2003:281–296.

73. McConnell SA, Gubbins PO, Anaissie EJ. Do antimicrobial-impregnated central venous catheters prevent catheter-related bloodstream infection? Clin Infect Dis 2003; 37:65–72.

74. Horan TC, Culver DH, Gaynes RP, Jarvis WR, Edwards JR, Reid CR. Nosocomial infections in surgical patients in the United States, January 1986–June 1992 Infect Control Hosp Epidemiol 1993; 14:73–80.

75. Haley RW, Culver DH, White JW, Morgan WM, Emori TG. The nationwide nosocomial infection rate: a new need for vital statistics Am J Epidemiol 1985; 121:159–167.

76. Mangram AJ, Horan TC, Pearson ML, Silver LC, Jarvis WR. The Hospital Infection Control Practices Advisory Committee. Guideline for the prevention of surgical site infection 1999 Infect Control Hosp Epidemiol 1999; 20:247–280.

77. Nichols RL. Postoperative wound infection N Engl J Med 1995; 307:1701–1702.

78. Nichols RL. Surgical wound infection Am J Med 1991; 91 (suppl 3B):54S–64S.

79. Nichols RL. Preventing surgical site infections: a surgeon's perspective Emerg Infect Dis 2001; 7:220–224.

80. Condon RE, Schulte WJ, Malangoni MA, Anderson-Teschendorf MJ. Effectiveness of a surgical wound surveillance program Arch Surg 1983; 118:303–307.

81. Mead PB, Pories SE, Hall P, Davis JH Jr, Gamelli RL. Decreasing the incidence of surgical wound infections: validation of a surveillance-notification program Arch Surg 1986; 121: 458–461.

82. McConkey SJ, L'Ecuyer PB, Murphy DM, Leet TL, Sundt TM, Fraser VJ. Results of a comprehensive infection control program for reducing surgical-site infections in coronary artery bypass surgery Infect Control Hosp Epidemiol 1999; 20: 553–558.

83. Burke JF. The effective period of preventive antibiotic action in experimental incision and dermal lesions Surgery 1961; 50: 161–168.

84. Larsen RA, Evans RS, Burke JP, Pestotnik SL, Gardner RM, Classen DC. Improved perioperative antibiotic use and reduced surgical wound infections through use of computer decision analysis Infect Control Hosp Epidemiol 1989; 10: 316–320.

85. Burke JP. Maximizing appropriate antibiotic prophylaxis for surgical patients: An update from LDS Hospital, Salt Lake City Clin Inf Dis 2001; 33(suppl 2):S78–S83.

86. Kluytmans JAJW, Mouton JW, Ijzerman EPF, Vanden-broucke-Grauls CA, Maat AW, Wagencourt J, Verbrugh HA. Nasal carriage of *Staphylococcus aureus* as a major risk factor for wound infections after cardiac surgery J Infect Dis 1995; 171:216–219.

87. Jarvis WR. Preventing the emergence of multidrug-resistant microorganisms through antimicrobial use controls: the complexity of the problem Infect Contol Hosp Epidemiol 1996; 17: 491–495.

88. Nicolle L. Infection control programmes to contain antimicrobial resistance. Available at: http://www.who.int/csr/resources/publications/drugresist/WHO_CDS_CSR_DRS_2001_7/en/ (accessed on August 15, 2003).

89. Muto CA, Jernigan JA, Ostrowsky BE, Richet HM, Jarvis WR, Boyce JM, Farr BM, Shea. SHEA guideline for preventing nosocomial transmission of multi-drug-resistant strains of *Staphylococcus aureus* and *Enterococcus* Infect Control Hosp Epidemiol 2003; 24:362–386.

90. Mayhall CG. Letter to the editor Infect Control Hosp Epidemiol. 2003; 24:311–312.

91. Hiramatsu K. Cui L, Kuroda M, Ito T. The emergence and evolution of methicillin-resistant *Staphylococcus aureus* Trends Microbiol; 2001:486–493.

92. Kreiswirth B, Kornblum J, Arbeit WE, Eisner W, Maslow JN, McGeer A, Low DE, Novick RP. Evidence for a clonal origin of methicillin-resistance in *Staphylococcus aureus*. Science 1993; 259:227–230.

93. Oliveira DC, Tomasz A, de Lencastre H. The evolution of pandemic clones of methicillin-resistant *Staphylococcus aureus*: identification of two ancestral genetic backgrounds and the associated mec elements Microb Drug Resist 2001; 7:349–361.

94. Musser J, Kapur V. Clonal analysis of methicillin-resistant *Staphylococcus aureus* from intercontinental sources: association of the mec gene with divergent phylogenetic lineages im-

plies dissemination by horizontal transfer and recombination J Clin Microbiol 1992; 30:2058–2063.

95. Givney R, Vickery A, Holliday A, Pegler M, Benn R. Evolution of an endemic methicillin-resistant *Staphylococcus aureus* population in an Australian hospital from 1967–1996 J Clin Microbiol 1998; 36:552–556.

96. Crisostomo MI, Westh H, Tomasz A, Chung M, Oliveria DC, de Lencastre H. The evolution of methicillin resistance in *Staphylococcus aureus*: similarity of genetic backgrounds in historically early methicillin-susceptible and resistant and contemporary epidemic clones Proc Natl Acad Sci U S A 2001; 98: 9865–9870.

97. Enright MC, Robinson DA, Randle G, Feil DJ, Grundmann H, Spratt BG. The evolutionary history of methicillin-resistant *Staphylococcus aureus* (MRSA) Proc Natl Acad Sci U S A 2002; 99:7687–7692.

98. Saïd-Salim B, Mathema B, Kreiswirth BN. Community-acquired methicillin-resistant *Staphylococcus aureus*: an emerging pathogen Infect Control Hosp Epidemiol 2003; 24:451–455.

99. Kreiswirth BN. Methicillin-resistant *Staphylococcus aureus* infections among competitive sports participants—Colorado, Indiana, Pennsylvania, and Los Angeles County, 2000–2003 MMWR Morb Mortal Wkly Rep 2003; 52:799–795.

100. Gold HS. Vancomycin-resistant enterococci: mechanisms and clinical observations Clin Infect Dis 2001; 33:210–219.

101. Bonten MJ, Willems R, Weinstein RA. Vancomycin-resistant enterococci: why are they here, and where do they come from? Lancet Infect Dis 2001; 1:314–325.

102. Murray BE. What can we do about vancomycin-resistant enterococci? Clin Infect Dis 1995; 20:1134–1136.

103. Martone WJ. Spread of vancomycin-resistant enterocci: why did it happen in the United States? Infect Control Hosp Epidemiol 1998; 19:539–545.

104. Morris JG, Shay DK, Hebden JN, McCarter RJ Jr, Perdue BE, Jarvis W, Johnson JA, Dowling TC, Polish LB, Schwalbe RS. Enterococci resistant to multiple antimicrobial agents includ-

ing vancomycin: establishment of endemicity in a university medical center Ann Intern Med 1995; 123:250–259.

105. Kim WJ, Weinstein RA, Hayden MK. The changing molecular epidemiology and establishment of endemicity of vancomycin resistance in enterococci at one hospital over a 6-year period J Infect Dis 1999; 179:163–171.

106. Donskey CJ, Chowdhry T, Hecker M, Hoyen CK, Hanrahan JA, Hujer AM, Hutton-Thomas RA, Whalen CC, Bonomo RA, Rice LB. Effect of antibiotic therapy on the density of vancomycin-resistant enterococci in the stool of colonized patients N Engl J Med 2000; 343:1925–1932.

107. Boyce JM, Potter-Bynoe G, Chenevert C, King T. Environmental contamination due to methicillin-resistant *Staphylococcus aureus*: possible infection control implications Infect Control Hosp Epidemiol 1997; 18:622–627.

108. Smith TL, Iwen PC, Olson SB, Rupp ME. Environmental contamination with vancomycin-resistant enterococci in an outpatient setting Infect Control Hosp Epidemiol 1998; 19:515–518.

109. Zachary KC, Bayne PS, Morrison V, Ford DS, Silver LC, Hooper DC. Contamination of gowns, gloves, and stethoscopes with vancomycin-resistant enterococci Infect Control Hosp Epidemiol 2001; 22:560–564.

110. Boyce JM, Opal SM, Chow JW, Zervos NJ, Potter-Bynoe G, Sherman CB, Romulc RL, Ford S, Medeiros AA. Outbreak of multi-drug resistant *Enterococcus faecium* with transferable vanB class vancomycin resistance J Clin Microbiol 1994; 32: 1148–1153.

111. Byers KE, Anglim AM, Anneski CJ, Germanson TP, Gold HS, Durbin LJ, Simonton BM, Farr BM. A hospital epidemic of vancomycin-resistant enterococcus: risk factors and control Infect Control Hosp Epidemiol 2001; 22:140–147.

112. Puzniak LA, Leet T, Mayfield J, Kollef M, Mundy L. To gown or not to gown: the effect on acquisition of vancomycin-resistant enterococci Clin Infect Dis 2002; 35:18–25.

113. Grundmann H, Hori S, Winter B, Tami A, Austin DJ. Risk factors for the transmission of methicillin-resistant *Staphylococcus aureus* in an adult intensive care unit: fitting a model to the data J Infect Dis 2002; 185:481–488.

114. Livornese LL, Dias S, Samel C, Romanowski B, Taylor S, May P, Pitsakis P, Woods G, Kaye D, Levison ME. Hospital-acquired infection with vancomycin-resistant *Enterococcus faecium* transmitted by electronic thermometers Ann Intern Med 1992; 117:112–116.

115. Smith MA, Mathewson JJ, Ulert IA, Scerpella EG, Ericsson CD. Contaminated stethoscopes revisited Arch Intern Med 1996; 156:82–84.

116. Singh D, Kaur H, Gardner WG, Treen LB. Bacterial contamination of hospital pagers Infect Control Hosp Epidemiol 2002; 23: 274–276.

117. Schulster L, Chinn RYW. Guidelines for environmental infection control in health-care facilities: recommendations of CDC and the Healthcare Infection Control Practices Advisory Committee (HICPAC) MMWR 2003; 52(RR-10):1–44.

118. Chinn RYW. National Nosocomial Infections Surveillance (NNIS) System report, data summary from January 1992–June 2001, issued August 2001 Am J Infect Control 2001; 29:404–421.

119. Calfee DP, Giannetta ET, Durbin LJ, Germanson TP, Farr BM. Control of endemic vancomycin-resistant *Enterococcus* among inpatients at a university hospital Clin Infect Dis 2003; 37: 326–332.

120. Ostrowsky BE, Trick WE, Sohn AH, Quirk SB, Holt S, Carson LA, Hill BC, Arduino MJ, Kuehnert MJ, Jarvis WR. Control of vancomycin-resitant *Enterococcus* in health care facilities in a region N Engl J Med 2001; 344:1427–1433.

121. Farr BM, Jarvis WR. Would active surveillance cultures help control healthcare-related methicillin-resistant *Staphylococcus aureus* infections? Infect Control Hosp Epidemiol 2002; 23: 65–68.

122. Harbarth S, Pittet D. Control of nosocomial methicillin-resistant *Staphylococcus aureus*: where shall we send our hospital director next time? Infect Control Hosp Epidemiol 2003; 24: 314–316.

123. Vriens MR, Fluit AC, Troelstra A, Verhoef J, Van Der Werken C. Are MRSA more contagious than MSSA in a surgical inten-

sive care unit? Infect Control Hosp Epidemiol 2002; 23: 491–494.

124. D'Agata EMC, Gautman S, Green WK, Tang Y. High rate of false-negative results of the rectal swab culture method in detection of gastrointestinal colonization with vancomycin-resistant enterococci Clin Infect Dis 2002; 34:167–172.

125. Francois P, Pittet D, Bento M, Pepey B, Vaudaux P, Lew D, Schrenzel J. Rapid detection of methicillin-resistant *Staphylococcus aureus* directly from sterile or nonsterile clinical samples by a new molecular assay J Clin Microbiol 2003; 41: 254–260.

126. Mayhall CG. Control of vancomycin-resistant enterococci: it is important, it is possible, and it is cost-effective Infect Control Hosp Epidemiol 2002; 23:420–423.

127. Muto CA, Giannetta ET, Durbin LJ, Simonton BM, Farr BM. Cost-effectiveness of perirectal surveillance cultures for controlling vancomycin-resistant *Enterococcus* Infect Control Hosp Epidemiol 2002; 23:429–435.

128. Edmund M. Letter to the editor Infect Control Hosp Epidedmiol.; 2003:309.

129. Dirrigl SN, Rogers G, Valenti AJ. A multifaceted approach to controlling the spread of methicillin-resistant *Staphylococcus aureus* and vancomycin-resistant enterococci in a multiple unit special care setting [abstr 138T], 30th Annual Educational Conference and International Meeting of Association of Practitioners of Infection Control, June 8–12, 2003, San Antonio, TX.

130. Bonten MJM, Austin DJ, Lipsitch M. Modeling endemic and epidemic infections. In: Wenzel RP, Ed Prevention and Control of Nosocomial Infections. Philadelphia: Lippincott Williams & Wilkins, 2003:136–144.

131. Thomson KS. Controversies about extended-spectrum and AmpC beta-lactamases Emerg Inf Dis 2001; 7:333–336.

132. Hanson ND. AmpC β-lactamases: what do we need to know for the future? J Antimicrob Chemother 2003; 52:2–4.

133. Hanson ND. Performance Standards for Antimicrobial Susceptibility Testing. NCCLS approved standard M100-S9. Wayne,

PA: National Committee for Clinical Laboratory Standards, 1999.

134. Steward CD, Wallace D, Hubert SK, Lawton R, Fridkin SK, Gaynes RP, McGowan JE Jr, Tenover FC. Ability of laboratories to detect emerging antimicrobial resistance in nosocomial pathogens: a survey of project ICARE laboratories Diagn Microbiol Infect Dis 2000; 38:59–67.

135. Tenover FC, Mohammed JM, Gorton T, Dembek ZF. Detection and reporting of extended-spectrum β-lactamase (ESBL)-producing organisms in Connecticut [abstr] Clin Infect Dis 1998; 27:1064.

136. Lautenbach E, Patel JB, Bilker WB, Edelstein PH, Fishman NO. Extended-spectrum beta-lactamase-producing *Escherichia coli* and *Klebsiella pneumonia*: risk factors for infection and impact of resistance on outcomes Clin Infect Dis. 2001; 32: 1162–1171.

137. D'Agata EMC, Thayer V, Shaffner W. An outbreak of *Acinetobacter baumannii*: the importance of cross transmission Infect Control Hosp Epidemiol 2000; 21:588–591.

138. Lucet JC, Decre D, Fichelle A, Joly-Guillou ML, Pernet M, Deblangy C, Kosmann MJ, Regnier B. Control of a prolonged outbreak of extended-spectrum beta-lactamase-producing enterobacteriaceae in a university hospital, Clin Infect Dis 1999; 29:1411–1418.

139. Paterson DL, Yu VL. Editorial response: extended-spectrum β-lactamases: a call for improved detection and control Clin Infect Dis 1999; 29:1419–1422.

140. Yu VL. Guidelines for preventing the transmission of Mycobacterium tuberculosis in health-care facilities, 1994 MMWR Morb Mortal Wkly Rep 1994; 43:1–32.

141. Construction-Related Nosocomial Infections in Care Facilities. Decreasing the risk of *Aspergillus*, *Legionella* and other infections Can Commun Dis Rep 2001; 27(suppl 2):1–46.

142. Cooper EE, O'Reilly MA, Guest DI, Dharmage SC. Influence of building construction work on *Aspergillus* infection in a hospital setting Infect Control Hosp Epidemiol 2003; 24:472–476.

143. Bartley JM and the 1997, 1998, and 1999 APIC Guidelines Committees. The role of infection control during construction in healthcare facilities Am J Infect Control 2000; 28:156–169.

144. Olsen MA, Fraser VJ. Proving your value in healthcare epidemiology and infection control Semin Infect Dis 2002; 2:26–50.

145. Fraser VJ, Olsen MA. The business of health care epidemiology: creating a vision for service excellence Am J Infect Control; 2002; 30:77–85.

146. Cosgrove SE, Carmeli Y. The impact of antimicrobial resistance on health and economic outcomes Clin Infect Dis 2003; 36:1433–1437.

147. Cosgrove SE, Perencevich EN, Sakoulas G, Schwaber MJ, Karchmer AW, Carmeli Y. Comparison of mortality related to methicillin-resistant and methicillin-susceptible *Staphylococcus aureus* bacteremia: a meta-analysis Clin Infect Dis 2003; 36:53–59.

148. Carmeli Y, Eliopoulos G, Mozaffari E, Samore M. Health and economic outcomes of vancomycin-resistanct enterococci Arch Intern Med 2002; 162:2223–2228.

149. Shlaes DM, Gerding DN, John JF Jr, Craig WA, Bornstein DL, Duncan RA, Eckman MR, Farrer WE, Greene WH, Lorian V, Levy S, McGowan JE Jr, Paul SM, Ruskin J, Tenover FC, Watanakunakorn C. Society for Healthcare Epidemiology of America and Infectious Diseases Society of America Joint Committee on The Prevention of Antimicrobial Resistance: guidelines for the prevention of antimicrobial resistance in hospitals Clin Infect Dis 1997; 25:584–599.

10

Antimicrobial Stewardship Initiatives: A Programmatic Approach to Optimizing Antimicrobial Use

GILLES L. FRASER

Department of Critical Care Medicine,
Maine Medical Center, Portland, and
Department of Medicine, University of
Vermont, College of Medicine,
Burlington, Vermont, U.S.A.

PATRICIA STOGSDILL

Division of Infectious Diseases, Maine Medical
Center, Portland, and Department of Medicine,
University of Vermont, College of Medicine,
Burlington, Vermont, U.S.A.

ROBERT C. OWENS, JR.

Department of Clinical Pharmacy Services and
Division of Infectious Diseases, Maine Medical
Center, Portland, and Department of Medicine,
University of Vermont, College of Medicine,
Burlington, Vermont, U.S.A.

We shall now discuss in a little more detail the struggle for existence.—*Charles Darwin, 1859*

Recognizing the importance of drug-resistant organisms, the Infectious Diseases Society of America (IDSA) and the Society of Healthcare Epidemiology of America (SHEA) in 1997 published recommendations for preventing and reducing antimicrobial resistance in hospitals (1). In 1999, the Interagency Task Force on Antimicrobial Resistance, a collective body co-chaired by the Centers of Disease Control and Prevention (CDC), Food and Drug Administration (FDA), and National Institutes of Health (NIH), assembled a more global document addressing the threat of increasing resistance (2). Both documents stress the importance of improving the use of antimicrobials, or antimicrobial stewardship, at the institutional level in combating antimicrobial resistance and have had success in serving as wake-up calls to clinicians and health care administrators alike. In addition, the United Kingdom's Antimicrobial Resistance Strategy and Action Plan has committed to "all options in the drive to promote prudent antimicrobial prescribing"(1,2). They further state that "Within the hospital setting, this includes the formation of multidisciplinary Antimicrobial Management Teams whose primary role is to coordinate the formulation, implementation, and assessment of antimicrobial policies".(3,4). However, while some still deliberate the need or strategy for a local response, antimicrobial resistance continues to accelerate. Fluoroquinolone-resistant pneumococci and gram-negative bacilli are becoming more prevalent in the community while in hospitals, extended-spectrum beta-lactamases (ESBLs) found in common organisms such as *Escherichia coli* and *Klebsiella* spp. are becoming more prolific, and finally vancomycin-resistant *Staphylococcus aureus* (VRSA) has emerged in the United States (5–7). This reality should further serve as a call to arms for health care systems to invest in programs that optimize the use of antimicrobial agents.

"*Antimicrobial Stewardship*", a term coined by Dale Gerding, is defined as the optimal selection, dose, and duration of an antimicrobial that results in the best clinical outcome for the treatment or prevention of infection, with minimal toxicity to the patient and minimal impact on subsequent resistance(3). Programmatic multidisciplinary antimicrobial stewardship programs (ASPs) instituted at hospitals both large and small have led to measurable benefits (4–9). Central to the argument for promoting good antimicrobial stewardship is the growing concern for antimicrobial resistance and patient safety. Peripheral to the central arguments, albeit important, is cost containment. Optimizing antimicrobial use has been shown to reduce pharmacy expenditures safely in patients, and is important to health care system viability in modern times. To this extent, we shall review the more recent literature surrounding the impact of ASPs on costs, outcomes, and resistance. In addition, important considerations for development, implementation, and monitoring of ASPs will be summarized.

THE ISSUE

Bacteria and other organisms account for 90% of the 10^{14} cells in the human body (15). Our primal beliefs about body integrity and invasion evoke the natural urge to use antibiotics to annihilate these interlopers (16). This must be balanced with an appreciation of the effect of antimicrobials on beneficial flora as well as their effect on the evolution of resistant organisms. Data suggest that prescribers may not fully value the importance of preserving these therapeutic resources. Twenty-five million pounds of antibiotics are produced yearly for human consumption and are administered to 30% to 50% of hospitalized patients, with nonhospitalized Americans receiving 160 million courses (17). All the while, studies and surveys suggest that as much as 50% of all antimicrobial use is inappropriate (8).

Rationale for Optimizing Antimicrobial Use

Optimizing antimicrobial use (by minimizing exposure to the drugs, performing dosing adjustments, reducing redundant therapy and targeting therapy to the likely pathogens) can be viewed as a strategy to enhance patient safety (18). In terms of its impact on antimicrobial resistance, however, the role of optimizing antimicrobial use can be more nebulous. The reason for this is that the factors promoting resistance are complex, numerous, and extend beyond the use of antimicrobial agents in humans; as such, it is not surprising that they do not allow for quick fixes(19,20). Although antimicrobial resistance has been present on Earth since the days of the primordial soup, its practical onset began in the 1920s with the observation that Pfeiffer's bacillus (now *Haemophilus influenzae*) showed a natural resistance to penicillin prior to its introduction to humans (21). In the 1930s, strains of *Neisseria gonorrhea* as well as pneumococcus were noted to have developed so-called insensitivity after the introduction of Gerhard Domagk's sulfa drugs (21). Observations from the laboratory moved to the clinic in the 1940s, shortly after the introduction of penicillin for the treatment of human infections. The miracle drug, penicillin, was now failing to treat infections caused by penicillinase-elaborating *S. aureus strains*. Even with the correlation of penicillin use with increasing staphylococcal resistance at the time, it is still not known whether penicillinase occurred naturally or if it was induced from a pharmacologic stimulus (21).

Since that time, studies have established a strong relationship between antimicrobial use and resistance. Levy and colleagues developed a biologic model that showed a clear relationship between antimicrobial use and the selection of resistance in humans, documenting biologic plausibility (22). Also, data derived from in vitro studies in which drug exposure selected for resistance, ecological studies that correlated drug exposure with resistance, controlled studies in which patients with prior use of antimicrobial drugs were more likely to be colonized or infected with resistant bacteria, and prospective studies in which drug use was associated with the development of resistant flora have provided sufficient evidence to take action (23–31).

Historically, time has shown us that all antimicrobial agents are not created equal with regard to their ability to induce resistance.

Among those with relatively strong *"use-versus–resistance"* relationships showing unfavorable ecologic impacts are penicillin with *S. aureus*, ciprofloxacin with MRSA, the third-generation cephalosporins with gram-negative bacilli, long–half-life macrolides with *S. pneumoniae*, and carbapenems with *Pseudomonas aeruginosa* and *Acinetobacter* spp. (32,33). On the other hand, other bug-drug combinations show a more favorable use-versus-resistance profile, such as vancomycin with glycopeptide-resistant *S. aureus* (34). In fact, despite the intensity of vancomycin use over a long period of time, it took nearly 30 years for *S. aureus* to develop resistance in the clinic. Programs designed to limit the utilization of agents that exert greater selective pressures, such as carbapenems and third-generation cephalosporins, have had success in reducing resistance rates in the institutional setting.

Can Appropriate Antibiotic Use Limit Health Care Resource Consumption?

Health care resource consumption associated with antibiotic use is staggering. Fifteen billion dollars are spent on this class of drugs yearly in the United States (16), and antibiotics historically account for 10% to 30% of hospital drug budgets. Antibiotic expenditures are only part of the picture. Infections caused by nosocomial antibiotic-resistant organisms cost an estimated $17,000 to $40,000 per case and result in an additional $1.3 billion to $4 billion in U.S. health care costs yearly (35–37).

A more complete representation of the economics of infectious disease (ID) therapeutics should consider factors such as clinical outcomes; length of hospital stay, including discharge placement barriers; cost of isolation for resistant organisms; and readmission rates, as well as the potential adverse sequelae of antibiotic use. Antibiotic use was associated with 23% of all adverse drug events in one hospital (38); adverse effects may range from rash, phlebitis, diarrhea, *Clostridium difficile* disease, intravenous line infection, bone marrow depression to organ damage. Antibiotics are the fourth most common class of drugs resulting in fatal adverse drug events in hospitalized medical patients (39). Finally, it is much more difficult to quantitate the clinical and financial impact of antibiotic failures due to inadequately treated infections and the potential for incapacitation due to illness (40).

Examining the Role of the Pharmaceutical Industry in Antibiotic Use

A recent report suggests that the cost of introducing a medicine to clinical practice now approaches $900 million (41). To insure a return on its investment, the pharmaceutical industry spent $9 billion in 2001 to market drugs, including antimicrobials, to physicians and consumers (42). Few, if any, marketing dollars were directed toward generic formulations. The impact of the lack of marketing for generic antibiotics was noted by Steinman et al. (43), who found that antibiotics that lost patent protection during the 8-year study period lost market share. For example, cefaclor accounted for 8% of antibiotic prescriptions during the years when it was a branded medication; after it became generically available, it accounted for only 1%. Today, the 1% market share is not ostensibly based upon the antibiotic's activity versus common respiratory tract pathogens but rather its palatable taste among children. In fact, with MIC_{90} values at 16 mg/L for *H. influenzae*, some have suggested the marketing phrase "tastes great, less killing." Clearly, the pharmaceutical industry has great interest (and great success) in marketing antibiotics, and sometimes these practices fall short in truthful representation of data (44).

On the other hand, the industry contributes in a very positive way to the struggle against microorganisms by producing effective medications, supporting research in this area, and underwriting educational efforts for professionals and the lay public (45). Our challenge is to harness the substantial personnel and monetary resources of pharmaceutical firms to help "pull" institution-initiated antibiotic directives. We believe that the industry can be involved in an institutional effort to optimize antibiotic use. If informed of the content and intent of antibiotic policies, restrictions, and guidelines, drug manufacturers can tailor their promotional efforts in ways that are consistent with the goals of the hospital. They can partner in other ways as well by helping with the financial burdens of producing locally written educational materials or with unrestricted educational grants to support antibiotic optimization programs.

Effective Strategies for Changing Prescribing Behaviors: Making It Easy to Do It Right

No one disputes the threat to humanity and the needless expenditures associated with inappropriate antibiotic use. However, even with universal recognition of the problem, physician prescribing patterns have been slow to change. A number of contributing factors have been identified: the belief that the pharmaceutical industry will always develop a new antibiotic to combat resistant strains; skepticism that efforts to optimize antibiotic use are rooted in cost savings and ignore individual patient needs; delays and difficulties in establishing ID diagnoses, prompting the initial (and often continued) use of broad-spectrum antibiotics; expectations of patients and their caregivers with attendant issues of satisfaction with provision of care; the perceived high risk of withholding antibiotics in patients with possible infections; lack of access to authoritative opinion leaders, such as ID specialists; industry marketing of newer agents; and the list goes on and on. There no longer should be any patience for excuses or explanations for prescribing practices that are capable of affecting societal health. We need to change the way antibiotics are used now. Every unnecessary antibiotic prescription written undermines the success of subsequent therapies.

Successful strategies that have been shown to help improve physician prescribing practices in other therapeutic areas have been applied to antibiotic optimization. Several methods have been used to effect change, including education, peer review, preadmission and concurrent review, consensus guidelines, data feedback, medical information system reminders, financial incentives such as withholds, and the use of opinion leaders (46,47). The use of opinion leaders in combination with data feedback has been one of the most successful mechanisms to change clinician behavior (48–51). We believe that multifaceted, nonregulatory, educationally based strategies that have direct impact on individual patient care are preferable alternatives to the micromanagement processes, such as prior authorization and preadmission certification, to which clinicians, by necessity, have become accustomed.

Changing prescribing behaviors is one thing, maintaining those changes is another. As an aid to sustaining any process improvement effect and to minimize the "antibiotic inspector" role, we employ point-of-use information imbedded within our computerized antibiotic ordering process, recognizing as Samuel Johnson did more than 200 years ago that "men more frequently need to be reminded than informed." The long-term effectiveness of this strategy has been confirmed in the literature and in our institution (52–55).

ANTIMICROBIAL STEWARDSHIP PROGRAMS

Overview of Published Antimicrobial Stewardship Programs

Because the practice of managing antimicrobial agents has changed significantly over the last two decades, our intent was not to re-review the epic ASP literature. John and Fishman did a noteworthy job of this in 1997 primarily focusing on cost savings and renumeration (56). Our review includes selected publications and presentations over the last few years that were selected to illustrate the diversity of methods and outcomes measured (9–13,57–63). **Table 1** summarizes several published ASPs, some of which are discussed in more detail in the text of this chapter. The use of the term ASP implies a multidisciplinary programmatic prospective interventional approach to optimizing the use of anti-infectives. A variety of prospective programmatic strategies have been proposed, but in reality, they can be simplified into one of two main categories, prior authorization and concurrent review with feedback. Of course the two are not mutually exclusive; hybrid programs using a blend of the central categories have been created. Why are programmatic multidisciplinary strategies important?

Table 1 Overview of Antimicrobial Stewardship Programs

Reference/ Hospital Size/ Primary Strategy	ASP Team Members	Outcomes				
		Patient Outcomes	Bacterial Resistance/ Infections	Impact on Antibiotic Use	Reduced Expenditures/ Costs (US dollars)	Comments/ Description
White et al.[13] 575 beds/ Prior authorization (24/7, dedicated pager)	ID physicians, Pharmacists	Outcomes (pre- and post-program implementation) were assessed for patients with Gram-negative bacteremia. • No difference in patient demographics, SAPSII score (all P values > 0.3) • No differences in survival (P = 0.49) • No differences in infection (bacteremia)- related length of stay (P > 0.05) • No differences in time to receipt of appropriate antibiotic (P > 0.05)	Reduction in resistance rates post-program implementation (P ≤ 0.01) for the following drug-organism pairings: • Ticarcillin/ clavulanate: *E. coli, P. aeruginosa, K. pneumoniae, E. cloacae, A. anitratus* • Imipenem: *E. coli, P. aeruginosa, K. pneumoniae* • Aztreonam: *E. coli, P. aeruginosa, K. pneumoniae, E. cloacae* • Ceftazidime: *E. coli, P. aeruginosa, E. cloacae, A. anitratus* • Amikacin: *E. coli* • Ciprofloxacin: *E. coli, P. aeruginosa*	Significant reductions in the use of the following restricted agents (P value not specified); overall appropriateness not assessed. • Aztreonam • Ceftazidime • Ciprofloxaicn • Imipenem • Ticarcillin/ clavulanate	• 1st year reduction in total antimicrobial expenditures: $803,910 • Antibiotic costs/ pt. Day: reduced from $18 to $14.4	Prospective before-and-after methodology used to study outcomes of a prior authorization program. Simultaneous Infection control efforts included three handwashing inservices for surgical ICU staff

(continued)

Table 1 *Continued*

Reference/ Hospital Size/ Primary Strategy	ASP Team Members	Outcomes				
		Patient Outcomes	Bacterial Resistance/ Infections	Impact on Antibiotic Use	Reduced Expenditures/ Costs (US dollars)	Comments/ Description
Gross et al.[10] 772-beds/ Prior authorization with dedicated pager	ID physician ID-trained PharmD	• No difference in patient demographics, MedisGroup score (all P values > 0.05) • Appropriateness of therapy defined as use of antimicrobial agent adheres to institution-specific guidelines for spectra of activity and route of delivery for each indication; Doses had to be correctly adjusted according to organ function; and known allergies had to be avoided. Results shown as: ASP vs. ID Fellows: Appropriateness: (87 vs. 47%, P < 0.001) Cure: (56 vs. 38%, P = 0.007) Failure: (15 vs. 28%, P = 0.03)	Not determined.	Factors contributing to inappropriate treatment (ASP vs. ID Fellows) (represented as #/total) Cost: 6/87 vs. 25/93 (P < 0.001) Spectrum too broad: 4/87 vs. 21/93 (P < 0.001) Spectrum too narrow: 1/87 vs. 5/93 (P = 0.11) Spectrum inappropriate: (other than reasons above) 1/87 vs. 14/93 (P < 0.001) Antimicrobial agents not indicated: 6/87 vs. 9/93 (P = 0.5) Route inappropriate: 0/87 vs. 2/93 (P = 0.17) Dose inappropriate: 0/87 vs. 2/93 (P = 0.17)	Median costs were compared between groups (ASP vs. ID fellow): Hospital cost after approval call: $6,468 vs. $7,864, P = 0.08 Cost attributable to infection: $3,510 vs. $4205, P = 0.10 Cost of antimicrobial agents: $79 vs. $122, P = 0.09	• Study prospectively compared the effectiveness of the ASP with that of the ID fellows covering the program (during off-hours) in terms of antimicrobial recommendations and clinical and economic outcomes. • Although costs were lower in the ASP group, they did not reach the traditional statistical significance breakpoint. • At the conclusion of the study, the ASP was reorganized to incorporate the ID fellows and the program director reviews their recommendations

| Bantar et al.[57] 250-bed/ Concurrent Review | ID physician, 2 pharmacists, clinical microbiologist, laboratory microbiologist, data analyst | Nosocomial infection rates: no difference Crude Mortality Rate: no difference Hospital length of stay: decreased significantly (P = 0.04) ICU length of stay: no difference | Correlation between consumption ratios of ≥ 2 antimicrobials and resistance over time was determined. The increase in cefepime use relative to the decreased use of the third-generation cephalosporins over time was associated with decreased resistance to *E. cloacae* (P = 0.03) and *P. mirabilis* (P = 0.05) Increased ampicillin/ sulbactam use relative to decreased 3rd generation cephalosporin use over time was associated with a reduction in *E. cloacae* resistance (P = 0.03) and MRSA (P = 0.04) | Only IV antimicrobial consumption was considered. Overall reduction in IV antimicrobial use from 430.89 DDD to 276.35 DDD/1000 pt. days (P < 0.0001) was documented. Significant reductions in consumption of carbapenems (P = 0.03), ceftriaxone (P < 0.0001), cephalothin (P < 0.0001), and clindamycin (P = 0.003), were noted. An increase in microbiologically-based prescribing intention occurred over the study period (from 27% to 62.8%, P < 0.0001. Interventions (n = 349): Reduced dose or duration: 11.5% | Only IV antimicrobial costs were considered • $913,236 savings during 18-month period | • Prospective comparative evaluation of a hospital-wide program to optimize antimicrobial use. • Study rolled out in 4 phases. • Primary inter-ventions and educational efforts were: 1.) to divert broad spectrum carbapenem and ceftriaxone use to effective, less resistance evoking agents (cefepime) and ampicillin/ sulbactam, 2.) to make an effort to document the microbiology of the infection prior to treatment • 44% of 450 patients in the pre-program group received carbapenems! • Primary driver of *(continued)* |

Table 1 Continued

Reference/ Hospital Size/ Primary Strategy	ASP Team Members	Outcomes				
		Patient Outcomes	Bacterial Resistance/ Infections	Impact on Antibiotic Use	Reduced Expenditures/ Costs (US dollars)	Comments/ Description
			Reduction of carbapenem use correlated with the reduction in *P. aeruginosa* resistant to carbapenems (P = 0.02) The increased use of cefepime was not associated with increased *P. aeruginosa* resistance.	Less expensive treatment: 86.1% Narrower spectrum of activity: 47%		cost reduction was shift in use from carbapenems to cefepime and ampicillin/ sulbactam.
Fraser et al.[9] 600-beds/ Concurrent review	ID fellow and Critical care PharmD	• No difference in patient demographics, Charlson Prognostic Comorbidity Index score (all P values > 0.1) Results shown as intervention group vs. non-intervention group:	Not determined.	• Fewer DDDs per patient were observed for the intervention group, but was not statistically significant: (10.16 DDDs vs. 13.59 DDDs, P = 0.09). • 50% of patients receiving targeted drugs had their treatment streamlined at	Antimicrobial charges were significantly less per patient in the intervention group: ($1287.17 vs. $1673.97, P < 0.04)	Prospective, randomized study of clinical, patient safety, and economic outcomes. Patients receiving ≥1 of 10 designated antibiotics for at least 3 days were randomized to the intervention group or control

Reference/Setting	Personnel	Study Description	Results	Comments
		…day 3 without negatively impacting outcomes.	Clinical response rates: 79.5% vs. 80.6%, P > 0.05 Microbiologic response rates: 9.4% vs. 5.1% (most were indeterminate, 87.4% vs. 89.8%) Measures of antimicrobial toxicity: no difference Length of stay: 20 days vs. 24.7 days, P = 0.11 Readmission rates antibiotics within 7 days of discontinuation: 4.7% vs. 13.3%, P = 0.02 Readmission rates within 30 days: no difference	(no intervention). Study demonstrated that interventions to optimize antimicrobial use could be done without adversely impacting short- and long-term clinical outcomes.
Stogsdill et al.[58]; Modjtabai et al.[59] 600-beds/ Concurrent review	ID physician, ID PharmD	5-year longitudinal study of changes in antibiotic use (influenced by computerized decision support and education) and the impact on resistance.	Not determined. Interventions (first six-months published): Dose optimization: (n = 239), Discontinuation of redundant therapy: (n = 94) Optimize Route: … Measured annual savings compared with pre-program expenditures: 2002: $67,356 2003: $227,028	Clinical program developed based on prospective, randomized study previously conducted at our institution (Fraser et al.).

(continued)

Table 1 Continued

Reference/ Hospital Size/ Primary Strategy	ASP Team Members	Outcomes				
		Patient Outcomes	Bacterial Resistance/ Infections	Impact on Antibiotic Use	Reduced Expenditures/ Costs (US dollars)	Comments/ Description
			Ceftazidime use diminished [36.6 to 10.4 antibiotic days (AD)/1000 patient days]. Cefepime use increased from 0 to 49 AD/1000 patient days over the same time period. In parallel, the susceptibility of *Serratia marcescens* and *E. cloacae* to the third-generation cephalosporins from 1998-2002 increased from 40 to 90% ($r^2 = 0.98$, $P = 0.0001$) and from 72 to 83% ($r^2 = 0.79$, $P = 0.04$), respectively.	(n = 88), Streamline therapy: (n = 55) Interventions (first 2-years, unpublished): Dose optimization: (n = 825), Discontinuation of redundant therapy: (n = 245) Optimize Route: (n = 220), Streamline therapy: (n = 210)		

| Camins et al.[11] large-sized hospital/ Concurrent review | Not determined. | Appropriate use defined as: (1) indication met hospital guidelines, (2) spectrum active against isolated or suspected pathogen, (3) use was necessary, and (4) no known allergy to prescribed antibiotic existed. Greater extent of appropriate antibiotic prescribing in the intervention group: 80% vs 60% (P < 0.005). Therapy was deemed inappropriate for the following reasons: (1) unnecessary treatment (contaminant or asymptomatic bacteriuria) in 43%, (2) overly broad or narrow spectrum in 30%, and (3) use outside hospital guidelines in 27%. | Not determined. | Not determined. | Randomized study of the impact of an ASP over a five month period, 12 medicine teams were randomized to (1) intervention group: teams received input on antimicrobial use from ASP, or (2) control group: teams used indication-based guidelines with no ASP input. Daily audits of targeted drug use (levofloxacin, piperacillin/ tazobactam, vancomycin) were tracked. |

(continued)

Table 1 *Continued*

Reference/ Hospital Size/ Primary Strategy	ASP Team Members	Outcomes				Reduced Expenditures/ Costs (US dollars)	Comments/ Description
		Patient Outcomes	Bacterial Resistance/ Infections	Impact on Antibiotic Use			
				The intervention group more likely to streamline therapy (79% vs. 59%, P<0.01) and had reduced exposure to inappropriate therapy (measured by median daily defined doses) (2 DDD vs 3 DDD, P = 0.006) and duration (3 days vs 5 days, P < 0.005).			
Srinivasan et al.[12] 1000-beds/ Concurrent review added to a prior authorization program.	ID physician, ID PharmD, Data analyst.	Not determined.	Not determined.	Not reported.		Costs for antimicrobial agents for the covered areas decreased by 6.4% the first year and 2.2% the second year. Authors factored in the inflation	Prior approval program at Johns Hopkins Hospital was supplemented by a more comprehensive strategy that published local treatment

				rate of 4.5%, reporting savings of $224,753 and $413,998 for fiscal years 2002 and 2003.	guidelines, offered educational sessions, and concurrent review of antimicrobial therapy. Cost savings justified program (ID physician, ID PharmD, and data analyst). A long-term successful impact on both costs and the hospital's ecology in terms of infection rates with problematic and/or drug-resistant organisms was demonstrated. Parenteral antibiotic use and expenditures were reduced in spite of a 15% increase in the Medicare Case Mix Index and a 56% increase in ICU patient-days throughout the 7-year period.
Carling et al.,[61] "medium-sized community hospital"/ Concurrent review	ID physician, ID PharmD	Not determined	Reductions in nosocomial infections caused by *C. difficile* (P = 0.002) and resistant enterobacteriaceae (P = 0.02) were reported. A 22% reduction in parenteral broad-spectrum antibiotics occurred during a seven-year period (P < 0.0001). Sustained reduction in ceftazidime use occurred (24.7 to 6.2 DDD/1,000 pt. days.	Comparing costs from 1990 to subsequent years demonstrated a reduction in annual antimicrobial expenditures between $200,000 and 250,000 each year.	

(continued)

Table 1 *Continued*

Reference/ Hospital Size/ Primary Strategy	ASP Team Members	Outcomes				Comments/ Description
		Patient Outcomes	Bacterial Resistance/ Infections	Impact on Antibiotic Use	Reduced Expenditures/ Costs (US dollars)	
Ruttiman et al.[60] 80-beds/ Concurrent rounding and prior authorization	Medicine department (13 medicine residents, 5 attending physicians) and Pharmacy Department (role not clarified)	• No difference in patient demographics. • Severity of illness scoring not determined. Results shown as intervention group vs. non-intervention group: Cured or improved: 81% vs. 84%, P = 0.52 Length of stay (median): 12 days vs. 13 days, P value not given Relapse during hospital stay: 1.4% vs. 1.7% days, P = 0.72 Infection-related mortality: 2.4% vs. 4.0% days, P = 0.15	Not determined.	Using DDD data: Reduction in overall antimicrobial use: 36% (P < 0.001) Reduction in intravenous antimicrobial use: 46% (P < 0.01)	Reduction in overall antimicrobial expenditures: 53% (P = 0.001)	"Quasi-experimental" before-and-after study conducted in a small Swiss hospital. Objectives were to evaluate the impact of their ASP on costs and clinical outcomes and to monitor the long-term impact on costs. Interventions: targeted antimicrobial restriction, education, feedback to staff on expenditures, provision of annual antibiogram.

Study	Outcomes		Interventions	Cost savings	Comments
LaRocco et al.[62] 120-beds/ Concurrent review. Concurrent review conducted 3 days/week for patients receiving multiple, prolonged, or high-cost antibiotic therapy. ID physician Clinical Pharmacist (Infection control and microbiology also represented)	Readmission rates within 30 days due to infection: 1.0% vs. 1.8%, P = 0.28 Not measured, but no adverse events attributable to the program were reported.	Not determined.	Dose optimization: (n = 20), Discontinuation due to redundant therapy, excessive duration, inappropriate use: (n = 127) Optimize Route: (n = 110) Add antimicrobial: (n = 77)	Antibiotic costs/pt. Day: reduced from $18.21 to $14.77 (19% reduction) Estimated annual savings: $177,000	Study showed durable value of ASP implementation at a small hospital. Relatively small hospital demonstrated that interventions aimed at optimizing antimicrobial use could be made, three days per week, and result in significant expenditure reductions.
Gentry CA, et al.[63] Veterens Affairs Medical Center/ Concurrent review of patients receiving restricted/non-formulary antimicrobials ID PharmD (Antimicrobial advisory group consisted of ID physicians, microbiology laboratory director, and ID PharmD)	• Patient demographics were similar, the intervention group was slightly older (63.8 vs 63.1 years, P = 0.049). • Severity of illness scoring not determined. Results shown as (pre- and post-program implementation):	Not determined.	Interventions (#first year/ #second year): Dose optimization: (87/140), Approved use of agent and recommended additional agent: (35/35) Approved use of agent while discontinuing current antibiotic:	Average annual reduction in intravenous antimicrobial expenditures was 30.8%, or $145,942/year	Retrospective study of patient outcomes and costs for two two-year periods (2 years pre- and 2 years post-program introduction). Clinical protocols were developed for the approval/denial of restricted/non-restricted antimicrobials

Table 1 *Continued*

Reference/ Hospital Size/ Primary Strategy	ASP Team Members	Outcomes				
		Patient Outcomes	Bacterial Resistance/ Infections	Impact on Antibiotic Use	Reduced Expenditures/ Costs (US dollars)	Comments/ Description
		Length of stay (mean): 13.2 days vs. 10.8 days, P < 0.0001. Infection-related Mortality: 8.28% vs. 6.61% days, P = 0.007 Readmission rates within 30 days due to infection: 10.96% vs. 10.42%, P = 0.46		(40/39) Initial order denied for an alternative regimen: (244/199)		formulary antimicrobials (indications, dose, alternative regimens). Restricted antimicrobials were allowed to be prescribed. The ID PharmD was notified of their use, followed the patients' courses, and approved or denied their continued use. For complex cases, the ID PharmD could facilitate ID consultation.

Carling et al. (64) demonstrated that among similarly matched hospitals, only the programmatic prospective interventional programs significantly impacted parenteral antimicrobial use patterns and costs, in contrast to those institutions that relied solely on passive strategies. These passive or adjunctive interventions, in our minds, may serve as tools to augment the two main strategies and include the use of stop orders, antibiotic order forms, closed formularies, selective susceptibility reporting, educational sessions, and restriction of pharmaceutical promotional activities.

Antibiotic streamlining was one of the first strategies to demonstrate the significant impact of a multidisciplinary programmatic approach on prescribing patterns of antimicrobials. Developed at the Hartford Hospital in the 1980s, this program focused on "converting from a more complex to a less complex regimen" using a multidisciplinary strategy (65). ID physicians and clinical pharmacists assessed antibiotic choices (in those receiving two or more antimicrobials) after 48 hours of therapy. Suggestions for antibiotic optimization were offered in verbal or written form (placed as a nonpermanent part of the medical record). Of the 625 patients reviewed over 7 months, 340 recommendations were made. The number of patients requiring intervention declined by 44.2% over the 7-month period, demonstrating the educational impact of the program. The acceptance rate for the interventions was 82.6%, of which almost all (97.2%) completed therapy with the recommended agent. At the time the study was conducted almost 15 years ago, the annualized cost savings for streamlining was $107,637.

Our initial work in the area involved a randomized study of a concurrent review program's impact on costs and patient outcomes (9). An ID physician fellow and a PharmD specializing in critical care reviewed therapy on adult inpatients receiving one of ten targeted parenteral antibiotics for more than 3 days. The intervention group (n = 141) received suggestions (written or verbally), whereas the control group did not (n = 111). The Charlson Prognostic Comorbidity Index was used to stratify patients' underlying illnesses. Outcomes were similar with respect to clinical and microbiologic response to therapy, adverse events, inpatient mortality, and readmission rates. Interventions included change to oral therapy (31%), regimen or dosing changes (42%), stopping therapy (10%), and ordering additional laboratory tests (18%); 85% of the suggestions were instituted. Multiple logistic regression models identified randomization of the intervention group as the sole predictor of lower antimicrobial expenditures. Annualized savings when converted from charges to costs were approximately $97,500. The intervention group also showed a trend toward reduced mean length of stay compared with controls (20 vs. 24 days, respectively). Fifty percent of patients receiving targeted regimens had their treatment refined at day 3, resulting in lower antimicrobial costs and importantly, without adversely impacting their outcomes.

The previously cited study by Fraser et al. (9), was modified and converted into a concurrent review program with minimal use of restrictive policies at Maine Medical Center (MMC) in 2000 (58). The MMC team consists of an ID physician (2 hours/day, 5 days/week) and an ID-trained PharmD (4 to 6 hours/day, 5 days/week). A steering committee was used to survey health care giver expectations and to identify/resolve barriers before launching the program (Fig. 1). Multiple components complement the primary concurrent review program. For example, education is facilitated by means of (i) academic detailing, (ii) making rounds with various services on an intermittent and as-requested basis, (iii) a widespread poster campaign providing clinicians with information on which infections and antimicrobials are amenable to transitional therapy as well as criteria for switching to oral therapy, including objective clinical stability measures, and (iv) provision of an antimicrobial formulary pocket guide that offers information on guidelines, restrictions, costs, and empirical/definitive treatment choices. A closed formulary is in place with a limited number of restricted agents. Our computerized physician order entry system also offers a limited number of point-of-care reminders that can be expanded on for further decision support assistance. The primary program revolves around daily audits of all adult patients receiving any antimicrobial agent, regardless of route of administration. Our belief is that

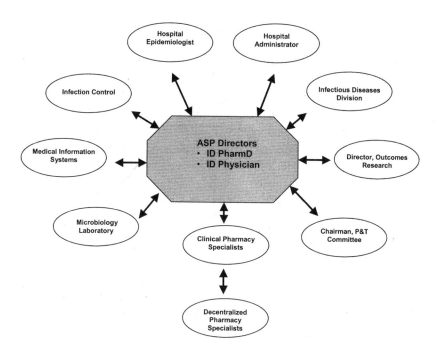

Figure 1 Figure 1. Organizational structure of an antimicrobial stewardship program (ASP). ID, infectious diseases; PharmD, doctor of pharmacy; P&T, pharmacy and therapeutics. (Adapted and modified from John JF Jr, Fishman NO. Programmatic role of the infectious diseases physician in controlling antimicrobial costs in the hospital. Clin Infect Dis 1997; 24:471–485.)

antimicrobials may be given unnecessarily, chosen discordant to susceptibility reports, and given in combination with other agents inappropriately, regardless of route of therapy or expense. We do not tend to play the armchair quarterback; rather, our intent is to supplement the decision making process by offering additional synthesis of data and knowledge. Interventions with educational explanations are left in the patient's medical record using a nonpermanent form (the form is slightly larger than the pages of the record so it can be removed at discharge) or by direct communication (phone or in person) if necessary. A copy of the form is used later to record interventions electronically into our physician order entry system, which can be downloaded into Excel from an Access database for tracking and reporting purposes. DDD data are used to quantify antimicrobial consumption, and purchase data are also used to track expenditures. We presented our initial 6-month evaluation (58). An average ($\pm$ standard deviation) of 105 ($\pm$ 27) patients were reviewed per day and 534 interventions were performed: pharmacodynamic dose optimization (n = 239), discontinuation of redundant therapy (n = 94), transitional therapy (n = 88), streamline therapy (n = 55), and a range of miscellaneous interventions (n = 55). The acceptance rate was 95%. Average monthly antibiotic expenditures decreased by $6,692. Antimicrobial costs prior to the ASP were $11.81/patient/day, which fell to $11.42/patient/ day (projected cost per patient day was $12.09).

Since that time (2.5 years later), our antimicrobial expenditures average $25,000 less per month compared with pre-ASP implementation, offering an annual expenditure reduction of $300,000 (Fig. 2). Targeted intravenous and oral antimicrobial use markers (e.g., fluconazole, ciprofloxacin, gatifloxacin) all showed large shifts toward increased oral utilization. For example, 60% to 70% of all fluconazole use prior to the ASP was administered via the intravenous route; this was reduced to an average of 40% in the postprogram period. The high rate of acceptance for this ASP is believed to be the result of the educational nature of the program rather than the use of draconian tactics, as well as the familiarity by our clinicians of such a program because of the study conducted at our own institution. Because our current program is not a randomized, controlled study, we are able to expend our efforts more efficiently (e.g., we do not have a control population) as reflected by the number of interventions in our clinical program compared with our previous study (increased by more than fivefold).

Camins et al. (11) at Emory University and Grady Memorial Hospital, a large urban teaching institution, studied the impact of an antibiotic utilization program on antimicrobial use in a randomized trial. Over a 5-month period, twelve medicine teams were randomized to one of two antibiotic use strate-

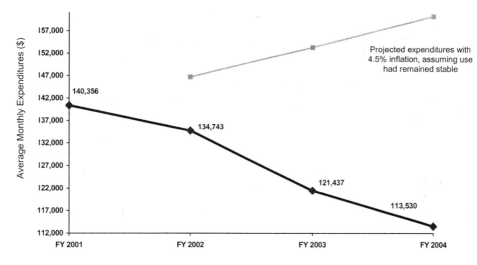

Figure 2 Figure 2. Durable reduction in antimicrobial expenditures associated with the antimicrobial stewardship program at Maine Medical Center. FY, fiscal year. (Figure provided courtesy of Robert C. Owens, Jr.)

gies: an intervention group, in which teams received input on antimicrobial use, or a control group, in which teams used indication-based guidelines. Daily audits of targeted drug use (levofloxacin, piperacillin/tazobactam, vancomycin) were used to determine appropriateness of use. Appropriate use was defined as the following: (i) the indication for use met hospital guidelines, (ii) the antibiotic was active against isolated or suspected pathogen, (iii) use was necessary, and (iv) no known allergy to the prescribed antibiotic existed. Over a period of 5 months, 508 prescriptions were evaluated: 270 in the control group and 230 in the intervention group. A greater proportion of prescriptions met the criteria for appropriate use (80% vs. 60%, $p < 0.005$) in the intervention group, and streamlining was more frequent in the intervention group (79% vs. 59%, $p < 0.01$). The intervention group also had reduced exposure to inappropriate therapy as measured by median DDD (2 DDD vs. 3 DDD, $p = 0.006$) and duration (3 days vs. 5 days, $p < 0.005$). The acceptance rate for the suggested recommendations in the intervention group was 90%. Therapy was deemed inappropriate for the following reasons: (i) unnecessary treatment (contaminant or asymptomatic bacteriuria) in 43%, (ii) overly broad or narrow spectrum in 30%, and (iii) use outside hospital guidelines in 27%.

Srinivasan et al. (12) studied the impact of an antimicrobial management program on antimicrobial expenditures at Johns Hopkins Hospital, a 1,000-bed teaching facility. Prior to the introduction of a comprehensive ASP, the hospital used a closed formulary system and employed prior-approval requirements on a number of antimicrobials. The ASP consisted of a hospital-funded ID physician, ID Pharm, and data analyst. The team concurrently reviewed antimicrobial therapy in all areas of the hospital except pediatrics and oncology. Their interventions included a survey, use of institution-specific guidelines, concurrent antimicrobial review, and educational sessions. A "knowledge, attitude, and beliefs" survey was used to determine awareness of antimicrobial use and resistance and sense deficiencies in knowledge that could lead to targeted education among house staff. Interestingly, only 18% viewed the program as an obstacle to patient care and 70% wanted additional feedback on antimicrobial choices. Hospital guidelines were published and updated annually. The publication included guidelines for treatment (both antimicrobial and non-antimicrobial) as well as diagnostic guidelines. In addition, the investigators included formulary and cost information. Initially, drafts were sent to more than twenty faculty members in various divisions to improve buy-in. Antimicrobial therapy interventions occurred prior to culture and susceptibility results being available only when actively solicited or when called for prior authorization of an antimicrobial agent. For all others, interventions were suggested at the time the microbiologic data became available. Compliance with suggested recommendations by the ASP was 79%. Costs for antimicrobial agents for the covered areas decreased by 6.4% the first year and 2.2% the second year. Assuming a steady inflation rate of 4.5%, savings translated to $224,753 and $413,998 for fiscal years 2002 and 2003.

Bantar et al. (57) demonstrated the impact of their interventional program on antimicrobial use, cost savings, and antimicrobial resistance at Hospital San Martin, a 250-bed hospital with ten ICU beds that cares for adult patients in Argentina. Their multidisciplinary team consisted of an ID physician, two pharmacists, a microbiologist and laboratory technologist, an internal medicine physician, and a computer systems analyst. In 6-month periods, four consecutive intervention strategies were unveiled. During the first 6 months, an optional antibiotic order form (ID diagnosis, pertinent epidemiologic data) was introduced and baseline data were collected (i.e., bacterial resistance, antibiotic use, prescribing practice, nosocomial infection, and crude mortality rates). In the second period, an "initial intervention" period consisted of transforming the optional order form to a compulsory form and providing feedback to clinicians based on a review of the data collected in the first period. In the third period, called the "education" period, clinicians were verbally engaged with each new antimicrobial order by members of the multidisciplinary team. It appears that the bulk of the discussions centered around antimicrobial selection, specifically the collateral resistance caused by third-generation cephalosporins and carbapenems. In the same discussion, the benefits with respect to collateral resistance of aminopenicillin/sulbactam combinations and cefepime were conveyed. The fourth or "active control" period was similar to the third period, but prescriptions were modified by the antimicrobial team if necessary. During the four periods, no antimicrobial agent was restricted. To estimate the rates of use of a particular drug in relation to other drugs, an index was calculated (e.g., rate of cefepime use to that for third-generation cephalosporins—ceftriaxone and ceftazidime—equaled cefepime/consumption of ceftriaxone and ceftazidime × 100). Consumption data were measured in DDD using the definitions set forth by the WHO. Expenditure data were collected only for parenterally administered antimicrobial agents. The ID physician collected data parallel to the antibiotic order form filled out by the clinician, with the addition of the modification(s) suggested by the antimicrobial team. Need for therapy was defined by Mandell's *Principles and Practice of Infectious Diseases* (66) and considered appropriate if mentioned as primary or alternative therapy in *The Sanford Guide to Antimicrobial Therapy* (67).

Not too surprising is that the antibiotic order form and education provided by the team with regard to avoidance of third-generation cephalosporins and carbapenems and their suitable replacements (aminopenicillin/sulbactam combinations, cefepime) were effective in shifting antimicrobial use between periods I and II, and this continued throughout the study. The program periods were associated with declining cost savings as time advanced (periods II, III, and IV were associated with a reduction of $261,955, $57,245, and $12,881, respectively). Comparing antibiotic order forms from period I (voluntary form and preintervention, n = 450) with period IV (mandatory form with active intervention, n = 349) noted an increase in microbiologically based treatment intent (27% vs. 62.8%, respectively, $p < 0.0001$). Twenty-seven percent of the period IV antibiotic order forms were intervened upon by the team. Of the interventions, either the dose or duration (not specified) was reduced in 11.5%, 86.1% were associated with cost reduction, and 47% involved streamlining therapy to a narrower choice. In terms of impact on nosocomial infection, length of hospitalization, and mortality, only length of stay was affected significantly ($p = 0.04$). The increased rate of cefepime use relative to third-generation cephalosporins was associated with declining third-generation cephalosporin resistance rates among *Proteus mirabilis* and *Enterobacter cloacae* but not to *E. coli* or *Klebsiella pneumoniae*. The increased rate of aminopenicillin/sulbactam use relative to the third-generation cephalosporins in conjunction with a sustained reduction in vancomycin use was associated with a reduction in MRSA rates. In addition, *P. aeruginosa* resistance rates to carbapenems declined to 0%. This was strongly associated with the reduction in carbapenem consumption over time.

This particular study is different from others in that it used a staggered approach to implementation. Though the cost reduction appeared to dwindle significantly with each newly introduced period, one cannot ignore the cumulative effect of the overall impact on cost. In addition, the final period offers a comprehensive mechanism for long-standing success and also serves as a template to introduce other initiatives as deemed necessary. Part of the success related to reduction in resistance rates noted by this program is related to the high rate of carbapenem and ceftriaxone use and the "seldom" ordered cefepime and aminopenicillin/sulbactam in conjunction with the types of problem pathogens noted at the investigators' hospital (e.g., ampC phenotypes and carbapenem-resistant *P. aeruginosa*). Penicillin-based inhibitor combinations and cefepime have been noted to more often "favorably" affect the environment in contrast to high usage rates of carbapenem and third-generation cephalosporins (68–70).

Ruttimann et al. (60) introduced a multidisciplinary program characterized by a blend of interventions including mild formulary restrictions, comprehensive education (direct communication, antibiograms, peer feedback every 6 months), making rounds with medical teams, and introduction of guidelines (appropriate initial empiric therapy, transitional therapy, duration of therapy). All adult patients admitted to the medicine service were consecutively evaluated before the introduction of the program (n = 500 patients) and postimplementation. Using DDD and hospital expenditure data, the investigators showed a 36% reduction in overall antimicrobial use ($p < 0.001$), intravenous antimicrobial use (46%, $p < 0.01$), and overall expenditures (53%, $p = 0.001$); all without compromising the quality of patient care (determined by inpatient survival, clinical improvement/cure, duration of hospitalization, and readmission rates within 30 days). These benefits were sustained for the 4-year period evaluated.

Carling et al. (69) published their 7-year experience in antimicrobial management. Their hospital is a medium-sized university-affiliated hospital academic center. Originally initiated in 1991 to control the use of third-generation cephalosporins, their multidisciplinary effort consists of a physician (one-quarter time support) and doctor of pharmacy (full-time support), both with specialty ID training. This concurrent review program has expanded to include a prospective evaluation of orders for imipenem, aztreonam, and parenteral quinolones, in addition to the previously targeted third-generation cephalosporins. Quantification of antimicrobial use is captured via DDD/1,000 patient days for these antimicrobial agents using the CDC's definition of DDD. The program is in operation on weekdays, and within the 8-hour day, new orders are typically evaluated within 4 hours of their entry. Orders falling outside the 8-hour day are reviewed as a priority the next time the doctor of pharmacy is on duty. Informal written notes are generated when the team identifies a problematic regimen and is then placed in the patient's chart. "Academic detailing" occurs as well between the doctor of pharmacy and the prescribing clinicians to supplement the written recommendations. The investigators evaluated their impact on VRE, MRSA, and *C. difficile* disease by means of internal benchmarking as well as by externally benchmarking themselves with like hospitals within the National Nosocomial Infections Surveillance System. A 22% reduction in parenteral broad-spectrum antibiotics occurred ($p < 0.0001$) in the face of a 15% increase in the acuity of their patient population over 7 years. Reductions in nosocomial infections caused by *C. difficile* ($p = 0.002$) and resistant Enterobacteriaceae ($p = 0.02$) were reported. MRSA rates remained unaffected, as would be anticipated by the very nature of its environmental presence in hospitals today. The study represents a long-term successful impact on both costs and the hospital's ecology in terms of infection rates with problematic and/or drug-resistant organisms.

Regardless of hospital size, antimicrobial agents are still used both appropriately and inappropriately. Although much of the published literature and research stems from larger, usually teaching institutions, it by no means should be implied that smaller, nonteaching facilities are not candidates for optimizing antimicrobial use. For example, a 120-bed community hospital successfully implemented an ASP using the concurrent antibiotic review methodology (62). The ASP involved an ID specialist physician and a clinical pharmacist as well as representatives from infection control and the microbiology laboratory. The time involvement of the ID physician was approximately 8 to 12 hours per week. The team reviewed antimicrobial therapy 3 days a week in patients receiving targeted drugs or prolonged durations of therapy. Recommendations were conveyed using a confidential form that was temporarily placed in the patient's chart, and by telephone if necessary. Physicians were not required to accept the team's recommendation. Barriers faced by the team included initial apprehension by fellow clinicians regarding the loss of prescriptive authority and those associated with relying on clinical information solely from the medical record to form clinical recommendations. Rather than tackling high-level or potentially controversial issues, they focused on the so-called low-hanging fruit. The end result showed that there was a lot of this low-hanging fruit, and clinicians appreciated their input. In addition to the prospective review process, clinicians now request the services of this ASP regularly. In terms of processes and outcomes, 488 recommendations were made over the course of a year, 69% were accepted, and a cost reduction of 19% was realized, with an estimated savings of $177,000. Common interventions were discontinuation of redundant antimicrobial therapy, discontinuation of treatment due to inappropriate use or excessive duration, transition from intravenous to oral therapy, and substitution or addition of an antibiotic to the regimen. The interventions were evidence based and have been shown in the published literature to be safe and effective, thus the investigators did not track clinical outcomes. This program is a good example of taking a template from an established, published program and customizing it to a hospital's size, needs, and resources.

Getting Started: The Groundwork

For those considering the initiation of a formal ASP, it is fundamentally important to appreciate the framework built by initial communications. Preliminary discussions should involve (i) developing goals and a formal plan, (ii) selection of the main strategy (*prior approval* or *concurrent review, or a hybrid of both*), (iii) determining of the members involved, their time commitment, and a funding stream for the program, (iv) assembling a multidisciplinary committee to provide a venue for ongoing dialogue, and (v) marketing the program to the clinicians.

Develop Goals and Practically Measure
Outcomes

In 1997, the Infectious Diseases Society of America and the
Society of Healthcare Epidemiology of America issued recommendations to hospitals to form multidisciplinary teams to
minimize antibiotic resistance, review antimicrobial usage
data, and increase efforts related to the surveillance of antimicrobial resistance in hospitals (1). The leaders of the ASP initiative should have an appreciation for local antibiotic patterns
of use relative to the published literature. Depending on the
hospital's size, it may be of value to distinguish utilization
further by hospital unit. Benchmarking data are available
from hospital consortiums and from the literature. In general,
relevant data to consider would be DDDs of target antibiotics
per 1,000 patient days or some quantifying *measure* of antimicrobial consumption, and dollars spent on antibiotics per patient day. Bhavnani discusses benchmarking in detail in her
chapter in this book.

   The next step is to understand local patterns of antimicrobial resistance, and if possible, to identify relationships with
antibiotic usage. Antibiograms are useful to identify trends in
antimicrobial resistance and may provide more useful information if community isolates are separated from organisms
collected from inpatients. If your hospital is served by an outside commercial laboratory, your antibiogram may be a collection of the laboratory's customers' isolates rather than your
specific organisms. Further, depending on the size of your institution, drilling down to specific units within the hospital
may be of value both in terms of educational feedback to specific units and in identifying areas of the hospital that can be
served by specific interventions to change resistance patterns.

Measuring Outcomes

Several studies have evaluated the impact of ASPs on a variety
of outcomes (**Table 1**). Although each has used a slightly different approach and outcome variables were not always defined uniformly (e.g., "appropriateness of therapy", antibiotic
consumption measurements), the resulting data obtained from

them has been valuable. For instance, oversight of antimicrobial use (be it restrictive or more subtle through concurrent review and feedback) has been shown to have a measurable impact on appropriateness of antimicrobial use, antimicrobial consumption and/or expenditures (9–13,57,58,60–63). Others have evaluated the impact of ASPs on resistance rates, infection rates, and clinical outcomes (9,10,13,57,59–61). Some have shown favorable results to widespread drug-organism combinations (13) and some efforts were more targeted. For example, two studies showed that reducing third generation cephalosporin use while simultaneously increasing fourth generation cephalosporin use through education, concurrent review and feedback, and computer physician order entry enhancements, resulted in significantly improved sus- ceptibilities among Gram-negative bacilli with AmpC beta-lactamase phenotypes (57,59). For comparative studies, some have used before-and-after methodologies (12,13,57–61) and some have used a control group (9–11). From these studies, ASPs have been created, some using a blend of strategies customized for local application.

For those interested in initiating an ASP, goals should be developed insuring that performance outcomes are easily measured and relevant. Economic issues never prevail over improving clinical outcomes, but remain important to measure (71). Measured outcomes and performance indicators in the literature include: recommendation acceptance rates, adherence rates with antibiotic usage guidelines, microbiologic and clinical response rates, frequency of antibiotic readministration within 7 days, adverse drug events, time to approve antimicrobials and time to their administration to the patient, hospital readmission rates related to infectious diagnoses, length of stay, mortality rates, antimicrobial resistance rates, infection rates, antibiotic expenditures and utilization rates measured in terms of DDD, associations between antimicrobial use and resistance or infection rates, overall costs of hospitalization and costs directly attributable to the infectious process. Outcome measurement should be customized to the institution and discussed (and agreed upon) prior to the implementation of the program. Surveys may be used prior to the introduction of an ASP or used as an ongoing tool to evaluate and assess clinician knowledge and attitude (12). For further reading on population-based antimicrobial usage measurement and resistance correlation, Madaras-Kelly has reviewed this in detail (72). It is important to remember that none of the above variables is perfect as benefits and limitations exist with each.

Studying the effects of an intervention on an outcome (e.g., antimicrobial use) is best conducted by using a matched control group in whom the intervention is not conducted. Another more commonly used (and perhaps "misinterpreted") method is the before and after study design. The recent introduction of interrupted time series with segmented regression analysis offers a more sophisticated means of measuring the true impact of before and after interventional studies (**Fig. 3**) (73,74). This type of analysis estimates how much an intervention impacted an outcome, immediately as well as over time and whether factors other than intervention could elucidate the change (74). Two parameters characterize each segment of a time series: the level and slope. A change in the level (rise or decline) post-intervention signifies an acute intervention effect (A) in **Figure 3** (74). A change in slope is signified by an increase or decrease in the slope following the intervention (compared with the slope before the intervention) and indicates a gradual change in either direction over time (B) in **Figure 3** (74). Adequate numbers of timepoints are necessary both pre- and post-intervention in order to adequately characterize a time series. The Cochrane Effective Practice and Organization of Care Group (EPOC) Data Collection Checklist suggests a minimum of three data points on both sides (pre- and post-intervention) (75). However, to adequately compensate for seasonal variation requires a minimum number of 24 data points pre- and post-intervention (74). Most before and after studies to date have not undergone such rigorous statistical analyses, but they should be applied to ongoing and future studies using such methodologies for proper characterization of the impact of interventions on outcomes.

Length of stay is commonly used to quantify the impact of interventions (e.g., clinical pathways, guidelines, transitional

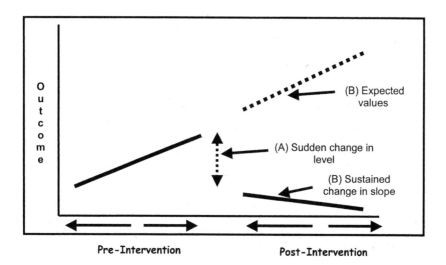

Figure 3   Figure 3. Segmented Regression Analysis of Interrupted Time Series Data. (Adapted from Ramsay C, Brown E, Hartman, Davey P. Room for improvement: a systematic review of the quality of evaluations of interventions to improve hospital antibiotic prescribing. J Antimicrob Chemother 2003;52:764-771.)

therapy programs, ASPs). Unfortunately, length of stay can be influenced by a variety of confounders, making this a difficult endpoint particularly when multiple interventions are simultaneously being introduced. Viewing the entire LOS distribution (**Fig. 4**) allows one to identify and compare populations of patients capable of being discharged "early" versus those whose discharge may not be directly affected by the implementation of a particular intervention or program(76). For example, we compared our lengths of stay pre- and post-introduction of our community-acquired pneumonia pathway using interrupted time series analysis. The latter tail of the distribution curve reflects patients whose care may not be impacted by early oral antibiotic therapy and whose length of stay is driven by other factors (e.g., short- and long-term care facility placement, stabilization of multiple comorbidities, etc.). Our so-called "dischargeable population" are defined as those with community-acquired pneumonia who were able to benefit from

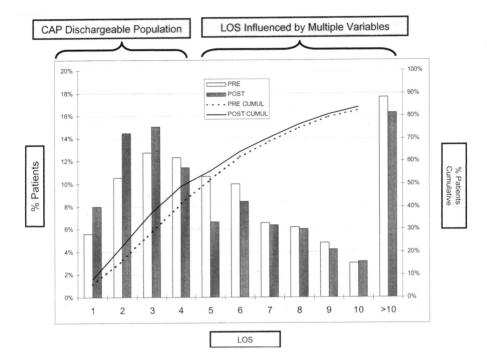

Figure 4 Figure 4. Length-of-stay distribution. (Figure provided courtesy of Robert C. Owens, Jr.)

the transition from intravenous to oral therapy (e.g., patients without significant and multiple comorbidites), resulting in subsequent discharge from the hospital. While our mean and median length of stay pre- and post-pathway introduction were 7.7 ($\pm$9.6) vs. 7.6 ($\pm$12.1), and 5 (1–132) and 5 (1–136) days, respectively ($P>0.05$); our "discharge efficiency" was improved in the post-pathway period ($p<0.001$), with a 7% increase in patients discharged within the first 3 days of admission. This method has also been employed in larger randomized controlled trial settings to assess the benefit of oral therapy (77).

The Choice of Program Strategy

In brief, two main programmatic, multidisciplinary strategies exist: prior authorization and concurrent review with feedback. The former relies on scheduled coverage (usually 24/7 or normal business hours with contingencies for off-hour antibiotic orders, typically through a dedicated pager and call system with a list of antimicrobial agents that require approval from the service prior to dispensation. Two programs serve as models for the prior authorization approach. White and colleagues (13) constructed a list of restricted antimicrobials based on cost and/or spectra of activity that included intravenous formulations of amikacin, ceftazidime, ciprofloxacin, ofloxacin, fluconazole, ticarcillin/clavulanate, piperacillin/tazobactam, and aztreonam, as an example. Members of the ID division were on call to receive approvals for these agents 24/7 via dedicated pager. Gross et al.,(10) initially employed a dedicated beeper schedule for weekdays, during normal business hours, which was covered by an antimicrobial management team (AMT) member (an ID doctor of pharmacy or ID physician). Second year ID fellows covered evenings and weekends. At night, restricted drugs were released pending next morning follow-up. Based on the results of the study, the ID fellows have been incorporated into the AMT and work with the PharmD and ID attending more directly. With regard to intranet/internet resources, they also have published their list of restricted antimicrobials and guidelines on a web site that can be accessed, at least in part, by outside institutions (www.uphs.upenn.edu/bugdrug). The list of restricted drugs can be large or small, based on cost, resistance evoking potential, and spectra of activity, as well as safety and tolerability.

The latter ASP strategy relies on less restrictive antimicrobial policies but reviews or makes rounds on patients identified from a computer generated list of those receiving specific (or all) antimicrobial agents (diagramed in **Fig. 5**) on scheduled days (e.g., Monday-Friday). The list can be modified to contain enough information to make general assessments related to appropriateness of combination therapy, dosing, selection (if culture and susceptibility information available), and route. Some programs wait until culture and susceptibility results are available, typically by the third day of treatment, to make recommendations. From the initial assessment, normally a chart review and/or discussion with other health care

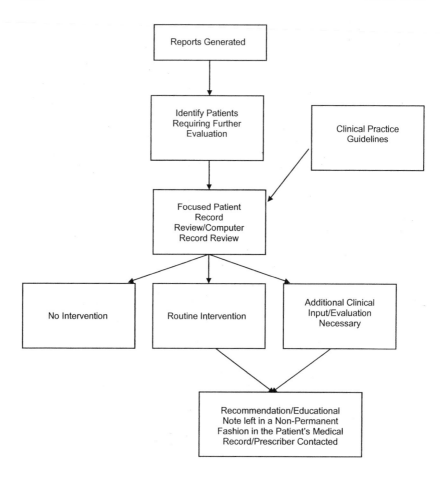

Figure 5   Figure 5. Concurrent review program workflow diagram. (Adapted from Stogsdill P, Claffey T, Bates P, et al. Antimicrobial stewardship program: from research to practice [abstr 583]. 40th Infectious Diseases Society of America Meeting, Chicago, Oct 24–27, 2002.)

team members ensues. When intervention is deemed necessary, nonpermanent notes are usually left in the medical record with educational vignettes, literature citations, and/or local guidelines, with verbal communication being utilized for more urgent matters. One of the more widely quoted published ASPs of this type originated as a randomized study of clinical and economic outcomes involving an ID physician and a doctor of pharmacy (9). Therapy was reviewed and intervened upon (when necessary) in adult inpatients receiving one of 10 targeted parenteral antibiotics (based on cost and spectrum of activity) for more than 3 days.

Interventions

The precise means for intervention varies to some degree but is, in general, limited to verbal and written communication. Briceland et al. (65) and Stogsdill et al. (59)-58 used nonpermanent notes left in the patient medical record along with verbal communication, depending on the need for immediate action; whereas, Bantar et al. (57) and Camins et al. (11) used verbal discussion exclusively with the prescriber teams. The timing of the intervention varies as well. In general, our program reviews all antimicrobial therapy, regardless of when it is initiated, as opposed to waiting for microbiologic data to intervene (usually 72 hours) (58). That being said, we tend not to split hairs either; if we do intervene, it is for good reason. Some programs do have a policy for the timing of the intervention that is usually after 72 hours of therapy (12).

Follow-up

Interventions should be followed for compliance. In our case, later the same day or on the following day, the copies of each intervention are used to guide the review of the patient's electronic medical records to determine the intervention's acceptance or rejection status. In the same computer system, documentation is made regarding the infection type, type of intervention (route change, streamlining, dose modification, drug addition, drug discontinuation, regimen change, drug interaction identification), acceptance (accepted, accepted in part, rejected, not applicable), a non–mutually exclusive impact assessment (improve medical quality, decrease potential for resistance, decrease cost), and a free text section to enter miscellaneous information. These data are downloaded into an access database and queried periodically for biannual reports to the pharmacy and therapeutics committee. We do not follow the clinical course of the patient after the intervention is made. However, if organ function or diet information changes after our initial intervention (e.g., dose adjustment or route change), we are able to identify this through a review of the daily list on the following days. Some data collection is necessary; however, at a certain point, it becomes crippling to the program's efforts and hinders the amount of patients that are able to be intervened upon each day.

Data collection is important for several reasons. In all likelihood, these data will be used for the purposes of internal and perhaps external benchmarking as well as to prepare reports to various committees (e.g., pharmacy and therapeutics, antibiotic subcommittee, infection control, executive committee), depending on the institution. Some form of impact assessment including intervention tracking and financial consequence needs to take place regardless of program strategy. It is critical to know, for instance, whether one's efforts are being accepted or not. Keep in mind that many programs from prominent institutions do not report 100% acceptance rates. In fact, one such program reported acceptance rates of 50%, which increased over a period of 3 years to 71% (78). Importantly, the reason for rejection and the individual or service associated with the rejection should be recorded in an effort to ascertain trends and rationale for rejection. Tactics can be customized and employed to correct nonadherence to protocols, pathways, or individual recommendations, such as a letter to the prescriber from a person with authority (e.g., department chief, pharmacy and therapeutics committee chair, infectious diseases representative). The type of recommendation should be categorized and longitudinally tracked, as this is useful to determine what type of interventions are being performed and whether there is variation from period to period. For example, we noticed that after a period of time, the number of transitional therapy interventions declined following a poster campaign to promote the logic of oral therapy. This allowed us to spend time on other aspects of our program, such as initiating new campaigns.

Barriers

The literature is helpful to point out some of the pitfalls those have experienced and concerns that need to be addressed. Delays in the approval for a necessary antimicrobial agent can be detrimental to critically-ill patients in need of initial broad-spectrum antimicrobial therapy. White and colleagues, showed no delay in the administration of antimicrobial agents prior to and after the introduction of their program; however, approval times and time to antibiotic administration should be monitored as an outcome variable (13). The perception of "threatened autonomy" can be a significant impediment to the effort. Previous studies, including the one by LaRocco and colleagues and in our experience, have shown the introduction of education and rationale at the point of communication diverts such emotion (9,62). Thus, some mechanism for education and consistent communication should be considered. Interestingly, the concept of *"gaming the system"* may be encouraged by more restrictive programs. For example, one program reported an outbreak of nosocomial infection following the introduction of their ASP (79). A 30% relative increase in documentation of infection in the medical record occurred (incidence of infection increased from 11 to 14.3 per 1000 patient care days, $P<0.05$) (79). After investigation, the outbreak was termed a "pseudo-outbreak", or in other words, the increased rate of infection represented clinicians attempting to justify the use of a particular restricted antimicrobial by documenting that infection existed in the medical record. The perception that ASPs are solely financially driven can also be an impediment. However, both national and international recommendations are helpful to point out that mechanisms need to be in place in hospitals to monitor the use of antimicrobial agents and provide feedback regarding their use in order to preserve their long-term utility. Program funding can be a barrier for some institutions, but as mentioned in the next section, the literature is helpful in pointing out that programs (in large or small hospitals) can usually pay for themselves as a side effect of promoting good antimicrobial stewardship.

Costs and Financial Support for the Program

Once the strategy has been selected and time commitments have been determined, the funding of the program needs to be discussed with the institution. Initial discussions with administrators may be better served with an informed principal clinical sponsor or advocate (without a vested interest in profiting financially) who understands the clinical benefit of optimal antimicrobial use, such as the chief of medicine. Salary support for a part-time ID physician and a full-time ID-trained PharmD is the minimal start-up cost for an ASP at most moderate-sized to large hospitals. However, smaller hospitals, such as those with 100 beds or fewer, may be able to get by with part-time support for both positions. The financial benefits from numerous published studies reviewed by John and Fishman (56) more than justify the cost of the program, and the authors have proposed three possible mechanisms for support: (i) defined compensation, (ii) payment on a time basis for consultation services, (iii) negotiation for a percentage of the cost savings.

Form a Multidisciplinary Steering Committee

Ideally, criteria for involvement in this group include a strong sense of commitment, cooperation, and, ideally, a high level of capability in the area of antibiotic use and ID. The reality is that not everyone shares such enthusiasm for appropriate antimicrobial use. The composition of the group will be unique to each institution, but the following should be considered for inclusion.

Infectious Disease Physicians

The involvement of ID physicians offers the ASP a level of expertise that insures the credibility of the program and facilitates its acceptance with physicians and other providers. As the ultimate opinion leaders in the field of antibiotic use, ID physicians can provide peer guidance to clinicians clinging to suboptimal prescribing practices. Unfortunately, not all institutions will have access to an ID specialist, yet this should not prevent development of an ASP. One alternative is to retain offsite ID specialists as consultants to review ASP policies and procedures and to provide a means of insuring quality of service. In these and other circumstances, trained clinical pharmacists have been able to effectively affect antibiotic prescribing in a manner similar to that of an ID physician (80).

Clinical Pharmacists

Clinical pharmacists trained in ID can offer insight into pharmacologic issues and expand the menu of antibiotics while identifying alternative approaches to ID management that are both clinically and fiscally responsible. These individuals should be familiar with the literature, and regarded as opinion leaders in their institutions. If a trained individual is not available, one should be sought, or at least a long-term mentorship with an experienced practitioner is necessary.

Microbiologists

The microbiology laboratory will serve as a critical resource for information necessary to any ASP effort and therefore should be at the table when related issues are discussed. In addition to providing antibiograms and breaking out data by hospital-unit, microbiologists may also assist with selective susceptibility reporting initiatives, customizing testing panels with regard to antibiotic choices, and exploration of novel diagnostic tests, to name a few.

Section Chiefs

The involvement of section chiefs is essential to the success of the program. They provide leadership to initiate and sustain changes in practice and forums to discuss the ASP during department meetings, at grand rounds, during morning report, and via written departmental communications. They may also provide insight on how to manage a predictably critical personality within their ranks.

Nurses

Nurses are patient advocates who share many of the same goals addressed by the ASP—more efficient delivery of health care that results in improved patient outcomes (such as earlier ambulation and reduced length of hospitalization). They are well placed to aid in the identification of patients who could benefit from the ASP. Nurse colleagues who serve in infection control positions or those who are involved in pathway production or discharge planning are natural fits for this committee. As the administrators of medications, their assistance with the implementation of concepts such as continuously infused beta-lactams can be helpful, given that policies and procedures and subsequent nursing education will need to take place.

Administrators

Administrators need to understand the issues and potential benefits of the ASP to the institution. Administrators can provide access to the institution's financial database and help to define (from their points of view) what end points the ASP should evaluate. They also control the purse strings of the hospital.

Introducing the Concept and Buy-In

Finally, each department affected by the ASP must be included and feedback sought. This may be the single most important aspects that determine the degree of success of any new program launched. Department meetings and specialty grand rounds provide venues for a presentation of the proposal. Because curmudgeons exist, be proactive. In other words, individual meetings to address specific concerns are better conducted before the launch of a program rather than placing the ASP in a reactive scenario following implementation. During the year of planning for our program, this marketing phase was concurrently conducted. Our intentions were discussed in a concise five- to ten-slide presentation to key departments. The Johns Hopkins group disseminated their program's antibiotic guidelines to more than twenty faculty members for review to gain consensus prior to it being published. Newsletters, independent of active communication, are insufficient to notify clinicians of ASP implementation.

Early in our consideration of initiating an ASP, we were concerned that we would be viewed as interlopers or armchair critics of antimicrobial choices for patients we were not invited to evaluate. We tried to develop a strategy to initiate and maintain a program that would be viewed in the spirit in which it was conceived—as an asset to patient care. Our goal was to develop a systematic approach to antibiotic utilization that would make it easy for prescribers to *do the right thing* in an educational, nonpunitive environment.

Essential Tools and Adjunctive Interventional Strategies for Antimicrobial Stewardship Programs

The following paragraphs provide some discussion related to key concepts used by successful ASPs to optimize antimicrobial use. In addition, examples of some adjunctive initiatives are provided.

Pharmacodynamic Dose Optimization

Dose optimization interventions are likely to be one of the most common interventions from an ASP. Intuitively, dose reductions for organ dysfunction would seem to predominate. Although common, dose reductions are almost matched at our institution by dose increase recommendations. Dose increases are common for infections in which difficulty in drug penetration is an issue (e.g., endocarditis, osteomyelitis, meningitis), in pathogens with elevated MICs (e.g., *P. aeruginosa*), and in obese patients. Unfortunately, drug dosing handbooks fail to account for 440-lb (200-kg) patients in their "usual dose" section; thus, obese patients may be significantly underdosed for their infection when fixed traditional doses are employed, which can contribute to clinical failure and resistance development (81–82). Andes and Craig provide a basic overview of pharmacodynamic concepts and Kuti et al. offer examples of pharmacodynamically based programs implemented at their hospital in their respective chapters within this book. In brief, continuously infused beta-lactams (e.g., piperacillin/tazobactam, cefepime), prolonged infusion (meropenem), extended-interval aminoglycoside dosing, and every-12-hour metronidazole regimens have been used successfully to maximize the killing properties of these agents while minimizing costs and adverse events.

Educational Efforts

Development and dissemination of pertinent information is the first step in any process leading to change. Early attempts at influencing prescribing behaviors relied heavily on educational efforts—it was simplistically believed that the reason physicians frequently inappropriately prescribed antibiotics was that they were "therapeutically undereducated" (83). The assumption was that misuse of antibiotics was more often the result of insufficient information rather than inappropriate behavior.

Over the years that we have taught antibiotic principles and specifics of therapy at MMC, we have been impressed by the intense interest both physicians-in-training and established practitioners have in learning more about antibiotics. But equally as impressive is the laissez-faire and even fatalistic attitude toward retaining and applying lessons learned in these educational sessions. Without direct application to current patients, prescribers often refer to antibiotics as "alphabet soup" and "impossible to understand." These impressions are supported in the literature. Educational efforts are the least effective, and certainly the shortest-lasting, way to affect prescriber behaviors. Some formats may, however, be more useful than others.

The pharmaceutical industry offers a clearly successful model for influencing prescribing behaviors. A cadre of trained representatives commonly offers one-on-one discussions with physicians to present data supportive of marketed drugs. Avorn and Soumerai (84) were early pioneers in borrowing this approach to provide a more impartial, objective discussion of therapeutics using educational visits by clinical pharmacists, termed *academic detailing*. Though effective, this approach requires a substantial investment in manpower for implementation. Variations on the theme of academic detailing have been employed to affect antimicrobial use. In a recent randomized, controlled trial, Soloman et al. (80) measured the influence of a targeted one-on-one educational program (academic detailing) on unnecessary levofloxacin or ceftazidime prescriptions. A 41% reduction in the rate of inappropriate use of these antibiotics was noted with the intervention. Other investigators using a combination of scheduled antibiotic educational conferences along with focused prescriber consultation showed a 43% reduction in the use of intravenous fluoroquinolones and a 16% reduction in inappropriate vancomycin prescriptions. The authors emphasize that the program offered personal, collegial contact to facilitate interactive discussions. This approach allows for an exchange of information that might not be available via review of the medical record, but its success depends on the ability and availability of the educators.

Computer-Assisted Decision Support Programs

Direct computer-based physician order entry is rapidly becoming the standard of care and has been adopted as one of the Leapfrog initiatives to avoid medication errors and improve the quality of care (85). The availability of computer technology offers an advantage over academic detailing because it can be accessed 24 hours a day when antibiotics are ordered. Extensions of this technology, computer-assisted decision support programs, have been designed to provide real-time integrated patient and institutional data including culture and susceptibility results (including results from the previous 5 years), laboratory measures of organ function, allergy history, contraindications, and drug interactions, as well as hospital microbial susceptibility and antibiotic information and cost data. They provide therapeutic choices for clinicians and allow for the incorporation of clinical judgment. Autonomy is preserved while insuring that important variables in the choice of antimicrobial therapy are considered.

Almost all published data on the effect of computer-assisted decision support programs on antibiotic use are from researchers at the LDS Hospital in Salt Lake City, Utah. This approach has been associated with reductions in antibiotic doses, inappropriate orders, costs, treatment duration, and associated adverse drug events (86-88). This degree of computer sophistication is not widely available, but that should not dissuade institutions from adapting their own computer systems to apply lessons learned from LDS. Waiting with a loaf of bread while the bread truck arrives is a better alternative than starving (15). Old-fashioned manipulation of available computer technology may be very useful in helping optimize antibiotic prescribing. For example, at MMC, we require that clinicians choose one of the CDC-recommended indications for vancomycin prior to computer ordering. We also capture patient-specific and real-time serum creatinine data to calculate creatinine clearance and guide appropriate dosing for antibiotics such as ciprofloxacin and cefepime. Laboratory tests to monitor therapy, such as serum creatinine and aminoglycoside levels—when this class of antibiotic is prescribed—are available on the drug ordering matrices as well.

Adaptation of Locally Customized Published Guidelines

Clinical pathways for various infectious conditions, such as community-acquired pneumonia and vascular catheter infections, have been developed using an evidence-based approach. The impact of guidelines or pathways on practice patterns has been disappointing. Part of the reason is the perception that guidelines concentrate on published results and are not readily applicable to specific patient care issues. Guidelines are helpful, though, because they identify contentious issues and offer a complete review of available data. The identification of the strengths and weaknesses of the recommendations, along with their adaptation pertinent to local antibiotic formulary and resistance patterns, foster buy-in and participation in the process. Comparing results in the literature with locally developed data can go a long way toward acceptance of the legitimacy and applicability of published guidelines. Conversely, if published guidelines are based largely on "expert opinion," this recognition gives the green light for a less dogmatic and more flexible approach. This strategy is team oriented and stresses consensus.

Formulary Interventions

A recent survey of teaching hospitals suggests that 80% limit prescriber access to antibiotics using a variety of mechanisms

(89). Formulary restriction is the most direct way to influence antimicrobial use. Most hospitals employ this strategy and offer prototypical antibiotic choices that satisfy the majority of clinical situations. Early examples were the preferential use of cefazolin for cephalothin and cefotetan for cefoxitin. This pattern of limiting formulary choice has extended to every category of antibiotic.

Barriers to the use of antibiotics in the form of utilization restriction based on indication are also commonly used. For example, vancomycin may be restricted to only CDC-recommended indications or amikacin may be reserved for multidrug-resistant *P. aeruginosa* infections. These efforts resulted in significant cost savings and were associated with a reduction in the frequency of nosocomial infections due to resistant organisms in a study by Frank et al. (90). Himmelberg et al. (91) found that ceftazidime and imipenem-cilastin use increased by 158% after a restriction policy was removed. This finding was also associated with increased inappropriate use of these antibiotics.

Pharmacodynamics can and should be employed in the formulary decision making process when possible. For example, it is possible to simulate clinical trials using Monte Carlo simulations for drugs with known pharmacokinetics, well-characterized local MIC data, and defined pharmacodynamic targets. This type of analysis can be used to customize antimicrobial choices available on the formulary to the organisms and their susceptibility profiles locally (92–95). We have incorporated pharmacodynamics in the routine evaluation of antimicrobials for formulary approval (81,92).

Antibiotic Order Forms

Other types of pharmacy-based antibiotic control procedures involve antibiotic order forms. This administrative hurdle typically offers educational messages designed to guide antibiotic choice and dose and requires documentation of appropriate indication for antibiotic use (96). It offers a consistent and effective approach (when prescribers are compliant), but suffers from paperwork stigma and is cumbersome to alter when formularies change. Most researchers who published success with this strategy years ago have moved on to other methods of antibiotic optimization (15). The transition to computerized drug order entry may soon make this strategy obsolete.

Evaluating Pricing Contracts

Periodic examination of drug pricing from wholesalers or individual companies is necessary to identify unexpected increases in drug costs. The purchasing department at our hospital employs a contract manager who works full time in the pharmacy department. Although it may be beyond the realm of an ASP's day-to-day function to review purchase history data daily, it is possible to evaluate alerts flagged by individuals who do review purchase data and contracts frequently. An example for our institution occurred during a formulary review for an antifungal agent. We discovered a 20% increase in lipid-based amphotericin B pricing that had already cost our institution an additional $30,000. This occurred as a result of the product being sold from one company to another, and through an oversight, our previously negotiated contract had been nullified. In response, we were able to recover the additional dollars spent on the drug because of the contract oversight as well as to return to the previous price. This alone resulted in more than $100,000 in recovered expenditures and expenditure avoidance over a 1-year period. Another example occurred as a result of reviewing antimicrobial expenditure data. We requested meetings with the companies who sold antimicrobial agents associated with the greatest expenditures. During these meetings, we were able to take advantage of certain programs that were available in terms of rebates and/or upfront pricing adjustments due to market share negotiations. Other mechanisms to reduce the purchase cost of antimicrobial agents through contracting include risk-sharing contracts, formulary changes to agents within the class that are more competitively priced (e.g., fluoroquinolones, lipid-based amphotericin B products), bundling strategies (ciprofloxacin and moxifloxacin vs. levofloxacin vs. gatifloxacin), combining related health care institutions to reflect the overall health care organization's market share as opposed to that of the single institution, and changing to generic antimicrobials (amoxicillin/clavulanate, and *upcoming*: ciprofloxacin–oral only, ceftriaxone, fluconazole). Some strategies may be better used by large health care organizations comprising several hospitals and by larger teaching institutions. The overall premise in negotiating leverage for many of the drugs used today is the fact that there are many decaffeinated beverages out there that are just as tasty as the original! In other words, there are a host of available antimicrobial agents that hospitals may use in place of certain agents. Often, this competition can be used to negotiate optimal pricing.

Managing Drug Shortages

Over the last several years, drug shortages have posed particular challenges to clinicians, as highlighted by surveys conducted by the Emerging Infections Network (97). The shortages of amphotericin B, piperacillin/tazobactam, meropenem, nafcillin, gentamicin, and vancomycin, to name a few, have forced institutions to develop strategies to provide therapeutic alternatives to patients requiring these agents. In many cases, the shortages have also caused administrators to perform "billfold biopsies" because of the several-fold cost increase of the therapeutic alternatives. The ASP may play a vital role in planning for a shortage by working with the pharmacy department to stock up while the drug is still available, if and when there is some advance notice. In addition, the development and distribution of therapeutic alternatives must be considered. The ASP can play a chief role in developing consensus with the users of these agents. For example, we met with our oncologists, our principle users of amphotericin B, as well as our ID colleagues and developed a plan for the use of alternative antifungals (e.g., intravenous and oral fluconazole, lipid-based amphotericin B, intravenous and oral voriconazole). If all our amphotericin B utilization was converted to lipid-based amphotericin B, we would face a $40,000-a-month increase in expenditures. Fortunately, this was pre-empted by the consensus development process and distribution of guidelines spearheaded by our ASP. Similarly, the piperacillin/tazobactam shortage was handled in a similar fashion, but with different players (e.g., surgery, pulmonary/critical care, and ID again). Infection-specific guidelines were developed and distributed. Instead of substituting imipenem for each piperacillin/tazobactam order, we were able to employ far less costly, equally therapeutic empiric treatment regimens, such as cefepime plus metronidazole or ciprofloxacin plus metronidazole or clindamycin for intra-abdominal infections. An Internet resource for updated information on drug shortages can be found on the Food and Drug Administration's website: www.fda.gov/cder/drug/shortages.

Optimizing Length of Stay

One key to a successful ASP is quarterbacking new initiatives. Because hospital length of stay is a primary driver of hospital expenditures, strategies to minimize length of stay can provide a substantial return on investment in resources. Dr. Ramirez's chapter discusses transitional therapy in detail and its ability to minimize hospital length of stay. In addition, Dr. Tice's chapter discusses home intravenous therapy that offers another mechanism to minimize expensive inpatient length of stay. Another opportunity for reducing length of stay involves taking advantage of new oral treatments for MRSA infections, specifically for nosocomial pneumonia and skin/skin-structure infections. Historically, patients with MRSA infections have a longer length of hospitalization than those infected with methicillin-susceptible strains of *S. aureus*. One reason for this is the historical lack of an acceptable oral alternative to vancomycin that has been proven effective in double-blinded, randomized, controlled trials. Figure 6 represents three current options institutions have for treating hospital-acquired pneumonia and skin and soft tissue infections: option A, keep the patient in the hospital for the entire 14-day treatment course; option B, treat the patient for some period of time intravenously, place a peripherally inserted central catheter (PICC) line, and treat for the remainder of time as an outpatient intravenously; and option C, treat the patient for some period of

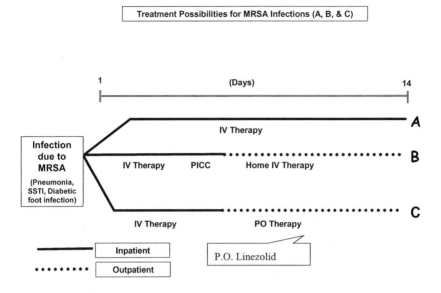

Figure 6 Figure 6. Treatment possibilities for methicillin-resistant *Staphylococcus aureus* (MRSA) infections **(A–C)**. IV, intravenous; PICC. peripherally inserted central catheter; PO, oral; SSTI, skin and soft tissue infection. (Figure provided courtesy of Robert C. Owens, Jr.)

time intravenously, do not place a PICC line, and transition to oral linezolid. Option C is associated with reduced length of stay simply because transition to the outpatient setting for oral treatment of infection is the path of least resistance (e.g., no need for skilled nursing services to administer intravenous medications, no visiting nursing care or home intravenous company to coordinate with). A knowledgeable care coordination and/or social services department to navigate the reimbursement methods (e.g., third-party payers, indigent care programs sponsored by the pharmaceutical industry) is vital to successful implementation. Involvement of the ASP can insure appropriate utilization of the drug and provide continuity across the diversity of potential prescribers. Supporting the shortened length-of-stay paradigm are the number of published studies that have demonstrated that patients with

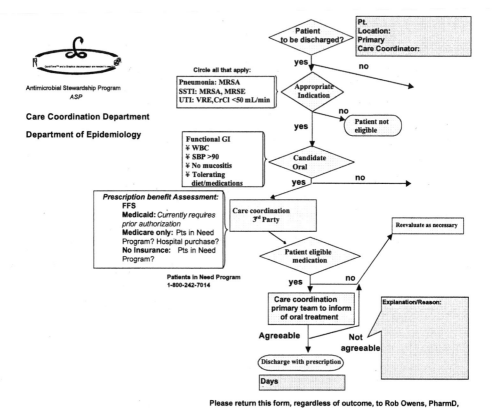

Figure 7 Figure 7. Multidisciplinary algorithm for optimizing length of stay for patients with methicillin-resistant *Staphylococcus aureus* (MRSA) infections. CrCl, creatinine clearance; FFS, fee for service; GI, gastrointestinal; MRSE, methicillin-resistant *Staphylococcus epidermis*; Pt, patient; SBP, systolic blood pressure; SSTI, skin and soft tissue infection; UTI, urinary tract infection; VRE, vancomycin-resistant enterococci; WBC, white blood cell. (Figure provided courtesy of Robert C. Owens, Jr.)

MRSA infections treated with linezolid have shorter lengths of stay than patients treated with vancomycin in comparative registration trials (98–100).

Based on these data, and the fact that options A and B are more expensive to the health care system than option C, we initiated a program to optimize these patients' length of hospitalization despite the cost of oral linezolid. Our algorithm is presented in Figure 7. Again, before implementation of this program, an exigent amount of time was invested in developing consensus among our ID, surgical, administrative, care coordination, and pharmacy colleagues. In addition, because some of our discharges were to skilled nursing facilities (SNFs), we invested time in discussing reimbursement strategies with them as well as assuring them that the drug cost (linezolid) was going to be incurred for only a defined, short period of time and that this was not a chronic medication. Coupled with the fact that Medicare patients qualify for a higher reimbursement rate if they have been on intravenous therapy within the last 14 days of hospitalization, barriers to accepting patients upon transfer from the hospital to the SNFs diminished. Outcomes measured are readmission rates, linezolid susceptibility monitoring, and days of hospitalization avoided. The ASP's role in this process was to again quarterback this initiative and coordinate the consensus process, education, and outcome measurement.

CONCLUSIONS

The problem of increasing antimicrobial resistance, due, in part, to suboptimal antimicrobial use, coupled with the fact that a growing number of pharmaceutical companies have abandoned anti-infective research and development, has resulted in a growing public health crisis (101). As hospitals are characterized by high-density antibiotic use, they are target-rich venues for proactive interventions to improve antimicrobial stewardship. ASP studies indicate that they can be effective in optimizing antimicrobial use, and that when implemented by ID-trained clinicians, the reduction in overall antibiotic use can occur without compromising clinical outcomes. Other proven benefits have included decreased rates of resistance for certain bug-drug combinations. ASPs thus provide an ideal partner to infection control efforts that are designed to reduce the horizontal spread of infection. A side effect of optimizing antimicrobial use has been a proven reduction in related expenditures, making these programs not only clinically necessary in the context of the current public health crisis, but financially possible. Dale Gerding has referred to good antimicrobial stewardship as being "akin to motherhood and apple pie"; to this end, the authors would agree. Kunin stated: "⋯ there are simply too many physicians prescribing antibiotics casually⋯ The issues need to be presented forcefully to the medical community and the public. Third-party payers must get the message that these programs can save lives as well as money (102)." Several areas for future research should be considered. These include standardization of outcome measures and their definitions, application of newer analytic methods (e.g., interrupted time series analysis) to distinguish significant changes in before and after studies, multicenter studies, and the determination of safety and efficacy of ASPs in pediatric populations, who are routinely excluded from published ASP studies.

REFERENCES

1. Schlaes DM, Gerding DN, John JF Jr, Craig WA, Bornstein DL, Duncan RA, Eckman MR, Farrer WE, Greene WH, Lorian V, Levy S, McGowan JE Jr, Paul SM, Ruskin J, Tenover FC, Watanakunakorn C. Society for Healthcare Epidemology of America and Infectious Diseases Society of America Joint Committee on the Prevention of Antimicrobial Resistance: Guidelines for the prevention of resistance in hospitals. Infect Control Hosp Epidemiol 1997; 18:275–91.

2. Bell D. Development of the *Public Health Action Plan to Combat Antimicrobial Resistance*, in The Resistance Phenomenon in Microbes and Infectious Disease Vectors: Implications for Human Health and Strategies for Containment–Workshop Summary Knobler SL, Lemon SM, Najafi M, Burroughs T, Eds

Forum on Emerging Infections.. Washington, DC: National Academy Press, 2003.

3. Department of Health NHS Executive. UK Antimicrobial Resistance Strategy and Action Plan, Crown Publishing, National Academy Press, June 2000.

4. Knox K, Lawson W, Dean B, Holmes A. Multidisciplinary antimicrobial management and the role of the infectious diseases pharmacist—a UK perspective J Hosp Infection; 2003; 53: 85-90.

5. Mohammed JM, Weigel L, Clark N, McDougal L, Raney P, Whitney A, McAllister S, Kellum M, Jevitt L, Tenover FC. High-level vancomycin resistance in a clinical isolate of Staphylococcus aureus. Abstract LB-7. Program and abstracts of the, 42nd Interscience Conference on Antimicrobial Agents and Chemotherapy, September 27-30, 2002, San Diego, California.

6. Paterson DL, Huejer KM, Hujer AM, Yeiser B, Bonomo MD, Rice LB, Bonomo RA. Extended-spectrum beta-lactamases in bloodstream isolates worldwide: Dominance of SHV type beta-lactamases and worldwide prevalence of CTX-M type enzymes. Abstract C2-1833. Program and abstracts of the, 42nd Interscience Conference on Antimicrobial Agents and Chemotherapy, September 27-30, 2002, San Diego, California.

7. Neuhauser MM, Weinstein RA, Rydman R, Danziger LH, Karam G, Quinn JP. Antibiotic resistance among gram-negative bacilli in US intensive care units JAMA; 2003; 289:885-888.

8. Gerding DN. The search for good antimicrobial stewardship Jt Comm J Qual Improv; 2001; 27:403-4.

9. Fraser GL, Stogsdill P, Dickens JD Jr, Wennberg DE, Smith RP Jr, Prato BS. Antibiotic optimization, an evaluation of patient safety and economic outcomes Arch Intern Med; 1997; 157:1689-1694.

10. Gross R, Morgan AS, Kinky DE. Impact of a hospital-based antimicrobial management program on clinical and economic outcomes Clin Infect Dis; 2001; 33:289-295.

11. Camins BC, Wells JB, Googe HL. The impact of an antibiotic utilization program on antibiotic use in a teaching hospital-

A randomized trial. Abstract 489. Program and abstracts of the, 41st Infectious Diseases Society of America Meeting, October 9-12, 2003, San Diego, California.

12. Srinivasan A, Patel A, Song X. Cost reductions in antimicrobial expenditures following implementation of a comprehensive antimcirobial management program. Abstract 488. Program and abstracts of the, 41st Infectious Diseases Society of America Meeting, October 9-12, 2003, San Diego, California.

13. White AC, Atmar RL, Wilson J, Cate TR, Stager CE, Greenberg SB. Effects of requiring prior authorization for selected antimicrobials: expenditures susceptibilities, and clinical outcomes Clin Infect Dis; 1997; 25:230-239.

14. Rahal JJ, Urban C, Horn D, Freeman K, Segal-Maurer S, Maurer J, Mariano N, Marks S, Burns JM, Dominick D, Lim M. Class restriction of cephalosporin use to control total cephalosporin resistance in nosocomial Klebsiella JAMA; 1998; 280: 1233-1237.

15. Schiff GD, Wisniewski M, Bult J, Parada JP, Aggarwal H, Schwartz DN. Improving inpatient antibiotic prescribing J Qual Improvement; 2001; 27:387-402.

16. Avorn J, Solomon DH. Cultural and economic factors that (mis) shape antibiotic use: the nonpharmacologic basis of therapeutics Ann Intern Med; 2000; 133:128-135.

17. Wenzel RP, Edmond MB. Multidrug-resistant Streptococcus pneumoniae N Engl J Med; 2001; 344:1331.

18. Glowacki RG, Schwartz DN, Itokazu GS, Wisniewski MF, Kieszkowski P, Weinstein RA. Antibiotic combinations with redundant antimicrobial spectra: clinical epidemiology and pilot intervention of computer-assisted surveillance Clin Infect Dis; 2003; 37:59-64.

19. McGowan JE. Do intensive hospital antibiotic control programs prevent the spread of antibiotic resistance? Infect Control Hosp Epidemiol; 1994; 15:478-483.

20. Phillips I. Prudent use of antibiotics: are our expectations justified? Clin Infect Dis; 2001; 23(Suppl 3):S130-S132.

21. Moberg CL. Rene Duos: A harbinger of microbial resistance to antibiotics Microbial Drug Resistance; 1996; 2:287-297.

22. Levy SB, Fitzgerald GG, Macone AB. Changes in the intestinal flora of farm personnel after introduction of tetracycline-supplemented feed on a farm N Engl J Med; 1976; 295:583-588.

23. Bell DM. Promoting appropriate antimicrobial drug use: perspective from the Centers for Disease Control and Prevention Clin Infect Dis; 2001; 33(Suppl 3):S245-S250.

24. McGowan JE Jr. Antimicrobial resistance in hospital organisms and its relation to antibiotic use Rev Infect Dis; 1983; 5: 1033-1048.

25. Dowell SF, Scwartz B. Resistant pneumococci: protecting patients through judicious antibiotic use Am Fam Physician; 1997; 55:1647-1654.

26. Scwartz B. Preventing the spread of antimicrobial resistance among bacterial respiratory tract pathogens in industrialized countries: the case for judicious antimicrobial use Clin Infect Dis; 1999; 28:211-213.

27. Diekema DJ, BootsMiller BJ, Vaughn TE. Antimicrobial resistance trends and outbreak frequency in United States hospitals Clin Infect Dis; 2004; 38:78-85.

28. Tenover FC, Weigel LM, Appelbaum PC. Vancomycin-Resistant Staphylococcus aureus Isolate from a Patient in Pennsylvania Antimicrob Agents Chemother.; 2004; 48:275-280.

29. Lautenbach E, Strom BL, Nachamkin I, Bilker WB, Marr AM, Larosa LA, Fishman NO. Longitudinal trends in fluoroquinolone resistance among enterobacteriaceae isolates from inpatients and outpatients, 1989-2000: differences in the emergence of resistance and epidemiology of resistance across organisms Clin Infect Dis; 2004; 38:655-662.

30. Chen DK, McGeer A, DeAzavedo JC, Low DE. Decreased susceptibility of Streptococcus pneumoniae to fluoroquinolones in Canada N Engl J Med; 1999; 341:233-239.

31. Bhavnani SM, Hammel JP, Jones RN, Ambrose PG. Relationship between increased levofloxacin use and decreased susceptibility of Streptococcus pneumoniae: Report from the AR-REST program. Abstract K-1397. Program and abstracts of the, 43rd Interscience Conference on Antimicrobial Agents and Chemotherapy, September 14-17, 2003, Chicago, Illinois.

32. Leibovici L, Berger R, Gruenewald T, Yahav J, Yehezkelli Y, Milo G, Paul M, Samra Z, Pitlik SD. Departmental consumption of antibiotic drugs and subsequent resistance: A quantitative link J Antimicrob Chemother; 2001; 48:535-540.

33. Jaccard C, Troillet N, Harbarth S, Zanetti G, Aymon D, Schneider R, Chiolero R, Ricou B, Romand J, Huber O, Ambrosetti P, Praz G, Lew D, Bille J, Glauser MP, Cometta A. Prospective randomized comparison of imipenem-cilastatin and piperacillin-tazobactam in nosocomial pneumonia or peritonitis Antimicrob Agents Chemother; 1998; 42:2966-2972.

34. Bernard L, Vaudaux P, Vuagnat A, Stern R, Rohner P, Pittet D, Schrenzel J, Hoffmeyer P;, Hoffmeyer P. Effect of vancomycin therapy for osteomyelitis on colonization by methicillin-resistant Staphylococcus aureus: lack of emergence of glycopeptide resistance Infect Control Hosp Epidemiol; 2003; 24: 650-54.

35. Pitout JDD, Sanders CS, Sanders WE. Antimicrobial resistance with focus on beta lactam resistance in gram-negative bacilli Am J Med; 1997; 103:51-59.

36. DiGiovine B, Chenoweth C, Watts C, Higgins M. The attributable mortality and costs of primary nosocomial bloodstream infections in the intensive care unit Am J Respir Crit Care Med; 1999; 160:976-981.

37. Cosgrove SE, Carmeli Y. The impact of antimicrobial resistance on health and economic outcomes Clin Infect Dis; 2003; 36:1433-1437.

38. Classen DC, Pestonik SL, Evans RS, Burke JP. Computerized surveillance of adverse drug events in hospital patients JAMA; 1991; 266:2847-2851.

39. Ebbesen J, Buajordet I, Erikssen J, Brors O, Hilberg T, Svaar H, Sandvik L. Drug-related deaths in a department of internal medicine Arch Intern Med; 2001; 161:2317-2323.

40. Petrak RM, Sexton DJ, Butera ML, Tenenbaum MJ, MacGregor MC, Schmidt ME, Joseph WP, Kemmerly SA, Dougherty MJ, Bakken JS, Curfman MF, Martinelli LP, Gainer RB. The value of an infectious disease specialist Clin Infect Dis; 2003; 36:1013-1017.

41. Projan SJ. Why is big pharma getting out of antibacterial drug discovery Curr Opin Microbiol; 2003; 6:427-430.

42. Besser RE. Antimicrobial prescribing in the United States: good news, bad news Ann Intern Med; 2003; 138:605-606.

43. Steinman MA, Gonzales R, Linder JA, Landefeld CS. Changing use of antibiotics in community-based outpatient practice, 1991-1999 Ann Intern Med; 2003; 138:525-533.

44. Zeigler MG, Lew P, Singer BC. Inaccuracy of drug information from pharmaceutical sales representatives JAMA; 1995; 273: 1296-1298.

45. Billstein SA. How the pharmaceutical industry brings an antibiotic drug to market in the United States Antimicrob Ag Chemother; 1994; 38:2679-2682.

46. Greco PJ, Eisenberg JM. Changing physicians' practices N Engl J Med; 1993; 329:1271-1274.

47. Davis DA, Thomason MA, Oxman AD, Haynes RB. Changing physician performance. A systematic review of the effect of continuing medical education strategies JAMA; 1995; 274: 700-705.

48. Fraser GL, Wennberg DE, Dickens JD Jr, Lambrew CT. Changing physician behavior in ordering digoxin assays Ann Pharmacother; 1996; 30:449-454.

49. Keller RB, Soule DN, Wennberg JE, Hanley DF. Dealing with geographic variations in the use of hospitals: the experience of the Maine Medical Assessment Foundation Orthopedic Study Group J Bone Joint Surg; 1990; 72A:1286-1293.

50. Soumerai SB, Avorn J. Principles of educational outreach (academic detailing) to improve clinical decision making JAMA; 1991; 263:549-556.

51. Garibaldi RA. Computers and the quality of care—a clinician's perspective N Engl J Med; 1998; 338:259-260.

52. Morris AH. Developing and implementing computerized protocols for standardization of clinical decisions Ann Intern Med; 2000; 132:373-383.

53. James BC. Making it easy to do it right N Engl J Med; 2001; 345:991-992.

54. Teich JM, Merchia PR, Schmiz JL, Kuperman GJ, Spurr CD, Bates DW. Effects of computerized physician order entry on prescribing practices Arch Intern Med; 2002; 160:2741-2747.

55. Fraser GL, Dickens JD, Wennberg DE. Changing Physician Digoxin Assay Ordering Behavior; a Five-Year Follow-up Study P&T; 1997; 22:385-392.

56. John JF Jr, Fishman NO. Programmatic role of the infectious diseases physician in controlling antimicrobial costs in the hospital Clin Infect Dis; 1997; 24:471-485.

57. Bantar C, Sartori B, Vesco E, Heft C, Saul M, Salamone F, Oliva ME. A hospitalwide intervention program to optimize the quality of antibiotic use: Impact on prescribing practice, antibiotic consumption, cost savings, and bacterial resistance Clin Infect Dis; 2003; 37:180-186.

58. Stogsdill P, Claffey T, Bates P. Antimicrobial Stewardship Program: From Research to Practice [Abstract 583]. In: Program and abstracts of the, 40th Infectious Diseases Society of America Meeting, October 24-27, 2003, Chicago, IL.

59. Modjtabai K, Prato BS, Stogsdill PB, Owens RC Jr. Impact of inpatient prescribing changes on antimicrobial susceptibilities: A five-year longitudinal study [Abstract 156]. In: Program and abstracts of the, 41st Infectious Diseases Society of America Meeting, October 9-12, 2003, San Diego, California.

60. Ruttimann S, Keck B, Hartmeier C, Maetzel A, Bucher HC. Long-term antibiotic cost savings from a comprehensive intervention program in a medical department of a university-affiliated teaching hospital Clin Infect Dis; 2004; 38:348-356.

61. Carling P, Fung T, Killion A, Terrin N, Barza M. Favorable impact of a multidisciplinary antibiotic management program conducted during 7 years Infect Control Hosp Epidemiol; 2003; 24:699-706.

62. LaRocco A Jr. Concurrent antibiotic review programs—A role for infectious diseases specialists at small community hospitals Clin Infect Dis; 2003; 37:742-743.

63. Gentry CA, Greenfield RA, Slater LN, Slater LN, Wack M, Huycke MM. Outcomes of an antimicrobial control program in a teaching hospital Am J Health-Syst Pharm; 2000; 57: 268-274.

64. Carling PC, Fung T, Coldiron JS. Parenteral antibiotic use in acute-care hospitals: a standardized analysis of fourteen institutions Clin Infect Dis; 1999; 29:1189-1196.

65. Briceland LL, Nightingale CH, Quintiliani RQ, Cooper BW, Smith KS. Antibiotic streamlining from combination therapy to monotherapy utilizing an interdisciplinary approach Arch Intern Med; 1988; 148:2019-2022.

66. Mandell GL, Bennett JE, Dolin R, Eds. New York: Churchill Livingstone, 1995.

67. Gilbert DN, Moellering RC, Sande MA. The Sanford Guide to Antimicrobial Therapy, 2002. Hyde Park Vermont.

68. Harris AD, Smith D, Johnson JA, Bradham DD, Roghmann MC. Risk factors for imipenem-resistant Pseudomonas aeruginosa among hospitalized patients Clin Infect Dis; 2002; 34: 340-345.

69. Ambrose PG, Owens RC Jr. New antibiotics in pulmonary and critical care medicine: focus on advanced generation quinolones and cephalosporins Seminars Resp Crit Care Med; 2000; 21:19-32.

70. Rice LB. Controlling antibiotic resistance in the ICU: Different bacteria, different strategies Cleveland Clinic J Med; 2003; 70:793-800.

71. Fraser GL. Antibiotic optimization: what are the costs associated with saving money? Pharmacoeconomics: Infectious Diseases 1997; 1:2-4.

72. Madaras-Kelly K. Optimizing antibiotic use in hospitals: the role of population-based antibiotic surveillance in limiting antibiotic resistance Pharmacotherapy; 2003; 23:1627-1633.

73. Ansari F, Gray K, Nathwani D, Phillips G, Ogston S, Ramsay C, Davey P. Outcomes of an intervention to improve hospital antibiotic prescribing: interrupted time series with segmented regression analysis J Antimicrob Chemother; 2003; 52:842-848.

74. Ramsay C, Brown E, Hartman E, Davey P. Room for improvement: a systematic review of the quality of evaluations of interventions to improve hospital antibiotic prescribing J Antimicrob Chemother; 2003; 52:764-771.

75. The Cochrane Effective Practice and Organization of Care Group (EPOC). The Data Collection Checklist. Cochrane Effective Practice and Organization of Care Group (EPOC) Methods Papers [Online.] 2002. http://www.epoc.uottawa.ca/ (accessed 14 March 2004).

76. Owens RC Jr, Bates P, Lerwick P. Effect of community-acquired pneumonia guidelines on discharge efficiency and initial antibiotic choices [Abstract 556]. Program and abstracts of the, 40th Infectious Diseases Society of America Meeting, October 24-27, 2002, Chicago, IL.

77. Vinken A, Li Z, Banan D, Rittenhouse B, Wilike R, Nathwani D. Economic evaluation of linezolid, flucloxacillin and vancomycin in the empirical treatment of cellulitis in UK hospitals: a decision analytical model J Hosp Infect; 2001; 49(Suppl A): S13-S24.

78. Pakyz A, Scheld WM, Schlag K. Evaluation of an antimicrobial surveillance team (AST) program after a three-year period. In Program and Abstracts of the, 39th Annual Infectious Diseases Society of America Meeting [abstract no. 810], October 25-28, 2001, Chicago, IL.

79. Calfee DP, Brooks J, Zirk NM, Giannetta ET, Scheld WM, Farr BM. A pseudo-outbreak of nosocomial infections associated with the introduction of an antibiotic management programme J Hosp Infect; 2003; 55:26-32.

80. Solomon DH, Van Houten L, Glynn RJ, Baden L, Curtis K, Schrager H, Avorn J. Academic detailing to improve use of broad-spectrum antibiotics at an academic medical center Arch Intern Med; 2001; 161:1897-1902.

81. Ambrose PG, Owens RC Jr, Grasela D. Antimicrobial Pharmacodynamics Medical Clinics North America; 2000; 84: 1431-1445.

82. Goldberg J, Owens RC Jr. Optimizing antimicrobial dosing in the critically ill patient Curr Opin Crit Care; 2002; 8:435-440.

83. Melmon KL, Blaschke TF. The undereducated physician's therapeutic decisions N Engl J Med; 1983; 308:1473-1474.

84. Avorn J, Soumerai SB. Improving drug-therapy decisions through educational outreach N Engl J Med; 1983; 308;:1457-1463.

85. http://www.leapfroggroup.org accessed 5/30/03.

86. Evans RS, Pestotnik SL, Classen DC, Burke JP. Evaluation of a computer-assisted antibiotic-dose monitor Ann Pharmacother; 1999; 33:1026-1031.

87. Pestotnik SL, Classen DC, Evans RS, Burke JP. Implementing antibiotic practice guidelines through computer-assisted decision support: clinical and financial outcomes Ann Intern Med; 1996; 124:884-890.

88. Evans RS, Pestotnik SL, Classen DC, Clemmer TP, Weaver LK, Orme JF Jr, Lloyd JF, Burke JP. A computer-assisted management program for antibiotics and other antiinfective agents N Engl J Med; 1998; 338:232-238.

89. Lesar TS, Briceland LL. Survey of antibiotic control policies in university-affiliated teaching institutions Ann Pharmacother; 1996; 30:31-34.

90. Frank MO, Batteiger BE, Sorensen SJ, Hartstein AI, Carr JA, McComb JS, Clark CD, Abel SR, Mikuta JM, Jones RB. Decrease in expenditures and selected nosocomial infections following implementation of an antimicrobial-prescribing improvement program Clinical Performance and Quality Health Care; 1997; 5:180-188.

91. Himmelgerg CJ, Pleasants RA, Weber DJ, Kessler JM, Samsa GP, Spivey JM, Morris TL. Use of antimicrobial drugs in adults before and after removal of a restriction policy Am J Hosp Pharm; 1991; 48:1220-1227.

92. Ambrose PG, Bhavnani SM, Owens RC Jr. Clinical Pharmacodynamics of Quinolones Infect Dis Clinics North America; 2003; 17:529-543.

93. Ambrose PG, Owens RC Jr, Russo R, Zoe-Powers A, Jones DT. Utilizing Pharmacodynamics in Formulary and Clinical Decision-Making. In: Nightingale CH, Murakawa T, Ambrose PG, Eds Antimicrobial Pharmacodynamics in Theory and Clinical Practice. New York: Marcel Dekker Publishers, 2001: 385-408.

94. Ambrose PG, Owens RC Jr, Garvey MJ, Jones RN. Pharmacodynamic Considerations in the Treatment of Moderate to Severe Pseudomonal Infections with Cefepime J Antimicrob Chemother; 2002; 49:445-453.

95. Ambrose PG, Bhavnani SM, Owens RC Jr. Clinical pharmaco-dynamics of quinolones Infect Dis Clin N Am; 2003; 17:529-543.

96. Avorn J, Soumerai J, Taylor W, Wessels MR, Janousek J, Weiner M. Reduction of incorrect antibiotic dosing through a structured educational order form Arch Intern Med; 1988; 148: 1720-1724.

97. Strausbaugh LJ, Jernigan DB, Liedtke LA. National shortages of antimicrobial agents: Results of 2 surveys from the Infectious Diseases Society of America Emerging Infections Network Clin Infect Dis; 2001; 33:1495-1501.

98. Li JZ, Willke RJ, Rittenhouse BE, Rybak MJ. Effect of linezolid versus vancomycin on length of hospital stay in patients with complicated skin and soft tissue infections caused by known or suspected methicillin-resistant Staphylococci: Results from a randomized clinical trial Surgical Infections; 2003; 4:57-70.

99. Li Z, Willke RJ, Pinto LA, Rittenhouse BE, Rybak MJ, Pleil AM, Crouch CW, Hafkin B, Glick HA. Comparison of length of hospital stay for patients with known or suspected methicillin-resistant Staphylococcus species infections treated with linezolid or vancomycin: A randomized, multicenter trial Pharmacotherapy; 2001; 21:263-274.

100. Wunderink RG, Rello J, Cammarata SK, Croos-Dabrera RV, Kollef MH. Linezolid vs vancomycin: Analysis of two double-blind studies of patients with methicillin-resistant Staphylococcus aureus nosocomial pneumonia Chest; 2003; 124:1789-97.

101. Projan SJ. Why is big pharma getting out of antibacterial drug discovery? Curr Opin Microbiol; 2003; 6:427-430.

102. Kunin CM. Editorial response: Antibiotic Armageddon Clin Infect Dis; 1997; 25:240-241.

11

Role of Computer-Assisted Programs in Optimizing the Use of Antimicrobial Agents

JOHN P. BURKE and RAJESH R. MEHTA

Department of Clinical Epidemiology
and Infectious Disease, LDS Hospital, and
Department of Medicine, University of
Utah School of Medicine,
Salt Lake City, Utah, U.S.A.

The *"iron triangle of health care"* refers to the inevitable trade-offs among quality, access, and cost containment (1). Health care policymakers say we can optimize any two of these goals but not the third. A similar iron triangle in infectious disease management may constrain efforts to optimize antimicrobial use, resistance, and costs. It is still unclear how the goals of optimal use of antimicrobials and reduced resistance are related to costs or if they are mutually reinforcing. Better use of antimicrobials in hospitals, for example, unquestionably could help to prevent resistance that, in turn, may decrease total costs.

Antimicrobial management programs in hospitals have been shown to be capable of improving use and preventing some types of microbial resistance in the short term (2,3). The resources to sustain these efforts, however, are usually formidable, and the methods have not been either practical or cost-effective for health care systems in general. Kunin (4) underscored the bleak outlook for control of antibiotic resistance: "There is only a thin red line of infectious disease practitioners who have dedicated themselves to rational therapy and the control of hospital infections."

A further question is whether "the juice will be worth the squeeze." That is, will methods to optimize the use of antimicrobials produce important benefits for patients and society? Many believe that computer-assisted programs can lower costs while retaining the benefits of more labor-intensive methods for antimicrobial optimization and even make programs feasible in settings without access to infectious disease pharmacists and physicians (5–7). Regardless, model programs employing computerized methods can reveal the limits of what is achievable with the current state of knowledge.

The continuing emergence of antimicrobial resistance has been attributed to two main factors: the extensive and often inappropriate use of antimicrobials and lapses in infection control measures such as hand hygiene and isolation. Computerized hospital information systems can help with both of these problems, but this chapter focuses on the former. Assessing the epidemiology of hospital-acquired infections and antibiotic use and providing regularly updated information about antimicrobial drug resistance in hospitals are essential first steps. Because antibiotic misuse more often results from inadequate information than from inappropriate behavior, providing access to useful information at the point of care and meeting the needs of physicians to use the data more efficiently in their daily work should become the focal point for optimizing antibiotic use. On the other hand, efforts to reduce the use of antibiotics by administrative means and formulary controls rather than by methods to optimize use for individual patients have been compared with squeezing a balloon: constraining one end causes the other end to bulge (8). Addressing the problems of antibiotic resistance by limiting the use of one class of compounds may be counteracted by corresponding changes in prescribing and drug resistance that are even more challenging (9).

Advanced computer systems can assist physicians in the use of antibiotics, for example, by recommending dosages and durations of therapy, providing susceptibility patterns for nosocomial pathogens from the local hospital, displaying the costs of the formulary antimicrobials, and triggering alerts for inappropriate antibiotic use, potential adverse drug events, and errors of commission or omission (10). Fishman (11) pointed out that the computer has the potential to be the ultimate method for antibiotic education and stewardship and that the lessons learned and approaches taken in developing the "Automated Antibiotic Assistant" at LDS Hospital in Salt Lake City should be a paradigm for the future design of such systems.

Physicians, especially the new generation of clinicians, readily accept and expect computer resources to help analyze and solve problems. Shea and Clayton (12) listed the various ways in which computers have affected clinical practice, for example, using online information sources and electronic communication (Table 1). Today's computer-based patient records vary widely in their ability to support clinical decision making, and vendors are aggressively competing to develop enhancements that include computerized physician order entry (CPOE) (13).

CLINICAL DECISION SUPPORT SYSTEMS

Although there is no single definition for a computerized clinical decision support system (CDSS), the term usually refers to medical logic that is encoded in a knowledge base (separate from the patient data) and that is applied to electronic patient records by an inference engine that generates real-time advice to clinicians (14) (Table 2). Thus, a CDSS usually requires a rule-based expert system, a type of artificial intelligence, that can be activated either on-demand at specific times or automatically by data capture, i.e., either time driven or data driven. The simple display of computerized guidelines or formatted laboratory

Table 1   Types of Clinical Information Systems

Function	Examples
Improve access to medical knowledge	Medline, Ovid, commercial websites such as UpToDate.com, Micromedex
Improve communication among providers and between patient and providers	E-mail notification, web alert, listserv
Improve documentation and access to clinical information	Computer-based patient records
Improve provider and patient decision making	Computerized clinical decision support systems such as Adult Antibiotic Assistant at LDS Hospital

From Shea S, Clayton PD. Computerized clinical decision support systems begin to come of age [editorial]. Am J Med 1999; 106:261–262.

data would not, therefore, be considered as a CDSS, and CPOE may or may not have expert system features.

The LDS Hospital's experience in developing CDSSs has led to recognition of the need to "manage the expectations" of the users. The most successful decision support programs meet these expectations by making the job of the physician easier. In addition, they educate the user, fit into the physician's workflow at the point of care, provide patient-specific information in real time and immediate online feedback from the user, present the physician with choices, and enhance clinical judgment, that is, the programs are "open-looped" (15) (Table 3). There is no expectation that the physician will accept the com-

Table 2   Definition of Computer-Assisted Clinical Decision Support Systems

Clinical consultation systems that use population statistics or encode expert knowledge to assist physicians in diagnosis and treatment planning.

From Wiederhold G, Shortliffe EH. System design and engineering. In: Shortliffe EH, Perreault LE, Wiederhold G, Fagan LM, eds. Medical Informatics: Computer Applications in Health Care and Biomedicine. 2d ed. New York: Springer-Verlag, 2001:180–211.

Table 3 Features of Successful
Computer-Assisted Clinical Decision
Support Systems

Makes the job easier
Educates
Is patient-specific
Is real-time oriented
Provides on-line feedback
Allows for choice/clinical judgment (open looped)

From Pestotnik SL, Classen DC, Evans RS, Burke JP.
Implementing antibiotic practice guidelines through
computer-assisted decision support: clinical and financial outcomes. Ann Intern Med 1996; 124:884–890.

puter's advice. The CDSS programs are designed to augment,
not replace, the clinician's judgment, and to inform rather than
to enforce clinical decisions. A computerized CDSS is non-
threatening to the user because the program does not primarily audit the performance of physicians, and because use of
the program is voluntary.

Whether computer applications in medicine can improve
the outcomes for patients is no longer contentious or in doubt;
open-looped CDSSs can be compared to the stethoscope as a
tool to enhance clinical judgment and to promote physicians'
autonomy. Physicians using a CDSS perform better than unaided physicians (16). On the other hand, many now seek to
use computers to control the behavior of physicians and to
restrict choices. This approach can reduce undesirable variation in care and make it more predictable, but it cannot lead
to continuous improvement in care. Another consequence of
this approach is that "ritual knowledge" or "cookbook medicine" may replace fundamental knowledge. Overreliance on
technology can cause atrophy and loss of important clinical
skills and reasoning.

Technologic solutions have great appeal and offer tools
that are transportable to different settings. They also may
have the ability to track and monitor processes of care. Though
the individual physician is not perfectible, the system of care
is. McDonald (17) predicted that the computer would play a

major part in the perfection of future care systems. Shortliffe (18) categorized computer decision support functions as (i) tools for information management (which facilitate access to patient data needed for clinical decision making), (ii) tools for focusing attention (clinical laboratory systems that flag abnormal values or pharmacy systems that alert providers to possible drug interactions), and (iii) tools for patient-specific consultations (provide customized assessments or advice based on sets of patient-specific data) (Table 4). The infrastructure to build such a system may not be easily developed, and some of the more sophisticated and well-known systems require intense integration of data sources from various components in a health care setting. For example, the different components of the database required to develop the Automated Antibiotic Assistant program at LDS Hospital included the patient's admission diagnosis, white cell count, temperature, body weight and height, surgical data, and information from pharmacy, radiology, pathology, serology, and microbiology, to determine the computer-suggested antimicrobial therapy (19). Such technology must also be built on a strong foundation of epidemiologic information, facts, and experience within a health care setting, i.e., both patient- and institution-specific information that also includes financial (cost) data.

Table 4   Types of Medical Decision Support Functions

Function	Examples
Tools for information management	Hospital information system, Medline
Tools for focusing attention	Pharmacy systems that alert providers to possible drug interactions, clinical laboratory systems that flag abnormal values
Tools for patient-specific consultation	Programs that provide customized assessments or advice based on sets of patient-specific data

From Shortliffe EH. Computer programs to support clinical decision making. JAMA 1987; 258:61–66.

OPTIMIZING ANTIMICROBIAL THERAPY USING A CLINICAL DECISION SUPPORT SYSTEM

The epidemiologic databases that are necessary for CDSS applications to support anti-infective use also have a fundamental role in guiding interventions by infection control practitioners and clinical pharmacists. These databases can be used to expand the range of collaboration and communication around patient care, a concept embraced by the term *"interventional epidemiology"* (20). By generating daily monitoring reports that are time driven, pharmacists, for example, can receive alerts of inappropriate antimicrobial use and bring relevant alerts to the attention of the caregivers. Inconsequential or trivial alerts can be filtered out so that only valid suggestions are brought to clinicians' attention by the antimicrobial management team. The face-to-face interaction humanizes the role of the computer system: Whenever possible, alerts are delivered by people. This process avoids information overload, for example, from a profusion of false-positive unedited alerts that might be sent by e-mail in some centers.

Surveillance programs in hospital epidemiology traditionally have been limited to tracking antibiotic resistance and influencing physician decision making by feedback after the fact rather than by real-time interventions (21). This use of epidemiology is thus archival or researching in nature, not interventional, and is insufficient. Although there have been some successes with various strategies, such as antimicrobial management programs, control/restriction programs, and antibiotic cycling programs, to name a few, having a direct impact on antimicrobial use and resistance rates, these strategies are intrusive for health care workers, do not address the needs for optimal therapy for individual patients, and are rather blunt instruments to force prescribing change. One way to improve antibiotic use, then, is computer-assisted decision support that provides timely information and guidance and encourages individualization and heterogeneity of antibiotic selection through a patient-centered approach (22).

Eliminating unnecessary variation in prescribing is a well-accepted goal of most quality improvement programs, but individualization of treatment that embraces individual patient variation is also necessary. This seeming contradiction is particularly important with regard to antibiotic use. The use of many different antibiotics according to individual circumstances may lead to heterogeneous prescribing patterns that may help to prevent antibiotic resistance.

CHALLENGES OF COMPLEX PRESCRIBING SYSTEMS

Antibiotic prescriptions are generated in many different settings: office- or clinic-based practice, special care and nursing units of acute care hospitals, rehabilitation facilities, long-term care units, and home care. Furthermore, many different types of health care professionals are now involved in prescribing: advanced practice nurses, physicians' assistants, and new types of clinical specialists, including hospitalists, emergent care specialists, critical care specialists, and even trainees such as medical and surgical house officers. In many teaching hospitals, the responsible attending physicians, i.e., the clinicians with the most clinical experience, are abjured from writing orders in order to assure that a single physician tracks all orders and to create an optimal learning experience for junior staff. These changes in the medical environment have created conditions that challenge all solutions to the problem of assuring optimal antibiotic prescribing. A complex system results in many different prescribers having differing levels of experience and training (23). Moreover, few of the prescribers have special training or experience with the management of infectious diseases. They have little or no formal training in the pharmacology, pharmacokinetics, and pharmacodynamics of newer antimicrobial drugs. They seldom have a clear understanding of the important main types of the indications for antibiotic therapy: prophylaxis, empiric therapy of suspected infections before the results of microbial cultures and other microbiologic tests are available to inform therapy, and pathogen-directed treatment of microbiologically confirmed infections. The implicit goals of antibiotic therapy are probably limited to achieving a clinical cure, with almost no attention paid to important secondary goals, such as achieving cure with minimal cost to the patient and minimal damage to the environment by avoiding the selection of resistant organisms, and ameliorating harm to the patient from unanticipated adverse drug events.

A common mind-set of today's prescribers leads to the liberal use of antibiotics, often in combination, with the belief that "they can't hurt and might help." This leads inexorably to two further problems: First, once antibiotics are started, they continue to be given, right up to the time of hospital discharge if the patient is doing well. Indeed, the landmark Pennsylvania study of antibiotic use in general hospitals found that the most frequent event predicting a stop order for antibiotics was hospital discharge (24). Second, antibiotics are changed frequently and others added without any additional information to drive changes in therapy simply because the patient remains sick and the prescribers are anxious that they may be "missing something" or they want to "cover" colonizing organisms. This pattern of antibiotic misuse has been called *"spiraling empiricism"* (25), and its practitioners frequently experience positive reinforcement. The patients either have a relentless downhill course to death "despite the fact that we did everything we could," or the patients have a gratifying response that is mistakenly attributed to the antibiotics. The current medicolegal environment adds another dimension of reinforcement, because lawsuits seldom, if ever, result from giving too many or unnecessary antibiotics. Excessive antibiotic use is also fanned by the pharmaceutical industry's encouragement to use the most broad-spectrum agents.

It should be no surprise that top-down administrative efforts to reduce and control antibiotic use have not been successful in a health care profession under siege. Nonetheless, professionalism remains the motivational force of greatest potential; physicians remain committed to better care of patients and believe that this offers them the "high ground" in their ongoing struggles with the health care changes that limit their autonomy and reduce their incomes (26). Furthermore, innovations that will increase their efficiency, make the job easier, and promote clinical autonomy would seem to have the best chances for success.

OPTIMIZING ANTIBIOTIC USE AT LDS HOSPITAL

At LDS Hospital, the clinical epidemiology team has demonstrated that computer-assisted decision support, based on the principles of epidemiology and the use of a flexible and dynamic medical informatics system, can be used to inform and improve antibiotic decisions rather than to enforce them (27). These patient-centered strategies may reduce the total amount of antibiotic use, promote unintentional random use of specific antimicrobials, and, thereby, stabilize antibiotic resistance. The key principle is that the individual physician retains control of antibiotic use on the basis of relevant information available at the bedside, using the computer system as a tool.

At LDS Hospital, a new treatment paradigm has been developed in which local epidemiologic surveillance data on antibiotic use, prescribing patterns, infection control, microbial susceptibility, and adverse drug events together with a knowledge base comprising local guidelines and expert opinion are combined in a computer program called the Automated Antibiotic Assistant. Its role is to assist physicians in the selection and use of antibiotics for prophylaxis or treatment at the patient's bedside. In using clinician-derived, patient-centered treatment guidelines and applying them at the point of care, the program represents a radical departure from the more traditional treatment paradigms based on national guidelines and administrative policies, such as restricted formularies, that aim to guide antibiotic selection (28).

New treatment paradigms, such as those developed by LDS Hospital, approach the problem of antibiotic prescribing from the perspective of the individual patient and the need for physicians to make decisions about patient care at the bedside (29). The goal of these new treatment paradigms is to improve, rather than simply reduce, antimicrobial use, a process that goes far beyond the initial antibiotic selected. The new treatment paradigms include dosage, route of administration, and duration of prophylaxis or treatment for the specific infection in a specific patient, taking into account the patient's physiologic status. For example, proper dosing using daily automated estimates of renal function has reduced the overall "tonnage" of the use of certain antibiotics by as much as 30%, with significant cost savings (30). The new paradigm also includes surveillance and prevention of adverse drug reactions (31), alerts to apply certain infection control practices (32), surveillance of hospital-acquired infections and reportable diseases, and decisions to obtain cultures and serum drug levels and perform laboratory tests (33).

At the heart of the LDS Hospital Automated Antibiotic Assistant is a system that can be accessed from any terminal within the hospital and from physicians' offices and homes via a personal computer and modem. It provides the physician with structured help during the prescribing process at a time when the treatment decisions are being made at the patient's bedside, not just with feedback after the event.

Central to the LDS Hospital antibiotic management program embodied in the Automated Antibiotic Assistant is the use of local epidemiologic data to help predict the most likely pathogens in given types of infection and the antibiotics that are most likely to be effective. With input from infectious disease specialists, infection control practitioners, and pharmacists, the database for the computer program includes information not only on the occurrence of infection but also resistance patterns within local areas of the hospital, such as different intensive care units (ICUs), and differences in drug usage for prophylaxis and therapy. The key to its effectiveness as a tool for improved antibiotic selection is continued monitoring of antibiotic use with intervention that makes useful information available at the point of care. As a practical tool to aid antibiotic prescribing, it has been applied to surgical prophylaxis (34–36), pathogen-directed treatment (5), and empiric therapy of hospital-acquired infections (37), with encouraging results. For each mode of antibiotic use, an integrated database with monitoring and reminder functions has been developed to assist clinicians with antibiotic prescribing (Table 5).

Table 5 Studies of Computerized Clinical Decision Support Systems (CDSSs) for management of antibiotic use and infectious diseases at LDS Hospital*

Function	CDSS	Outcomes/conclusions	Preference/year
Assisting	Implementing antibiotic practice guidelines	Local clinician-derived practice guidelines can improve antibiotic use, reduce associated costs, and stabilize the emergence of antibiotic-resistant pathogens.	(15)/1996
	Timing of prophylactic use of antibiotics	Administration of surgical antibiotic prophylaxis on time reduces the risk of wound infection.	(36)/1992
	Reminders of perioperative antibiotic use	Improved prescribing and a concurrent decline in postoperative wound infections.	(34)/1989
	Selecting appropriate empiric antibiotics	Information from computer-based medical records helped to improve physicians' selection of empiric antibiotics for infections.	(37)/1994
Alerting	Adapting disease specific isolation guidelines	Improved and more accurate use of isolation.	(32)/1986
	Reducing the duration of prophylactic antibiotic use	Improved usage of antibiotic prophylaxis by monitoring all antibiotics given to surgical patients and identifying patients receiving antibiotic prophylaxis longer than necessary.	(35)/1990

Interpreting	Surveillance of hospital-acquired infections and antibiotic use	Computer screening helped focus the activities and improved the efficiency of hospital surveillance personnel.	(33)/1986
	Identifying patients at high risk for hospital-acquired infection	Computerized regression equations to identify patients at risk of having hospital-acquired infections helped focus prevention efforts.	(46)/1992
Critiquing	Therapeutic antibiotic monitoring	Efficient method to assure the appropriate use of therapeutic antibiotics and to identify and correct errors in antimicrobial prescribing.	(5)/1990
	Prospective surveillance of imipenem/cilastatin use and associated seizures	Monitoring of imipenem/cilastatin dosages in relation to renal function resulted in a reduced incidence of seizures.	(47)/1993
	Monitoring and adjusting daily antibiotic dose for changes in renal function	Reduced the excessive use and cost of antibiotic therapy and the number of adverse drug events secondary to antibiotics.	(30)/1999
Managing	Computer physician order entry program for antibiotics	Improved quality of patient care and reduced costs and length of stay.	(10)/1998

* Functions listed according to categories suggested by Pryor; "diagnosing" was also listed as a function by Pryor but is not included here because none of the antimicrobial management programs focuses on this function.
From Pryor TA. Development of decision support systems. Int J Clin Monit Comput 1990; 7:137–146.

CLINICAL DECISION SUPPORT SYSTEMS FOR
SURGICAL ANTIBIOTIC PROPHYLAXIS

For surgical prophylaxis, local guidelines have been developed for case selection, selection of antibiotic agents by surgical subspecialty, appropriate delivery time for selected agents, intraoperative dosing, and duration of antibiotic prophylaxis.

Implemented over the past decade, the use of the Automated Antibiotic Assistant for surgical prophylaxis and definitive treatment has led to significant improvements in overall antibiotic use at the LDS Hospital. Between 1988 and 1998, the period during which computer-based decision support was first introduced, optimal timing of antibiotic prophylaxis for surgical patients improved from 40% to over 99% while rates of surgical site infection were also reduced (38). Computer-assisted interventions accompanied these improvements and achieved significantly shorter durations of prophylaxis, a reduction in the proportion of patients receiving prophylaxis for more than 24 hours (from 30% in 1988 to less than 6% in 1998) and a 50% reduction in the mean number of antibiotic doses over the 10-year period.

CLINICAL DECISION SUPPORT SYSTEMS FOR
DIRECTED ANTI-INFECTIVE THERAPY

For definitive or therapeutic use of antibiotics, a relatively simple set of guidelines has been developed. The foci of these guidelines include patients with positive microbial cultures identified in the laboratory that meet computerized criteria as probable pathogens and for which treatment has not been given; infections for which therapy would be inappropriate because of resistance; cases in which therapy with a less costly antibiotic would be appropriate; or cases in which incorrect dosage, route of administration, or treatment intervals or inappropriate serum levels and laboratory monitoring have been found.

Corresponding improvements were seen with therapeutic antibiotic use following the introduction of computer-based decision support. Appropriate antibiotic use increased, as reflected by reductions in the mean number of daily alerts from 2.95 in 1988 to 1.38 in 1998, as did the rate of physician compliance, which rose from 42.2% in 1988 to 99.8% in 1998.

CLINICAL DECISION SUPPORT SYSTEMS FOR EMPIRIC ANTIBIOTIC USE

Extension of the Automated Antibiotic Assistant to the empiric therapy of hospital-acquired infections represents the most sophisticated application of the computer-based decision-support system. It uses a local epidemiologic database containing 5 years of nosocomial infection surveillance data, updated monthly to reflect changes in site-specific pathogens and susceptibility patterns, and is based on logistic regression models. Physicians can access a computer display at bedside terminals that suggests a suitable empiric regimen for a specific patient based on the likelihood of coverage in relation to cost, antibiotic allergies, and renal function. Because the suggested empiric treatment is selected according to patient-specific information such as allergies and renal function and institution-specific information such as cost of different regimens, taking into account the effect of individualized dosing on cost, this method of selecting both directed and empiric therapy assures a more-or-less random use of different antimicrobials and avoids repetitive use of a favored broad-spectrum antimicrobial.

To access this information, the physician need only identify (from a menu screen) the patient and site of infection. The physician can also access information that shows the computer logic that was used in making the therapeutic suggestion. Other menu options can be used to review antibiotic susceptibility patterns for both community-acquired and hospital-acquired pathogens for both 5-year and the most recent 1-year periods, as well as the cost for each antibiotic, adjusted for the individual patient's needs, and formulary monographs containing key prescribing information. The LDS program demonstrates how computers can be used to collect the large amount of patient data that are presented to physicians each day and gather them in a logical context that can assist physicians in administering patient care.

The appropriateness of empiric antibiotic therapy suggested by the Automated Antibiotic Assistant was evaluated with reference to the actual results of antibiotic susceptibility tests and treatment selected by physicians. The actual empiric prescribing was found to be appropriate 94% of the time when physicians accessed the computerized decision support program, as compared with 77% of the time when selected by unaided physicians ($p < 0.001$). Furthermore, physicians prescribed appropriate antibiotics (to which all pathogens were susceptible) within 12 hours of culture significantly more often when using the Automated Antibiotic Assistant compared with the control period ($p < 0.035$). When interviewed about the usefulness of computer-aided support, 88% of physicians stated they would recommend the program to other physicians, 85% felt it improved their selection of empiric therapy, and 81% felt it contributed to improved patient care.

THE IMPACT OF CLINICAL DECISION SUPPORT SYSTEMS ON ANTIBIOTIC USAGE, RESISTANCE, ADVERSE EVENTS, AND COST

Since its introduction over a decade ago, the Automated Antibiotic Assistant has made a significant contribution to antibiotic use within LDS Hospital (Table 6). No antibiotic can be used at LDS Hospital without being affected by these programs, even if some clinicians never use the voluntary program themselves. Between 1988 and 1998, antibiotic usage has been significantly reduced while more patients have received empiric therapy for shorter duration. Over the period since the Automated Antibiotic Assistant's introduction into clinical practice, the number of defined daily doses of antibiotics per 100 bed-days used each year declined by more than 30%, contributing to per-patient reductions in cost of nearly 70% in inflation-adjusted dollars (39,40). The proportion of adverse events due to antibiotics also declined over this period,

Table 6 Quality of Antibiotic Use

Homogeneous	Heterogeneous
Drug formulary	Open access
Restrictive policies	Choice
Forced consultation	Clinician-initiated consultation
Controlled information	Patient-/institution-specific information
Static guidelines/protocols	Dynamic guidelines/protocols
Monosynaptic decision	Polysynaptic decision
Epidemic resistance	Stable resistance
Control resistance	Manage resistance
Regulatory policy	Quality improvement
Component management	Clinical management
Component costs	Total costs
Enforced decision making	Informed decision making

From Burke JP, Pestotnik SL. Computer-assisted prescribing and its impact on resistance. In: Andremont A, Brun-Buisson C, McGowan JE Jr, eds. Antibiotic Therapy and Control of Antimicrobial Resistance in Hospitals. Paris: Elsevier; 1999:89–95.

whereas mortality from nosocomial infections decreased at a time when the underlying risk factors for mortality were increasing in the inpatient population. These changes have occurred in parallel with marked increases in the number of patients receiving antibiotics as well as the more frequent use of broad-spectrum agents. No single measure of antibiotic use is a definitive marker of the quality of prescribing, but the rate of adverse drug events is an additional useful and sensitive indicator of quality. Systems for surveillance of adverse drug events are, therefore, an important component of the epidemiologic infrastructure required for optimal use of computerized CDSSs.

Moreover, no upsurge in antimicrobial resistance (which can be considered a type of adverse drug event and one that is compounded by inadequate infection control) was observed during this period, in contrast to the picture that has been seen in many hospitals and especially ICUs over the past decade. With few exceptions, susceptibility to the main antibiotics used empirically at LDS Hospital to treat suspected nosocomial infections showed little change. There was evidence of reduced susceptibility to ciprofloxacin among isolates of *Pseu-*

domonas aeruginosa, consistent with trends reported in recent National Nosocomial Infections Surveillance System surveys, and of reduced susceptibility of coagulase-negative staphylococci and *Staphylococcus aureus* to methicillin, reflecting the universal challenge posed by methicillin-resistant staphylococci. Importantly, no evidence of vancomycin-resistant enterococci or extended-spectrum beta-lactamase-producing strains of gram-negative bacilli emerged to any significant degree during this period.

LIMITATIONS OF CLINICAL DECISION SUPPORT SYSTEMS

As our experience has shown, the use of a computer-assisted decision-support system may not only improve physicians' selection of empiric antibiotics for treatment of nosocomial infections but may also help to stabilize the development of antimicrobial resistance. However, it is imperative to stress that it is only an aid to prescribing and should not replace clinical judgment. Although decision support software such as the Automated Antibiotic Assistant can help in the selection of antibiotics and guide decisions regarding the dosage, route, interval. and duration of therapy, computer programs cannot decide whether the patient should receive antibiotic therapy in the first place. Such a decision requires the assimilation of information from many diverse sources and is still best performed by the clinician. In a 1-year study in the LDS Hospital ICU, when antibiotic ordering through the computer was required, physicians selected the computer-recommended antibiotics only about 50% of the time but selected the computer-suggested dosages more than 90% of the time. These results were taken to mean that the CDSS programs were being used thoughtfully to enhance clinical judgment and not being blindly followed.

THE FUTURE: DATA MINING, MONITORING, AND COMPUTER PROVIDER ORDER ENTRY

Many strategies have been shown to be capable of reducing inappropriate prescribing of antimicrobials. Multifaceted interventions, including formulary restrictions, ongoing education, and guidelines, and supervision by qualified health care professionals have also led to net cost savings, even without computer assistance. Nonetheless, these programs have not been widely implemented, perhaps, in part, because of insufficiently trained and supported professionals, especially in smaller and community hospitals.

Exalted claims and overly optimistic projections have regularly accompanied discussions about computer applications in health care. Some of the disconnect results from the failure to distinguish clinical from operational computer programs. Clinical applications depend on electronic medical records (EMRs) that are still not widely available and, when fully integrated with coded data based on a data dictionary, enable a wide range of decision-support functions. Operational computer systems capture the billing records and basic demographic data from hospital discharge summaries. Such systems are more widely available and have been used to create "data warehouses." These systems enable operational decision support to monitor quality of care and evaluate physician performance and can be used for "data mining" to generate research hypotheses, but they do not lead to bedside tools at the point of care (41).

Computer monitoring can help structure interventional epidemiology by defining specific trigger tools for interventions and outcome measures to track progress. Many experts believe that computer-assisted antibiotic prescribing may supplement or replace such strategies in the future. Moreover, traditional treatment paradigms may not be suitable and new treatment paradigms, such as those embodied in the LDS Hospital program that uses patient- and institution-specific data to tailor treatment to individual patient circumstances, will be necessary. A survey at the 4th Decennial International Conference on Healthcare-Associated Infections highlighted CPOE as the most promising approach to reduce antibiotic resistance (42). A recent review notes that CPOE is a complex undertaking and should not be the first computer clinical system attempted by an organization (13).

Claims are now being made that CPOE can substantially decrease the overuse, underuse, and misuse of health care services, decrease costs, shorten lengths of stay, decrease medical errors from handwritten orders, and improve compliance with several types of guidelines. The strongest force in health care today is the pressure to control costs. The Institute of Medicine's 1999 report *"To Err Is Human"* galvanized the U.S. media and Congress (43). This has created funding opportunities centered on the issue of patient safety, which in turn, has raised expectations that CPOE is just around the corner. There is, of course, the danger of disillusionment if this goal proves elusive. A consortium of large employers, called the Leapfrog Group (www.leapfroggroup.org), has made CPOE a centerpiece in the strategies to eliminate errors in prescribing. An aroused public and enhanced funding could align the incentives for CPOE that will serendipitously benefit the infectious disease community. The unanticipated consequence of the campaign to reduce medical errors could advance the computer systems and infrastructure needed to optimize antibiotic treatment and prevent resistance.

To take advantage of these larger trends in health care, infectious disease professionals must consider the lessons of quality improvement theory by focusing on controlling the processes of care and not on controlling physicians. These lessons are paradigmatically removed from those that have been developed by noncomputer-assisted antibiotic management programs, which aim to control decisions by individual prescribers through administrative and educational means. In addition, there are many stages of computer development short of CPOE that may be exploited to improve prescribing. For example, a computer-generated operative schedule can be used to monitor and improve the use and timing of surgical antibiotic prophylaxis, a strategy that may foster a "virtuous" cycle of reduced postoperative infections due to resistant microorganisms, and, in turn, reduced antibiotic use (44).

Computerized physician order entry is being touted as a means to prevent errors by blocking inappropriate orders; it can certainly help to avoid errors caused by poor handwriting. However, "smart" CPOE could constitute a "closed-looped" medical device that would require Food and Drug Administration approval and extensive evaluation. A closed-looped device would not support physician choice and would not learn from experience, one of the principal advantages of advanced computer systems that exploit artificial intelligence. Furthermore, such a computer program may "industrialize" errors; amplification of errors across large populations is a concern for all computer applications but especially for closed-looped CDSSs. A more practical approach would emphasize open-looped decision support and enhance physician choice and options by providing treatment suggestions, reminders, and mechanisms for on-line feedback.

CONCLUSIONS

The main lessons of these early experiences with computer-assisted CDSS are that computer screen displays provide a way to focus attention on simple relationships in a complex environment, they enable active interventions by antimicrobial management and infection control teams, and in a world of uncertainty, they can help clinicians make better decisions. Information technology clearly has the potential to be a major weapon in the war on antibiotic resistance. Even if the Internet and wireless handheld devices make the technology widely available, effective use will depend on epidemiologic support. The development of electronic medical record systems has enabled the creation of improved patient information databases, which together with local epidemiologic data on antibiotic use, prescribing patterns, infection control, microbial susceptibility, and adverse drug events can be used to develop software to assist the decision-making process. If and when these services can deliver information customized to a specific patient at the time of clinical decision making, the claims for the powerful role computers can play in health care may be realized.

The approach at LDS Hospital has been broad based and focused on improving all types of antibiotic use, whether prophylactic, empiric, or pathogen-directed therapy. Indeed, all antibiotic use is under continuous review, with real-time feedback of important "triggers" from the medical knowledge base and elements from the electronic patient records. Clinical pharmacists follow up on triggers, such as improper dosing or potential adverse drug events, so that the computer system encourages increased communication among caregivers. The Automated Antibiotic Assistant system has shown that patient- and institution-specific data can be used to tailor therapy to individual patient circumstances. Such an approach avoids mandatory controls or restrictions on antibiotics inherent in traditional treatment paradigms and helps preserve physician choice and strengthen the patient-physician relationship, the most important venue for preventing antibiotic misuse and resistance.

Programs to optimize the use of antibiotics and other anti-infective drugs in health care organizations are better positioned now than ever before to capture the institutional support and resources that are now required to assure patient safety, prevent medication errors, and develop computerized provider/physician order entry (45). All health care organizations are now required to demonstrate a commitment to quality improvement. Optimizing antibiotic use should be a major focus of quality improvement—and the best chance of success depends on integrating and interweaving antibiotic management with these other quality and patient safety programs.

REFERENCES

1. Kissick WL. Medicine's Dilemmas: Infinite Needs vs. Finite Resources. New Haven. CT: Yale University Press, 1994.

2. Struelens MJ. Multidisciplinary antimicrobial management teams: the way forward to control antimicrobial resistance in hospitals [editorial review]. Curr Opin Infect Dis; 2003; 16: 305–307.

3. Ohl C. Antimicrobial stewardship as a means to control drug-resistant pathogens. Sem Infect Control; 2001; 1:210–221.

4. Kunin CM. Editorial response: antibiotic Armageddon. Clin Infect Dis; 1997; 25:240–241.

5. Pestotnik SL, Evans RS, Burke JP, Gardner RM, Classen DC. Therapeutic antibiotic monitoring; surveillance using a computerized expert system. Am J Med; 1990; 88:43–47.

6. Barenfanger J, Short MA, Groesch AA. Improved antimicrobial interventions have benefits. J Clin Microbiol; 2001; 39: 2823–2828.

7. Glowacki RC, Schwartz DN, Itokazu GS, Wisniewski MF, Kieszkowski P, Weinstein RA. Antibiotic combinations with redundant antimicrobial spectra: clinical epidemiology and pilot intervention of computer-assisted surveillance. Clin Infect Dis; 2003; 37:59–64.

8. Burke JP. Antibiotic resistance—squeezing the balloon [editorial]? JAMA; 1998; 280:1270–1271.

9. Rahal JJ, Urban C, Horn D, Freeman K, Segal-Maurer S, Maurer J, Mariano N, Marks S, Burns JM, Dominick D, Lim M. Class restriction of cephalosporin use to control total cephalosporin resistance in nosocomial *Klebsiella*. JAMA; 1998; 280: 1233–1237.

10. Evans RS, Pestotnik SL, Classen DC, Clemmer TP, Weaver LK, Orme JF Jr, Lloyd JF, Burke JP. A computer-assisted management program for antibiotics and other antiinfective agents. N Engl J Med; 1998; 338:232–238.

11. Fishman NO. Antimicrobial management and cost containment. In: Mandell GL, Bennett JE, Dolin R, Eds Mandell, Douglas, and Bennett's Principles and Practice of Infectious Diseases. 5th ed. Philadelphia: Churchill Livingstone, 2000: 539–546.

12. Shea S, Clayton PD. Computerized clinical decision support systems begin to come of age [editorial]. Am J Med; 1999; 106: 261–262.

13. Kuperman GJ, Gibson RF. Computer physician order entry: benefits, costs, and issues. Ann Intern Med; 2003; 139:31–39.

14. Wiederhold G, Shortliffe EH. System design and engineering. In: Shortliffe EH, Perreault LE, Wiederhold G, Fagan LM, Eds Medical Informatics: Computer Applications in Health Care and Biomedicine. 2nd ed. New York: Springer-Verlag, 2001: 180–211.

15. Pestotnik SL, Classen DC, Evans RS, Burke JP. Implementing antibiotic practice guidelines through computer-assisted decision support: clinical and financial outcomes. Ann Intern Med; 1996; 124:884–890.

16. Hunt DL, Haynes RB, Hanna SE, Smith K. Effects of computer-based clinical decision support systems on physician performance and patient outcomes. A systematic review. JAMA; 1998; 280:1339–1346.

17. McDonald CJ. Computer reminders, the quality of care and the non-perfectibility of man. N Engl J Med; 1976; 295:1351–1355.

18. Shortliffe EH. Computer programs to support clinical decision making. JAMA; 1987; 258:61–66.

19. Evans RS, Pestotnik SL, Classen DC, Burke JP. Development of an automated antibiotic consultant. MD Comput; 1993; 10: 17–22.

20. Burke JP, Pestotnik SL. Antibiotic resistance—the combat zone [editorial review]. Curr Opin Infect Dis; 1998; 11:441–443.

21. Burke JP. Surveillance, reporting, automation, and interventional epidemiology [editorial]. Infect Control Hosp Epidemiol; 2003; 24:10–12.

22. Karam GH, Niederman MS. How do we achieve adequate therapy for severe infection? Crit Care Med; 2003; 31:648–650.

23. Burke JP, Pestotnik SL. The pharmacy and drug usage. In: Wenzel RP, Ed Assessing Quality Health Care: Perspectives for Clinicians. Baltimore: Williams & Wilkins, 1991:509–520.

24. Shapiro M, Townsend TR, Rosner B, Kass EH. Use of antimicrobial drugs in general hospitals: patterns of prophylaxis. N Engl J Med; 1979; 301:351–355.

25. Kim JH, Gallis HA. Observations on spiraling empiricism: its causes, allure, and perils, with particular reference to antibiotic therapy. Am J Med; 1989; 87:201–206.

26. ABIM Foundation. American Board of Internal Medicine; ACP-ASIM Foundation. American College of Physicians-American Society of Internal Medicine; European Federation of Internal Medicine. Medical professionalism in the new millennium: a physician charter. Ann Intern Med; 2002; 136:243–246.

27. Kassirer JP. The quality of care and the quality of measuring it [editorial]. N Engl J Med; 1993; 329:1263–1265.

28. Dunagan WC, Medoff G. Formulary control of antimicrobial usage. What price freedom? Diagn Microbiol Infect Dis; 1993; 16:265–274.

29. Garibaldi RA. Computers and the quality of care—a clinician's perspective [editorial]. N Engl J Med; 1998; 338:259–260.

30. Evans RS, Pestotnik SL, Classen DC, Burke JP. Evaluation of a computer-assisted antibiotic-dose monitor. Ann Pharmacother; 1999; 33:1026–1031.

31. Classen DC, Pestotnik SL, Evans RS, Burke JP. Computerized surveillance of adverse drug events in hospital patients. JAMA; 1991; 266:2847–2851.

32. Jacobson JT, Johnson DS, Ross CA, Conti MT, Evans RS, Burke JP. Adapting disease-specific isolation guidelines to a hospital information system. Infect Control; 1986; 7:411–418.

33. Evans RS, Larsen RA, Burke JP, Gardner RM, Meier FA, Jacobson JA, Conti MT, Jacobson JT, Hulse RK. Computer surveillance of hospital-acquired infections and antibiotic use. JAMA; 1986; 256:1007–1011.

34. Larsen RA, Evans RS, Burke JP, Pestotnik SL, Gardner RM, Classen DC. Improved perioperative antibiotic use and reduced surgical wound infections through use of computer decision analysis. Infect Control Hosp Epidemiol; 1989; 10:316–320.

35. Evans RS, Pestotnik SL, Burke JP, Gardner RM, Larsen RA, Classen DC. Reducing the duration of prophylactic antibiotic use through computer monitoring of surgical patients. DICP Ann Pharmacother; 1990; 24:351–354.

36. Classen DC, Evans RS, Pestotnik SL, Horn SD, Menlove RL, Burke JP. The timing of prophylactic administration of antibiotics and the risk of surgical-wound infection. N Engl J Med; 1992; 326:281–286.

37. Evans RS, Classen DC, Pestotnik SL, Lundsgaarde HP, Burke JP. Improving empiric antibiotic selection using computer decision support. Arch Intern Med; 1994; 154:878–884.

38. Burke JP. Maximizing appropriate antibiotic prophylaxis for surgical patients: an update from LDS Hospital, Salt Lake City. Clin Infect Dis; 2001; 33(suppl 2):S78–S83.

39. Burke JP, Pestotnik SL. Computer-assisted prescribing and its impact on resistance. In: Andremont A, Brun-Buisson C, McGowan JE Jr., Eds Antibiotic Therapy and Control of Antimicrobial Resistance in Hospitals. Paris: Elsevier, 1999:89–95.

40. Burke JP, Pestotnik SL. Antibiotic use and microbial resistance in intensive care units: impact of computer-assisted decision support. J Chemother; 1999; 11:530–555.

41. Avorn J, Solomon DH. Cultural and economic factors that (mis)-shape antibiotic use: the nonpharmacologic basis of therapeutics. Ann Intern Med; 2000; 133:128–135.

42. Coignard B, Siegel JD, Weinstein RA, Sohn AH, Sinkowitz-Cochran RL, Jarvis WR. Reality check: how should we control antimicrobial use? Current practices and controversies. Infect Control Hosp Epidemiol; 2000; 21:792–795.

43. Kohn LT, Corrigan JM, Donaldson MS, EdsTo Err Is Human: Building a Safer Health System. Washington. DC: National Academy Press, 1999.

44. Burke JP, Pestotnik SL. Antibiotic resistance—systems thinking, chaos, and complexity theory [editorial review]. Curr Opin Infect Dis; 1999; 12:317–319.

45. Burke JP. Infection control: a problem for patient safety [health policy report]. N Engl J Med; 2003; 348:651–656.

46. Evans RS, Burke JP, Classen DC, Gardner RM, Menlove RL, Goodrich KM, Stevens LE, Pestotnik SL. Computerized identification of patients at high risk for hospital-acquired infection. AJIC Am J Infect Control; 1992; 20:4–10.

47. Pestotnik SL, Classen DC, Evans RS, Stevens LE, Burke JP. Prospective surveillance of imipenem/cilastatin use and associated seizures using a hospital information system. Ann Pharmacother; 1993; 27:497–501.

48. Pryor TA. Development of decision support systems Int J Clin Monit Comput; 1990; 7:137–146.

12

Application of Pharmacodynamic Principles: From Theory to Practice

JOSEPH L. KUTI and DAVID P. NICOLAU

Center for Anti-Infective Research and
Development, Hartford Hospital,
Hartford, Connecticut, U.S.A.

As outlined throughout this book, the pharmacodynamic concepts behind how antimicrobials kill bacteria have been well described. For instance, we know that aminoglycoside antimicrobials kill bacteria best when their peak concentrations are relatively high in relation to the minimum inhibitory concentration (MIC) of the pathogen (1–4). These theories support administering these agents in high doses with extended dosing intervals. Yet, despite the plethora of *in vitro* and *in vivo* animal and human data to support such doses, a standard randomized, double-blind, controlled trial has not been conducted (5). Therefore, as approved by the Food and Drug Administration (FDA), aminoglycosides (gentamicin, tobramycin) should still be administered as 1 to 2 mg/kg doses every 8 to 12 hours. Similar situations are apparent for other antimicrobial classes because at the time these agents were under development, knowledge of pharmacodynamic concepts was limited and not yet accepted (6). Thus, the most effective method of administering specific antimicrobials may not be the FDA-approved regimens, and most pharmacodynamically influenced dosing strategies never go further than simply being documented in the literature.

Despite these realities, clinicians can still use their prescriptive authorities to modify doses and administration methods as supported by pharmacodynamic concepts or choose agents based on high probabilities of achieving critical pharmacodynamic breakpoints. Such measures have led to anecdotal case reports of treatment successes (7–10). However, additional benefits of applying pharmacodynamic concepts to dosing regimens, such as reductions in toxicity and costs, cannot be realized until the dosing strategy is standardized at one's institution and many patients have received it. This is best accomplished by developing institution-specific clinical programs that consider not only pharmacodynamic concepts, but also the patient populations most often treated and one's microbiology antibiogram. In this chapter, we provide examples of improving antimicrobial dosing by employing pharmacodynamic principles and demonstrate methods to develop clinical programs based on these concepts.

CLINICAL PROGRAMS

The application of antimicrobial pharmacodynamics to daily clinical practice is derived from early implementation of clinical pharmacy services, specifically pharmacokinetic consulting (6). Because much of pharmacodynamics depends on evaluating the pharmacokinetics of an antibiotic in a specific patient and optimizing the dose, it is clear why this was the first step in applying these principles in the clinical practice setting. Over the past decade, the percentage of hospitals providing pharmacy-based pharmacokinetic consultations increased from 40% in 1989 to 80% in 1998 (11). The majority of consultations were for antimicrobials such as aminoglycosides and vancomycin. Additionally, drug therapy protocol management, defined as allowing pharmacists to order laboratory tests and adjust dosages to obtain desired therapeutic outcomes based upon a preapproved protocol, increased from 25% in 1989 to 70% in 1998. Again, aminoglycosides (91%) as well as other antibiotics (48%) were among the most common drugs managed by pharmacists.

Adjusting antibiotic doses based on therapeutic drug monitoring allows for physicians and pharmacists to target specific serum drug concentrations that are expected to correlate with a positive outcome or prevent toxicity from occurring. These therapeutic ranges or targets for antibiotics were derived from pharmacodynamic studies in *in vitro* and animal models of infection as well as from clinical trials in humans (12).

Not all antimicrobials require pharmacokinetic assessment during treatment to apply pharmacodynamic concepts. For instance, the fluoroquinolones are available in fixed doses and clinical drug assays are unavailable. Thus, the key to applying pharmacodynamic concepts with this class is to choose the agent that gives the highest probability of obtaining optimal pharmacodynamic exposures versus a specific pathogen. The use of Monte Carlo simulation has been employed to evaluate and compare the many fluoroquinolones available (13,14). Monte Carlo simulation is an analytic technique that generates random numbers based on assumptions provided to a computer program. This procedure allows for simulation of antibiotic exposure while considering variability in patient-specific pharmacokinetic and bacteria susceptibility data. Further discussion on the role of Monte Carlo simulation in comparing the pharmacodynamics of fluoroquinolones and other antimicrobials is available in the next chapter of this textbook. In addition to results from Monte Carlo simulations, an institution's pharmacy and therapeutics committee should consider safety and cost data when choosing a fluoroquinolone for formulary inclusion.

As will be discussed later in this chapter, for most uses, beta-lactams also do not require pharmacokinetic monitoring to apply pharmacodynamic concepts. Moreover, clinical drug assays for these agents are limited, but available for certain agents. For instance, at the time of writing, the authors of this chapter offer clinical assays for cefepime, meropenem, and piperacillin/tazobactam, but depending on the number of samples to be run, results may be available the day after receiving samples or on a weekly or monthly basis.

For antimicrobials that do not require pharmacokinetic evaluation, pharmacodynamic concepts can be applied to patient care based on a nomogram or protocol, which attempts to provide optimal exposure for patients who are treated. These clinical protocols often incorporate a fixed dose of an antimicrobial for specific uses or bacterial pathogens, for example, the use of continuous-infusion piperacillin/tazobactam at a dose of 9 g over 24 hours for patients with community-acquired infections and 13.5 g over 24 hours for patients with nosocomial infections or those suspected of infection with *Pseudomonas aeruginosa* (15).

PHARMACODYNAMIC PRINCIPLES

The concepts of antimicrobial pharmacodynamics are discussed in great detail earlier in this textbook. Briefly, antimicrobials exhibit two primary patterns of bacterial killing: concentration-dependent and concentration-independent, or time-dependent, killing (16). Concentration-dependent antibiotics are characterized by a greater rate and extent of bacterial killing as drug concentrations are increased. This pattern is observed with aminoglycosides, fluoroquinolones, and metronidazole (16). In contrast, for concentration-independent drugs, bacterial killing is seldom affected by increasing drug concentrations once the concentration is above four to five times the MIC. Instead, these agents are commonly referred to as *displaying time-dependent bactericidal activity* because the extent of bacterial killing is primarily dependent on the duration of exposure above the MIC. This pattern is observed with beta-lactams (penicillins, cephalosporins, monobactams, and

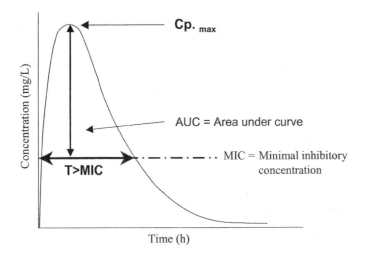

Figure 1   Figure 1. Pharmacokinetic/pharmacodynamic parameters. Cp, peak concentration; T>MIC, time above minimum inhibitory concentration.

carbapenems), glycopeptides, macrolides, clindamycin, tetracyclines, and oxazolidinones (16).

The concepts of antimicrobial killing characteristics can be further quantified by the use of pharmacodynamic parameters (Fig. 1), which include the area under the curve (AUC) to MIC ratio, the peak concentration (Cp) to MIC ratio, and the time above the MIC (T>MIC) (12). These parameters mathematically reference the concentration of drug (i.e., pharmacokinetics) to its MIC versus a given pathogen. Depending on whether an antimicrobial displays concentration-dependent or time-dependent killing at the doses administered, different pharmacodynamic parameters can be employed as a means to target antimicrobial therapy.

OPTIMIZING PHARMACODYNAMICS OF CONCENTRATION-DEPENDENT ANTIBIOTICS

Aminoglycosides

Owing to their concentration-dependent bacterial killing, increasing aminoglycoside concentrations to achieve a Cp/MIC ratio of approximately 10 to 12 is coupled with a greater rate and extent of bacterial kill, potentially leading to improved clinical outcomes (2–4). This characteristic, along with a prolonged postantibiotic effect against most bacteria, promotes administration of these compounds as high bolus doses separated by extended intervals of 12 to 24 hours or longer, depending on a patient's renal function. This dosing technique has been termed once-daily, high-dose, or extended-interval administration and is in direct contrast to the older, conventional method of aminoglycoside administration, in which low doses were given numerous times a day in order to maintain drug concentrations in excess of the MIC.

Several studies in humans have supported extended-interval dosing of the aminoglycosides (2–4,17–21). Compared with conventional dosing, all of these studies have demonstrated equal or greater clinical outcomes when a high-dose, extended-interval administration is employed. As a secondary end point, the majority of these studies have attempted to determine if a reduction in nephrotoxicity with extended-interval dosing is realized. Aminoglycoside-associated nephrotoxicity is caused by accumulation of the drug molecule in the proximal renal tubular epithelial (PRTE) cells, inducing cellular toxicity and necrosis (22,23). The uptake of aminoglycosides into the PRTE cell is limited to the luminal border, where the drug molecule binds to the cell surface and is taken up by pinocytosis, a rate-limited and saturable step (24). Consequently, no matter how much aminoglycoside is present on the outside of the PRTE cell, only a finite amount can be taken up over a period of time. This method of uptake is perhaps linked to the rationale of why high-dose, extended-interval aminoglycoside dosing delays the onset of nephrotoxicity. The administration of larger doses early on provides for maximum concentrations at the PRTE cell, which overwhelm and saturate the uptake mechanism. Thus, the same amount of aminoglycoside will be taken up into the cell as with conventional dosing. When the uptake mechanism is ready to transport more drug, much of the aminoglycoside has already bypassed the kidney with the high, infrequent dose. Conversely, the shorter dosing intervals associated with conventional dosing will likely assure small amounts of drug are continuously present for uptake into the PRTE cells, and thus the aminoglycoside will accumulate inside the PRTE cell quicker. Unfortunately, inappropriate power, confounding variables, and differing definitions of nephrotoxicity in clinical trials have made assessment of this outcome more difficult. Several meta-analyses, designed to address the inappropriate power with previous studies, demonstrated that trends for decreased toxicity are actually borne out in clinical practice when extended-interval dosing is used (25–28).

Together, all of the available human data suggest that a pharmacodynamic approach to the dosing and administration of aminoglycosides is at least equal to, if not better than, the conventional dosing methodology in terms of clinical effectiveness and nephrotoxicity. Moreover, this concept for the dosing of aminoglycosides has become the standard approach for administration (29).

Although the theory of concentration-dependent bacterial killing with the aminoglycosides is no longer debatable, trepidation continues regarding the ideal approach to administration of these extended-interval doses. Individualized pharmacokinetic monitoring has been proposed as the most accurate method of achieving the dynamic Cp/MIC target of 10 to 12 (30,31). These investigators initiate therapy with a gentamicin or tobramycin dose of 7 mg/kg and then collect serum concentration samples to determine patient-specific pharmacokinetic parameters and an individualized dose and schedule. Although certainly the most accurate method for obtaining a Cp/MIC ratio of 10, this approach is limited by the cost of multiple drug samples, the potential for impractical dosing schedules (e.g., every 31 hours), the requirement for a significant understanding of pharmacokinetic principles by the clinician, and the expertise and time associated with using pharmacokinetic computer software to calculate kinetic parameters. Moreover, the denominator in the Cp/MIC ratio is seldom available to the practicing clinician, thus the economic benefit of potentially administering lower doses for bacteria with a lower aminoglycoside MIC is rarely realized. This individualized approach, however, is the most appropriate method for administering the agent to patients with unusual pharmacokinetics, such as pregnant women, burn patients, or patients with ascites.

Another approach to extended-interval aminoglycoside administration has been through the use of population kinetics and institution-specific dosing nomograms (32–35).The largest report of this kind was in more than 2,000 patients at Hartford Hospital in Hartford, Connecticut (32). The authors reported the use of a 7 mg/kg dose to achieve a peak concentration of approximately 20 (g/mL, which at that time was ten times the MIC_{90} (2 (g/mL) for gentamicin against *P. aeruginosa*. The dosing interval was subsequently chosen based on a single serum concentration sample collected between 6 and 14 hours after the initiation of the first dose. This concentration was plotted on a nomogram (Fig. 2) to determine an every-24-hour, every-36-hour, every-48-hour, or longer dosing interval. The dosing interval was designed based on pharmacokinetic data from previous experiments, which allowed the investigators to estimate trough values and a drug-free interval based on the single point

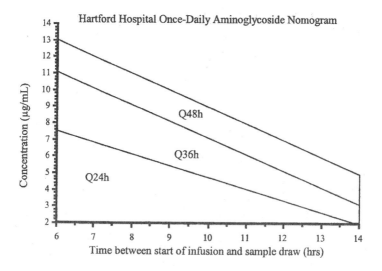

Figure 2   Figure 2. Hartford Hospital once-daily aminoglycoside nomogram for the assessment of dosing interval using a 7 mg/kg dose of gentamicin or tobramycin.

estimate. When this estimate was too high, as in patients with renal dysfunction, the nomogram would jump up to the next dosing interval to allow for a similar drug-free interval, thus preventing drug accumulation.

Outcome data collected during the use of this program suggested no alterations in clinical response rates after implementation. Application of this pharmacodynamic dosing regimen did, however, result in a reduction in the incidence of nephrotoxicity to 1.2% compared with a historical control of 3% to 5% (32). Additionally, the once-daily aminoglycoside (ODA) program demonstrated a 58% reduction in aminoglycoside-associated hospital cost, primarily because of a reduction in the number of therapeutic drug samples measured and costs associated with the management of nephrotoxicity (36).

The ideal dose used in a nomogram should be one that is based on the aminoglycoside MIC_{90} for the most common pathogen targeted at that specific institution (e.g., *P. aeruginosa*). Other nomograms have suggested doses of 5 mg/kg instead of 7 mg/kg once daily. In many instances, a dose of 5 mg/kg is more than adequate to achieve a Cp/MIC ratio of 10 to 12. In other cases, a dose higher than 7 mg/kg may be necessary if the MIC is greater than 2 (g/mL. For instance, the MIC_{90} for gentamicin against *P. aeruginosa* is no longer 2 (g/mL at Hartford Hospital (personal communication, Hartford Hospital, Department of Microbiology). However, the tobramycin MIC_{90} remains between 1 and 2 (g/mL, thus this agent has replaced gentamicin in serious gram-negative infections and the 7 mg/kg dose is still appropriate. Continued monitoring of MIC distribution changes is necessary to assure appropriate use of nomogram dosing.

Metronidazole

Like the aminoglycosides, metronidazole displays concentration-dependant bactericidal activity (16). Although approved at doses of 250 mg to 500 mg every 6 to 8 hours, metronidazole's concentration-dependent pharmacodynamics, along with its long half-life (6 to 8 hours) and an active metabolite, justify administering this agent at a dose of 1,000 mg every

24 hours or 500 mg every 12 hours. Studies conducted with metronidazole administered 1,000 mg once daily or 500 mg twice daily observed bactericidal activity for the entire dosing regimen against *Bacteroides fragilis* (37–39). As a result, investigators concluded that metronidazole can be administered as a 1,000 mg dose given every 24 hours, with an alternate dose of 500 mg every 12 hours in patients who cannot tolerate the high once-daily dosing regimen. This dosing regimen would, in turn, decrease the number of nursing administrations per day, thereby reducing resource utilization and cost, important considerations in this era of health care reform.

Accordingly, at Hartford Hospital, twice-daily dosing of metronidazole combined with a third-generation cephalosporin such as ceftizoxime or ceftriaxone has replaced the use of the cephamycins (cefotetan and cefoxitin) in intra-abdominal procedures. Through this automatic conversion, these investigators reported a projected annual cost avoidance of $25,567 (1997 U.S dollars) (40). The twice-daily dosing regimen of metronidazole can also be employed in the treatment of *Clostridium difficile*–associated diarrhea, as the MIC is similar to that of *B. fragilis* (41).

OPTIMIZING PHARMACODYNAMICS OF TIME-DEPENDENT ANTIBIOTICS

Beta-lactams, when administered at doses commonly used in clinical practice, exhibit time-dependent or concentration-independent killing. Thus, the extent of bacterial death is correlated with the percent of the dosing interval that drug concentrations are maintained above the MIC (%T>MIC) of the pathogen. In general, concentrations at the site of the infection for these antimicrobials need to exceed the MIC for 50% of the dosing interval (50% T>MIC). However, greater exposure may lead to additional benefits, such as better rates of response (i.e., earlier defervescence or normalization of white blood cell count) and a decreased potential for reducing resistance.

Several administration techniques have been employed to optimize the %T>MIC for beta-lactam antibiotics. One may give larger doses over the same dosing interval; however, this approach is not efficient because by doubling the dose, acquisition costs are doubled while the %T>MIC is only increased by approximately one half-life, commonly 1 hour or less for the beta-lactams. Additionally, more frequent doses may be given throughout the day. Once again, this strategy substantially increases the cost of therapy. Beta-lactams with long half-lives, such as ceftriaxone or ertapenem, may be used to provide adequate %T>MIC while administered only once a day against targeted pathogens. Alternatively, for some beta-lactams, simultaneously decreasing the dose and dosing interval over a period of 24 hours can maximize the %T>MIC. This strategy generally uses less drug over 24 hours, thereby reducing costs while increasing the %T>MIC or at least providing similar exposure. Lastly, for beta-lactams that maintain stability over 24 hours, continuous infusion may be employed, which also commonly allows for the use of a reduced dose over a period of 24 hours.

Piperacillin/Tazobactam

Piperacillin/tazobactam has become a popular antimicrobial in the treatment of nosocomial infectious processes and is used frequently in the institutional setting. As a result, this agent is often responsible for a large percentage of antimicrobial expenditures; therefore, any opportunity to maximize its effectiveness while reducing cost would be of interest to institutions with the drug on formulary.

In the United States, piperacillin/tazobactam is approved as a 30-minute intermittent infusion of 3.375 g every 6 hours (42). Additionally, more frequent dosing, 3.375 g every 4 hours, in combination with an aminoglycoside is suggested for nosocomial pneumonia in which *P. aeruginosa* is suspected. Considering this agent's linear pharmacokinetics and its time-dependent pharmacodynamics, similar %T>MIC exposure can be achieved by increasing the dose and extending the dosing interval (i.e., administering 4.5 g every 8 hours) (43,44). This regimen has demonstrated clinically equivalent bactericidal activity to 3.375 g every 6 hours against *B. fragilis, Escherichia coli, Enterococcus faecalis,* and *P. aeruginosa* while providing one less dose per day, thus reducing labor expenses associated with administering the antibiotic (45). Likewise, a regimen of 4.5 g every 6 hours achieves similar pharmacodynamic exposure to 3.375 g every 4 hours and also allows for the use of less drug over a 24-hour dosing period (46).

Applying the same theories as above via increasing the dose and extending the dosing interval, investigators at Hartford Hospital have studied piperacillin/tazobactam doses as high as 6.75 g and 9 g infused over 1 hour and administered every 12 hours (47). Piperacillin pharmacokinetics continued to be linear and dose proportional as compared with the standard regimens; however, the tazobactam clearance was reduced, likely through competitive inhibition with piperacillin for renal secretion (Fig. 3). Both high-dose regimens were well

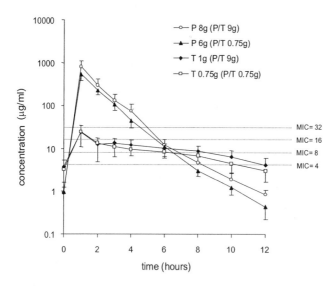

Figure 3 Figure 3. Serum concentrations of piperacillin (P) and tazobactam (T). Subjects were administered multiple-dose regimens of P/T 9.0 g every 12 hours and 6.75 g every 12 hours, and concentrations were measured around the administration of the third dose. Values are means ± standard deviation of ten subjects. MIC, minimum inhibitory concentration.

tolerated in healthy volunteers and achieved similar pharmacodynamic exposure to 3.375 g and 4.5 g regimens (Table 1). These infrequent regimens should further lead to reduced labor costs associated with preparation and administration. Additionally, twice-daily regimens would simplify the use of intravenous piperacillin/tazobactam in the outpatient setting.

Although the above methods for optimizing the pharmacodynamics of piperacillin/tazobactam are applicable, administration by continuous infusion would be the ideal method to maximize this antibiotic's pharmacodynamics while simultaneously resulting in an economic benefit. The pharmacokinetics of piperacillin/tazobactam administered by continuous infusion have been demonstrated in several healthy-volunteer studies (48,49). Average steady-state serum concentrations using 9 g piperacillin/tazobactam and 13.5 g given by continuous infusion were 14.58 ± 5.19 µg/mL and 28 ± 6.9 µg/mL, respectively. Burgess and Waldrep (50) observed similar mean steady-state concentrations of 37.2 ± 6.8 µg/mL for the 13.5 g continuous infusion piperacillin/tazobactam dose in a recent healthy-volunteer study. The majority of these steady-state concentrations were higher than the current breakpoints for most susceptible Enterobacteriaceae, *Bacteroides* species, and *Staphylococcus aureus*, which are 16/4 µg/mL or less, 16/4 µg/mL or less, and 8/4 µg/mL or less, respectively. Although the

Table 1 Percent Time above Minimum Inhibitory Concentration (%T>MIC) of the Study Regimens and Calculated %T>MIC of Conventional Regimens from Literature Pharmacokinetic Parameters

MIC	Conventional dosage regimens			Study regimens	
	3.375 g q6h	4.5 g q8h	4.5 g q6h	6.75 g q12h	9.0 g q12h
2	89.98	80.48	92.60	78.04	86.98
4	76.14	68.86	79.10	68.39	76.83
8	62.31	57.23	65.60	58.62	66.67
16	48.47	45.60	52.09	48.84	56.62
32	34.63	33.97	38.59	39.04	46.37
64	20.79	22.35	25.09	29.29	36.22

susceptibility breakpoint for *P. aeruginosa* is 64/4 μg/mL or less, most isolates in the United States and Canada have lower MICs, ranging from 4 to 8 μg/mL, of which drug concentrations are well in access (51,52). Additionally, steady-state concentrations from these studies were derived in healthy volunteers with excellent renal function and are expected to be higher in infected patients because of reduced clearance. To confirm this, we employed population pharmacokinetics and Monte Carlo simulation to demonstrate that the probability of achieving piperacillin concentrations above the MIC for *P. aeruginosa* at our institution would be 97% (53,54).

Based on results from these pharmacokinetic studies as well as pharmacodynamic concepts, an automatic substitution of continuous for intermittent infusion of piperacillin/tazobactam was approved by the pharmacy and therapeutics committee at Hartford Hospital and a clinical program was instituted (15). The clinical protocol allowed pharmacists to automatically modify orders for intermittent infusion to the continuous infusion based on the protocol in Table 2. After a bolus loading dose of 2.25 g over 30 minutes, the choice of piperacillin/tazobactam dose was based on the patient's renal function and clinical utility. Accordingly, for nosocomial infections in which *P. aerugi-*

Table 2 Protocol for Administration of Piperacillin/Tazobactam by Continuous Infusion at Hartford Hospital*

	Standard regimen	Nosocomial regimen†
Loading dose	2.25 g over 30 min	2.25 g over 30 min
Continuous infusion	CrCl ≥ 20 mL/min:	If CrCl ≥ 40 mL/min:
	8 g/1 g in 150 mL	12 g/1.5 g in 150 mL NS
	Normal Saline	@ 7 mL/h
	@7 mL/h	If CrCL = 20–40 mL/min:
		8 g/1 g in 150 mL NS
		@ 7 mL/h

* Exclusions: patients with creatinine clearance (CrCl) < 20 mL/min or limited intravenous access.
† Nosocomial infection: infection developing 48 h after admission or suspected *Pseudomonas aeruginosa*.
NS,.

nosa was suspected, a higher dose was initiated. Clinical and economic data were collected prospectively on the program and compared with a historic control of 4 g/0.5 g administered by intermittent infusion every 8 hours. This analysis demonstrated that the continuous-infusion regimen was no different from the intermittent one in terms of clinical and microbiologic efficacy (94% vs. 82%, $p = 0.081$, and 91% vs. 75%, $p = 0.092$, respectively) when treating infections such as nosocomial pneumonia, skin/soft tissue infections, and intra-abdominal infections. Moreover, days to normalization of fever (temperature less than 101.0(F) were significantly less for the continuous-infusion regimen (1.2 ± 0.8 days vs. 2.4 ± 1.5 days, $p = 0.012$), suggesting an increase in the rate of response to therapy. The drug acquisition, preparation, supply, and administration costs were also significantly less for the continuous-infusion regimen ($p = 0.028$) (15).

Other administration strategies, such as prolonging the infusion of piperacillin/tazobactam over 4 hours, have also been investigated, with favorable results (55). Accordingly, doses of 3.375 g infused over 4 hours and administered every 8 hours provided equivalent probability of achieving adequate %T>MIC compared with standard intermittent regimens while offering cost savings because of the use of less piperacillin/tazobactam over a 24-hour period.

Cefepime

Cefepime, a broad-spectrum fourth-generation cephalosporin antibiotic, is approved at a dose of 1 g every 12 hours for mild infections and 2 g every 12 hours for more moderate to severe infections, specifically where *P. aeruginosa* is of concern (56). As previously discussed, one method to optimize the %T>MIC for beta-lactams is to reduce the dose while shortening the dosing interval. Accordingly, Paterson et al. (57) demonstrated with the use of Monte Carlo simulation that 1 g every 8 hours of cefepime results in drug exposures similar to that obtained with 2 g every 12 hours while using less drug daily and reducing drug-associated acquisition costs (i.e., half the dose administered more frequently throughout the day). Based on these concepts and observations, the dosing protocol shown in Table 3 has been implemented at our institution, as well as at the University of Pittsburgh Medical Center and others, for empiric and targeted dosing of cefepime. Currently, clinical and economic outcomes of this program have yet to be collected.

Table 3 Cefepime Dosing Protocol at Hartford Hospital

Empiric therapy or documented *Pseudomonas aeruginosa* infections in non-neutropenic hosts:

- 1 g q8h will be the usual dose for most patients with CrCl $\geq$50 mL/min, as calculated by the Cockcroft-Gault equation.
- 1 g q12h will be the usual dose for patients with CrCl 30–49 mL/min.
- 1 g q24h will be the usual empiric dose for patients with CrCl <30 mL/min.
- 2 g doses should use similar dosing intervals as above and are only appropriate for the following:
  - Extremely obese patients (actual body weight >1.5 times ideal body weight)
  - Edematous patients, such as those with ascites, third space fluid losses, or other complications
  - Pancreatitis patients
  - Patients with CNS or eye infection
  - **Neutropenic hosts (ANC <500 or between 500 and 1,000 but presumed to proceed under 500), regardless of infecting pathogen**

Documented infections other than *P. aeruginosa* in non-neutropenic hosts:

- 1 g q12h will be the usual dose for patients with CrCl $\geq$50 mL/min.
- 1 g q24h will be the usual dose for patients with CrCl <50 mL/min.
- 2 g doses should use similar dosing intervals as above and are only appropriate for the following:
  - Extremely obese patients (actual body weight >1.5 times ideal body weight)
  - Edematous patients, such as those with ascites, third space fluid losses, or other complications
  - Pancreatitis patients
  - Patients with CNS or eye infection

ANC, absolute neutrophil count; CNS, central nervous system; CrCl, creatinine clearance.

Meropenem

Meropenem, a broad-spectrum intravenous carbapenem antibiotic, is commonly administered at a dose of 1,000 mg every 8 hours in the United States (58). A recent analysis using Monte Carlo simulation showed that meropenem 500 mg every 6 hours resulted in similar %T>MIC exposure compared with 1,000 mg every 8 hours (59). Additionally, a significant reduction in the daily drug acquisition cost with 500 mg every 6 hours was demonstrated. Based on these observations, a clinical program allowing pharmacists to automatically adjust the meropenem dose based on the protocol in Table 4 was implemented. Preliminary outcomes data comparing the 500 mg every 6 hours regimen to the standard 1,000 mg every 8 hours

Table 4 Meropenem Dosing Protocol at Hartford Hospital

Non-neutropenic hosts:

- 500 mg q6h will be the usual dose for most patients with CrCl ≥50 mL/min, as calculated by the Cockcroft-Gault equation, including infections caused by *Pseudomonas aeruginosa.**
- 500 mg q8h will be the usual dose for patients with CrCl = 25–49 mL/min.
- 500 mg q12h will be the usual dose for patients with CrCl = 10–24 mL/min.
- 500 mg q24h will be the usual dose for patients with CrCl <10 mL/min.
- 1,000 mg doses should use similar dosing intervals as above and are only appropriate for the following:

  - Patients with actual body weight >2× their calculated ideal body weight
  - Patients with CNS or eye infection
  - Cystic fibrosis patients

Neutropenic hosts (ANC <500 or <1,000 with high suspicion of declining below 500):

- When used as monotherapy, 1 g q6h will be the dose for most patients with CrCl ≥50 mL/min.
- For patients with CrCl <50 mL/min, similar percent dosage reduction and dosing interval extensions apply as listed above.

ANC, absolute neutrophil count; CNS, central nervous system; CrCl, creatinine clearance.

revealed similar clinical and microbiologic outcomes, with a significant reduction in the amount used (mg per patient) and cost of meropenem (Hartford Hospital, data on file).

As with other beta-lactams, the maximization of T>MIC for the carbapenems is best achieved through continuous infusion. Because meropenem's stability at room temperature (approximately 4 to 10 hours) limits this administration technique (60), prolonging the infusion of meropenem over 3 hours, as previously described for piperacillin/tazobactam, has been proposed to optimize the pharmacodynamic profile while maintaining drug stability. A recent study conducted in healthy volunteers demonstrated that the 3-hour prolonged infusion of meropenem optimized the pharmacodynamic profile by maintaining adequate drug exposure while working within the constraints of room temperature stability and total daily dosage (61). This concept was further supported in a Monte Carlo simulation, revealing that 500 mg over 3 hours administered three times daily had a high probability of achieving a bactericidal pharmacodynamic target against clinically relevant pathogens such as Enterobacteriaceae and would reduce costs associated with drug therapy because of the use of less drug over the 24-hour period. Higher doses, such as 2,000 mg over 3 hours three times daily, would optimize pharmacodynamics against *Acinetobacter* spp. and *P. aeruginosa* (62). At the time of writing, a clinical program infusing meropenem 1,000 mg over 3 hours every 8 hours was under way at Albany Medical Center in Albany, New York. The clinicians will be collecting data on the outcomes and economics of this program shortly.

Additionally, the pharmacokinetics of meropenem when administered as a continuous infusion have been reported in critically ill patients and adults with cystic fibrosis (63,64). In the first study, Thalhammer et al. (63) administered 1,000 mg of meropenem by continuous infusion at a rate of 125 mg/hr. New solutions were prepared and administered every 8 hours to account for the stability of the agent at room temperature. Steady-state concentrations in the study patients were 11.9 ± 5.0 μg/mL, thus providing 100% T>MIC for all susceptible pathogens according to the NCCLS susceptibility breakpoint of 4 μg/mL.

The investigators concluded that continuous-infusion meropenem was equivalent to 30-minute intermittent infusions of 2,000 mg every 8 hours and would be suitable for treating critically ill patients. To address the stability concerns with meropenem, Grant and et al. (65) evaluated *in vitro* concentrations of meropenem in a CADD pump surrounded by two frozen bags; meropenem concentrations remained stable over 24 hours utilizing this methodology. Employing the same delivery system, we found the pharmacokinetics of continuous-infusion meropenem at a dose of 3,000 mg over 24 hours achieved a steady-state serum concentration of 8.31 ± 0.68 μg/mL in adults with cystic fibrosis (64). Although slightly lower than concentrations found in critically ill patients, likely because of differences in volume of distribution and clearance, concentrations in the cystic fibrosis patients were also maintained above the susceptibility breakpoint for 100% of the dosing interval. Furthermore, because of the use of the frozen bags, meropenem stability was preserved over 24 hours.

Clindamycin

Clindamycin, a lincosamide antimicrobial, is still widely used in the treatment of mild to moderate skin infections caused by *S. aureus* and *Streptococcus* spp. The common intravenous dose for these infections is 600 to 900 mg every 6 to 8 hours. Because clindamycin has demonstrated time-dependent bactericidal activity and its primary adverse event, diarrhea, is dose dependent, investigators have evaluated alternative dosing regimens to optimize its pharmacodynamics and reduce its adverse events (66). Bactericidal activity against two strains each of *S. aureus* and *B. fragilis* were achieved with clindamycin doses of 300 mg every 8 hours, as the concentrations were maintained over the MIC for greater than 80% of the dosing interval (67). Against strains of *Streptococcus pneumoniae*, bactericidal activity was achieved with doses of 300 mg every 12 hours (67). Similar findings supporting these doses were reported in an *in vitro* dynamic model (68). Accordingly, clindamycin 300 mg administered every 8 to 12 hours has become the standard dose to treat bacterial infections at our institution.

IMPLEMENTING A CLINICAL PROGRAM

Implementation of a clinical program that incorporates pharmacodynamic concepts may commonly encounter resistance and barriers from other health care practitioners. Often, physicians and other clinical staff are so accustomed to dosing or administering an antibiotic in the usual or FDA-approved way that it is quite difficult to change their practices. Furthermore, the suggestion of such a program may be interpreted only as a method of reducing the drug budget, and not what is best for the patient Accordingly, the key to implementation of a successful program is a combination of providing evidence-based science, gaining support of key opinion leaders at the institution, providing education to the entire health care staff, and then following the results of the program and reporting back to the staff.

A clear example of this was implementation of the ODA program at Hartford Hospital (69). In addition to program innovations at the time concerning the selected dose and dosing interval, the program included the automatic conversion of all adult patients to the ODA dosing regimen by the hospital pharmacists. The success of this program, initially, was dependent on the joint development and approval by the members of the Department of Pharmacy and the Division of Infectious Diseases. In addition to the hospital Division of Infectious Diseases, the opinions of several private-practice infectious disease specialists were garnered to secure the best opportunity for a successful implementation. Support from the director of the clinical chemistry section of the hospital laboratory was sought because of the effect such a program was expected to have on normal therapeutic ranges for aminoglycosides and the number and timing of blood sampling. Lastly, the general views and concerns of the pharmacists were particularly important, as they would be the health care members ultimately responsible for rolling out the program. After approval by these members, the program was presented to the pharmacy and therapeutics committee. Although ODA dosing was being used by many of the infectious disease physicians already, final approval by the therapeutics committee allowed hospital-wide use in all adults meeting inclusion criteria.

As with the implementation of any institutional program, the education of the involved members of the hospital staff was paramount for program success. For the ODA program, an aggressive 3-month educational approach was undertaken before introduction. This included frequent in-services to the medical and surgical house staff, pharmacy staff, and chemistry section of the clinical laboratory. To reach other members of the health care team, such as the nursing staff, several poster sessions were held in the hospital's main cafeteria. Finally, a thorough explanation of the theory, potential benefits, and implementation of the ODA program was distributed in several sources of written material, such as hospital newsletters and signs at each physician charting area on every nursing unit.

After program implementation, data were collected both prospectively and retrospectively for all patients receiving the ODA dosing regimen. The results and experience of the clinical program were distributed to all members of the health care staff in newsletters as well as published in several peer-reviewed journals. This final part of clinical program implementation is perhaps the most difficult, yet it is the most important. Significant time is needed to collect and analyze these data and then report back to the staff; however, this technique has been associated with the highest rates of program acceptance and adherence. This analysis also allows for identification of problems encountered after implementation, which may have never been addressed.

Such a process has been conducted for the majority of programs discussed in this chapter, including the continuous-infusion piperacillin/tazobactam program, and has been met with great success. It is important to realize that for many of the described programs, institution-specific patient populations (i.e., pharmacokinetics) as well as antibiograms (pathogen MICs) were considered when optimizing doses; thus if one is implementing a clinical program in one's institution, each program should be tailored to the medical center or even the unit in which it will be used.

CONCLUSION

Knowledge and application of pharmacodynamic principles to dosing and administration of antibacterials can optimize clinical and bacteriologic efficacy while potentially reducing toxicity and costs associated with therapy. Although the majority of data supporting these concepts have been gathered from *in vitro* and *in vivo* animal models of infection, human clinical data are accumulating, predominantly because of a number of small uncontrolled trials, case reports, and hospital clinical programs. For example, based on the preliminary results of our continuous-infusion piperacillin/tazobactam clinical program, a randomized, multicenter clinical trial assessing the efficacy, safety, and economic benefit of continuous infusion in patients with complicated intra-abdominal infections has been initiated. The results from well-designed studies such as these should provide the data necessary to confirm that the application of pharmacodynamics to antimicrobial dosing truly does provide a benefit.

In conclusion, the concepts outlined within this chapter may be used as a guideline to create a strategic approach to implementation of clinical programs based on pharmacodynamic principals in one's practice setting. Accordingly, consideration of the potential patient population in which the program is to be used and the institution- or unit-specific antibiogram will be essential for success. Finally, after implementing such a program, outcomes—whether they are clinical, economic, or both—should be collected and reported back to the staff to ensure continued compliance.

REFERENCES

1. Craig WA, Ebert SC. Killing and regrowth of bacteria in vitro: a review Scand J Infect Dis; 1991; 74(suppl):63–70.

2. Moore RD, Lietman PS, Smith CR. Clinical response to aminoglycoside therapy: importance of the ratio of peak concentration to minimal inhibitory concentration J Infect Dis; 1987; 155: 93–99.

3. Moore RD, Smith CR, Lietman PS. Association of aminoglycoside plasma levels with therapeutic outcome in gram-negative pneumonia Am J Med; 1984; 77:657–762.

4. Moore RD, Smith CR, Lietman PS. The association of aminoglycoside plasma levels with mortality in patients with gram-negative bacteremia J Infect Dis; 1984; 149:443–448.

5. Gilbert DN. Meta-analyses are no longer required for determining the efficacy of single daily dosing of aminoglycosides Clin Infect Dis; 1997; 24:816–819.

6. Rodvold KA. Pharmacodynamics of anti-infective therapy: taking what we know to the patient's bedside Pharmacotherapy; 2001; 21(11 pt 2):319S–330S.

7. Daenen S, de Vries-Hospers H. Cure of *Pseudomonas aeruginosa* infection in neutropenic patients by continuous infusion of ceftazidime Lancet; 1988; 1:937.

8. Mekonen ET, Noskin GA, Hacek DM, Peterson LR. Successful treatment of persistent bacteremia due to vancomycin-resistant, ampicillin-resistant *Enterococcus faecium* Microb Drug Resist; 1995; 1:249–253.

9. Tam VH, McKinnon PS, Levine DP, Brandel SM, Rybak MJ. Once-daily aminoglycoside in the treatment of *Enterococcus faecalis* endocarditis: case report and review Pharmacotherapy.; 2000; 20:1116–1119.

10. Domenig C, Traunmuller F, Kozek S, Wisser W, Klepetko W, Steininger R, Spiss C, Thalhammer F. Continuous beta-lactam antibiotic therapy in a double-lung transplanted patient with a multi-drug resistant *Pseudomonas aeruginosa* infection Transplantation; 2001; 71:744–745.

11. Raehl CL, Bond CA. 1998 National Clinical Pharmacy Services Study Pharmacotherapy; 2000; 20:436–460.

12. Craig WA. Pharmacokinetic/pharmacodynamic parameters: rationale for antibacterial dosing of mice and men Clin Infect Dis; 1998; 26:1–12.

13. Ambrose PG, Grasela DM. The use of Monte Carlo simulation to examine pharmacodynamic variance of drugs: fluoroquinolone pharmacodynamics against *Streptococcus pneumoniae* Diagn Microb Infect Dis; 2000; 38:151–157.

14. Montgomery MJ, Beringer PM, Aminimanizani A, Louie SG, Shapiro BJ, Jelliffe R, Gill MA. Population pharmacokinetics and use of Monte Carlo simulation to evaluate currently recommended dosing regimens of ciprofloxacin in adult patients with cystic fibrosis Antimicrob Agents Chemother; 2001; 45: 3468–3473.

15. Grant EM, Kuti JL, Nicolau DP, Nightingale CH, Quintiliani R. Clinical efficacy and pharmacoeconomics of a continuous infusion piperacillin-tazobactam program in a large community teaching hospital Pharmacotherapy; 2002; 22:471–483.

16. Craig WA. Pharmacodynamics of antimicrobials: general concepts and applications. In: Nightingale CH, Murakawa T, Ambrose PG, Eds Antimicrobial Pharmacodynamics in Theory and Clinical Practice. New York: Marcel Dekker Inc, 2002:1–22.

17. Maller R, Ahrne H, Eilard T, Eriksson I, Lausen I. Efficacy and safety of amikacin in systemic infections when given as a single daily dose or in two divided doses J Antimicrob Chemother; 1991; 27:121S–128S.

18. Prins JM, Buller HR, Kuijper EJ, Tange Ra, Speelman P. Once versus thrice daily gentamicin in patients with serious infections Lancet; 1993; 341:335–339.

19. Efficacy and toxicity of single daily doses of amikacin and ceftriaxone versus multiple daily doses of amikacin and ceftazidime for infection in patients with cancer and granulocytopenia Ann Intern Med; 1993; 119:584–593.

20. Marik PE, Lipman J, Kobilski S, Scribante J. A prospective randomized study comparing once- versus twice-daily amikacin dosing in critically ill adult and pediatric patients J Antimicrob Chemother; 1991; 28:753–764.

21. Gilbert DN, Lee BL, Dworkin RJ, Leggett JL, Chambers HF, Modin G, Tauber MG, Sande MA. A randomized comparison of the safety and efficacy of once-daily gentamicin or thrice-daily gentamicin in combination with ticarcillin-clavulanate Am J Med; 1998; 105:182–191.

22. Mingeot-Leclerq M, Tulkens PM. Aminoglycosides: nephrotoxicity Antimicrob Agents Chemother; 1999; 43:1003–1012.

23. Tulkens P. Experimental studies on nephrotoxoicty of aminoglycosides at low doses Am J Med; 1986; 80:105–114.

24. Giuliano RA, Verpooten GA, Verbist L, Wedeen RP, De Broe ME. *In vivo* uptake kinetics of aminoglycosides in the kidney cortex of rats J Pharmacol Exp Ther; 1986; 236:470–475.

25. Galoe AM, Graudal N, Christensen HR, Kampmann JP. Aminoglycosides: single or multiple daily dosing? A meta-analysis on efficacy and safety Eur J Clin Pharmacol; 1995; 48:39–43.

26. Freeman CD, Strayer AH. Mega-analysis of meta-analysis: an examination of meta-analysis with an emphasis on once-daily aminoglycoside comparative trials Pharmacotherapy; 1996; 16: 1093–1102.

27. Hatala R, Dinh T, Cook D. Once-daily aminoglycoside dosing in immunocompromised adults: a meta-analysis Ann Intern Med; 1996; 124:717–725.

28. Munckhof WJ, Grayson JL, Turnidge JD. A meta-analysis of studies on the safety and efficacy of aminoglycosides given with once daily or as divided doses J Antimicrob Chemother; 1996; 37:645–663.

29. Chuck SK, Raber SR, Rodvold KA, Areff D. National survey of extended-interval aminoglycoside dosing Clin Infect Dis; 2000; 30:433–439.

30. Kashuba ADM, Bertino JS, Nafziger AN. Dosing of aminoglycosides to rapidly attain pharmacodynamic goals and hasten therapeutic response by using individualized pharmacokinetic monitoring of patients with pneumonia caused by gram-negative organisms Antimicrob Agents Chemother; 1998; 42: 1842–1844.

31. Wallace AW, Jones M, Bertino JS. Evaluation of four once-daily aminoglycoside dosing nomograms Pharmacotherapy; 2002; 22: 1077–1083.

32. Nicolau DP, Freeman CD, Belliveau PP, Nightingale CH, Ross JW, Quintiliani R. Experience with a once-daily aminoglycoside program administered to 2,184 adult patients Antimicrob Agents Chemother; 1995; 39:650–655.

33. Infrequent Aminoglycoside Dosing, from Barnes-Jewish Hospital at Washington University Medical Center. Available from http://internalmed.wustl.edu/divisions/house_staff/aminoglyco sides.html (accessed September 2002).

34. Anaizi N. Once daily dosing of aminoglycosides: a consensus document Int J Clin Pharmacol Ther; 1997; 35:223–226.

35. Gilbert DN, Moellering RC Jr, Sande MA, EdsThe Sanford Guide to Antimicrobial Therapy 2001. 31st ed. Hyde Park. VT: Antimicrobial Therapy, Inc., 2001.

36. Hitt CM, Klepser ME, Nightingale CH, Quintiliani R, Nicolau DP. Pharmacoeconomic impact of once-daily aminoglycoside administration Pharmacotherapy; 1997; 17:810–814.

37. Freeman CD, Nightingale CH, Nicolau DP, Belliveau PP, Quintiliani R. Serum bactericidal activity of ceftriaxone plus metronidazole against common intra-abdominal pathogens Am J Hosp Pharm; 1994; 51:1782–1787.

38. Freeman CD, Nightingale CH, Nicolau DP, Belliveau PP, Tessier PR, Fu Q, Xuan DW, Quintiliani R. Bactericidal activity of low-dose ceftizoxime plus metronidazole compared with cefoxitin and ampicillin-sulbactam Pharmacotherapy; 1994; 14: 185–190.

39. Sullivan MC, Nightingale CH, Quintiliani R, Sweeney KR. Comparison of the pharmacodynamic activity of cefotaxime plus metronidazole with cefoxitin and ampicillin plus sulbactam Pharmacotherapy; 1995; 15:479–486.

40. Quintiliani R, Hitt CM, Ambrose PG, Nicolau DP, Nightingale CH. Ceftizoxime/metronidazole replace cefotetan for intra-abdominal infections Formulary; 1997; 32:740–745.

41. Barbut F, Decre D, Burghoffer B, Lesage D, Delisle F, Lalande V, Delmee M, Avesani V, Sano N, Coudert C, Petit JC. Antimicrobial susceptibilities and serogroups of clinical strains of *Clostridium difficile* isolated in France in 1991 and 1997 Antimicrob Agent Chemother; 1999; 43:2607–2611.

42. Zosyn Package Insert. Lederle Piperacillin, Inc., Carolina, Puerto Rico, 2002.

43. Occhipinti DJ, Pendland SL, Schoonover LL, Rypins EB, Danziger LH, Rodvold KA. Pharmacokinetics and pharmacodynamics of two multiple-dose piperacillin-tazobactam regimens Antimicrob Agent Chemother; 1997; 41:2511–2517.

44. Kim MK, Capitano B, Mattoes HM, Xuan D, Quintiliani R, Nightingale CH, Nicolau DP. Pharmacokinetic and pharmaco-

dynamic evaluation of two dosing regimens for piperacillin-tazobactam Pharmacotherapy; 2002; 22:569–577.

45. Klepser ME, Marangos MN, Zhu Z, Nicolau DP, Quintiliani R, Nightingale CH. Comparison of the bactericidal activities of piperacillin-tazobactam, ticarcillin-clavulanate, and ampicillin-sulbactam against clinical isolates of *Bacteroides fragilis*, *Enterococcus faecalis*, *Escherichia coli*, and *Pseudomonas aeruginosa* Antimicrob Agent Chemother; 1997; 41:435–439.

46. Mattoes HM, Capitano B, Kim MK, Xuan D, Quintiliani R, Nightingale CH, Nicolau DP. Comparative pharmacokinetic and pharmacodynamic profile of piperacillin/tazobactam 3.375g q4h and 4.5 g q6h. 75g q4h and 4.5 g q6h Chemotherapy; 2002; 48:59–63.

47. Kim MK, Xuan D, Quintiliani R, Nightingale CH, Nicolau DP. Pharmacokinetic and pharmacodynamic profile of high dose extended interval piperacillin-tazobactam J Antimicrob Chemother; 2001; 48:259–267.

48. Hitt CM, Patel KB, Nicolau DP, Zhu Z, Nightingale CH. Influence of piperacillin-tazobactam on pharmacokinetics of gentamicin given once daily Am J Health Syst Pharm; 1997; 54: 2704–2708.

49. Richerson MA, Ambrose PG, Bui KQ, Grant E, Nicolau DP, Nightingale CH, Quintiliani R. Pharmacokinetic and economic evaluation of piperacillin/tazobactam administered as either continuous or intermittent infusion with once-daily gentamicin Infect Dis Clin Pract; 1999; 8:195–200.

50. Burgess DS, Waldrep T. Pharmacokinetics and pharmacodynamics of piperacillin/tazobactam when administered by continuous infusion and intermittent dosing Clin Ther; 2002; 24: 1090–1104.

51. Jones RN, Croco MA, Kugler KC, Pfaller MA, Beach ML. Respiratory tract pathogens isolated from patients hospitalized with suspected pneumonia: frequency of occurrence and antimicrobial susceptibility patterns from the SENTRY Antimicrobial Surveillance Program (United States and Canada, 1997) Diagn Microbiol Infect Dis; 2000; 37:115–125.

52. Kuti JL, Grant EM, Sutherland CA, Ye M, Zhou W, McCarter Y, Nightingale CH, Nicolau DP. Divergence in MIC distribu-

tions of Pseudomonas aeruginosa for piperacillin and piperacillin/tazobactam. C distributions of *Pseudomonas aeruginosa* for piperacillin and piperacillin/tazobactam J Infect Dis Pharmacother; 2001; 5:41–51.

53. Facca BF, Triesenberg SN, Barr LL. Population pharmacokinetics of continuous infusion piperacillin-tazobactam J Infect Dis Pharmacother; 2002; 5:51–67.

54. Kuti JL, Nightingale CH, Quintiliani R, Nicolau DP. Pharmacodynamic profiling of continuously infused piperacillin/tazobactam against *Pseudomonas aeruginosa* using Monte Carlo analysis Diagn Microbiol Infect Dis; 2002; 44:51–57.

55. Lomaestro BM, Rodvold KA, Danziger LH, Drusano GL. Pharmacodynamic evaluation of extending the infusion time of piperacillin/tazobactam doses using Monte Carlo analysis [abstr]. In: Programs and Abstracts of the 41st Interscience Conference on Antimicrobial Agents and Chemotherapy (Chicago). Washington. DC: American Society for Microbiology, 2001:36.

56. Maxipime package insert. Dura Pharmaceuticals, Inc., San Diego, CA, 2002.

57. Paterson DL, Clarke L, Ndirangu MW, Kuznetsov D. Use of pharmacodynamic principles and stochastic modeling to choose an optional empiric cefepime dose for suspected *Pseudomonas aeruginosa* infections within a single institution [abstract]. In: Programs and Abstracts of the 42nd Interscience Conference on Antimicrobial Agents and Chemotherapy (San Diego). Washington. DC: American Society for Microbiology, 2002:9.

58. Merrem package insert. AstraZeneca Pharmaceuticals, LP, Wilmington, DE, 2001.

59. Kuti JL, Maglio D, Nightingale CH, Nicolau DP. Economic benefit of a meropenem dosing strategy based on pharmacodynamic concepts Am J Health Syst Pharm; 2002; 60:565–568.

60. Patel RP, Cook SE. Stability of meropenem in intravenous solutions Am J Health Syst Pharm; 1997; 54:412–421.

61. Dandekar PK, Maglio D, Sutherland CA, Nightingale CH, Nicolau DP. Pharmacokinetics of meropenem 0.5g and 2g every 8h administered as a 3h infusion [abstr]. In: Program and Abstracts of the 42nd Interscience Conference on Antimicrobial

Agents and Chemotherapy (San Diego). Washington. DC: American Society for Microbiology, 2002:18.

62. Kuti JL, Dandekar PK, Nightingale CH, Nicolau DP. Pharmacodynamic comparison of prolonged and traditional infusions of meropenem in gram negative bacteria [abstr]. In: Programs and Abstracts of the 42nd Interscience Conference on Antimicrobial Agents and Chemotherapy (San Diego). Washington. DC: American Society for Microbiology, 2002:8.

63. Thalhammer F, Traunmuller F, El Menyawi I, Frass M, Hollenstein UM, Locker GJ, Stoiser B, Staudinger T, Thalhammer-Scherrer R, Burgmann H. Continuous infusion versus intermittent administration of meropenem in critically ill patients J Antimicrob Chemother; 1999; 43:523–527.

64. Kuti JL, Nightingale CH, Knauft R, Nicolau DP. Pharmacokinetics of continuously infused meropenem in adults with cystic fibrosis [abstr] Am J Resp Crit Care Med; 2003; 167:A372.

65. Grant EM, Zhong MK, Ambrose PG, Nicolau DP, Nightingale CH, Quintiliani R. Stability of meropenem in a portable infusion device in a cold pouch Am J Health Syst Pharm; 2000; 57: 992–995.

66. Klepser ME, Banevicius MA, Quintiliaqni R, Nightingale CH. Characterization of bactericidal activity of clindamycin against *Bacteroides fragilis* via kill curve methods Antimicrob Agent Chemother; 1996; 40:1941–1944.

67. Klepser ME, Nicolau DP, Quintiliani R, Nightingale CH. Bactericidal activity of low-dose clindamycin administered at 8- and 12-hour intervals against *Staphylococcus aureus*, *Streptococcus pneumoniae*, and *Bacteroides fragilis* Antimicrob Agents Chemother; 1997; 41:630–635.

68. Lewis RE, Klepser ME, Ernst EJ, Lund BC, Biedenbach DJ, Jones RN. Evaluation of low-dose, extended-interval clindamycin regimens against *Staphylococcus aureus* and *Streptococcus pneumoniae* using a dynamic *in vitro* model of infection Antimicrob Agents Chemother; 1999; 43:2005–2009.

69. Nicolau DP, Belliveau PP, Nightingale CH, Quintiliani R, Freeman CD. Implementation of a once-daily aminoglycoside program in a large community-teaching hospital Hosp Pharm; 1995; 30:674–680.

13

The Antimicrobial Formulary: Reevaluating Parenteral Cephalosporins in the Context of Emerging Resistance

ROBERT C. OWENS, JR.

Division of Infectious Diseases and Department of Clinical Pharmacy Services, Maine Medical Center, Portland, and Department of Medicine, University of Vermont, College of Medicine, Burlington, Vermont, U.S.A.

PAUL G. AMBROSE

Division of Infectious Diseases, Cognigen Corporation, Buffalo, New York, U.S.A.

RONALD N. JONES

The JONES Group/JMI Laboratories, North Liberty, Iowa, and Tufts University School of Medicine, Boston, Massachusetts, U.S.A.

The primary goal in the treatment of infections is to provide the best possible clinical outcome for our patients while minimizing associated drug-related adverse events, including the possibility of collateral resistance developing during therapy. In order for these to occur, one must consider and evaluate a tremendous amount of data, much of it changing continually. Now, more important than ever, it is critical to select (and dose) initial empiric therapy so that it has the highest probability of eradicating the suspected pathogens for a given infection type. Because the utility of some cephalosporins has been diminished over the last decade or so, in part because of resistance to them and also owing to their adverse ecologic impact on host and institutional flora, it is important to reevaluate their strengths and weaknesses.

Institutionally acquired infections affect approximately 2 million people in the United States annually (1). Resistance varies geographically, but we as a population are extremely mobile, thus so is our microbial enemy. Because of continued breaks in infection control practice and relatively close quarters in hospital and long-term care environments, the horizontal transmission of resistant organisms still occurs. The gross tonnage of antimicrobial use, with an unacceptably high percentage being inappropriate, combined with an increasingly immunologically impaired host population provides bacteria with an ideal milieu for promiscuous growth and mutation.

Over the last decade, antimicrobial-resistant organisms have led clinicians to discuss and debate the optimal methods to treat and prevent infections caused by them. Often-discussed gram-positive organisms include multidrug resistant pneumococci, methicillin-resistant *Staphylococcus aureus* (MRSA), vancomycin-resistant enterococci (VRE), and in more limited but challenging terms, vancomycin-resistant *S. aureus* (VRSA) (2). None of the currently marketed cephalosporins has activity against MRSA, VRSA, or VRE; however, there are some in various phases of development with activity against these resistant gram-positive organisms (3). For example, BAL9141 and RWJ-54428 are investigational cephalosporins that target the penicillin-binding protein (PBP) 2a of MRSA strains, their primary mechanism of resistance to all current beta-lactams;

whereas RWJ-54428 targets PBP5, which is associated with resistance to penicillins in the enterococci. *Streptococcus pneumoniae* is a pathogen that has separated the cephalosporins further because of the continued upward creep in minimum inhibitory concentrations (MICs). Cefepime, ceftriaxone, cefotaxime, and ceftizoxime remain active against the majority of multidrug-resistant pneumococci in contrast to older drugs in the class or to ceftazidime (4). Among the gram-negative organisms, *Pseudomonas aeruginosa, Stenotrophomonas maltophilia, Burkholderia cepacia, Acinetobacter* spp, and Enterobacteriaceae harboring extended-spectrum beta-lactamases (ESBLs) and AmpC beta-lactamases pose the greatest challenges to clinicians (5,6).

Optimizing antimicrobial use should be viewed as a strategy to minimize the development and dissemination of resistant organisms in general, and as a complementary partner to infection control efforts. However, some organisms have been demonstrated to respond better to antimicrobial optimization strategies and typically involve those that are selected from patients' endogenous flora during antimicrobial therapy (7). This includes many of the gram-negative organisms listed above and, to a degree, VRE. Once a resistant organism is selected during antimicrobial therapy, opportunities arise for its horizontal spread. Some organisms, such as MRSA and *B. cepacia* in the cystic fibrosis population, appear to be spread via horizontal transmission and can be best managed by infection control strategies (8). Ultimately, the methods for prevention and treatment of infection due to resistant organisms are hindered by the many complexities associated with "bug-drug-host" interactions that are not easily measured. Discussed within this chapter are some of those complexities, the diversity of beta-lactamases found among organisms causing clinical infection that have limited the use of many cephalosporins, and collateral resistance issues contributing to some of their demises.

BETA-LACTAM RESISTANCE: A HISTORICAL PERSPECTIVE

The evolving process of bacterial resistance has not changed since Alexander Fleming's discovery of penicillin, which revolutionized the treatment of infectious diseases. Today, it is difficult to imagine that penicillin was actually a useful anti-staphylococcal agent that resulted in many cures for serious staphylococcal infections circa 1945 (9). A short time after the widespread introduction of penicillin and its availability as an oral dosage form, once routinely susceptible staphylococci progressively resisted the effects of this powerful agent. Ominously, Fleming predicted this in an interview with the *New York Times* in 1945, in which he proclaimed that the misuse of penicillin would lead to the selection of mutant strains untreatable by penicillin, a situation he had already simulated in his laboratory (10). Resistance would be amplified when an oral formulation became available, Fleming predicted, because unlike in the controlled hospitalized environment, appropriate outpatient use would be unmonitored and unmanageable. Unfortunately, still today, the appropriate use of anti-infective agents, both in inpatient and outpatient venues, is often difficult to control despite educational efforts regarding the continual increase in bacterial resistance (6).

The less sophisticated beta-lactamases (penicillinases) produced by mutant staphylococci, over time, disallowed the use of penicillin for the treatment of staphylococcal infections. Similar situations subsequently occurred in *Haemophilus influenzae* and *Neisseria gonorrhea* isolates in the decades that followed. In current times, we now discuss far more sophisticated and difficult-to-treat beta-lactamases that continue to rapidly evolve, requiring molecular experts to monitor and classify (and re-classify) them. This is often burdensome and confusing for the practicing clinician treating these infections. Therefore, the following sections are dedicated to the newer beta-lactamases and their clinical implications.

PROBLEMATIC BETA-LACTAMASES AND BETA-LACTAMS

General resistance mechanisms to beta-lactam antimicrobials include alteration of target binding sites (e.g., PBPs), decreased permeability into the bacterial cell (e.g., altered membrane porin channels), efflux pumps, and most commonly, the production of a heterogenous group of beta-lactamases. Beta-lactamases enzymatically cleave the amide bond in the beta-lactam ring structure, thus inactivating its activity. Similar to the earlier-described penicillin–*Staphylococcus* situation, many clinically important Enterobacteriaceae have developed resistance to beta-lactams through the elaboration of more complex chromosomal and/or plasmid-mediated beta-lactamase. The result of these increasingly common mutants has seriously limited the use of the third-generation cephalosporins (e.g., ceftazidime) in many institutions and has unfortunately led to the increased use of carbapenems (e.g., imipenem, meropenem) in some hospitals. Among the most common and challenging to treat are the chromosomally mediated AmpC beta-lactamases and the typically plasmid-mediated ESBLs.

AmpC Beta-Lactamases

The AmpC beta-lactamase, also known as a type of molecular class C or Bush group 1 beta-lactamase (Table 1), was first documented following the introduction of the potent beta-lactamase inducer cefoxitin in 1978 and is particularly worrisome because its expression confers resistance to all cephalosporins (except the newer fourth-generation agents), all penicillins, aztreonam, and beta-lactamase inhibitor combinations (e.g., tazobactam, clavulanate, sulbactam) (11). The gene encoding the AmpC beta-lactamase is naturally present in many species of Enterobacteriaceae and some nonfermentative gram-negative bacilli that some call the SPICE organisms: *Serratia marcescens*, *P. aeruginosa*, *indole-positive proteae (e.g., Morganella* spp), *Citrobacter spp, and Enterobacter spp—organisms that are responsible for many hospital-acquired infections of the respiratory tract, gastrointestinal tract, wounds, and the urinary tract (12). Although the AmpC* gene is present in all of the aforementioned bacteria, clinical expression of the beta-lactamase does not always occur. The dormant (repressed) gene may be activated by induction or the selection of a permanently activated (stably derepressed) mutant that occurs naturally in bacterial populations at a frequency of approximately one in 10^6 to one in 10^7 organisms (12).

Table 1 Classification of Beta-Lactamases

Functional group (Bush et al. [42])	Subgroups	Molecular class	Estimated numbers of enzymes through 2000	Characteristics
1	None	C	51	Includes AmpC beta-lactamases Most commonly chromosomally mediated
2	2a	A, D	256	Penicillinases
	2b		23	(staphylococcal
	2be (ESBLs)		16	and enterococcal)
	2br		119	TEM-1 and SHV-1 from
	2c		24	gram-negative bacteria
	2d		19	ESBLs, conferring
	2e		31	resistance to oxyimino
	2f		20	beta lactams Inhibitor-
			4	resistant TEM beta-lactamases, one SHV derivative Carbenicillin-hydrolyzing enzymes Cloxacillin/oxacillin-hydrolyzing enzymes Cephalosporinases inhibited by clavulanic acid Carbapenem-hydrolyzing enzymes, inhibited by clavulanate
3	3a, 3b, 3c	B	24	Metallo-beta-lactamases that confer resistance to all beta-lactams, including carbapenems and inhibitors (e.g., tazobactam). Monobactams retain susceptibility.
4	None	?	9	Miscellaneous category

ESBL, extended-spectrum beta-lactamase.
Adapted from Bush K. New beta-lactamases in gram-negative bacteria: diversity and impact on the selection of antimicrobial therapy. Clin Infect Dis 2001; 32:1085–1089.

Induction, or the temporary expression of the AmpC beta-lactamase resulting in a mild elevation in MIC from baseline, occurs as a result of burdening the amp D enzyme that is responsible for recycling cell wall fragments (Fig. 1)(12). Potent inducers of the AmpC beta-lactamase include cefoxitin, cefotetan, clavulanate, and the carbapenems (13–15). Induction may be reversible, i.e., once the inducing agent is removed, the MIC values may return to baseline (15). Permanent production of this beta-lactamase occurs when the amp D enzyme undergoes a significant mutational event, allowing the buildup of murein cell wall fragments within the bacterial cell, leading to the subsequent unrelenting production of the AmpC beta-lactamase (e.g., stably derepressed mutant) (12).

It used to be relatively simple, the SPICE organisms were associated with chromosomal beta-lactamase production (e.g., AmpC beta-lactamases), and *Escherichia coli* and *Klebsiella pneumoniae* were primarily associated with plasmid-mediated beta-lactamases (e.g., ESBLs) or other enzymes. As we have come to learn from our bacterial teachers, evolution is eternal. Now, *E. coli* and *Klebsiella* spp have been detected harboring plasmid-mediated AmpC beta-lactamases and *Enterobacter* spp have been observed to possess plasmid-mediated TEM- or SHV-derivative ESBLs (16–18). Also, multiple enzymes may be isolated from a single organism; hence, phenotypic recognition of the type of beta-lactamase (AmpC beta-lactamase vs. ESBL) by the practicing clinician may be confusing. AmpC beta-lactamase genes found on plasmids in organisms such as *E. coli* thus far have generally originated ("borrowed") from strains of *Enterobacter cloacae* (MIR-1), *Citrobacter freundii* (CMY-2A, LAT-1, BIL-1), and *P. aeruginosa* (MOX-1, FOX-1) (19). For example, Odeh et al. (19) identified the AmpC beta-lactamase (CMY-2) in two multidrug-resistant *E. coli* strains isolated from urinary specimens.

Identification

The hydrolytic characteristics of AmpC beta-lactamases are similar despite their genetic origin (15). AmpC enzymes can be recognized phenotypically and are, as a general rule, resistant to all cephalosporins (with the exception of the fourth-

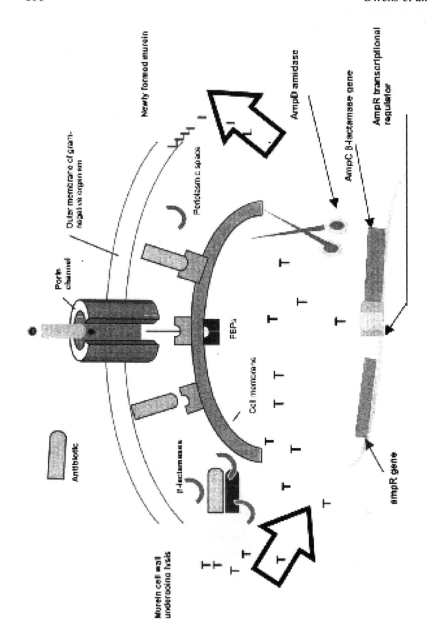

generation agents [e.g., cefepime, cefpirome]), monobactams (e.g., aztreonam), penicillin–beta-lactamase inhibitor combinations (e.g., ampicillin/sulbactam, ticarcillin/clavulanate, piperacillin/tazobactam). Cephamycins (e.g., cefoxitin and cefotetan) are typically susceptible to hydrolysis by AmpC enzymes and can be used to differentiate AmpC phenotypes from ESBL phenotypes because the latter often show *in vitro* susceptibility to the cephamycins. However, identification may be clouded by the presence of multiple enzymes in a single organism, the presence of ACT-1 (an AmpC-like plasmid-mediated beta-lactamase with increased affinity toward the cephamycins but less so toward ceftazidime) overproduction of the enzyme, and the loss of outer membrane porin channels that restrict the access of the drug to the periplasmic space (15).

Antimicrobial Use, Selective Pressure, and Clinical Outcomes

Although correlating antimicrobial use with resistance does not always indicate definitive causality (because of the many complexities that are uncommonly accounted for), there are data from a variety of sources that denote strong associations. The use of third-generation cephalosporins has been associated with the development of resistance during therapy and clinical failures in patients (20–27). Clinical failures associated with AmpC resistance mechanisms are important for several reasons, the most compelling being that organisms such as *E. cloacae* and *P. aeruginosa* have been associated with a high mortality rate and limited treatment options, as well as surviving organisms that may be transmissible to other patients (12).

◄────────────────────────────────────

Figure 1   Regulation of chromosomally mediated AmpC beta-lactamase production. PBP, penicillin-binding protein. (Adapted from Medeiros AA. Evolution and dissemination of β-lactamases accelerated by generations of β-lactam antibiotics. Clin Infect Dis 1997; 24(suppl 1):41–55; and Ambrose PG, Owens RC Jr. New antibiotics in pulmonary and critical care medicine: focus on advanced generation quinolones and cephalosporins. Semin Resp Crit Care Med 2000; 21: 19–32.)

   Studies have demonstrated that the selective pressure exerted by antimicrobial agents may be different, i.e., all antimicrobials are not created the same. With respect to organisms with inducible resistance characteristics (*E. cloacae* and *P. aeruginosa*), Aronoff and Shlaes (28) established that the frequency of bacterial mutation under antimicrobial pressure was directly related to the ratio of drug concentration to the MIC of the bacteria. Serial passage studies have also indicated that *Enterobacter* spp become resistant to antimicrobials at different rates (29). As presented in Figure 2, resistance occurs faster to ceftriaxone and ceftazidime (3 and 4 days, respectively) in contrast to cefepime and meropenem (8 days). Clinically, this is important and may explain why AmpC-mediated resistance seems to occur during therapy with third-generation cephalosporins and not for the fourth-generation cephalosporins or carbapenems, because by day 8, most if not all of the infecting organisms have long been eradicated.

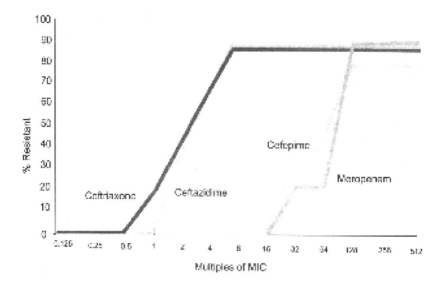

Figure 2 Development of resistance following exposure to third-generation cephalosporins, cefepime, and meropenem. MIC, minimum inhibitory concentration. (Figure provided courtesy of Robert C. Owens, Jr.)

A prospective study by Chow et al. (27) evaluated *Enterobacter* spp bacteremias and showed a strong association between third-generation cephalosporin use and the emergence of resistant *Enterobacter* spp during therapy. In this study, multidrug-resistant *Enterobacter* spp strains were associated with significantly higher mortality rates than their susceptible counterparts, an association that was confirmed via multivariate regression analysis. Also important from this study was the fact that combination therapy failed to prevent the emergence of resistance during treatment (in contrast to the circulating dogma that combination therapy protects against resistance). Johnson and Ramphal (22) also reported substantial mortality associated with ceftazidime-resistant *Enterobacter* spp infections compared with infection due to susceptible strains in a different population, cancer patients with fever and neutropenia.

During one of Kollef's (30) scheduled antimicrobial class change (or "cycling") studies, it was noted that a decreased likelihood of inadequate therapy (defined as an empiric treatment choice that was not active against the organisms eventually cultured) occurred in the cefepime arm in contrast to the ceftazidime arm (4.4 vs. 1.6%, $p < 0.001$). More than 1,000 patients were treated in each arm of the study. This reduction in inadequate therapy led to an increased survival rate for patients treated with cefepime ($p < 0.001$) with Acute Physiology and Chronic Health Evaluation (APACHE) II scores greater than 15 (severely ill patients).

Kollef's results, as well as the others mentioned above, support the strategy suggested by Paterson and Rice (31) in a recent review. They stated that it is time to limit or remove the availability of antimicrobials associated with a high probability of bug-drug mismatches, because they result in greater probabilities of inadequate empiric therapy, ultimately resulting in poorer clinical outcomes in patients.

Resistance Reversal Strategies

Because of their propensity to stimulate resistance, the third-generation cephalosporins have been a target for formulary removal or restriction (32,33). Likewise, optimizing the cephalosporin formulary has been recently shown to have a favorable impact on the susceptibilities of problematic gram-negative bacilli in several institutions. For instance, restriction of ceftazidime use in a pediatric intensive care unit (ICU) resulted in a small but not significant reduction in ceftazidime-resistant gram-negative bacteria overall. However, if one looks at the organisms associated with AmpC beta-lactamase production, in which one would expect to see a difference, resistance decreased from 68.2% to 45.9%, $p < 0.05$ (34). Improved susceptibilities appear to be even greater when ceftazidime has been replaced completely by a fourth-generation cephalosporin. Goldman et al. (35) showed a dramatic increase in *E. cloacae* susceptibilities to a variety of antimicrobial classes following a formulary conversion from ceftazidime to cefepime in six ICUs at the Cleveland Clinic Foundation. Likewise, Mebis et al. (36) replaced ceftazidime-based combination regimens with cefepime-based combination therapy in the treatment of fever and neutropenia. This conversion was in response to *E. cloacae* resistance rates of 75% (ceftazidime), 52.5% (ciprofloxacin), and 36% (amikacin). Ten months after a single cephalosporin change, resistance rates decreased to 35% (ceftazidime), 24% (ciprofloxacin), and 18% (amikacin). Orrick et al. (37) also showed significant improvements in susceptibilities for four AmpC-producing organisms following a formulary conversion from ceftazidime to cefepime (Table 2).

Table 2 Susceptibilities to Ceftazidime and Ticarcillin/Clavulanate Pre–and Post–Formulary Conversion from Ceftazidime to Cefepime for AmpC-Producing Organisms

	Preconversion*/ % susceptible	1-Year postconversion*/ % susceptible
Enterobacter aerogenes	61/53	87/83
Enterobacter cloacae	59/52	82/74
Serratia marcescens	89/86	95/82
Pseudomonas aeruginosa	86/—	93/—

* Listed as percent susceptible to ceftazidime/ticarcilllin-clavulanate.
Data from Orrick J, Ramphal R, Johns T, Russell W. Improving antibiotic susceptibility of type-1 beta-lactamase producing organisms after formulary replacement of ceftazidime with cefepime [abstr 731]. 39th Interscience Conference on Antimicrobial Agents and Chemotherapy, San Francisco, Sept 26–29, 1999.

Following the introduction of cefepime to the formulary at Maine Medical Center (Portland, ME), ceftazidime was not removed or restricted as in the aforementioned studies, but rather its use was guided by education and computerized physician order entry decision support (33). A significant shift in utilization patterns correlated with a reduction in resistance rates. Ceftazidime use diminished over the years from 1998 to 2002 (36.6 to 10.4 antimicrobial days [AD]/1,000 patient days), and cefepime use increased from 0 to 49 AD/1,000 patient days over the same time period (Fig. 3). In parallel, the susceptibility of *S. marcescens* and *E. cloacae* to the third-

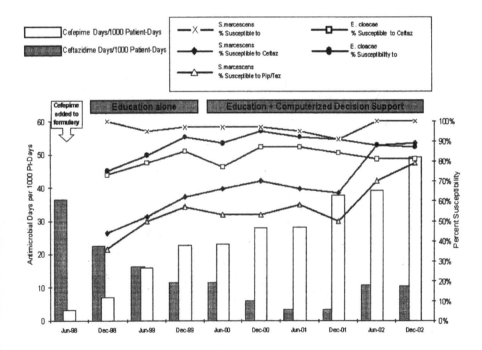

Figure 3 Ecologic impact of cefepime replacement of ceftazidime use over a 5-year period. (Figure provided courtesy of Robert C. Owens, Jr., from Modjtabai K, Prato BS, Stogsdill PB, Owens RC Jr. Impact of inpatient prescribing changes on antimicrobial susceptibilities: a five-year longitudinal study [abstr 156]. 41st Infectious Diseases Society of America Meeting, San Diego, Oct 9–12, 2003.)

generation cephalosporins from 1998 to 2002 increased from 40% to 90% ($r^2 = 0.98$, $p = 0.0001$) and from 72% to 83% ($r^2 = 0.79$, $p = 0.04$), respectively. The minimization of ceftazidime use and replacement by cefepime showed positive and, importantly, durable changes in AmpC phenotypic gram-negative bacilli susceptibility. As expected, cefepime maintained susceptibility at or near 100% to all of the AmpC phenotypic organisms studied over the 5-year period. This study is atypical from many others evaluating resistance changes following significant modification in antimicrobial use patterns, as most studies evaluate pre-and post-periods of 1 year or less.

Bantar et al. (38) employed a multidisciplinary antimicrobial stewardship program to correct patterns of observed antimicrobial misuse. In particular, they targeted the carbapenems and third-generation cephalosporins (ceftazidime and ceftriaxone), replacing them with cefepime and ampicillin/sulbactam. The increased rate of cefepime use relative to third-generation cephalosporins was associated with declining third-generation cephalosporin resistance rates among *Proteus mirabilis* and *E. cloacae*. The increased rate of ampicillin/sulbactam use relative to the third-generation cephalosporins in conjunction with a sustained reduction in vancomycin use was associated with a reduction in MRSA rates. In addition, *P. aeruginosa* resistance rates to carbapenems declined to 0%, which was strongly associated with the reduction in carbapenem consumption over time.

Extended-Spectrum Beta-Lactamases

Extended-spectrum beta-lactamases, first described in Germany two decades ago, followed the introduction of cefotaxime to clinical use, and these enzymes are mutant plasmid-mediated derivatives of the basic and well-described TEM-1 and -2 as well as SHV-1 penicillinases (see Table 1) (39). These TEM- and SHV-origin ESBLs, so called for their extended-spectrum hydrolysis beyond penicillins, now have more than 130 card-carrying members, with most being ceftazidimases (40). For the purposes of familiarizing readers to the nomenclature of these lineages, TEM was named after a little girl (patient's first name) and SHV stands for sulfhydryl variant (41). ESBLs are a diverse group of so-called molecular class A beta-lactamases and fall into the functional group 2be family of the classification scheme, as proposed by Bush et al. (42). The Bush group 2be ESBLs can be further differentiated by their hydrolytic preference toward either ceftazidime or cefotaxime (40). Although they have been described in numerous Enterobacteriaceae, they are most commonly associated with *E. coli* and *K. pneumoniae* in clinical infections. In contrast to the AmpC beta-lactamase–producing organisms, bacteria expressing ESBLs typically acquire the ability to produce such enzymes via plasmids that are often exchanged by bacteria to one another via conjugation, rather than by uniformly possessing the chromosome that encodes the beta-lactamase. ESBL rates, although stable for many years, may be increasing in prevalence (in North America), with recently reported rates of ceftazidime-resistant *Klebsiella* spp. (used as a marker) ranging from 5% to 13% (6). Their worldwide distribution is variable, and in some areas, such as Latin America, Eastern Europe, and parts of Southeast Asia, their prevalence may be far in excess of that seen in the United States. Of alarming concern is the fact that these enzymes do not show a penchant for extinction; rather, they continue to evolve and to be isolated in both clinical and research laboratories worldwide.

An emerging group of cefotaximases is gaining attention: the CTX-M enzymes (40). These ESBLs confer resistance to the aminopenicillins, carboxypenicillins, ureidopenicillins, first- and second-generation cephalosporins (except cefoxitin, cefotetan), cefotaxime, and ceftriaxone; variable resistance to the fourth-generation cephalosporins; and elevated (but in the susceptible range) MIC values to aztreonam and ceftazidime (40).

Characteristically, plasmids encoding ESBLs may also contain additional resistance determinants that result in aminoglycoside (e.g., via aminoglycoside-modifying enzymes), tetracyclines, and trimethoprim/sulfamethoxazole (TMP-SMX). Fluoroquinolone resistance (e.g., via efflux pumps) may also reside on the mobile genetic element. Alarmingly, plasmids containing the chromosomal AmpC beta-lactamase have recently been identified conferring resistance to additional agents (43).

Identification

Because unfortunately, not all clinical laboratories have acceptable contemporary practice despite recommendations to do so, clinicians practicing at institutions served by them are left to distinguish potential ESBL-producing Enterobacteriaceae (44). Two reasons for this have been identified: either clinical laboratories have difficulty detecting resistance or they fail to test for ESBLs at all, usually because their commercially produced testing systems do not offer clear guidance (44,45). Culture and susceptibility reports may be somewhat helpful to clinicians in the phenotypic identification of suspect Enterobacteriaceae (e.g., ceftazidime- or cefotaxime-resistant *E. coli* or *Klebsiella* spp). ESBL-producing isolates typically retain susceptibility to the cephamycins (e.g., cefoxitin, cefotetan); however, AmpC beta-lactamases may also be present in the organism in question, which would cause resistance to the cephamycins. In addition, the loss of outer membrane porins often results in pan-resistance to beta-lactams and some other antimicrobial classes. Identifying these organisms based on the susceptibility report from the laboratory may be insensitive, as the MIC of the oxyimino cephalosporin to the ESBL-producing organism may be below the susceptibility breakpoint. Therefore, the National Committee for Clinical Laboratory Standards (NCCLS) (46) has suggested implementation of screening tests, such as using cefpodoxime or other third-generation agents (e.g., cefotaxime, ceftazidime, ceftriaxone) at low concentrations (MIC 2 μg/mL or greater) to detect possible ESBLs. Alone, the cefpodoxime test results in an unacceptably high rate of false-positive tests, so it is necessary to subsequently perform an appropriate synergy test to confirm the results (47). Several confirmatory tests are available (Fig. 4), including the double-disk diffusion assay, the ESBL E-test strip (AB BIODISK, Solna, Sweden)™, and multiple automated susceptibility-testing systems (e.g., Vitek and Vitek 2 [bioMérieux, Hazelwood MO]™, MicroScan [Dade Behring,

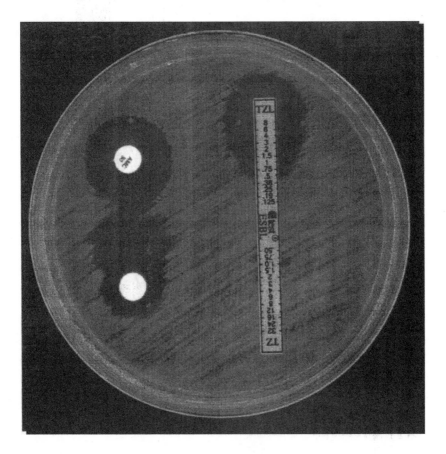

Figure 4 Disk approximation method (*left*) and the E-test extended-spectrum beta-lactamase (ESBL) strip (*right*). The disk approximation method (between ceftazidime and amoxicillin/clavulanate disks) will result in a 5 mm or greater increase around the test disk in the presence of clavulanic acid. The E-test strips (with and without 4 μg/mL of clavulanic acid) will result in an ellipse around the strip containing the inhibitor and a minimum inhibitory concentration eightfold or more lower than the cephalosporin alone. (Figure provided courtesy of Ronald N. Jones, MD)

Inc Microscan, West Sacramento, CA]®). In these tests, enhanced oxyimino cephalosporin (e.g., ceftazidime, cefotaxime, ceftriaxone) or monobactam activity by clavulanic acid inhibition suggests the presence of an ESBL enzyme. Currently, the NCCLS calls for the microbiology laboratory to report ESBL-producing organisms as resistant to all penicillins, cephalosporins, and aztreonam, regardless of the susceptibility test result.

Because plasmids are notorious for containing resistance determinants to other classes of antimicrobials, ESBL-producing Enterobacteriaceae may demonstrate clinical resistance to quinolones, tetracyclines, TMP-SMX, and aminoglycosides. These plasmids may be prevalent in geographic areas with higher target-mutation rates. For example, a recent study showed that fluoroquinolone resistance was 55% among ESBL-producing *E. coli* and *K. pneumoniae* (48). Risk factors for fluoroquinolone resistance among ESBL-producing isolates were noted to be fluoroquinolone and aminoglycoside use (odds ratio [OR], 11.20 and 5.83, respectively), and long-term care facility residence (OR, 3.39). Because ESBLs represent more than 100 actual enzymes with differing hydrolyzing affinities, it is prudent under outbreak or epidemic situations to determine the type (e.g., TEM-10) of ESBL being encountered locally to direct interventions.

Antimicrobial Use and Selective Pressure

The use and/or overuse of the oxyimino group–containing beta-lactams (e.g., cefuroxime, cefotaxime, ceftriaxone, ceftazidime, aztreonam) have been associated with outbreaks of ESBL-producing *E. coli* and *K. pneumoniae* (49–53). Data continue to support these associations, such as the study by Paterson et al. (54), who also showed a strong correlation between oxyimino beta-lactam use and bacteremias caused by ESBL-producing *K. pneumoniae* (risk ratio, 3.9 [95% CI, 1.1-13.8]) (54). In Donskey's biologic model, antianaerobic agents (e.g., clindamycin) were also shown to promote the overgrowth of ESBL-producing *K. pneumoniae* in stool (55). When larger inoculum densities of ESBL-producing strains were already present as colonizing organisms in the gastrointestinal tract, the administration of agents such as piperacillin/tazobactam, ceftriaxone, and ceftazidime promoted persistent high-density colonization. Higher densities of these organisms may increase the probability of horizontal transmission of ESBL-producing organisms.

The ongoing saga at New York Hospital Queens, a 500-bed urban teaching facility in the heart of a working-class community, has successfully illustrated the antimicrobial use-resistance selection relationship (56–58). The effects of various countermeasures used to contain both the endogenous selection and horizontal transmission of resistant gram-negative bacilli were also documented. An initial series of infections caused by *Acinetobacter baumannii* (multidrug resistant but ceftazidime susceptible) led to the increased use of ceftazidime. From this reliance on ceftazidime, significant numbers of infections due to both ceftazidime-resistant *A. baumannii* (in 1988) and ceftazidime-resistant (ESBL-producing) *K. pneumoniae* (in 1993) arose, requiring the greater use of imipenem. To gain perspective, in 1993, 37% of all *K. pneumoniae* strains isolated were ESBL producers. The resultant increased imipenem use and continued selective pressure exerted by ceftazidime and cefotetan culminated with the development of *A. baumanni* strains resistant to imipenem and ceftazidime, *K. pneumoniae* now resistant to ceftazidime (an ESBL), cefotetan (ACT-1 plasmid-mediated AmpC-type beta-lactamase), and imipenem (outer membrane porin loss), as well as imipenem-resistant *P. aeruginosa*. Selective pressure exerted by both ceftazidime and imipenem undoubtedly contributed to the genesis of these resistant organisms, and once established, horizontal transmission amplified their dissemination.

Quale et al. (53) reported that an advanced outbreak was occurring in 2002 in the New York City area as they collected 281 ESBL-producing isolates of *K. pneumoniae* from fifteen hospitals in Brooklyn. Isoelectric points suggested a predominance of SHV-5 enzymes mixed with smaller numbers of other enzymes, including the plasmid-mediated AmpC beta-lactamase ACT-1. Percent susceptibilities to several antimicrobials were reported for the isolates, including ceftazidime (13%), cefoxitin

(34%), ciprofloxacin (42%), ceftriaxone (48%), piperacillin/tazo-bactam (55%), amikacin (57%), cefepime (86%), and imipenem (99%). The high rate of cephamycin resistance (66%) and low rate of resistance to cefepime strongly suggests the co-presence of AmpC and ESBL enzymes. Antimicrobial utilization data indicated that the use of cephalosporins as a group and aztreonam correlated strongly with the prevalence of ESBL-producing strains at each institution via multivariate analysis ($p = 0.014$).

As experienced by the New York Hospital Queens, the neighboring hospitals in Brooklyn also experienced significant ESBL-producing Enterobacteriaceae and *Acinetobacter* spp outbreaks. From their experience arose a case-control study of their clinical outcomes. Longer lengths of stay following the infection were noted for patients with ESBL-producing *K. pneumoniae* infections compared with controls (median, 29 vs. 11 days, $p = 0.03$; mean, 37 ± 25 vs. 15 ± 10 days, $p = 0.04$) (59). ESBL cases had a higher but not statistically significant mortality rate when compared with controls (44% vs. 34%).

Imipenem has demonstrated a negative effect on hospital ecology in other well-conducted studies, primarily resulting in the emergence of resistance among strains of *P. aeruginosa* during therapy (60–62). Once an outbreak of ESBL-producing strains has been effectively managed at the hospital level, it is important to recognize that these organisms have likely disseminated into the surrounding community, including long-term care facilities (48,56,63). Strains may be reintroduced to the hospital from these venues, further emphasizing the importance of effective and prospective infection control programs for ESBL.

Clinical Outcomes

Paterson et al. (64) reviewed more than 400 consecutive isolates of *K. pneumoniae* and their resulting infections, eighty of which were associated with ESBL-producing strains. The primary end point was mortality, a crude estimate of efficacy, which may or may not be associated with drug efficacy, depending on various other factors, such as underlying disease.

Carbapenems (e.g., imipenem, meropenem) were used to treat the majority of cases, resulting in the lowest mortality rate (5%). The mortality rate of patients receiving ciprofloxacin was 21%. Only eight patients were treated with either cefepime or piperacillin/tazobactam—four each. Two of four patients treated with cefepime died. The majority of all isolates tested during the study period were susceptible to cefepime (87%). Two of four patients who were treated with piperacillin/tazobactam died as well, and interestingly, only 38% of *Klebsiella* spp isolates were susceptible to this agent. Several important limitations exist with this study, including the retrospective nature of the study, the end point used to evaluate antimicrobial efficacy (crude, not attributable mortality), the absence of antimicrobial exposure information (e.g., dose, interval, duration, organ dysfunction), and limited patient sample sizes (e.g., two to four patients) treated with various noncarbapenem regimens.

Einhorn et al. (65) retrospectively determined the frequency, risk factors, and outcomes associated with "presumed" ESBL-producing *E. coli* and *K. pneumoniae* (resistance to ceftazidime used as a phenotypic marker) in a nonoutbreak setting in an urban teaching hospital. From 1991 to 1999, *E. coli* and *K. pneumoniae* resistant to ceftazidime increased from 0% to 4% and 2% to 6%, respectively, according to antibiogram data. This study is important in that it described the epidemiology of presumed ESBL-producing Enterobacteriaceae in a nonoutbreak setting and that it captured potential community-cultured cases, though inherent limitations to this investigation also existed. Perhaps because of the endemic setting, the patients were generally younger (median 56.5 years, range 26 to 79 years) than those reported in other studies and some isolates appear to have originated in the community (isolates cultured as outpatients). Four of the eight patients with community-acquired organisms were seen as outpatients in settings where their phenotypically identified ESBL-producing isolates were cultured; the other four were identified on admission. Only three of the eight patients had prior antimicrobial exposure histories, with TMP-SMX being most common. Four of the eight had at least two significant comorbidities (median APACHE II score of the four admitted patients was 16, range 5 to 27). Considering the group of patients whose isolates were recovered in the hospital or long-term care facility, their risk factors were similar to those identified from other published studies. Overall, 74% had documented histories of antimicrobial use, with 19% and 35% receiving third-generation cephalosporins and fluoroquinolones, respectively. This study points out the fact that the fluoroquinolones have reduced susceptibilities (24%) against some ESBL-producing organisms, similar to other studies. In terms of outcomes, empiric therapy with active agents did not appear to correlate with improved outcomes; this, perhaps, was because the source of infection in 62% of patients was the urinary tract, a site that is easier to penetrate, affording better opportunities to maximize drug exposure.

Resistance Reversal Strategies

In part, strategies for containing or reversing the resistance trend for AmpC- and ESBL-producing organisms are probably not very different. Antimicrobial control or stewardship, infection control efforts, administrative support for resources, and education must work in concert to produce positive change. From the experience of New York medical centers, knowledge has been gained in terms of potential strategies to reverse outbreak and endemic resistance situations. The solutions of Go et al. (66) involved a concerted approach integrating changes in antimicrobial utilization patterns and infection control efforts with the sound backing of hospital administration. With regard to the multidrug-resistant *A. baumanni*, contact isolation, patient cohorting, and local application of polymixin resulted in the elimination of carbapenem-resistant clones (66). Restriction of second- and third-generation cephalosporins, including the cephamycins, resulted in a 44% reduction in ESBL-producing *K. pneumoniae* housewide (87% reduction in ICUs) (57). As of 2002, continued contact isolation and local polymyxin application are being used to reduce the endemic spread of the imipenem-resistant *P. aeruginosa* strains (56).

Although it is evident from the overwhelming data that infection and colonization with ESBL-producing organisms may be strongly influenced by the use of particular antimicrobial agents, infection control strategies are also critical to preventing the horizontal spread from these resistant variants. Paterson et al. (67) successfully controlled an outbreak due to ESBL-producing *E. coli* organisms by means of gut decontamination with norfloxacin, contact isolation, and feedback on hand hygiene in a liver transplantation unit. In their case, genotypic relatedness of all recovered isolates indicated horizontal transfer of the ESBL-positive strains. Patients were isolated in individual rooms with sinks and nonmedicated soap. Nurses and other health care providers were stopped after leaving each room and asked to participate in a "teaching exercise" by the infection control department. The glove juice sampling procedure indicated that nurses and physicians were culture positive (32% and 23%, respectively) for organisms such as MRSA and VRE, but not ESBL-producing *E. coli*. Staff were confidentially informed of their culture positivity and educated regarding the significance of hand washing. Contact precautions (gloves and gowns) were required for all ESBL-positive patients and their environments, which lasted for their current and all future admissions. Norfloxacin (400 mg every 12 hours for 5 days) was used to reduce the density of ESBL organisms in the stool of identified patients. The results of the decontamination effort were fleeting, as 40% of patients had positive cultures 14 days after receiving the last dose of norfloxacin, and 60% at 30 days. The strategy was successful in curtailing the outbreak of ESBL-producing isolates; however, caution was suggested by the authors in using so-called fluoroquinolone decontamination regimens, because of the potential for high percentages of these organisms being quinolone resistant.

Minimizing the use and availability of offending/selecting agents has been central to most strategies. For instance, Empey et al. (68) affected their hospital's cephalosporin use by using the formulary to reduce the utilization of third-generation cephalosporins (both ceftazidime and cefotaxime) and to replace their use with the fourth-generation cephalosporin cefepime. The use of ceftazidime and cefotaxime was reduced by 89%. As a result, infections caused by certain resistant organisms decreased from the pre– to the post–formulary change periods, as exemplified by ceftazidime-resistant *K. pneumoniae* (13% to 3%), piperacillin-resistant *P. aeruginosa* (22% to 14%), and ceftazidime-resistant *P. aeruginosa* (25% to 15%), $p < 0.05$ for all. As expected, MRSA rates were unchanged; however, an unexpected increase in the rate of VRE was noted. The authors, however, were unable to find a correlation between antibiotic use and the frequency of VRE by using regression models. Additionally, the biologic model expanded on by Donskey et al. (69) does not support the fact that cefepime would increase rates of VRE.

Rice et al. (70) reported a TEM-6–producing *K. pneumoniae* outbreak caused by the widespread use of ceftazidime at a Veterans Affairs facility. Utilization of ceftazidime was replaced by piperacillin/tazobactam, resulting in a dramatic reduction in the isolation of ceftazidime-resistant *K. pneumoniae*. Similar reductions were subsequently reported by others in the literature (71,72).

From these experiences, it would appear that the fourth-generation cephalosporins and some beta-lactam/beta-lactamase inhibitor combinations positively affect institutional ecology whereas carbapenems and third-generation cephalosporins should be reserved for limited use. Replacement of the latter with the former has successfully been used to reverse resistance trends in these outbreak situations in both the short- and long-terms, without sacrificing treatment spectrum or potency.

Controversy

An area of *in vitro* controversy exists surrounding the clinical relevance of the so-called inoculum effect. To understand this, standardized susceptibility testing occurs in the laboratory using a bacterial inoculum of approximately 5×10^5 colony-forming units (CFU)/mL. A fixed concentration of antimicrobial is placed in the well containing the organisms. Simply, the amount of organisms used determines the amount of beta-lactamase produced, and when the drug in the well is hydrolyzed, the organisms will not be inhibited, resulting in regrowth and a possible increased MIC. *In vitro* testing using higher inocula (e.g., 10^7 CFU/mL) naturally results in a higher quantity of beta-lactamase, which, if the same fixed amount of antibiotic is used, will predictably result in elevated MIC (and is termed the *inoculum effect*).

A recent criticism of the *in vitro* inoculum test is the fact that fixed drug concentrations are used, a scenario that is not generalizable to the treatment of infection in *vivo*. In humans and animals, drug concentrations change over time and are replenished with new drugs on each newly administered dose (as opposed to a one-time lump addition to a tube or broth microdilution test well). Also, the inoculum size at the site of infection changes over time because of the contribution of host defenses and the antibacterial effects of the drug, which cannot collectively be characterized by any *in vitro* test. Although it has been formulated as a central argument to label all cephalosporins, aztreonam, and penicillins, regardless of their individual susceptibilities, as resistant to ESBL-producing organisms isolated in the clinical laboratory by the NCCLS, it should be remembered that the inoculum effect is also a characteristic of non–ESBL-producing organisms. Bedenic et al. (73) showed that the *in vitro* inoculum effect is strain dependent and present in both ESBL- and non–ESBL-producing Enterobacteriaceae. Indeed, if the inoculum effect is a credible argument to declare classes of drugs resistant to ESBL-producing organisms, it would appear that *all E. coli* and *Klebsiella* spp, regardless of ESBL production, should be declared "resistant" to all cephalosporins!

Several *in vivo* studies have called into question the validity of the inoculum effect. Maglio et al. (74) studied the *in vivo* impact of cefepime dosing regimens on various TEM-producing and non–ESBL-producing *E. coli* isolates at standard and increased inocula (10^5 and 10^7 CFU/mL). A significant increase in cefepime MIC results with increased inocula were observed for *E. coli* isolates, denoting the inoculum effect (*in vitro*). This effect was noted regardless of ESBL production in the *E. coli* strains. Interestingly, the magnitude of the *in vitro* inoculum effect appeared to be greater among ESBL-negative strains of *E. coli*. The dose-response curves for the ESBL isolates indicate that similar milligram-per-kilogram doses would achieve similar reductions in *in vivo* bacterial density at both inocula. These data support the use of conventional MIC determinations in the pharmacodynamic assessment of cefepime against ESBL-producing organisms.

Others have noted the paradox of microbiologic effectiveness in the face of *in vitro* resistance when higher inocula are used. For example, cefepime was effective in a rat abscess model because of infection with a high inoculum (greater than 10^7) of *K. pneumoniae* that harbored the TEM-26 enzyme, an ESBL presumed to be common in the United States (75). Cefepime MICs were in the susceptible range at 10^5 CFU/mL but fit the criteria for "resistant" at a 10^7 CFU/mL inoculum concentration. Using simulated human exposures, the authors noted that the greater efficacy observed with cefepime compared with the other beta-lactams tested was surprising given that cefepime appeared least potent *in vitro* at 10^7 CFU/mL in comparison with the other agents. However, efficacy would seem to be explained in this study by MIC results obtained at 10^5 CFU/mL, a concentration at which cefepime was most potent in comparison with other agents.

Andes and Craig (76) evaluated the impact of ESBL-producing *K. pneumoniae* and *E. coli* with various TEM- and SHV-derived ESBLs in the neutropenic murine-thigh infection model. Mice were infected with high inocula (e.g., 10^7 and 10^8 CFU/thigh). Non–ESBL-producing organisms of the same genus and species were used as controls. High-density inocula made no difference in terms of the amount of time above the MIC (T>MIC) necessary for *in vivo* cefepime efficacy. This, again, points to the fact that the MIC appears to capture the information required to predict bacterial eradication when combined with the magnitude of drug exposure.

Pharmacodynamics as a Predictor of Efficacy

Based on data suggesting that the MIC obtained at standard inoculum sizes may, in fact, be used as a successful surrogate, Ambrose et al. (77) conducted a study to compare target attainments for piperacillin/tazobactam and cefepime against ESBL-producing organisms. The probability of T>MIC target attainment for these agents against 105 *K. pneumoniae* and *E. coli* with ESBL phenotypes (e.g., ceftazidime and/or ceftriaxone and/or aztreonam MICs 2 µg/mL or greater) obtained from the SENTRY Antimicrobial Surveillance Program in 2000 were compared (77). The *in vitro* susceptibility of cefepime and piperacillin/tazobactam to *K. pneumoniae* (92.5% and 62.5%, respectively) and *E. coli* (98.5% and 89.1%, respectively) were reported. In terms of conservative T>MIC targets in humans (T>MIC for 70% of the dosing interval), cefepime dosed 1 g every 12 hours achieved optimal target attainments of 93% to 96% against *K. pneumoniae* and *E. coli*, respectively. Whereas for piperacillin/tazobactam, using the same T>MIC target and employing 3.375 g every 4 and every 6 hours, the target attainments were poor at 16% and 48% for *K. pneumoniae* and 28% and 77% for *E. coli*, respectively. These data are important in that treatment options for ESBL-producing pathogens are often limited, and although laboratories suspecting ESBL enzymes in a clinical isolate may report it to be resistant to all cephalosporins according to the NCCLS, not all cephalosporins should be considered equally unusable.

Treatment Implications

To date, there have been no prospective randomized, controlled trials conducted for the treatment of infections caused by ESBL-producing organisms. Based on *in vitro* data, clinically unsubstantiated theories related to the purported inoculum effect, and a limited number of uncontrolled clinical studies, the carbapenems have laid claim as the "treatments of choice" for infections caused by ESBL-producing organisms. In support of the carbapenems, there are anecdotal case series that have demonstrated efficacy against ESBL-producing organisms; however, failures involving imipenem therapy have also been reported (78). Moreover, with little data to suggest that the use of certain cephalosporins leads to treatment failures for infections caused by susceptible ESBL-producing organisms, it may be time to reevaluate the class resistance reporting of cephalosporins by the NCCLS and to rethink the current breakpoints for the Enterobacteriaceae overall.

The presence of ESBL-producing Enterobacteriaceae in hospitals poses vexing empiric treatment situations, as illustrated by a case report of a patient with spontaneous bacterial peritonitis (SBP) and end-stage liver disease (79). Though treated empirically with piperacillin/tazobactam that was eventually determined to be susceptible (MIC, 8 μg/mL), the patient developed intractable septic shock and died 4 days into therapy. The isolate was cultured from both blood and ascitic fluid, and determined to be an ESBL-producing *E. coli* upon confirmatory testing. The isolate was resistant to ceftazidime (MIC greater than 256 μg/mL), intermediate to cefotaxime and ceftriaxone (MICs16 μg/mL and 32 μg/ml, respectively), and susceptible to cefepime (MIC 1 μg/mL). Cefotaxime is commonly used as an empiric treatment choice for SBP, and this case should raise concerns about its empiric use in those patients at risk for ESBLs.

A recent study elegantly demonstrated favorable clinical responses to nonceftazidime extended-spectrum cephalosporin regimens for the treatment of pathogens that produced certain ESBLs (80). The investigators evaluated the largest number of bloodstream infections (n = 36) caused by *K. pneumoniae* and *E. coli* with ceftazidime MICs 2 μg/mL or greater to date that were not associated with an outbreak. Five types of ESBLs were identified: TEM-6, TEM-12, TEM-71, SHV-5, and SHV-12. Nonceftazidime extended-spectrum cephalosporins were most successful in treating TEM-6 or TEM-12 ESBLs, whereas ceftazidime was associated with failures to all five types of ESBLs isolated from patients. This study challenges the current paradigm that only carbapenems will be useful for the treatment of ESBL infections.

Although currently impractical in most hospital settings, knowing the identity of the specific ESBL and whether or not it is accompanied by other beta-lactamases in a clinical isolate may give hope for optimizing therapy directed against these organisms in real time. For now, if ESBL-producing isolates are suspected to have infiltrated a health care facility, it would be prudent to determine the enzyme being encountered from both an epidemiologic and potentially a treatment perspective. Knowing the specific enzyme, in conjunction with knowing its MIC and the probability of pharmacokinetic-pharmacodynamic (PK-PD) target attainment in a particular patient, would allow for optimal selection and dosing of the antimicrobial(s).

LIMITATIONS OF CLINICAL TRIALS TO DIFFERENTIATE ANTIMICROBIAL THERAPIES

Why can't we rely on clinical trial data to differentiate beneficial outcomes in comparative registration trials? Aside from studies being powered to show only equivalence, there exists another significant limitation in the design of blinded clinical studies conducted for registration purposes. Historically, if an organism is cultured, the protocol specifies that it must be susceptible to both study agents. The obvious limitation of this design is that it fosters equivalence among comparative regimens and does not allow for the evaluation of regimens against organisms with higher MIC values. To this end, Sanders et al. (81) reported outcomes of infections for patients excluded from trials with infections due to *Enterobacter* spp (ceftazidime-resistant strains) that were treated with cefepime. To clarify, these patients were randomized to receive cefepime in comparative trials with ceftazidime. Upon the clinician's receipt of the susceptibility information indicating ceftazidime resistance, the patients were excluded from the registration trials per protocol. Included in this group were patients with bacteremia, pneumonia, urinary tract infection, and intra-abdominal infection as well as chronically infected patients who had responded poorly to imipenem, aminoglycosides, and ciprofloxacin. The success rate of cefepime in this group of patients was 88.2%, and the development of resistance to cefepime was not reported to occur during therapy. As a result of the exclusion criteria, patients with infections due to organisms with ESBLs and AmpC as mechanisms of resistance are rarely, if ever, studied among protocol evaluable patients. Thus, patient populations evaluated in studies may more or less be artificial and data obtained from them may not be readily generalizable.

FORMULARY SELECTION OF CEPHALOSPORINS

From the cited data and from what has been previously suggested, it appears that managing beta-lactam (cephalosporin) components of formularies to provide antimicrobials with high probabilities of initial bacterial eradication may improve outcomes as well as reduce the probability of selecting for certain problematic organisms (31,82). Because changes in susceptibility have occurred over the past decade, hospitals may benefit from a regular reevaluation of their formularies as a part of their strategy to optimize antimicrobial use (83). Overall, certain generalizations apply to the cephalosporin class of antimicrobials: (i) they are well tolerated (an increasing concern with modern antimicrobial therapy) and are devoid of drug interactions (with the exception of probenecid), (ii) most are relatively inexpensive (all are below, and most are well below the acquisition price of piperacillin/tazobactam, imipenem, and meropenem), and (iii) most offer less-frequent dosing schedules compared with piperacillin/tazobactam, imipenem, and meropenem. In addition, all of these agents can be pushed intravenously at a relatively rapid rate (less than 5 minutes), and some can be administered intramuscularly (84). The most serious safety issue is anaphylaxis in the beta-lactam allergic patient. As a class, the cephalosporins are less likely than the penicillins and carbapenems to cause serious, life-threatening anaphylactic reactions (85). Seizures and nephrotoxicity are very rare complications and may occur in patients who are not properly dose-adjusted for renal impairment. Patients requiring these agents for therapy can be desensitized using a dose-escalation protocol. For the purposes of this review, only commonly used parenteral cephalosporins are discussed below.

First-Generation Cephalosporins

Cefazolin is a traditional workhorse cephalosporin that has the benefit of a narrow spectrum of activity, an inexpensive purchase price, and an every-8-hour dosing schedule. It is active against methicillin-susceptible *Staphylococcus aureus* (MSSA), penicillin-susceptible streptococci, and a very limited number of gram-negative organisms. The gram-negative organisms can be remembered by the acronym *PECK* for *Proteus spp, E. coli, and Klebsiella spp. Thus, the utility of this agent fits specific indications, such as surgical prophylaxis for many procedures, skin and soft tissue infections, community-acquired urinary tract infections, and as a narrow-spectrum streamlining choice when culture and susceptibility results become available. First-generation cephalosporins are not active against H. influenzae* or *Moraxella catarrhalis*, precluding their use for the empiric treatment of respiratory tract infections. Also, these agents do not penetrate into the cerebrospinal fluid (CSF), thus they are not useful for the treatment of meningitis or other central nervous system infections. Cefazolin is a cornerstone in the institutional formulary for the aforementioned indications.

Second-Generation Cephalosporins

The primary respiratory second-generation parenteral cephalosporin (cefuroxime sodium) is active against the same pathogens as cefazolin, but adds activity against *H. influenzae, M. catarrhalis*, and *Neisseria* spp. Interestingly, at the time cefuroxime was launched, it was used and indicated for the treatment of meningitis owing to its good penetration into the CSF and spectrum of activity. Over time, failures due to *S. pneumoniae* were reported with increasing frequency and when ceftriaxone and cefotaxime were marketed, it became obsolete as a treatment for meningitis (86). Similarly, for respiratory tract infections, this generation of cephalosporins has been decimated by the rise in its MIC value for *S. pneumoniae*. Because of this, many hospitals have abandoned cefuroxime for inpatient treatment in favor of more potent antipneumococcal cephalosporins, such as ceftriaxone, cefepime, and cefotaxime (87). The inclusion of a respiratory second-generation cephalosporin in a modern formulary has become unnecessary.

Among the second-generation agents are the cephamycins cefoxitin and cefotetan, which differ from the others in that they have some activity against anaerobic organisms and possess strong beta-lactamase induction characteristics. It is likely the use of these agents stimulated the isolation of the first stably derepressed AmpC beta-lactamases found among Enterobacteriaceae. Their activity against anaerobes has waned over the past two decades. Because of this as well as their documented negative effects on host flora, they are rarely used for the treatment of infection, but rather serve as surgical prophylactic agents for procedures requiring some antianaerobic activity. Even with prophylactic use, however, negative effects on gram-negative bacilli can be traced to the use of these agents. The debate between which of these two agents should be positioned on formulary has, after more than a decade, been reduced to a mild brawl. Cefoxitin is the least favored agent, primarily because of its every-6-hour dosing schedule compared with cefotetan's every-12-hour schedule. Because of the rare therapeutic use of these agents today, usually a single dose of either would suffice in most surgical prophylaxis settings.

Third-Generation Cephalosporins

The third-generation cephalosporins are relatively heterogenous in terms of their spectra of activity; however, a common theme among them also exists. They can be broken down in terms of their spectra of activity (antistreptococcal vs. antipseudomonal) and primary utilities. Cefotaxime, ceftriaxone, and ceftizoxime are active against many Enterobacteriaceae (though they have been implicated in selecting for resistant strains when used to treat them) as well as MSSA and streptococci. Their antipneumococcal activity has stood the test of time (cefotaxime = ceftriaxone > ceftizoxime) and may be viewed as their primary strength. They are best fitted in modern times for the treatment of hospitalized patients with community-acquired respiratory tract infections and for the treatment of meningitis. In 2002, the NCCLS introduced new a breakpoint for *S. pneumoniae* for ceftriaxone, cefotaxime, and the fourth-generation agent cefepime to compensate for their activity outside of the CNS (88). The previous "one size fits all" breakpoints for susceptible, intermediate, and resistant of 0.5 μg/mL or less, 1 μg/mL, and 2 μg/mL or greater now apply only to CNS infections, for which they were initially developed, whereas infections outside the CNS now have different breakpoints of 1 μg/mL or less, 2 μg/mL, and 4 μg/mL or greater. Most laboratories should be reporting these body site–specific breakpoints for pneumococcal infections. All these agents penetrate into the CNS adequately to treat related infections. Ceftriaxone carries the unique distinction among all cephalosporins in that it does not require renal dosing adjustments unless both hepatic and renal systems are compromised. Institution-specific purchase prices may simply be the best separating factor for these agents. Ceftriaxone's patent-life is ending, which, if the price is reduced, will make it more favorable because of its once-daily dosing schedule. Hospitals with home intravenous infusion centers tend to favor daily-dosed agents for their outpatient population.

The antipseudomonal third-generation agents include ceftazidime and cefoperazone. The increased activity against *P. aeruginosa* is countered by their diminished susceptibility to ESBL- and AmpC-producing Enterobacteriaceae and gram-positive organisms (MSSA and streptococci). The common theme among them appears to be their association with so-called collateral damage to host and institutional flora. Associations between their use and the selection of VRE, ESBL- and AmpC-producing Enterobacteriaceae, and *Clostridium difficile* disease have been reported (89,90). In addition to the vast clinical data, Donskey's model demonstrates the ability of third-generation cephalosporins to select for and sustain VRE and ESBL-producing organisms (55,91).

Fourth-Generation Cephalosporins

Cefepime and cefpirome comprise the only so-called fourth-generation cephalosporins, with the former being the only compound available in the United States. These agents combine the beneficial characteristics seen with other generations (e.g., retain gram-positive activity equivalent to ceftriaxone, including multidrug-resistant pneumococci) and gram-negative activity including *P. aeruginosa* and AmpC-producing Enterobacteriaceae (92,93). In addition, activity against some ESBL-producing Enterobacteriaceae has been demonstrated both *in vitro* and *in vivo*. In contrast to the third-generation cephalosporins, cefepime has not been shown to adversely affect institutional ecology when used as a workhorse empiric treatment option and has shown survival benefits compared with ceftazidime (30,94). Cefepime is somewhat unique among cephalosporins in that it is a zwitterionic (net neutral) compound (similar to the carbapenems), allowing it to penetrate through porin channels more rapidly than ionically charged oxyimino cephalosporins. Lastly, these agents are more stable in the presence of most clinically important beta-lactamases (92).

In most instances, cefepime is administered every 12 to 24 hours. Renal dosing adjustment from every 12 hours to every 24 hours for cefepime takes place at a relatively high creatinine clearance (60 mL/minute or less) for most infections. Infections in which an every-8-hour interval (assuming good renal function) may be preferred include meningitis, osteomyelitis, endocarditis, and *P. aeruginosa* infections caused by organisms with higher MIC values (in the susceptible to intermediate range), such as 8 to 16 μg/mL, in which a more frequent dosing interval may optimize the pharmacodynamic profile of the agent at the site of infection (95,96).

Some experts suggest cefepime be dosed every 8 hours for fever and neutropenia also; however, it has been studied and shown to be as effective when dosed every 12 hours for this indication (97–99). Based on its activity against probable pathogens, cefepime has been studied and shown to be effective for the following infections: nosocomial-, nursing home-, and community-acquired pneumonia; complicated urinary tract infections; bacteremias; neutropenic fever in cancer patients; meningitis; skin and soft tissue infections; and intraabdominal infections (in combination with metronidazole) (100–103). The cefepime activity against *S. pneumoniae* has remained at least as effective as that demonstrated by ceftriaxone (101).

Finally, several studies have shown the benefit of the fourth-generation cephalosporins on the institutional ecology, in contrast to the negative data surrounding the use of third-generation cephalosporins as previously reviewed. These agents, based on a large amount of compiled data, are worth considering as workhorse therapies for empiric therapy of a variety of infections and to treat problematic organisms, replacing other-generation cephalosporins.

COST-EFFECTIVENESS STUDIES

In addition to the assessment of the clinical impact of such failures, the costs associated with these instances because of resistant bacteria have been evaluated (26,104). The chapter by Scott et al. in this book provides an excellent overview and perspective of this subject. Although problematic to quantify, costs associated with bacterial resistance may be significant. It has been shown that for community- and hospital-acquired infections caused by drug-resistant organisms, mortality, the likelihood of hospital admission, and lengths of hospital stay were commonly twofold greater compared with infection caused by the same, but drug-susceptible, bacteria (104). Ambrose et al. (26) evaluated the efficacy of cefepime compared with ceftazidime for the treatment of nosocomial pneumonia. A cost-effectiveness analysis demonstrated a reduction in total costs (e.g., drug acquisition, supplies, additional antibiotics required for treatment failures, hospitalization costs) when cefepime was utilized (cefepime cost/cure = $235.89 and cost/failure = $375.44 vs. ceftazidime cost/cure = $319.81 and cost/failure = $520.11). Significantly more treatment failures occurred in patients receiving ceftazidime (40%) compared with patients who received cefepime (20%) (p = 0.04), requiring the use of additional antimicrobials to treat these failures.

CONCLUSION

Infection control programs and antimicrobial stewardship efforts provide our only defense against the creation and dissemination of many multidrug-resistant organisms. Insufficient efforts of either strategy are detrimental to local and global battles being fought against these microbial evolutionary forces. Reasons for suboptimal infection control and antimicrobial use programs are similar: insufficient resources—both human and monetary—apathy, and ignorance (105).

With respect to optimizing the use of antimicrobials, the literature is now replete with the negative effect of certain agents (e.g., third-generation cephalosporins) on the ecology of hospital and institutional flora. This has led many institutions to remove these agents from formulary or to place restrictions on their use, as well as to introduce more heterogeneity into their antimicrobial prescriptive habits. An increasing amount of information has also suggested that the use of antianaerobic agents promotes intestinal colonization with drug-resistant organisms, including ESBLs and VRE. Although the use of antianaerobic agents may be unavoidable for some infections, their routine use for infections not caused by anaerobes should be avoided. It has also become clear that all cephalosporins are not created equal with regard to their inherent resistance selection potential and their utility in treating resistant organisms. Currently, cefazolin still provides the narrowest spectrum of activity and has enjoyed workhorse status for years for narrow-spectrum infections and surgical prophylaxis. Although some of the third-generation cephalosporins (e.g., ceftriaxone, cefotaxime, ceftizoxime) and cefepime remain highly active and useful for the treatment of resistant pneumococcal infections, negative collateral effects have been observed when third-generation agents, as well as ceftazidime, have been overused. The fourth-generation cephalosporins appear to be capable of being commonly used for the empiric treatment of serious community-acquired infections (e.g., pneumonia) as well as those that are institutionally acquired, without adversely affecting resistance profiles or the environment. They share the distinction of being the only cephalosporins, as well as being mentioned on the short list of antimicrobials, that are useful for the treatment of AmpC-producing gram-negative bacilli.

Currently, there are not enough data to suggest that nonceftazidime cephalosporins should be totally abandoned as treatment options for ESBL-producing organisms once susceptibilities are known. Thus, more data are needed before the cephalosporins as a class can be excluded from the clinician's armamentarium for the treatment of ESBL-producing infections. To pretend that we know the absolute method for the treatment of the evolving beta-lactamase crisis within the world of the gram-negative bacilli is the antithesis of science. We must continue to be proactive and study strategies for the containment and treatment of infections caused by them, as well as to modify and expand our approaches when more information becomes available.

REFERENCES

1. Centers for Disease Control and Prevention. 1992. Public health focus: surveillance, prevention and control of nosocomial infections MMWR Morb Mortal Wkly Rep; 1992; 41: 783–787.

2. Tenover FC, Weigel LM, Appelbaum PC, McDougal LK, Chaitram J, McAllister S, Clark N, Killgore G, O'Hara CM, Jevitt L, Patel JB, Bozdogan B. Vancomycin-resistant *Staphylococcus aureus* isolate from a patient in Pennsylvania Antimicrob Agents Chemother; 2004; 48:275–280.

3. Abbanat D, Macielag M, Bush K. Novel antibacterial agents for the treatment of serious gram-positive infections Expert Opin Investig Drugs; 2002; 12:379–399.

4. Gordon KA, Beidenbach DJ, Jones RN. Comparison of *Streptococcus pneumoniae* and *Haemophilus influenzae* susceptibilities from community-acquired respiratory tract infections and hospitalized patients with pneumonia: five-year results for the SENTRY Antimicrobial Surveillance Program Diagn Microbiol Infect Dis; 2003; 46:285–289.

5. Neuhauser MM, Weinstein RA, Rydman R, Danziger LH, Karam G, Quinn JP. Antibiotic resistance among gram-negative bacilli in US intensive care units JAMA; 2003; 289: 885–888.

6. Diekema DJ, BootsMiller BJ, Vaughn TE, Woolson RF, Yankey JW, Ernst EJ, Flach SD, Ward MM, Franciscus CL, Pfaller MA, Doebbeling BN. Antimicrobial resistance trends and outbreak frequency in United States hospitals Clin Infect Dis; 2004; 38:78–85.

7. Rice LB. Controlling antibiotic resistance in the ICU: different bacteria, different strategies Cleve Clin J Med; 2003; 70: 793–800.

8. Ledson MJ, Gallagher MJ, Corkill JE, Hart CA, Walshaw MJ. Cross infection between cystic fibrosis patients colonized with *Burkholderia cepacia* Thorax; 1998; 53:432–436.

9. Anderson DG. The treatment of infections with penicillin (concluded) N Engl J Med; 1945; 232:421–429.

10. Levy SB. The Antibiotic Paradox. How Miracle Drugs Are Destroying the Miracle. New York: Plenum Publishing, 1992.

11. Sanders CC, Sanders WE Jr. Emergence of resistance to cefamandole: possible role of cefoxitin-inducible β-lactamases Antimicrob Agents Chemother; 1979; 15:792–797.

12. Sanders WE Jr, Sanders CC. *Enterobacter* spp.: pathogens poised to flourish at the turn of the century Clin Microbiol Rev; 1997; 10:220–241.

13. Jones RN. Important and emerging beta-lactamase mediated resistances in hospital-based pathogens: the AmpC enzymes Diagn Microbiol Infect Dis; 1998; 31:461–466.

14. Minami S, Yotsuji A, Inoue M, Mitsuhashi S. Induction of beta-lactamases by various beta-lactam antibiotics in *Enterobacter cloacae* Antimicrob Agents Chemother; 1980; 18: 382–385.

15. Hanson ND. AmpC beta-lactamases: what do we need to know for the future? J Antimicrob Agents Chemother; 2003; 52:2–4.

16. Moland ES, Black JA, Ourada J, Reisbig MD, Hanson ND, Thomson KS. Occurrence of newer beta-lactamases in *Klebsiella pneumoniae* isolates from 24 U.S. hospitals Antimicrob Agents Chemother; 2002; 46:3837–3842.

17. Crowley B, Ratcliffe G. Extended-spectrum beta-lactamases in *Enterobacter cloacae*: underestimated but clinically significant! J Antimicrob Chemother; 2003; 51:1316–1317.

18. Arpin C, Labia R, Dubois V, Noury P, Souquet M, Quentin C. TEM-80, a novel inhibitor-resistant beta-lactamase in a clinical isolate of *Enterobacter cloacae* Antimicrob Agents Chemother; 2002; 46:1183–1189.

19. Odeh R, Kelkar S, Hujer AM, Bonomo RA, Schreckenberger PC, Quinn JP. Broad resistance due to plasmid-mediated AmpC beta-lactamases in clinical isolates of *Escherichia coli* Clin Infect Dis; 2002; 35:140–145.

20. Sanders CC, Sanders WE Jr. Emergence of resistance during therapy with the newer β-lactam antibiotics: role of inducible

β-lactamases and implications for the future Rev Infect Dis; 1983; 5:639–648.

21. Sanders CC, Sanders WE Jr. β-lactam resistance in gram-negative bacteria: global trends and clinical impact Clin Infect Dis; 1992; 15:824–839.

22. Johnson MP, Ramphal R. β-lactam resistant *Enterobacter* bacteremia in febrile neutropenic patients receiving monotherapy J Infect Dis 1990; 162:981–983.

23. Fussle R, Biscoping J, Behr R, Sziegoleit A. Development of resistance by *Enterobacter cloacae* during therapy of pulmonary infections in intensive care patients Clin Investig; 1994; 72:1015–1019.

24. Burwen DR, Banerjee SN, Gaynes RP. Ceftazidime resistance among selected nosocomial gram-negative bacilli in the United States J Infect Dis; 1994; 170:1622–1625.

25. Quinn JP. Clinical problems posed by multiresistant nonfermenting gram-negative pathogens Clin Infect Dis; 1998; 27(suppl 1):S117–S124.

26. Ambrose PG, Richerson MA, Bui K, Nightingale CH, Quintiliani R. Cost-effectiveness analysis of cefepime versus ceftazidime in ICU patients with hospital-acquired pneumonia. Clin Infect Dis; 1998; 27:1046.

27. Chow JW, Fine MJ, Shlaes DM, Quinn JP, Hooper DC, Johnson MP, Ramphal R, Wagener MM, Miyashiro DK, Yu VL. *Enterobacter* bacteremia: Clinical features and emergence of antibiotic resistance during therapy Ann Intern Med; 1991; 115:585–590.

28. Aronoff SC, Shlaes DM. Factors that influence the evolution of β-lactam resistance in β-lactamase-inducible strains of *Enterobacter cloacae* and *Pseudomonas aeruginosa* J Infect Dis; 1987; 155:936–941.

29. Chan WC, Li RC, Ling JM, Cheng AF, Schentag JJ. Markedly different rates and resistance profiles exhibited by seven commonly used and newer beta-lactams on the selection of resistant variants of Enterobacter cloacae J Antimicrob Chemother; 1999; 43:55–60.

30. Kollef MH. The clinical impact of scheduled antibiotic class changes for the empiric treatment of nosocomial gram-nega-

tive bacterial infections in the intensive care unit setting
[abstr 701], 39th Interscience Conference on Antimicrobial
Agents and Chemotherapy, San Francisco, Sept 26–29, 1999.

31. Paterson DL, Rice LB. Empirical antibiotic choice for the seriously ill patient: are minimization of selection of resistant
organisms and maximization of individual outcome mutually
exclusive? Clin Infect Dis; 2003; 36:1006–1012.

32. Safdar N, Maki DG. The commonality of risk factors for nosocomial colonization and infection with antimicrobial-resistant
Staphylococcus aureus, enterococcus, gram-negative bacilli,
Clostridium difficile, and *Candida* Ann Intern Med; 2002; 136:
834–844.

33. Modjtabai K, Prato BS, Stogsdill PB, Owens RC Jr. Impact of
inpatient prescribing changes on antimicrobial susceptibilities: a five-year longitudinal study [abstr 156], 41st Infectious
Diseases Society of America Meeting, San Diego, Oct 9–12,
2003.

34. Toltzis P, Yamashita T, Vilt L, Green M, Morrissey A, Spinner-
Block S, Blumer J. Antibiotic restriction does not alter endemic colonization with resistant gram-negative rods in a
pediatric intensive care unit Crit Care Med; 1998; 26:
1893–1898.

35. Goldman M, Adelman MH, Thompson CE. Impact of a conversion from ceftazidime to cefepime on ICU resistance patterns
of *Enterobacter cloacae*, 8th International Congress of Infectious Diseases, Boston, May 1998.

36. Mebis J, Goossens H, Bruyneel P, Sion JP, Meeus I, Van
Droogenbroeck J, Schroyens W, Berneman ZN. Decreasing antibiotic resistance of Enterobacteriaceae by introducing a new
antibiotic combination therapy for neutropenic fever patients
Leukemia; 1998; 12:1627–1629.

37. Orrick J, Ramphal R, Johns T, Russell W. Improving antibiotic
susceptibility of type-1 beta-lactamase producing organisms
after formulary replacement of ceftazidime with cefepime
[abstr 731], 39th Interscience Conference on Antimicrobial
Agents and Chemotherapy, San Francisco, Sept 26–29, 1999.

38. Bantar C, Sartori B, Vesco E, Heft C, Saul M, Salamone F,
Oliva ME. A hospitalwide intervention program to optimize

the quality of antibiotic use: impact on prescribing practice, antibiotic consumption, cost savings, and bacterial resistance Clin Infect Dis; 2003; 37:180–186.

39. Knothe H, Shah P, Krcmery V, Antal M, Mitsuhashi S. Transferable resistance to cefotaxime, cefoxitin, cefamandole and cefuroxime in clinical isolates of *Klebsiella pneumoniae* and *Serratia marcescens* Infection; 1983; 11:315–317.

40. Bonnet R. Growing group of extended-spectrum beta-lactamases: the CTX-M enzymes Antimicrob Agents Chemother; 2004; 48:1–14.

41. Rice LB. Evolution and clinical importance of extended-spectrum beta-lactamases Chest; 2001; 119(suppl):391S–396S.

42. Bush K, Jacoby GA, Medeiros AA. A functional classification scheme for beta-lactamases and its correlation with molecular structure Antimicrob Agents Chemother; 1995; 39: 1211–1213.

43. Bush K. New beta-lactamases in gram-negative bacteria: diversity and impact on the selection of antimicrobial therapy Clin Infect Dis; 2001; 32:1085–1089.

44. Bush K. Laboratory capacity to detect antimicrobial resistance, 1998 MMWR Morb Mortal Wkly Rep; 2000; 48: 1167–1171.

45. Steward CD, Wallace D, Hubert SK, Lawton R, Fridkin SK, Gaynes RP, McGowan JE Jr, Tenover FC. Ability of laboratories to detect emerging antimicrobial resistance in nosocomial pathogens: a survey of project ICARE laboratories Diagn Microbiol Infect Dis; 2000; 38:59–67.

46. Tenover FC. Performance Standards for Antimicrobial Susceptibility Testing. Document M100-S14. Wayne. PA: NCCLS, 2004.

47. Bradford PA. Extended-spectrum beta-lactamases in the 21st century: characterization, epidemiology, and detection of this important resistance threat Clin Microbiol Rev; 2001; 14: 933–951.

48. Lautenbach E, Strom BL, Bilker WB, Patel JB, Edelstein PH, Fishman NO. Epidemiological investigation of fluoroquinolone resistance in infections due to extended-spectrum

beta-lactamase-producing *Eschericia coli* and *Klebsiella pneumoniae* Clin Infect Dis; 2001; 33:1288–1294.

49. Quinn JP. Clinical significance of extended-spectrum beta-lactamases Eur J Clin Microbiol Infect Dis; 1994; 13(suppl 1): 39–42.

50. Naumovski L, Quinn JP, Miyashiro D, Patel M, Bush K, Singer SB, Graves D, Palzkill T, Arvin AM. Outbreak of ceftazidime resistance due to extended spectrum beta-lactamase in isolates from cancer patients Antimicrob Agents Chemother; 1992; 36:1991–1996.

51. Meyer KS, Urban C, Eagan JA, Berger BJ, Rahal JJ. Nosocomial outbreak of *Klebsiella* infection resistant to late generation cephalosporins Ann Intern Med; 1993; 119:353–358.

52. Rice LB, Willey SH, Papanicolaou GA, Medeiros AA, Eliopoulos GM, Moellering RC Jr, Jacoby GA. Outbreak of ceftazidime resistance caused by extended-spectrum beta-lactamases at a Massachusetts chronic-care facility Antimicrob Agents Chemother; 1990; 34:2193–2199.

53. Quale JM, Landman D, Bradford PA, Visalli M, Ravishankar J, Flores C, Mayorga D, Vangala K, Adedeji A. Molecular epidemiology of a citywide outbreak of extended-spectrum beta-lactamase-producing *Klebsiella pneumoniae* infection Clin Infect Dis; 2002; 35:834–841.

54. Paterson DL, Ko WC, Von Gottberg A, Mohapatra S, Casellas JM, Goossens H, Mulazimoglu L, Trenholme G, Klugman KP, Bonomo RA, Rice LB, Wagener MM, McCormack JG, Yu VL. International prospective study of *Klebsiella pneumoniae* bacteremia: implications of extended-spectrum beta-lactamase production in nosocomial infections Ann Intern Med; 2004; 140:26–32.

55. Hoyen CK, Pultz NJ, Paterson DL, Aron DC, Donskey CJ. Effect of parenteral antibiotic administration on establishment of intestinal colonization in mice by *Klebsiella pneumoniae* strains producing extended-spectrum beta-lactamases Antimicrob Agents Chemother; 2003; 47:3610–3612.

56. Rahal JJ, Urban C, Segal-Maurer S. Nosocomial antibiotic resistance in multiple gram-negative species: experience at

one hospital with squeezing the resistance balloon at multiple sites Clin Infect Dis; 2002; 34:499–503.

57. Rahal JJ, Urban C, Horn D, Freeman K, Segal-Maurer S, Maurer J, Mariano N, Marks S, Burns JM, Dominick D, Lim M. Class restriction of cephalosporin use to control total cephalosporin resistance in nosocomial *Klebsiella* J Amer Med Assoc; 1998; 280:1233–1237.

58. Burke JP. Antibiotic resistance—squeezing the balloon? JAMA; 1998; 280:1270–1271.

59. Burke JP. The cost of antibiotic resistance: effect of resistance among *Staphylococcus aureus*, *Klebsiella pneumoniae*, *Acinetobacter baumannii*, and *P. aeruginosa* on length of hospital stay Infect Control Hosp Epidemiol; 2002; 23:106–108.

60. Lepper PM, Grusa E, Reichl H, Hogel J, Trautmann M. Consumption of imipenem correlates with beta-lactam resistance in *P. aeruginosa* Antimicrob Agents Chemother; 2002; 46: 2920–2925.

61. Jaccard C, Troillet N, Harbarth S, Zanetti G, Aymon D, Schneider R, Chiolero R, Ricou B, Romand J, Huber O, Ambrosetti P, Praz G, Lew D, Bille J, Glauser MP, Cometta A. Prospective randomized comparison of imipenem-cilastatin and piperacillin-tazobactam in nosocomial pneumonia or peritonitis Antimicrob Agents Chemother; 1998; 42:2966–2972.

62. Harris AD, Smith D, Johnson JA, Bradham DD, Roghmann MC. Risk factors for imipenem-resistant *Pseudomonas aeruginosa* among hospitalized patients Clin Infect Dis; 2002; 34: 340–345.

63. Wiener J, Quinn JP, Bradford PA, Goering RV, Nathan C, Bush K, Weinstein RA. Multiple antibiotic-resistant *Klebsiella* and *Escherichia coli* in nursing homes JAMA; 1999; 281: 517–523.

64. Paterson DL, Ko W, Von Gottberg A, Casellas JM, Mulazimoglu L, Klugman KP, Bonomo RA, Rice LB, McCormack JG, Yu VL. Outcome of cephalosporin treatment for serious infections due to apparently susceptible organisms producing extended-spectrum beta-lactamases: implications for the clinical microbiology laboratory J Clin Micro; 2001; 39:2206–2212.

65. Einhorn AE, Neuhauser MM, Bearden DT, Quinn JP, Pendland SL. Extended-spectrum beta-lactamases: frequency, risk factors, and outcomes Pharmacotherapy; 2002; 22:14–20.

66. Go E, Urban C, Burns J, Kreiswirth B, Eisner W, Mariano N, Mosinka-Snipas K, Rahal JJ. Clinical and molecular epidemiology of *Acinetobacter* infections sensitive only to polymixin B and sulbactam Lancet; 1994; 344:1329–1332.

67. Paterson DL, Singh N, Rihs JD, Squier C, Rihs BL, Muder RR. Control of an outbreak of infection due to extended-spectrum beta-lactamase-producing *Escherichia coli* in a liver transplantation unit Clin Infect Dis; 2001; 33:126–128.

68. Empey KM, Rapp RP, Evans ME. The effect of an antimicrobial formulary change on hospital resistance patterns Pharmacotherapy; 2002; 22:81–87.

69. Donskey CJ, Hanrahan JA, Hutton RA, Rice LB. Effect of parenteral antibiotic administration on persistence of vancomycin-resistant *Enterococcus faecium* in the mouse gastrointestinal tract J Infect Dis; 1999; 180:384–390.

70. Rice LB, Eckstein EC, DeVente J, Shlaes DM. Ceftazidime-resistant *Klebsiella pneumoniae* isolates recovered at the Cleveland Department of Veterans Affairs medical center Clin Infect Dis; 1996; 23:118–124.

71. Pena C, Pujol M, Ardanuy C, Ricart A, Pallares R, Linares J, Ariza J, Gudiol F. Epidemiology and successful control of a large outbreak due to *Klebsiella pneumoniae* producing extended-spectrum beta-lactamases Antimicrob Agents Chemother; 1998; 42:53–58.

72. Piroth L, Aube H, Doise J-M, Vincent-Martin M. Spread of extended-spectrum beta-lactamase-producing *Klebsiella pneumoniae*: are beta-lactamase inhibitors of therapeutic value? Clin Infect Dis; 1998; 27:76–80.

73. Bedenic B, Beader N, Zagar Z. Effect of inoculum size on the antibacterial activity of cefpirome and cefepime against *Klebsiella pneuminae* strains producing SHV extended-spectrum beta-lactamases Clin Microbiol Infect; 2001; 7:626–635.

74. Maglio D, Ong C, Banevicius MA, Geng Q, Nightingale CH, Nicolau DP. Determination of the in vivo pharmacodynamic

profile of cefepime against extended-spectrum beta-lactamase producing *Escherichia coli* at various inoculum Antimicrobial Agents Chemother 2004; In press.

75. Thauvin-Eliopoulos C, Tripodi M, Moellering RC Jr, Eliopoulos GM. Efficacies of piperacillin-tazobactam and cefepime in rats with experimental intra-abdominal abscesses due to an extended-spectrum beta-lactamase producing strain of *Klebsiella pneumoniae* Antimicrob Agents Chemother; 1997; 41:1053–1057.

76. Andes D, Craig WA. Impact of extended-spectrum beta-lactamase production on the activity of cefepime in a murine-thigh infection model [abstr A-1099], 41st Interscience Conference on Antimicrobial Agents and Chemotherapy, Chicago, Sept 22–25, 2001.

77. Ambrose PG, Bhavnani SM, Jones RN. Pharmacokinetics-pharmacodynamics of cefepime and piperacillin-tazobactam against *Escherichia coli* and *Klebsiella pneumoniae* strains producing extended-spectrum beta-lactamases: report from the ARREST program Antimicrob Agents Chemother; 2003; 47:1643–1646.

78. Wong-Beringer A. Therapeutic challenges associated with extended-spectrum, beta-lactamase-producing *Escherichia coli* and *Klebsiella pneumoniae* Pharmacotherapy; 2001; 21: 583–592.

79. Paterson DL, Singh N, Gayowski T, Marino IR. Fatal infection due to extended-spectrum beta-lactamase-producing *Escherichia coli*: implications for antibiotic choice for spontaneous bacterial peritonitis Clin Infect Dis; 1999; 28:683–684.

80. Wong-Beringer A, Hindler J, Loeloff M, Queenan AM, Lee N, Pegues DA, Quinn JP, Bush K. Molecular correlation for the treatment outcomes in bloodstream infections caused by *Escherichia coli* and *Klebsiella pneumoniae* with reduced susceptibility to ceftazidime Clin Infect Dis; 2002; 34:135–146.

81. Sanders WE Jr, Tenney JH, Kessler RE. Efficacy of cefepime in the treatment of infections due to multiply resistant *Enterobacter* species Clin Infect Dis; 1996; 23:454–461.

82. Rice LB. Editorial response: a silver bullet for colonization and infection with methicillin-resistant *Staphylococcus aureus* still eludes us Clin Infect Dis; 1999; 28:1067–1070.

83. Ambrose PG, Owens RC Jr. New antibiotics in pulmonary and critical care medicine: focus on advanced generation quinolones and cephalosporins Semin Resp Crit Care Med; 2000; 21:19–32.

84. Ambrose PG, Owens RC Jr, Grasela D. Antimicrobial pharmacodynamics Med Clin North Am; 2000; 84:1431–1446.

85. Wilson DL, Owens RC Jr, Zuckerman JB. Successful meropenem desensitization in a patient with cystic fibrosis Ann Pharmacother; 2003; 37:1424–1428.

86. Schaad UB, Suter S, Gianella-Borradori A, Pfenninger J, Auckenthaler R, Bernath O, Cheseaux JJ, Wedgwood J. A comparison of ceftriaxone and cefuroxime for the treatment of bacterial meningitis in children N Engl J Med; 1990; 322: 141–147.

87. Owens RC Jr, Tessier P, Nightingale CH, Ambrose PG, Quintiliani R, Nicolau DP. Pharmacodynamics of ceftriaxone and cefixime against community-acquired respiratory tract pathogens Int J Antimicrob Agents; 2001; 17:483–489.

88. Mandell LA, Bartlett JG, Dowell SF, File TM Jr, Musher DM, Whitney C Infectious Diseases Society of America. Update of practice guidelines for the management of community-acquired pneumonia in immunocompetent adults Clin Infect Dis; 2003; 37:1405–1433.

89. Quale J, Landman D, Saurina G, Atwood E, DiTore V, Patel K. Manipulation of a hospital antimicrobial formulary to control an outbreak of vancomycin-resistant enterococci Clin Infect Dis; 1996; 23:1020–1025.

90. Handwerger S, Raucher B, Altarac D, Monka J, Marchione S, Singh KV, Murray BE, Wolff J, Walters B. Nosocomial outbreak due to *Enterococcus faecium* highly resistant to vancomycin, penicillin, and gentamicin Clin Infect Dis; 1993; 16: 750–755.

91. Donskey CJ, Hanrahan JA, Hutton Ra, Rice LB. Effect of parenteral antibiotic administration on the establishment of colonization with vancomycin-resistant *Enterococcus faecium* in the mouse gastrointestinal tract J Infect Dis; 2000; 181: 1830–1833.

92. Sanders CC. Cefepime: the next generation? Clin Infect Dis; 1993; 17:369–379.

93. Ambrose PG, Owens RC Jr, Quintiliani R, Yeston N, Crowe HM, Cunha BA, Nightingale CH. Antibiotic use in the critical care unit Crit Care Clin; 1998; 14:283–308.

94. Owens RC Jr, Ambrose PG, Quintiliani R. Ceftazidime to cefepime formulary switch: pharmacodynamic and pharmacoeconomic rationale Conn Med; 1997; 61:225–227.

95. Ambrose PG, Owens RC Jr, Garvey MJ, Jones RN. Pharmacodynamic considerations in the treatment of moderate to severe pseudomonal infections with cefepime J Antimicrob Chemother; 2002; 49:445–453.

96. Goldberg J, Owens RC Jr. Optimizing antibiotic dosing in the critically ill patient Curr Opin Crit Care; 2002; 8:435–440.

97. Owens RC Jr. Maximizing antibiotic effectiveness while minimizing costs Infect Dis Clin Pract; 2000; (suppl):14–16.

98. Owens RC Jr, Owens CA, Holloway WJ. Comparative evaluation of the cefepime Q12 hour dosing schedule as empirical monotherapy in febrile neutropenic patients Pharmacotherapy; 1999; 19:496–497.

99. Biron P, Fuhrmann C, Cure H, Viens P, Lefebvre D, Thyss A, Viot M, Soler-Michel P, Rollin C, Gres JJ. Cefepime versus imipenem-cilastatin as empirical monotherapy in 400 febrile patients with short duration neutropenia J Antimicrob Chemother; 1998; 42:511–518.

100. Raad II, Escalante C, Hachem RY, Hanna HA, Husni R, Afif C, Boktour MR, Whimbey EE, Kontoyiannis D, Jacobson K, Kantarjian H, Levett LM, Rolston KV. Treatment of febrile neutropenic patients with cancer who require hospitalization: a prospective randomized study comparing imipenem and cefepime Cancer; 2003; 98:1039–1047.

101. Saez-Llorens X, O'Ryan M. Cefepime in the empiric treatment of meningitis in children Pediatr Infect Dis J; 2001; 20: 356–361.

102. Grossman RF, Campbell DA, Landis SJ, Garber GE, Murray G, Stiver HG, Saginur R, McIvor RA, Laforge J, Rotstein C, Dubois J, Rivard M, Boulerice F. Treatment of community-

acquired pneumonia in the elderly: the role of cefepime, a fourth-generation cephalosporin J Antimicrob Chemother; 1999; 43:549–554.

103. Barie PS, Vogel SB, Dellinger EP, Rotstein OD, Solomkin JS, Yang JY, Baumgartner TF. A randomized, double-blind clinical trial comparing cefepime plus metronidazole with imipenem-cilastatin in the treatment of complicated intra-abdominal infections Arch Surg; 1997; 132:1294–1302.

104. Holmberg SD, Solomon SL, Blake PA. Health and economic impacts of antimicrobial resistance Rev Infect Dis; 1987; 9: 1065–1078.

105. Sefton AM. Mechanisms of antimicrobial resistance: their clinical relevance in the new millennium Drugs; 2002; 62: 557–566.

106. Medeiros AA. Evolution and dissemination of β-lactamases accelerated by generations of β-lactam antibiotics Clin Infect Dis; 1997; 24(suppl 1):41–55.

14

Early Discharge Strategies: Role of Transitional Therapy Programs

JULIO RAMIREZ

Division of Infectious Diseases, Department of
Medicine, University of Louisville
School of Medicine,
Louisville, Kentucky, U.S.A.

In hospitalized patients with infections, the length of hospital stay is one of the primary factors that contribute to the cost of care. The cost of antimicrobial therapy for these patients may range from as low as $10 per day for a hospitalized patient with a community-acquired cellulitis that is treated with a first-generation cephalosporin to more than $200 per day for a patient with a serious nosocomial infection treated with triple antibiotic therapy. On the other hand, the cost for a hospital stay in a general ward bed in the United States averages $1,000 per day (1).

When cost of hospital stay is compared with antibiotic cost, it is clear that decreasing 1 day of hospitalization will have a bigger impact on total hospital savings than any streamlined technique that can be applied to the antimicrobial regimen.

During recent years, several modalities have been studied with the goal of decreasing the length of stay (LOS) for hospitalized patients with infections while maintaining good outcomes. The early switch from intravenous to oral antibiotics, or switch therapy, is an approach incorporated into the management of hospitalized patients with infectious diseases that is considered one of the most important early discharge strategies. After initiation of empiric intravenous therapy, a significant number of patients will be candidates for switch therapy and hospital discharge. These patients can continue therapy of the infection in the outpatient setting with oral antibiotics (Fig. 1, group A). A group of hospitalized patients with infections will clinically improve with intravenous therapy but will not be able to be switched to oral therapy due to a lack of oral antibiotics to treat a resistant organism or because of the site

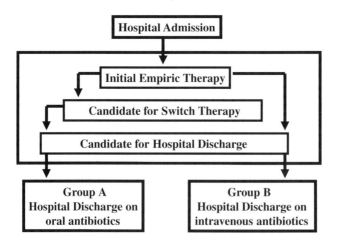

Figure 1   Early discharge with oral antibiotics after switch therapy (group A), and early discharge with intravenous antibiotics in patients that are not candidates for switch therapy (group B)

of infection (e.g., endocarditis, meningitis). If these patients are candidates for hospital discharge, their infection can be managed in the outpatient setting with intravenous therapy (Fig. 1, group B). This practice, referred to as *outpatient parenteral antimicrobial therapy*, is another approach to safely decreasing LOS and is discussed in Chapter 9 of this book.

THE CLINICAL COURSE OF HOSPITALIZED PATIENTS WITH INFECTIONS

It is unusual today to have a hospitalized patient who is being treated for an infectious disease of mild or moderate severity. Almost all patients with an infection who are treated in the hospital setting have a severe infection. Patients with community-acquired infections are hospitalized only when the infection is considered severe. Patients who are hospitalized for other medical problems and develop a nosocomial infection usually have multiple medical comorbidities or immunologic abnormalities that predispose them to severe infections. Because of severity of disease, patients in the hospital setting are treated initially with intravenous antibiotics with the goal of securing maximal serum levels. In these patients, it is recommended to start empiric intravenous therapy as soon as appropriate cultures have been obtained, because delayed antibiotic administration may decrease outcomes. Empiric therapy is defined as the use of antibiotics after a clinical diagnosis of infection is reached, but before the microbiologic etiology and susceptibilities are known. After initiation of empiric antibiotics, hospitalized patients with infections should be carefully monitored to evaluate clinical response to therapy.

Considering the patient's clinical response at day 3 and day 7 of antimicrobial therapy, the clinical course of hospitalized patients with infections can be classified in five groups (Fig. 2) (2). After 3 days of antimicrobial therapy, some patients will have evidence of early clinical improvement, (Fig. 2, group 1), others will have evidence of early clinical deterioration (Fig. 2, group 3), and others will remain clinically unchanged (Fig. 2, point B). By day 7 of therapy, some patients

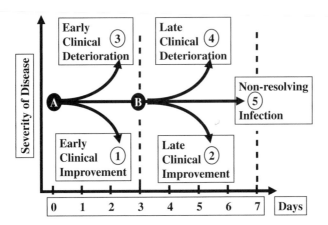

Figure 2 The clinical course of hospitalized patients with infections (Adapted from reference 1)

will have evidence of late clinical improvement (Fig. 2, group 2), others will have evidence of late clinical deterioration (Fig. 2, group 4), and others will remain clinically unchanged and will be considered to have a nonresolving infection (Fig. 2, group 5). Patients with evidence of early or late clinical deterioration should be completely reexamined to define the etiology of deterioration and to evaluate whether a change of antimicrobial therapy is necessary.

The Clinical Recovery Curve

Patients with early or late clinical improvement after initiation of empiric therapy will enter the recovery phase of infection (Fig. 2, groups 1 and 2). The recovery phase of hospitalized patients with infections can be represented with a curve divided into three different periods (3,4). The first period starts with the initiation of intravenous empiric antibiotic therapy (Fig. 3, point A). Despite appropriate empiric antibiotic therapy, the majority of patients will remain clinically unstable for at least 48 hours. Because of this, it is not recommended to change the initial empiric antibiotic regimen during the first 48 hours unless there is evidence of clinical deterioration. The

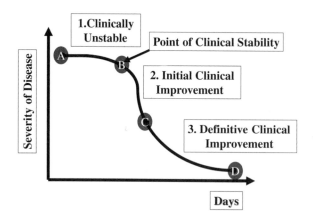

Figure 3 The curve of clinical response for hospitalized patients with serious infections (From references 2 and 3)

second period starts when the patient reaches the point of clinical stability (Fig. 3, point B). During this second period, the signs, symptoms, and laboratory abnormalities caused by the infection will begin to normalize and the patient will show evidence of initial clinical improvement. During the third period of recovery, the signs, symptoms, and laboratory abnormalities will be greatly improved or resolved. This third period will end at the point at which the patient is clinically cured of the infection (Fig. 3, point D).

SWITCH THERAPY IN HOSPITALIZED PATIENTS WITH INFECTIONS

Until recently, the most common approach to the treatment of hospitalized patients with severe infections was the use of intravenous antibiotics during the recovery phase until the patient reached the third period of recovery and definitive clinical improvement was documented. The switch therapy strategy is based on the identification of the point of clinical stability, when the patient is moving from the first to the second period of recovery (Fig. 4, point B). Once there is evidence of

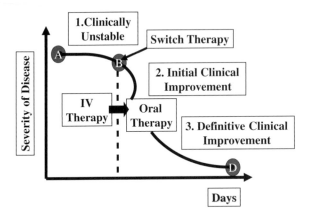

Figure 4 The switch therapy approach during the recovery phase of hospitalized patients with serious infections

initial clinical improvement, the intravenous antibiotics are switched to oral (3,4). Then, switch therapy can be defined as the switch from intravenous to oral antibiotics at the time the patient reaches clinical stability and is entering the period of initial clinical improvement.

Switch Therapy Criteria

In an attempt to objectively identify the point of clinical stability during the recovery phase of infections, we defined concrete criteria to consider when a patient has reached stability and can be considered a switch therapy candidate (4,5). The first criterion indicates that the patient needs to have subjective and objective evidence of improvement from the local inflammatory response produced by the infection. The local signs and symptoms of infection that will need to improve to fulfill the first criterion will change according to the site of infection. For example, in a patient with pneumonia, the local signs and symptoms will include cough, sputum production, and shortness of breath. On the other hand, in a patient with cellulitis, the local signs and symptoms will include pain, redness, and swelling. The second criterion indicates that the patient should be afebrile for at least 8 hours. The third criterion indicates that the white blood cell count should be trending toward a normal value. Because the normalization of the white blood cell count occurs days after initial clinical improvement, the patient fulfills the third criterion when the white blood cell count is normalizing, without waiting for a return to a normal value. The fourth criterion indicates that oral intake and gastrointestinal absorption need to be adequate. Determination of gastrointestinal absorption is based on clinical evidence. Patients who are taking food by mouth without severe diarrhea are considered to have adequate absorption. A significant number of hospitalized patients may not have normal absorption because of impaired splanchnic circulation as a consequence of hypoxemia, hypotension, congestive heart failure, diabetes, or atherosclerosis. Even though at the time of switch therapy some patients may not have "normal" gastrointestinal function, from a clinical point of view, a patient who is taking food by mouth without vomiting or severe diarrhea, is considered to have "adequate" oral intake and gastrointestinal absorption.

A patient is considered clinically stable and ready to discontinue intravenous antibiotics on the day that the four switch therapy criteria are met (Table 1). Because the time for initial clinical improvement for hospitalized patients with infections is variable, it is not wise to recommend switching from intravenous to oral antibiotics on a specific day (e.g., switch therapy on day 3). As previously described, some patients with infections may have a rapid clinical response to empiric antibiotic therapy, allowing the implementation of switch therapy during the first 72 hours after admission (Fig.

Table 1   Criteria to Define a Patient as a Candidate to be Switched From Intravenous to Oral Therapy

1. Local signs and symptoms of infection are improving
2. Patient is afebrile for at least 8 hours
3. White blood cell count is normalizing
4. Oral intake and gastrointestinal absorption are adequate

2, group 1). Because of host or pathogen factors, some patients will have a delayed clinical improvement and will need to be switched beyond day 3 of therapy (Fig. 2, group 2). For patients with clinical deterioration or lack of improvement, the switch to oral therapy will not be indicated.

Selection of Oral Antibiotics

When a patient is a switch therapy candidate, if cultures are negative and the etiology of the infection is unknown, the switch to oral therapy is performed from intravenous empiric therapy (4,5). This clinical scenario can be referred to as *empiric switch therapy* (Fig. 5, point A). If the etiology of the infection is identified, the initial broad-spectrum empiric therapy can be streamlined to pathogen-directed therapy. In these patients, the switch to oral therapy is performed from intravenous pathogen-directed therapy. This clinical scenario can be referred to as *pathogen-directed switch therapy* (Fig. 5, point B). When pathogen-directed switch therapy is performed, the selection of the oral antibiotic is based on the susceptibility of the isolated organism. In some patients, the identification of an organism resistant to all oral antibiotics will preclude the implementation of switch therapy. When empiric switch ther-

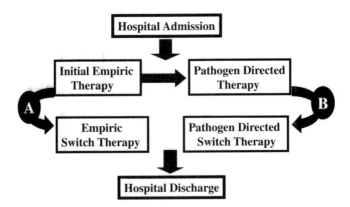

Figure 5   Selection of oral antibiotics for switch therapy based on microbiological report (Adapted from reference 5)

apy is performed, the selection of oral antibiotics should take into consideration the spectrum of activity of the intravenous empiric regimen. The spectrum of activity of the oral regimen should reproduce the spectrum of activity of the intravenous regimen. Patients who are clinically responding to broad-spectrum intravenous combination therapy are likely to need a switch to combination oral therapy to reproduce the antimicrobial spectrum of the intravenous regimen. If more than one antibiotic is available with the required spectrum of activity, then other important characteristics to consider in the selection of oral therapy include the antibiotic bioavailability, the potential toxicity, and cost.

Considering that the intravenous formulation of an antibiotic will achieve 100% of predicted blood level, after the switch to an oral formulation, some antibiotics will achieve a blood level in a range similar to the level achieved intravenously. The switch to oral therapy with antibiotics with this type of bioavailability is also called *sequential therapy* (Fig. 6, point A) (6). Switching to an oral antibiotic that will reach a significantly lower percentage of the blood level achieved intravenously is also referred to as *step-down therapy* (Fig. 6,

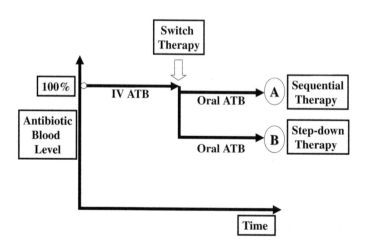

Figure 6 Classification of oral antibiotics used for switch therapy based on their bioavailability

point B) (6). Commonly used oral antibiotics for switch therapy with sequential bioavailability include all the quinolones, linezolid, metronidazole, clindamycin, and trimethoprim-sulfamethoxazole. Commonly used oral antibiotics for switch therapy with step-down bioavailability include the penicillins, cephalosporins, macrolides, and tetracyclines. It should be remembered that interactions with food and other drugs in the gastrointestinal tract might reduce the absorption of some oral antibiotics. For example, the concomitant oral administration of a quinolone with multivitamins, calcium, or antacids will significantly decrease the absorption of quinolone antibiotics. Good clinical outcome after switch therapy has been documented with the sequential or step-down approach.

The selected oral antibiotic is regularly used at the recommended daily dosage. In some clinical scenarios, e.g., in a patient with potentiality decreased gastrointestinal absorption, the total daily dose of the oral antibiotic may need to be increased. Oral antibiotics can be classified into two pharmacodynamic classes based on whether their antibacterial killing effect are concentration dependent (e.g., quinolones, metronidazole) or time dependent (e.g., penicillins, cephalosporins, clindamycin) (7). The total daily dose of an oral antibiotic with concentration-dependent killing is increased primarily by raising the dose and maintaining the frequency of administration. The total daily dose of an oral antibiotic with time-dependent killing is increased primarily by decreasing the frequency of administration while maintaining the dose.

Clinical Outcomes

Several clinical studies have been performed to evaluate the clinical outcome of patients after switch therapy. The most common clinical trial design includes a group of patients who, after reaching clinical stability, were switched to oral therapy (Fig. 7, group 1) versus a group of patients who, after reaching stability, were continued on intravenous therapy (Fig. 7, group 2).

The largest amount of data from clinical trials is in the areas of respiratory tract and urinary tract infections, but sev-

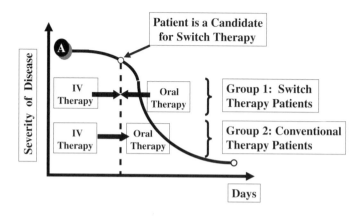

Figure 7 Study design of clinical trials to evaluate switch therapy versus conventional therapy in hospitalized patients with infections

eral other infectious sites have been studied. All clinical trials indicate that the clinical cure rate for patients treated with switch therapy is equivalent to that obtained with continuation of intravenous therapy (8–18).

By decreasing the duration of hospitalization, switch therapy can decrease the risk of serious hospital-associated infections. Because line-related infection and sepsis is a nosocomial infection that is associated with significant morbidity, one can speculate that by discontinuation of intravenous lines and favoring early hospital discharge, switch therapy has the potential to improve patient outcome. Although we were not able to prove cause and effect, the mortality for hospitalized patients with community-acquired pneumonia at our institution decreased soon after we initiated a pneumonia switch therapy program (16).

CORRELATION OF SWITCH THERAPY WITH HOSPITAL DISCHARGE

Criteria for Hospital Discharge

Once a patient has been switched to oral therapy, immediate consideration should be given to the possibility of hospital dis-

Table 2 Criteria to Define a Patient as a Candidate
for Hospital Discharge

---

1. Patient reached clinical stability
2. No need for in-hospital treatment of comorbidities
3. No need for in-hospital diagnostic work-up
4. No necessity to resolve social needs

---

charge. Figure 1 depicts the relationship of empiric therapy,
switch therapy, and hospital discharge. One should bear in
mind that switching a patient to oral therapy is not the only
necessary step in safely discharging a patient from the hospital. A patient may reach clinical stability and still require in-
hospital treatment of comorbidities, diagnostic workup, or resolution of social needs. In our institution, we define four criteria to consider a patient as a candidate for hospital discharge
(Table 2).

Length of Stay "Related" or "Unrelated" to Infection

In patients reaching clinical stability in whom there is no need
to treat comorbidities, no need for diagnostic workup, and no
social needs, hospital discharge should be performed within
the 24-hour period after patients meet switch therapy criteria.
In these types of patients, the length of hospital stay is considered related to the infection. However, in clinical practice, it
is not unusual to have a patient who is clinically stable from
an infection point of view, meets switch therapy criteria, and
was switched to oral therapy, but needs to remain in the hospital for the treatment of a noninfectious problem, the diagnostic
work-up of a new medical condition, or the necessity to resolve
a social need. In these types of patients, the length of hospital
stay is considered unrelated to infection.

Interventions directed toward improving the management of infection, such as the implementation of a switch therapy program, will be expected to decrease LOS related to infection. When comparing LOS before and after a particular
intervention, it is important to remember that LOS unrelated

to infection will not be affected by interventions directed to the management of infection.

In a clinical trial of hospitalized patients with community-acquired pneumonia, we investigated what proportion of patients would be candidates for switch therapy during the first 3 days of intravenous therapy and from this group of patients, what proportion would be candidates for hospital discharge within 24 hours after the patients had met switch therapy criteria. From a total of 200 consecutive patients hospitalized with pneumonia, 133 patients (67%) were candidates for switch therapy during the first 3 days of hospitalization and ninety-nine patients (44%) were discharged during the 24 hours after they became switch therapy candidates. The study indicated that early switch and early discharge may be safely performed in a significant proportion of hospitalized patients with community-acquired pneumonia (2).

Cost Savings and Patient Satisfaction

In patients with infection-related LOS, switch therapy reduces cost of treatment primarily by allowing an early hospital discharge. Besides the savings associated with decreased LOS, switch therapy is associated with savings related to the costs of intravenous versus oral antibiotics, intravenous antibiotic preparation and administration time, and intravenous lines and their care.

We investigated whether early hospital discharge may negatively affect patient satisfaction with care because with early switch and early discharge, patients are sent home when they are still symptomatic from the original infection. A group of patients who were managed with switch therapy followed by rapid hospital discharge were asked the following questions: (i) Are you satisfied with the care that you received? (ii) Do you think you were sent home too soon? (iii) Did you have adequate follow-up? The results of the interview, performed 30 days after discharge, indicated that more than 95% of patients were satisfied with the care they had received and did not think they were sent home too soon (2).

CORRELATION OF INITIAL EMPIRIC THERAPY
WITH HOSPITAL DISCHARGE

The outcomes most frequently used to evaluate the effect of antibiotics in hospitalized patients with infections include the patient's clinical response to therapy during the last follow-up visit. These outcomes may be referred to as *late outcomes* because they are usually measured days after the patient completed the antibiotic regimen. Presently, there is an increased recognition that although late outcomes are very important, it is also critical to measure early outcomes when evaluating antibiotic therapy.

As previously mentioned, in patients with infection related LOS, hospital discharge should occur within 24 hours after a patient is considered a switch therapy candidate. Figure 8 is a schematic representation of the correlation of time to hospital discharge, with the curves representing clinical, immunologic, and microbiologic response for a patient with LOS related to infection. After initiation of appropriate em-

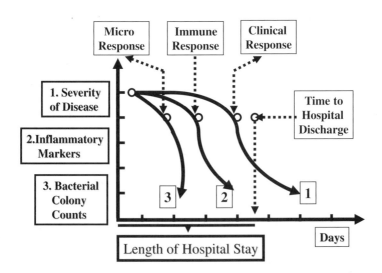

Figure 8   Correlation of microbiological, immunological, and clinical response with time to hospital discharge

piric intravenous therapy, initially there is a rapid microbiologic response. The decreased bacterial inoculum is followed
by a decrease in proinflammatory cytokine production by
macrophages and lymphocytes at the site of infection. The decreased level of cytokines in the systemic circulation is followed by an improvement in the patient's signs, symptoms,
and laboratory abnormalities. The patient reaches clinical stability and meets the criteria for switch therapy after an appropriate microbiologic and immunologic response has occurred.
At this time, the patient is switched to oral therapy and discharged from the hospital.

There is a clear correlation among the microbiologic, immunologic, and clinical response curves. It would be expected
that an antibiotic with poor bactericidal activity will shift the
curve for microbiologic response to the right, and as a consequence, will shift the immunologic and clinical response curves
to the right, with delayed time to hospital discharge. On the
other hand, the initiation of an intravenous antibiotic with a
rapid bactericidal activity will shift the microbiologic response
to the left, with a consequent shift of the immunologic and
clinical response curves, with decreased time to hospital discharge.

If the evaluation of two antibiotics in a clinical trial is
based only on late outcomes, very important differences between the antibiotics may be missed. Figure 9 represents the
evaluation of two antibiotics for the management of hospitalized patients with infections. Both antibiotics have the same
clinical cure rate but significantly different early outcomes. In
this example, patients treated with antibiotic A will have a
shorter time to switch therapy and shorter duration of hospitalization.

Examples of early outcomes include microbiologic response, time to clinical stability, time to switch therapy, time
to hospital discharge, and duration of hospitalization. When
comparisons are performed regarding time to hospital discharge or duration of hospitalization, it is important to determine whether length of hospital stay is related or unrelated
to infection. Incorporating these early outcomes in antibiotic
trials will greatly improve our ability to evaluate the most cost-

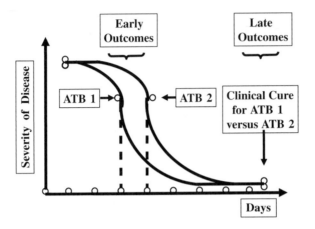

Figure 9   Early and late outcomes in hospitalized patients with serious infections

effective antibiotic for therapy of hospitalized patients with serious infections.

IMPLEMENTING A PROGRAM FOR EARLY SWITCH/EARLY HOSPITAL DISCHARGE

A common strategy used in hospitals to facilitate the identification of patients who are candidates for switch therapy and to promote the use of oral antibiotics is to develop a local hospital antimicrobial program. This program is typically run by a hospital antimicrobial team composed of members from the pharmacy, infectious diseases, microbiology, and nursing departments. The creation of a hospital antimicrobial team was originally suggested in 1988 by the Infectious Diseases Society of America as a mechanism for improving the use of antimicrobial agents in hospitals (19). Following these recommendations, in 1989, we developed a multidisciplinary hospital program to optimize antimicrobial use and implement switch therapy. We presented our switch therapy and antibiotic review (STAAR) program as one of the workshops of the Interscience Conference on Antimicrobial Agents and Chemotherapy during the meetings held from 1994 to 1999 (20). The collaborative efforts of the multidisciplinary team are a key factor in the program's success (21). Several institutions have demonstrated the accomplishment that can be achieved with the approach of shortening patient stay and decreasing cost of care while maintaining optimal outcome in hospitalized patients with respiratory, urinary, skin and soft tissue, and intra-abdominal infections (11–14,22–24).

REFERENCES

1. American Hospital Association. American Hospital Association Hospital Statistics. Chicago: American Hospital Association, 1998:3.

2. Ramirez JA, Vargas S, Ritter GW, Brier ME, Wright A, Smith S, Newman D, Burke J, Mushtaq M, Huang A. Early switch from intravenous to oral antibiotics and early hospital discharge. A prospective observational study of 200 consecutive patients with community-acquired pneumonia Arch Intern Med 1999; 159:2449–2454.

3. Quintiliani R, Cooper BW, Briceland LL, Nightingale CH. Economic impact of streamlining antibiotic administration Am J Med 1987; 82(suppl 4A):391–394 .

4. Ramirez JA. Switch therapy in community-acquired pneumonia Diagn Microbiol Infect Dis 1995; 22:219–223 .

5. Ramirez JA. Advances in antibiotic use: switch therapy Curr Ther Res 1994; 55(suppl A):30–34 .

6. Niederman MS, Bass JB Jr, Campbell GD, Fein AM, Grossman RF, Mandell LA, Marrie TJ, Sarosi GA, Torres A, Yu VL. Guidelines for the management of adults with community-acquired pneumonia. American Thoracic Society Am J Respir Crit Care Med 2001; 163:1730–1754.

7. Ebert SC, Craig WA. Pharmacodynamic properties of antibiotics: application to drug monitoring and dosage regimen design Infect Control Hosp Epidemiol 1990; 11:319–326 .

8. Grasela TH, Paladino JA, Schentag JJ, Huepenbecker D, Rybacki J, Purcell JB, Fiedler JB. Clinical and economic impact

of oral ciprofloxacin as follow-up to parenteral antibiotics DICP 1991; 25:857–862 .

9. Hendrickson JR, North DS. Pharmacoeconomic benefit of antibiotic step-down therapy: converting patients from intravenous ceftriaxone to oral cefpodoxime proxetil Ann Pharmacother 1995; 29:561–565 .

10. Ahkee S, Smith S, Newman D, Ritter W, Burke J, Ramirez J. Early switch from intravenous to oral antibiotics in hospitalized patients with infections: a 6-month prospective study Pharmacotherapy 1997; 17:569–575 .

11. Ehrenkranz NJ, Nerenberg DE, Shultz JM, Slater KC. Intervention to discontinue parenteral antimicrobial therapy in patients hospitalized with pulmonary infections: effect on shortening patient stay Infect Control Hosp Epidemiol 1992; 13: 21–32 .

12. Frighetto L, Nickoloff D, Martinusen SM, Mamdani FS, Jewesson PJ. Intravenous-to-oral stepdown program: four years of experience in a large teaching hospital Ann Pharmacother 1992; 26:1447–1451 .

13. Ehrenkranz NJ, Nerenberg DE, Slater KC, Shultz JM. Intervention to discontinue parenteral antimicrobial therapy in patients hospitalized with urinary tract infection, skin and soft tissue infection, or no evident infection Infect Control Hosp Epidemiol 1993; 14:517–522.

14. Okpara AU, Maswoswe JJ, Stewart K. Criteria-based antimicrobial IV to oral conversion program Formulary 1995; 30: 343–348 .

15. Rhew DC, Tu GS, Ofman J, Henning JM, Richards MS, Weingarten SR. Early switch and early discharge strategies in patients with community-acquired pneumonia. A meta-analysis Arch Intern Med 2001; 161:722–727 .

16. Ramirez JA. Switch therapy in adult patients with pneumonia Clin Pulm Med 1995; 2:327–333 .

17. Terg R, Cobas S, Fassio E, Landeira G, Rios B, Vasen W, Abecasis R, Rios H, Guevara M. Oral ciprofloxacin after a short course of intravenous ciprofloxacin in the treatment of spontaneous bacterial peritonitis: results of a multicenter, randomized study J Hepatol 2000; 33:564–569.

18. Solomkin JS, Reinhart HH, Dellinger EP, Bohnen JM, Rotstein OD, Vogel SB, Simms HH, Hill CS, Bjornson HS, Haverstock DC, Coulter HO, Echols RM. Results of a randomized trial comparing sequential intravenous/oral treatment with ciprofloxacin plus metronidazole to imipenem/cilastatin for intraabdominal infections Ann Surg 1996; 223:303–315.

19. Marr JJ, Moffet HL, Kunin CM. Guidelines for improving the use of antimicrobial agents in hospitals: a statement from the Infectious Diseases Society of America J Infect Dis 1988; 157: 869–876.

20. Ramirez JA. A program for improving the use of antimicrobials and preventing bacterial resistance in hospitals, Workshop presented at 34th, 35th, 36th, 37th, 38th, and 39th Interscience Conference on Antimicrobial Agents and Chemotherapy, 1994–1999.

21. Burke JD, Ahkee S, Ritter GW, Ramirez JA. Development for interdisciplinary anti-microbial team: elements for success Hosp Pharm 1996; 31:361.

22. Ramirez J. Antibiotic streamlining: development and justification of an antibiotic streamlining program Pharm Pract Manag Q 1996; 16:19–34 .

23. Briceland LL, Lesar TS, Lomaestro BM, Lombardi TP, Gailey RA, Kowalsky SF. Streamlining antimicrobial therapy through pharmacists' review of order sheets Am J Hosp Pharm 1989; 46:1376–1380 .

24. Pastel DA, Chang S, Nessim S, Shane R, Morgan MA. Department of pharmacy–initiated program for streamlining empirical antibiotic therapy Hosp Pharm 1992; 27:596–603.

15

Impact of Guidelines on Antimicrobial Treatment of Respiratory Tract Infections

THOMAS M. FILE, JR.
Northeastern Ohio Universities College of
Medicine, Rootstown, and
Summa Health System,
Akron, Ohio, U.S.A.

Respiratory tract infections (RTIs) are the most common type of infection managed by health care providers and are of potentially great consequence (1). Overall, RTIs are the greatest single cause of death in children worldwide (4.3 million deaths in 1992), whereas lower RTIs are the most common cause of death due to infectious disease in the United States. RTIs are also the source of most antibiotic use. Approximately three-fourths of all outpatient antimicrobial use is for respiratory infections (2). Although many RTIs require antimicrobial therapy for optimal management, respiratory viruses, for which antibiotic use is not warranted, cause most outpatient respiratory infections (i.e., acute bronchitis, nasal pharyngitis, cold, nonspecific upper respiratory tract infection [URI]). Use of antibiotics for these conditions is a source of great antibiotic abuse and increases the likelihood of further hindering the already high level of antibiotic resistance. Paradoxically, the progress previously made in dealing with the most common bacterial cause of respiratory infections, *Streptococcus pneumoniae*, is now associated with a global explosion of drug resistance that has made treatment decisions very difficult.

To address the appropriate use of antibiotics and to improve care of patients with RTIs who warrant antibiotics, various professional groups have developed numerous guidelines. The primary purposes of these guidelines are to standardize care and ultimately improve outcome of patients. Promoting the appropriate use of antibiotics through the development and application of such treatment guidelines and educational efforts aimed at clinicians as well as patients should not only optimize clinical outcomes, but also help curb inappropriate prescribing and misuse of antibiotics, decrease treatment costs, and increase patient satisfaction.

This chapter considers recommendations for judicious antibiotic use for RTIs, reviews guidelines for specific infections (with a greater emphasis on community-acquired pneumonia), and reviews their impact on outcome.

PRINCIPLES OF JUDICIOUS USE OF ANTIBIOTICS TO TREAT RESPIRATORY TRACT INFECTIONS

The discovery of potent antimicrobial agents was one of the greatest contributions to medicine in the twentieth century. Unfortunately, the emergence of antimicrobial-resistant pathogens now threatens these advances. The increase in resistance is a result of several factors, but a major factor driving resistance is the overall volume of antimicrobial prescribing—particularly for indications that do not warrant such therapy (3). It is vitally important that judicious use of antimicrobials be encouraged in order to curb this overuse and, hopefully, minimize resistance emergence. One way to promote the appropriate use of antibiotics is through the development and application of treatment guidelines, which are based on sound scientific evidence.

Antimicrobial-Resistant *S. pneumoniae*

Antibiotic overuse and inappropriate antibiotic selection have been associated with increased drug resistance among several respiratory pathogens—most notably *S. pneumoniae,* the most common bacterial pathogen in RTI. However, the clinical significance of antimicrobial-resistant *S. pneumoniae* is not clear for all RTIs. Although there is adequate information to indicate penicillin-resistant *S. pneumoniae* is important when treating meningitis or otitis media, the relevance for lower RTIs, especially pneumonia, is unsettled (4). Presently, the level of resistance of *S. pneumoniae* to beta-lactams and macrolides does not result in clinical treatment failures in most patients with pneumonia; however, as a shift in minimum inhibitory concentration (MIC) occurs (i.e., higher prevalence of *S. pneumoniae* with penicillin MIC 4 μg/mL or greater), it is anticipated that an adverse clinical impact of resistance among the pneumococci will become more apparent. Risk factors for penicillin-resistant *S. pneumoniae* have been identified (i.e., age younger than 2 years or older than 65 years, beta-lactam therapy within 3 months, alcoholism, medical comorbidities, immunosuppressive illness or therapy, and exposure to a child in a day care center), although it is not clear whether these are specific enough for individual patients to be clinically reliable (5)

The clinical relevance of macrolide-resistant *S. pneumoniae* (MRSP) may be dependent on the type of resistance expressed by a particular strain. The most common mechanisms of resistance include methylation of a ribosomal target encoded by the *erm* gene and an efflux of the macrolides by cell membrane protein transporter, encoded by the *mef* gene (6). *S. pneumoniae* strains with *mef* are resistant at a lower level (with

MICs generally 1 to 16 μg/mL) than erm-resistant strains, and it is possible that such strains (particularly with MIC less than 8 μg/mL) may be inhibited if sufficiently high levels of macrolide can be obtained within infected tissue (as may occur with a newer macrolide such as clarithromycin or azithromycin) (7–12). However, there is recent evidence that the MICs of these strains are increasing, and this may affect the efficacy of these macrolides (12). The "*mef*-resistant" strains are usually susceptible to clindamycin. Most *erm*-resistant isolates have an MIC greater than 32 μg/mL for erythromycin and are considered highly level resistant for all macrolides and clindamycin. Until recently, reports of failure of community-acquired pneumonia (CAP) treated with macrolides has been rare, particularly for patients at low risk for drug-resistant strains. However, since 2000, anecdotal reports and one controlled study have documented failures due to MRSP in patients treated with an oral macrolide who have subsequently required admission to the hospital with *S. pneumoniae* bacteremia (13–16). Currently *mef*-associated resistance predominates in North America. *Erm*-associated resistance predominates in Europe and is common in Japan.

Although the worldwide prevalence of pneumococcal resistance to the newer fluoroquinolones (levofloxacin, gatifloxacin, moxifloxacin) remains low (less than 2%), in some countries, resistance has increased markedly (17–19). The overall prevalence of fluoroquinolone resistance (levofloxacin greater than 4 mcg/mL) in Hong Kong in 2000 had increased to 13.3% as a result of the dissemination of a fluoroquinolone-resistant clone (18). Treatment failures have already been reported, mostly in patients who have previously been treated with fluoroquinolones (20,21). Risk factors for levofloxacin resistance were identified as prior exposure to a fluoroquinolone, nursing home residence, nosocomial infection, and chronic obstructive pulmonary disease (COPD) (22).

Principles of Judicious Antimicrobial Use

Because of the increase in resistance, it is increasingly important that recommendations for judicious use of antibiotics for RTI be reviewed. Several organizations have published guidelines for appropriate antimicrobial usage (23–26). When recommendations from such guidelines are applied to select an appropriate empiric agent, the clinical outcome is hopefully optimized and the costs associated with incorrect prescribing and multiple courses of antibiotics can be avoided. Principles of optimized therapy should be promoted and utilized by prescribing clinicians in order to result in the best outcomes for our patients and reduce the emergence of antibiotic resistance; this is the recently published conclusion of a consensus group on resistance and prescribing in RTI. Recently, an independent multinational interdisciplinary group was established to identify fundamental principles that should form the basis of prescribing in RTI and of guideline formulation, with particular emphasis on countering bacterial resistance and maximizing beneficial patient outcomes (27).

The consensus group listed several core principles of antibiotic therapy that should provide optimal benefit for patients as well as minimize resistance; among these are:

1. Use antibacterial therapy only in those patients with bacterial infection.
2. Utilize diagnostic and other measures to reduce prescribing.
3. Therapy should maximally reduce or eradicate the bacterial load.
4. Use antimicrobial agents with optimal pharmacodynamics to achieve eradication.
5. Use locally relevant resistance data in the decision process.
6. Understand that antimicrobial acquisition cost may be insignificant compared with therapeutic failure.

Reduction of Unnecessary Antimicrobials

The consensus group identified inappropriate prescribing to be the major influence on developing resistance and increasing costs, and called for antibiotic therapy to be limited to infections in which bacteria are the predominant cause. Although this principle certainly seems self-evident, it is one to which adherence seems very difficult. The reasons for overprescribing antibiotics are multifactorial. Patients may consult clinicians expecting an antibiotic to be prescribed for an acute respiratory infection for which the etiology is most likely viral; as a result, clinicians may feel pressured to write antibiotic prescriptions to satisfy patients and to maintain good doctor-patient relationships. Receiving an antibiotic reinforces the patient's perception that antibiotics are warranted in similar situations. Thus, patients may continue to consult clinicians each time similar symptoms occur, expecting that antibiotics are again needed. Clinicians also may prescribe antibiotics as a rapid means of treating patients' symptoms rather than taking the time to educate patients that antibiotics are not always necessary, especially if a viral infection is suspected. However, clinicians should recognize that patient satisfaction is not compromised by the absence of an antibiotic prescription, provided patients understand the reasons. Hamm et al. (28) demonstrated that patient satisfaction was influenced by patient perceptions that the clinician spent enough time discussing the illness and by patient knowledge about the treatment choice. Moreover, clinicians may prescribe antibiotics as part of a defensive approach to avoid the potential sequelae of not prescribing for patients with bacterial infection.

Unfortunately, most patients and many clinicians view "unnecessary" antibiotic prescribing as at worst a neutral intervention (i.e., cannot harm, but may help). It is imperative that patients understand this is not the case. In fact, the unnecessary use of antibacterials has several possible harmful effects in addition to selection of resistance, such as increased cost and exposure to unnecessary adverse reactions. Decreasing excess antibiotic use is an important strategy for combating the increase in community-acquired antibiotic-resistant infections. Several studies have documented a benefit of combining physician intervention and patient education that has resulted in decreased use of antimicrobials and reduction of resistance (Table 1) (29–34).

Correct diagnosis to differentiate viral from bacterial infection is a key to limiting unnecessary antimicrobials. Unfortunately, there is a lack of rapidly available, cost-effective diagnostic tests that reliably differentiate self-limiting viral from bacterial infection. However, practice guidelines can offer

Table 1   Impact of Guideline Interventions on Antimicrobial Use and Resistance

Study	Country	Intervention	Observations
Kristinsson et al. (29)	Iceland	Reduction in antibiotic use	Overall reduction in antibiotic use (penicillin from 20% to <15%), associated with reduction of drug-resistant *Streptococcus pneumoniae.*
Seppala et al. (30)	Finland	Reduction in macrolide use for certain infections	Resistance of *Streptococcus pyogenes* decreased from 19% to 9%.
Pestotnik et al. (31)	U.S.	Evaluation of antibiotic practice guidelines through computer-assisted decision support	Antibiotic use decreased by 22.8%, rate of antibiotic adverse events decreased by 30%, anti-biotic resistance remained stable.
Petersen et al. (32)	U.S.	Provider and community education for prescribing antibiotics for RTIs in Alaska	Education of health care providers and patients substantially decreased the number of visits and antimicrobial prescriptions for RTI and the carriage of PRSP.
Gonzales et al. (23)	U.S.	Use of household and/or office-based patient educational materials as well as clinician detailing compared with controls	Antibiotic prescription rates declined at sites implementing both use of office-based patient educational materials and clinician detailing.
Guillemot et al. (34)	France	Educational interventions aimed at parents, physicians, and pharmacists designed to reduce reduce antibiotic use for upper RTIs	Antibiotic sales fell 32%–37%, depending on the intervention. The rate of colonization with PRSP was seen in intervention groups.

PRSP, penicillin-resistant *S. pneumoniae*; RTI, respiratory tract infection.

pragmatic criteria for better antimicrobial use. For example, restriction of antibiotic therapy in otitis media to those children with acute bacterial disease and avoidance in otitis media with effusion could reduce unnecessary use by two-thirds (35). The consensus group concluded that antibiotics that maximize bacterial eradication, improve both short- and longer-term clinical outcomes, reduce overall costs—particularly those relating to treatment failure and consequent hospital admission—and assist in the minimization of resistance emergence and dissemination. They believe that a radical reevaluation of RTI therapy, incorporating these principles, is long overdue and would more accurately guide the decisions of both individuals and formulary and guideline committees.

In addition to reducing antimicrobial use, more effective use of pneumococcal vaccines offers the promise of decreasing the burden of this pathogen and resistance in both pediatric and adult populations. Preliminary data indicate significant reductions in hospitalization and mortality from use of these vaccines, suggesting an associated reduced necessity of prescribing (36). However, of primary importance, is the continued promotion of principles of judicious antibiotic use when they are warranted.

GUIDELINES FOR RESPIRATORY TRACT INFECTIONS

The Value of Guidelines

In general, clinical guidelines have been shown to improve medical practice (37). The use of clinical practice guidelines may be an effective means of changing behavior, such as promoting the appropriate use of antibiotics. Effective clinical guidelines should improve patient care while enhancing cost savings. However, cost savings should not be the primary motivating factor. A recent example reported by Beilby et al. (38) described a government intervention in Australia intended to decrease costs by reducing the use of amoxicillin-clavulanate. As a result, costs increased through the occurrence of adverse outcomes in patients with otitis media, sinusitis, lower RTI, and acute exacerbation of chronic bronchitis (AECB).

To maximize effectiveness and applicability, antibiotic use guidelines should be evidence based. The guidelines should also reflect data on resistance, recognizing that local patterns of resistance often differ across geographic regions. Hence, effective guidelines should be readily adaptable for implementation locally. Primary objectives of guidelines for treating RTIs should be to discourage antibiotic use to treat viral illness, to outline diagnostic criteria, and to avoid the use of ineffective antimicrobials.

Unfortunately, a meta-analysis of relevant studies has shown that there are numerous barriers to adherence to practice guidelines (Table 2) (39). For example, clinicians may not

Table 2 Barriers to Clinician Adherence to Clinical Practice Guidelines

Barrier	Explanation
Lack of awareness	Clinician is unaware that the guidelines exist.
Lack of familiarity	Clinician is aware of guidelines but unfamiliar with specifics.
Lack of agreement	Clinician does not agree with a specific recommendation made in guideline or is averse to the concept of guidelines in general.
Lack of self-efficacy	Clinician doubts whether he/she can perform the behavior.
Lack of outcome expectancy	Clinician believes the recommendations will be unsuccessful.
Lack of motivation	Clinician is unable/unmotivated to change previous practices.
Guideline-related barriers	Guidelines are not easy or convenient to use.
Patient-related barriers	Clinician may be unable to reconcile guidelines with patient preferences.
Environmental barriers	Clinician may not have control over some changes (e.g., time, resources, organizational constraints).

Adapted from Cabana MD, Rand CS, Powe NR, Wu AW, Wilson MH, Abboud PA, Rubin HR. Why don't physicians follow clinical practice guidelines? A framework for improvement. JAMA 1999; 282:1458–1465.

be aware of all of the available guidelines or may not be well versed in how to apply specific recommendations appropriately. In addition, clinicians may not agree with some or all of the recommendations made or, as a general principle, may resist the concept of guidelines. If clinicians are doubtful that they can perform the task called for in the guidelines or harbor a belief that the recommendations will be unsuccessful, they probably will not follow the guidelines. Time constraints or health care organization requirements may impose restrictions that hamper the clinician's ability to implement the guidelines. Furthermore, the clinician may not have control over some changes called for in guidelines, such as the acquisition of new resources to perform diagnostic tests. Patient preferences for alternatives not recommended in guidelines also may obstruct adherence to clinical practice guidelines. To be successful, educational efforts and interventions aimed at improving adherence to practice guidelines—such as the use of checklists and reminder systems—should address all the identified barriers.

Antimicrobial Recommendations in Respiratory Tract Infections Guidelines—General Approach

Guidelines are usually evidence based, as assessed by a panel of experts. Guidelines for the management of specific RTIs have been developed by numerous professional organizations. For their development, most groups have relied on information obtained from prospectively performed studies on which to base recommendations. Thus, published data and expert opinion have served as major influences in the formulation of these documents.

The selection of specific antimicrobial agents in the guidelines is usually based on multiple factors, including the most likely pathogens and pathogen-susceptibility patterns; the patient's age, comorbidities, and ability to tolerate side effects; and cost. Dosing frequency and side effects play a significant role in promoting or deterring patient adherence to therapy. Selecting agents that have more favorable side-effect profiles and less-frequent dosing requirements may aid in achieving adherence. Epidemiologic information that may indicate the likelihood of a particular pathogen (such as recent epidemics of influenza, recent travel, and recent exposure to animals or other patients with specific infections) and disease severity (i.e., outpatient vs. inpatient) also significantly influences therapeutic choices.

The following represents brief descriptions of the major guidelines published in North America concerning the most common RTIs.

The Use of Treatment Recommendations/ Guidelines in Respiratory Tract Infections Other Than Pneumonia

Acute Otitis Media

Treatment for bacterial acute otitis media (AOM) must take into account pathogens most commonly implicated in this condition (i.e., *S. pneumoniae, Haemophilus influenzae, Moraxella catarrhalis*) as well as their resistance patterns. AOM treatment recommendations have been developed in the context of increasing levels of drug-resistant bacteria and selecting the appropriate antibiotic agents. In 1999, guidelines were published from a multidisciplinary group coordinated by the Centers for Disease Control and Prevention (CDC) (40). After reviewing the data, the Drug-Resistant *S. pneumoniae* Therapeutic Working Group of the CDC recommended that amoxicillin (standard dose, 40 to 45 mg/kg/day; or high dose, 80 to 90 mg/kg/day) should be used as first-line therapy in AOM (Fig. 1). If factors associated with the likelihood of resistance are present, the recommendations suggest using high-dose amoxicillin, high-dose amoxicillin-clavulanate, or cefuroxime axetil as first-line therapy. These factors include day care attendance, age, and recent prior exposure to antibiotics (e.g., within 4 to 6 weeks). Amoxicillin-clavulanate, cefuroxime axetil, and intramuscular (IM) ceftriaxone are recommended for treatment if amoxicillin fails after 3 days of therapy (Fig. 1). Although a single injection of IM ceftriaxone achieves high concentrations in middle ear fluid for several days, the clinical outcome is not improved compared with a 10-day course of

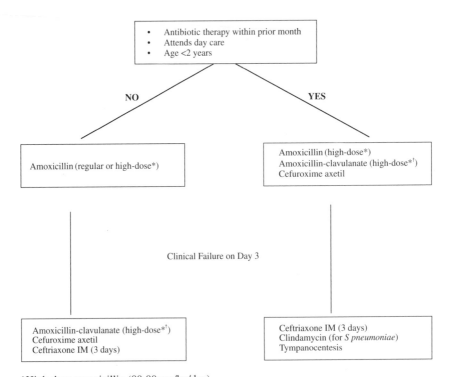

*High-dose amoxicillin (80-90 mg/kg/day).

†80-90 mg/kg/day of the amoxicillin component, with 6.4 mg/kg/day of clavulanate.

Figure 1 Algorithm outlining Centers for Disease Control and Prevention recommendations for treating acute otitis media. IM, intramuscularly. (From Meehan TP, Fine MJ, Krumholz HM, Scinto JD, Galusha DH, Mockalis JT, Weber GF, Petrillo MK, Houck PM, Fine JM. Quality of care, process, and outcomes in elderly patients with pneumonia. JAMA 1997; 278:2080–2084.)

amoxicillin-clavulanate (41). Furthermore, a series of daily injections given for 3 days may be needed to improve the effectiveness of ceftriaxone against penicillin-resistant *S pneumoniae* (40). Other agents, such as cefprozil, cefpodoxime, cefaclor, cefixime, ceftibuten, loracarbef, trimethoprim-sulfamethoxazole, and the macrolides, are not included in the list of preferred antimicrobials for a variety of reasons, including inadequate pharmacokinetic properties and decreased activity against beta-lactamase enzymes and drug-resistant *S. pneumoniae* (DRSP).

Patients who are allergic to penicillin may be treated with a newer macrolide or trimethoprim-sulfamethoxazole. However, these agents have less activity against DRSP. Fluoroquinolones, although effective against common respiratory pathogens, are not approved for use in children.

Acute Bacterial Rhinosinusitis

Similar to the CDC's recommendations for AOM, the guidelines issued by the Sinus and Allergy Health Partnership recommend empiric choices for treating acute bacterial rhinosinusitis (ABRS) (42). As in AOM, *S. pneumoniae* and *H. influenzae* are frequently implicated in ABRS. However, *M. catarrhalis* is less likely to be the infectious cause of this condition compared with its role in AOM (2% vs. 12%).The guidelines recognize that patients exposed to an antibiotic within 4 to 6 weeks of their current infection are likely to be infected with a resistant pathogen. In developing its antimicrobial guidelines, the panel employed the Poole Therapeutic Outcome Model to predict the therapeutic effectiveness of various antimicrobial agents. Recognizing that resistance rates may change over time and may vary from community to community, the panel intends to revise the guidelines as resistance rates change and as new antibiotics are introduced. The model is available at the Sinus and Allergy Health Partnership's website (http://www.sahp.org), where clinicians may input local resistance rates and develop their own optimal treatment recommendations.

Agents recommended for the treatment of ABRS are listed in Table 3. The antibiotic selections listed in the table are stratified by disease severity, age of the patient, and recent antibiotic exposure. The preferred agents are those that are active against the pathogens commonly implicated in acute sinusitis—*S. pneumoniae, H. influenzae,* and *M. catarrhalis.* Switching to a second agent is suggested if, after 72 hours, the patient's condition does not clinically improve or worsens.

Table 3 Agents Recommended for Treatment of Acute
Bacterial Rhinosinusitis

Population	Mild disease	Moderate disease
Adults If no antibiotics in past 4–6 wk	Amoxicillin (high dose)* Amoxicillin-clavulanate Cefpodoxime proxetil Cefuroxime axetil *Alternatives—limited* *effectiveness, bacterial* *failure rates 20%–25%:* • Cefprozil • Clarithromycin† • TMP/SMX† • Doxycycline† • Azithromycin† • Erythromycin†	Amoxicillin (high dose)* Amoxicillin-clavulanate Cefpodoxime proxetil Cefuroxime axetil *Alternatives:* • Gatifloxacin • Levofloxacin • Moxifloxacin
Adults If antibiotics in past 4–6 wk	Amoxicillin (high dose)* Amoxicillin-clavulanate Cefpodoxime proxetil Cefuroxime axetil *Alternatives:* • Gatifloxacin • Levofloxacin • Moxifloxacin	Amoxicillin-clavulanate Gatifloxacin Levofloxacin Moxifloxacin Combination therapy: gram- positive coverage (amoxicillin or clindamycin) + gram-negative coverage (cefixime or cefpodoxime proxetil)
Children If no antibiotics in past 4–6 wk	Amoxicillin (high dose)* Amoxicillin-clavulanate Cefpodoxime proxetil Cefuroxime axetil *Alternatives—limited* *effectiveness, bacterial* *failure rates 20%–25%:* • TMP/SMX • Azithromycin • Clarithromycin • Erythromycin	Amoxicillin (high dose)* Amoxicillin-clavulanate Cefpodoxime proxetil Cefuroxime axetil
Children If antibiotics in past 4–6 wk	Amoxicillin (high dose)* Amoxicillin-clavulanate Cefpodoxime proxetil Cefuroxime axetil	Amoxicillin-clavulanate Combination therapy: gram- positive coverage (amoxicillin or clindamycin) + gram-negative coverage (cefixime or cefpodoxime proxetil)

* High-dose amoxicillin (80–90 mg/kg/day).
† For penicillin allergy.
TMP/SMX, trimethoprim/sulfamethoxazole.
Adapted from Sinus and Allergy Health Partnership. Antimicrobial treatment guidelines for
acute bacterial rhinosinusitis. Otolaryngol Head Neck Surg 2000; 123(Suppl):S1–S32.

Selection of the appropriate antibiotic may help prevent the development of chronic sinusitis, decrease costs associated with multiple treatment failures, and curtail the development of resistance.

First-line therapy for adult patients with mild disease and no antibiotic therapy during the previous 4 to 6 weeks is limited to high-dose amoxicillin, amoxicillin-clavulanate, cefpodoxime proxetil, and cefuroxime axetil. The guidelines note that cefprozil may have a bacterial failure rate of up to 25%. Similarly, although clarithromycin, trimethoprim-sulfamethoxazole, doxycycline, azithromycin, or erythromycin may be considered for patients with beta-lactam allergies, they are generally less active for DRSP. The use of trimethoprim-sulfamethoxazole also has been associated with potentially fatal toxic epidermal necrolysis. For adults with mild disease who have had recent antibiotic therapy or for those with moderate disease with no recent antibiotic therapy, first-line treatment recommendations include amoxicillin-clavulanate, high-dose amoxicillin, cefpodoxime proxetil, and cefuroxime axetil. Appropriate agents for beta-lactam–allergic or –intolerant patients include gatifloxacin, levofloxacin, and moxifloxacin. In adult patients with moderate disease and recent antibiotic use, the indicated agents are amoxicillin-clavulanate, gatifloxacin, levofloxacin, moxifloxacin, or combination therapy ß3/4 amoxicillin or clindamycin for gram-positive coverage plus cefixime or cefpodoxime proxetil for gram-negative coverage.

In pediatric patients with mild disease and no antibiotic use in the previous 4 to 6 weeks, first-line therapy includes amoxicillin-clavulanate, high-dose amoxicillin, cefpodoxime proxetil, or cefuroxime axetil. In patients with a history of immediate type I hypersensitivity to beta-lactams, the use of trimethoprim-sulfamethoxazole, azithromycin, clarithromycin, or erythromycin is recommended, although bacterial failure rates of 20% to 25% are possible with these agents. For children with moderate disease who have had no recent antibiotic therapy or for those with mild disease who have had recent antibiotic therapy, indicated treatment agents are high-dose amoxicillin, amoxicillin-clavulanate, cefpodoxime proxetil, and cefuroxime axetil. In children with moderate disease who have received recent antibiotic therapy, the recommended treatment is amoxicillin-clavulanate or combination therapy—amoxicillin or clindamycin for gram-positive coverage plus cefixime or cefpodoxime proxetil for gram-negative coverage.

Pharyngitis (Strep Throat)

The primary use of antibiotics in pharyngitis is to treat infection due to group A streptococcus (GAS). GAS is the most common bacterial agent causing acute pharyngitis and accounts for approximately 15% to 30% of cases in children and 5% to 10% of adults (43,44). However, streptococcal pharyngitis is difficult to differentiate from other causes (such as viral etiology) on clinical grounds (44).

Definitive diagnosis of streptococcal pharyngitis is based on the identification of GAS in the throat by culture, by rapid antigen detection test, or by serologic means. Results of culture and serologic testing are not available at the time of clinical decision making and are therefore not timely. The rapid antigen detection test provides the result to the clinician within minutes. However, the sensitivity varies from 60% to 90%, thus a false test does not rule out the diagnosis.

Intramuscular penicillin and oral penicillin V or oral amoxicillin continue to be the recommended first-line drugs by most guidelines. Table 4 shows the most recent antimicrobial agents recommended for the treatment of streptococcal pharyngitis and prevention of rheumatic fever from recent guidelines (45–47). GAS continues to be highly sensitive to penicillin and amoxicillin, and these agents have been the first-line recommended therapy. In patients with penicillin allergy, an oral cephalosporin or a macrolide is recommended. An oral cephalosporin may be used in patients who do not have immediate-type hypersensitivity to beta-lactam agents. Macrolide antibiotics may be used in patients who are allergic to penicillin, regardless of the type of reaction. However, the increasing resistance of group A beta-hemolytic streptococci to macrolide worldwide is of major concern (48). Macrolide resistance may reside in the *erm* gene or *mef* gene. Cross-resistance to all the

Table 4   Recommendations for Antimicrobial Therapy for Group
A Streptococcal Pharyngitis*

Route	Antimicrobial agent, dosage	Duration
Oral	Children: 250 mg b.i.d. or t.i.d.	10 d
	Adolescents and adults: 250 mg t.i.d. or q.i.d.	10 d
	Adolescents and adults: 500 mg b.i.d.	10 d
Oral	Amoxicillin may be used in place of penicillin V using a 50 mg dose or 750 mg dose.	10 d
IM	Benzathine penicillin G 1.2 million U	1 dose
	Benzathine penicillin G 600,000 U (children <27 kg)	1 dose
		1 dose
	Mixtures of benzathine and procaine penicillin (dose should be based on benzathine penicillin)	
Oral	Erythromycin (dose varies with formulation)	10 d
	Erythromycin ethylsuccinate 40 mg/kg/d (maximum 1.5 g/d) t.i.d.†	
	Erythromycin estolate 20–240 mg/kg/d (maximum 1.5 g/d) t.i.d.†	
	Erythromycin stearate 1 g/day in 2 or 4 divided doses‡	
Oral	First-generation cephalosporins (should not be used to treat patients with immediate-type hypersensitivity to beta-lactam antibiotics)	10 d
Oral	Cefadroxil	5 d
Oral	Cefixime	5 d
Oral	Cefdinir	5 d
Oral	Cefpodoxime	5 d
Oral	Azithromycin 500 mg first day followed by 250 mg daily for 4 more days	5 d
Oral	Clarithromycin 500 mg daily	5 d

* Based mainly on the Practice Guideline from the Infectious Diseases Society. (Bisno AL, Gerber MA, Gwaltney Jr. JM, Kaplan EL, Schwartz RH. Practice guideline for the diagnosis and management of group A streptococcal pharyngitis. Clin Infect Dis 2002; 35:113–125.)
† Based on WHO recommendation (Division of Drug Management and Policies (World Health Organization). WHO Model Prescribing Information. Drugs Used in the Treatment of Streptococcal Pharyngitis and Prevention of Rheumatic Fever. Geneva: World Health Organization, 1999.).
‡ Based on Bisno AL. Acute pharyngitis. N Engl J Med 2001; 344:205–211.
IM, intramuscular; b.i.d., twice daily; t.i.d., three times daily, q.i.d., four times daily.

macrolide antibiotics is the rule. Streptococci with a low level of macrolide resistance are commonly associated with the *mef* gene, which is responsible for the efflux of the antibiotic out of the bacterial cells. These bacteria are usually susceptible to clindamycin. Streptococci that are highly macrolide resistant are usually not susceptible to clindamycin as well, and the *erm* gene commonly mediates this resistance.

Acute Exacerbations of Chronic Bronchitis

Timely and accurate diagnosis and treatment of AECB remain challenges to clinicians because of the indefinite beginnings and uncertain treatment modalities of the condition. Because patients with AECB have chronic bronchitis as an underlying disease and because the definition of AECB is subjective, it is sometimes difficult to determine when an exacerbation has begun or ended.

The most common bacterial pathogens associated with AECB are *H. influenzae, M. catarrhalis*, and *S. pneumoniae* (49,50). Gram-negative pathogens, including *Pseudomonas aeruginosa*, may be significant pathogens in patients with more severe underlying COPD. Because as many as 50% of AECB episodes may be nonbacterial in origin and because there is no reliable method of distinguishing bacterial episodes from nonbacterial episodes based on clinical criteria, the appropriateness of antimicrobial therapy is controversial, particularly in light of current trends in resistance. However, because recurrent episodes of AECB can impair pulmonary function and can severely affect quality-of-life, many clinicians choose to treat the condition with antibiotics in order to address those cases that are bacterial in origin. To help decide whether antimicrobial therapy is warranted, clinicians may also stratify patients by type of exacerbation and by presence of risk factors associated with poor outcome. Several randomized, placebo-controlled trials have shown that antibiotic treatment is beneficial in selected patients with AECB. Specifically, studies show that patients with more severe exacerbation (type I) are more likely to experience benefit than are those with less severe disease (51). Patients with type I exacerbation have all three cardinal symptoms: increased dyspnea, increased sputum volume, and increased sputum purulence, whereas patients with type II exacerbation have two symptoms and patients with type III have only one. In comparison, patients with moderate exacerbation (type II) experienced less benefit from antibiotics compared with those who received placebo, and patients with mild episodes (type III) did not appear to benefit from antibiotic treatment compared with the placebo group. In the study by Anthonisen et al. (51), patients with AECB who received antibiotic therapy had a more rapid return of peak flow, were more likely to achieve clinical success, and experienced clinical failure less frequently than patients given placebo. Other studies also have shown the benefit of antibiotic therapy in AECB (52). A clinical practice guideline for management of AECB formulated by the American College of Physicians–American Society of Internal Medicine and the American College of Chest Physicians was recently published; this position paper recommends the use of antibiotics in patients with severe exacerbation (such as type I) of COPD (53).

In addition to stratification by type, patients at high-risk for poor outcome of AECB have been identified and include patients with a history of repeated infections (more than four per year), comorbid illnesses (e.g., diabetes, asthma, coronary heart disease), or marked airway obstruction (less than 50% forced expiratory volume at 1 second [FEV_1]) (54).

In patients with AECB of bacterial origin, antibiotics may have the long-term benefit of decreasing the amount of bacteria chronically colonizing the airway once the patient is clinically stable, thus helping to prevent progression to parenchymal lung infection.(49). Antibiotic treatment may also prevent progressive airway injury due to persistent infection and may prolong the duration between exacerbations.

Agents with activity against the most commonly encountered pathogens in AECB—*S. pneumoniae, H. influenzae,* and *M. catarrhalis*—should be selected for treatment. An appropriate agent also should be resistant to beta-lactamase destruction, have good penetration into bronchial tissue and sputum, promote patient adherence through convenient dosing, and have a favorable side-effect profile. The specific choice of antibiotic for AECB remains controversial. Most previously published trials have demonstrated a benefit of narrow-spectrum antibiotics (i.e., amoxicillin, trimethoprim-sulfamethoxazole, and tetracycline) as initial treatment (53). However, most of these studies were done before the emergence of multidrug-resistant pathogens. Many experts recommend stratifying antibiotics on the basis of severity of disease and on the presence of risk factors of outcome. Table 5 lists agents recommended for AECB treatment according to one classification scheme (54).

Table 5 Proposed Classification and Therapy of Acute Bronchitis and Acute Exacerbations of Chronic Bronchitis

Class	Clinical status	Criteria/risk factors	Pathogens	Treatment
1	Acute bronchitis	No underlying chronic inflammatory lung disease	Viral	None
2	Simple chronic bronchitis	FEV_1 >50%, increased sputum volume and purulence	*Haemophilus influenzae, Moraxella catarrhalis, Streptococcus pneumoniae*	Amoxicillin, doxycycline, newer macrolide (azithromycin or clarithromycin), cephalosporin
3	Complicated chronic bronchitis	As for class 2, plus: FEV_1 <50%, advanced age, >4 exacerbations/year, or significant comorbidity	As for class 2; concern for resistant strains	Quinolone, amoxicillin-clavulanate
4	Chronic bronchial infection	As for class 3, plus continuous sputum through year	As for class 3, plus Enterobacteriaciae, *Pseudomonas aeruginosa*	Ciprofloxacin

FEV_1, forced expiratory volume in 1 second.
Modified from Adams and Anzueto. Antibiotic therapy in acute exacerbations of chronic bronchitis. Semin Respir Infect 2000; 15:234–247.

Guidelines for Community-Acquired Pneumonia

Community-acquired pneumonia is a common disorder that is potentially life threatening, especially in older adults and those with comorbid disease. Despite substantial progress in therapeutic options, CAP remains a significant cause of morbidity and death worldwide and continues to have major controversies concerning antimicrobial management. Guidelines from numerous international organizations have been developed over the past decade. For this chapter, however, only those from North American organizations are reviewed. Recent recommendations for empiric antimicrobial therapy are summarized in Table 6 (55–58). Although the different guidelines vary somewhat in their emphasis on the importance of defining the etiologic agents so that directed therapy can be implemented, it is acknowledged that the majority of patients will be treated empirically. This is particularly the case for outpatients in whom diagnostic testing is not cost efficient and is not emphasized. Moreover, even at tertiary-level university centers where multiple diagnostic testing methods are used for patients who require hospitalization, an etiologic agent is found in only (approximately) 50% of cases.

Although numerous pathogens have been associated with the etiology of CAP, a limited range of key pathogens causes the majority of CAP, with *S. pneumoniae* being the most common. Other common etiologic agents to which empiric therapy is usually directed according to the North American guidelines include *H. influenzae* (and *M. catarrhalis*) and the "atypical pathogens" (*Mycoplasma pneumoniae, Chlamydia pneumoniae,* and *Legionella* spp). Other pathogens considered important for empiric therapy under selected conditions include *Staphylococcus aureus, Chlamydia psittaci, Coxiella burnetii,* gram-bacteria bacilli, fungi, *Mycobacterium* spp, anaerobes (aspiration pneumonia), and respiratory viruses.

The North American guidelines place significant emphasis on the potential role of the atypical organisms. The rationale is that these organisms are becoming more commonly recognized in recent studies as the etiology of CAP, and in several observational studies of therapy for patients who re-

Table 6 Comparison of Recommendations of Recently Published North American Guidelines for Empiric Antimicrobial Therapy of Community-Acquired Pneumonia in Adults

Guideline (reference)	Outpatient	General ward	ICU/severe
North America Centers for Disease Control Drug-Resistant *Streptococcus pneumoniae* Therapeutic Working Group (55)	Favored: Macrolide **or** doxycycline Also listed: Beta-lactams* (i.e., cefuroxime, amoxicillin, amoxicillin/clavulanate)—not effective for "atypical" pathogens; **or** antipneumococcal fluoroquinolone† (Not first line because of concerns for emerging resistance)	Beta-lactam‡ *plus* macrolide; **or** anti-pneumococcal fluoroquinolone† (Not first line because of concerns for emerging resistance)	IV beta-lactam‡ *plus* IV macrolide; **or** IV beta-lactam *plus* antipneumo-coccal fluoro-quinolone†; **or** antipneumo-coccal fluoro-quinolone†
Canadian Infectious Diseases Society/ Canadian Thoracic Society (57)	Without modifying factors: 1. Macrolide 2. Doxycycline With modifying factors—COLD (no recent antibi-otics or steroids): 1. New macrolide§ 2. Doxycycline COLD (recent anti-biotics or steroids): 1. Antipneumo-coccal fluoro-quinolone‖ 2. Amoxicillin-clavulanate	1. Antipneumococcal fluoroquinolone‖ 2. Second-, third-, or fourth-generation cephalosporin *plus* macrolide	*Pseudomonas aeruginosa* not suspected: 1. IV antipneumo-coccal fluoro-quinolone *plus* cefotaxime, ceftriaxone, or beta-lactam/beta-lactamase inhibitor IV macrolide plus cefotaxime, ceftriaxone, or beta-lactam/beta-lactamase inhibitor

Table 6 *Continued*

Guideline (reference)	Outpatient	General ward	ICU/severe
	or second-generation cephalosporin; and macrolide		*P. aeruginosa* suspected: 1. Antipseudomonal fluoroquinolone (e.g., ciprofloxacin) *plus* antipseudomonal beta-lactam# or aminoglycoside 2. Triple therapy with antipseudomonal beta-lactam# *plus* aminoglycoside *plus* macrolide
Infectious Diseases Society of America (56)	Doxycycline **or** macrolide **or** antipneumococcal fluoroquinolone# Selection considerations: choice should be by regional antibiotic susceptibility patterns for *S. pneumoniae* and the presence of risk factors for PRSP. For older patients or those with underlying disease, antipneumococcal fluoroquinolones may be preferred; some authorities prefer to reserve fluoroquinolones for such patients.	Macrolide *plus* cefotaxime, ceftriaxone, or a beta-lactam/ beta-lactamase inhibitor (ampicillin-sulbactam or piperacillin-tazobactam) **or** Antipneumococcal fluoroquinolone	IV antipneumococcal fluoroquinolone or IV macrolide, *plus* cefotaxime, ceftriaxone, or a beta-lactam/ beta-lactamase inhibitor (ampicillin-sulbactam or piperacillin-tazobactam) If structural lung disease: antipseudomonal agents with activity for *S. pneumoniae* (i.e., cefepime, imipenem, meropenem, piperacillin) plus a fluoroquinolone (including ciprofloxacin)

Table 6 *Continued*

Guideline (reference)	Outpatient	General ward	ICU/severe
American Thoracic Society (58)	**No cardiopulmonary disease, no modifying factors****: azithromycin or clarithromycin (doxycycline if allergic or intolerant of macrolides) **Modifying factors****: beta-lactam (cefpodoxime, cefuroxime, high-dose amoxicillin, amoxicillin-clavulanate; or parenteral ceftriaxone followed by oral cefpodoxime) *plus* Macrolide or doxycycline; **or** antipneumococcal fluoroquinolone‖	**No modifying factors****: IV azithromycin; doxycyline *plus* a beta-lactam; **or** Monotherapy with an antipneumococcal fluoroquinolone‖ **Modifying factors****: IV beta-lactam (cefotaxime, ceftriaxone, ampicillin-sulbactam, high-dose ampicillin) *plus* IV or oral macrolide or doxycycline; **or** IV antipneumococcal fluoroquinolone	**No risk for *P. aeruginosa*:** IV beta-lactam (cefotaxime, ceftriaxone) *plus* IV macrolide (azithromycin) or IV antipneumococcal fluoroquinolone **Risk for *P. aeruginosa:*** IV antipseudomonal beta-lactam (cefepime, imipenem, meropenem, piperacillin-tazobactam) *plus* IV antipseudomonal quinolone (ciprofloxacin) IV antipseudomonal beta-lactam plus IV aminoglycoside plus either IV azithromycin or IV nonpseudomonal fluoroquinolone

* Cefuroxime axetil, amoxicillin, amoxicillin-clavulanate, cefpodoxime, cefprozil; does not cover atypical pathogerns.
† Levofloxacin, sparfloxacin; not first line because of concerns about emerging resistance.
‡ Ceftriaxone, cefotaxime.
§ Clarithromycin, azithromycin.
‖ Levofloxacin, gatifloxacin, or moxifloxacin; trovafloxacin is restricted because of potential severe hepatotoxicity.
For example, ceftazidime, piperacillin-tazobactam, imipenem, meropenem.
** Modifying factors: elderly, multiple comorbidities, risk factors for drug resistance.
COLD, chronic obstructive lung disease; ICU, intensive care unit; IV, intravenous; PRSP, penicillin-resistant *S. pneumoniae.*

quire hospitalization, antimicrobial regimens that have activity against the "atypicals" have been associated with better outcomes. In addition, it is now well recognized that it is difficult in most cases to differentiate the etiology of CAP (i.e., atypical vs. *S. pneumoniae*) from the clinical and radiographic findings at presentation of the patient.

Recommendations for Empiric Therapy of Community-Acquired Pneumonia Outpatients

All the new North American guidelines variably recommend macrolides, doxycycline, or an antipneumococcal fluoroquinolone (i.e., levofloxacin, gatifloxacin, and moxifloxacin) as treatment options for patients who are mildly ill and can be treated as outpatients. In general, the North American guidelines recommend a macrolide or doxycycline as first-line treatment for outpatients with no comorbidity or risk factors for DRSP. The rationale for positioning the macrolides as prominent first-line agents for mild CAP in otherwise healthy hosts is partly based on the perception that the newer macrolides (azithromycin or clarithromycin) may be effective against MRSP strains in which lower-level resistance results from increased drug efflux with a resulting MIC of 1 to 8 μg/mL. This partly explains the difference between the North American and European positioning of macrolides because the majority of resistance in North America is efflux (often with an MIC greater than 16 μg/mL) whereas it is ribosomal (with MICs greater than 32 μg/mL) in most locations within Europe. In addition, at the time of the development of the North American guidelines, cases of macrolide failure for outpatients, especially for cases not associated with risks for DRSP, had been infrequent. However, the trend in increasing MICs of the efflux-associated resistant strains in the United States is of significant concern. As these strains become more prominent, additional treatment failures may be expected and reconsideration of the North American recommendations may be required.

In the Canadian statement, outpatients are stratified into those without modifying factors, for whom a macrolide or doxycycline may be used, and those with modifying factors (such as chronic obstructive lung disease or use of recent antibiotics or steroid—for which there may be a greater likelihood of DRSP), for whom fluoroquinolones are considered more appropriate as first-line empiric therapy. The Infectious Diseases Society of America's statement indicates that selection considerations among the three options should be influenced by regional antibiotic susceptibility patterns for *S. pneumoniae* and the presence of risk factors for DRSP (such as the use of antimicrobial agents within the previous 3 months). The statement further indicates that "for older patients or those with underlying disease, a fluoroquinolone may be a preferred choice; some authorities prefer to reserve fluoroquinolones for such patients," thus implying macrolide as first-line therapy for those patients without comorbidity or risk factors for DRSP. The CDC statement is similar but stresses that macrolides should be used first-line and fluoroquinolones should be reserved for cases associated with failure of or allergy to other agents or for cases due to documented DRSP. The rationale is that fear of widespread use may lead to the development of fluoroquinolone resistance among the respiratory pathogens (as well as other pathogens colonizing the treated patients). Similar to the Canadian statement, the revised American Thoracic Society (ATS) guidelines recommend stratifying outpatients into two categories (Table 6), with macrolides being recommended as first-line therapy for patients with no cardiopulmonary disease and no risks for DRSP, aspiration, or enteric gram-negatives. Doxycycline is a second choice (because of less reliable activity against *S. pneumoniae*) if patients are intolerant of or allergic to macrolides. The statement indicates that if *H. influenzae* is not likely, any macrolide may be used, including erythromycin. For more complex outpatients, the ATS statement recommends a beta-lactam plus macrolide (or doxycycline) combination or monotherapy with an antipnuemococcal fluoroquinolone. The rationale is to treat the possibility of DRSP with the fluoroquinolone or an appropriate beta-lactam (i.e., higher dose amoxicillin or amoxicillin-clavulanate) plus the atypical organisms (which can be effectively treated by the macrolide, doxycycline, or fluoroquinolone).

Recommendations for Empiric Therapy of
Community-Acquired Pneumonia Inpatients

All the North American guidelines recommend treatment with a beta-lactam plus a macrolide or monotherapy with a fluoroquinolone for patients admitted to the general ward. The rationale for recommending these regimens is based on studies showing these regimens were associated with a significant reduction in mortality compared with administration of cephalosporin alone. For patients with severe CAP who require admission to an intensive care unit, all guidelines recommend comprehensive antimicrobial therapy to cover *S. pneumoniae* (including DRSP), *Legionella*, and the possibility of *Pseudomonas* in selected cases. For this group of patients with severe disease, azithromycin is the preferred macrolide over erythromycin by the ATS statement because of difficulties in administration and tolerance with erythromycin (parenteral clarithromycin is not available in the United States).

Impact of Community-Acquired Pneumonia Guidelines on Outcomes

For guidelines to be of value, they must be shown to be associated with an improvement of care for the patient. The efficacy of the management recommendations of guidelines can be evaluated by analyzing several parameters, including clinical outcomes, influence on antimicrobial prescribing, effect on bacterial resistance, and cost. Audits of practice guidelines and care pathways for patients with CAP have shown they can improve the quality of care and reduce cost (Table 7) (59–67). In a national evaluation of Medicare patients treated in hospitals from 1997 to 1999, Jencks et al. (68) found that 79% of patients were treated with antimicrobial therapy consistent with current recommendations in the guidelines.

Several studies have attempted to evaluate the validity of the published treatment guidelines for CAP. Gleason et al. (61) evaluated the therapies and outcomes of 864 outpatients with CAP from the Patients Outcomes Research Trial database. Most patients were treated with an oral macrolide, including older patients and those with comorbid conditions. Although monotherapy with a macrolide was not recommended by the guidelines for patients with more complex illness, they appeared to have good outcomes as well. However, the number of patients treated according to the guidelines was small and the patients were more severely ill compared with

Table 7   Impact of Guideline Interventions on Outcome of
Community-Acquired Pneumonia

Study (reference)	Country	Intervention	Outcome
Meehan et al. (59)	U.S.	Observational evaluation of timing of antimicrobials for older inpatients	30-d mortality less if first dose given within 8 h of presentation
Bratzler et al. (60)	U.S.	Observational evaluation of timing of antimicrobials for older inpatients	30-d mortality less if first dose given within 4 h of presentation
Gordon et al. (62)	U.S.	Examined initial choice of antimicrobial therapy of approx. 4,500 patients admitted to general ward	Therapy according to ATS guidelines was associated with lower mortality than if nonrecommended therapy was used.
Menendez et al. (63)	Spain	Examined initial choice of antimicrobial therapy in 295 patients admitted to a hospital	Adherence to antibiotics of ATS guidelines was associated with decreased mortality when compared with nonadherent treatments
Gleason et al. (61)	U.S.	Evaluated 864 patients treated as outpatients	Recommended antimicrobials for younger, healthier patients in 1993 ATS guidelines were cost effective; for more complex outpatients, the recommendations were more costly, without increased benefit
Gleason et. al. (65)	U.S.	Observational study of 12,945 inpatients ($\geq$ 65 years of age)	Second- or third-generation cephalosporin plus a macrolide, or fluoroquinolone monotherapy, had reduced 30-d mortality

Table 7 *Continued*

Study (reference)	Country	Intervention	Outcome
Dudas et al. (66)	U.S.	Observational study of 10,000 inpatients from 72 nonteaching hospitals	Beta-lactam plus a macrolide, or a fluoroquinolone, associated with decreased mortality and decreased length of stay
Stahl et al. (64)	U.S.	Prospective evaluation of 100 inpatients at single hospital	Patients receiving macrolides as part of initial therapy had shorter hospital stay
Houck et al. (67)	U.S.	Observational study of 10,000 Medicare patients admitted to hospital	Depending on the time period, beta-lactam plus a macrolide, or fluoroquinolone, was associated with lower mortality

ATS, American Thoracic Society.

those treated by non-guideline therapy. Gordon et al. (62) evaluated more than 4,000 patients admitted to the general wards of a hospital and found that therapy according to the ATS guidelines (1993 version) was associated with a lower mortality than if non-guideline therapy was used. In a more recent study, Menendez et al. (63) studied 295 patients admitted to a hospital from February 1998 to March 1999 and compared the outcomes in relation to the initial antimicrobial therapy. In a multivariate analysis, adherence to the ATS guidelines was independently associated with decreased mortality.

Several observational studies have found that antimicrobial regimens as listed in the guidelines are associated with decreased mortality and shorter length of stay (LOS) for patients who require hospitalization. Stahl et al. (64) evaluated 100 prospective patients hospitalized with CAP. Patients were stratified according to the antibiotic received. Patients who received macrolides (usually intravenous erythromycin or oral clarithromycin) within the first 24 hours of admission had a markedly shorter LOS (2.8 days) than those not so treated. The investigators speculated that the direct antimicrobial effect against atypical pathogens, as well as a beneficial immunologic or anti-inflammatory effect, may be responsible for the advantage of the macrolides. In a study of 12,945 Medicare patients (65 years of age or older), Gleason et al. (65) found that the addition of a macrolide to a second- or third-generation cephalosporin resulted in a significantly reduced 30-day mortality for elderly patients hospitalized with pneumonia. The authors suggested that this finding of better outcome may be related to the better activity for the common typical and atypical bacterial pathogens. Dudas et al. (66) in an observational study of 3,035 patients hospitalized with pneumonia in one of seventy-two nonteaching hospitals with a national group purchasing organization, found the addition of a macrolide to either a second- or third-generation cephalosporin or a beta-lactam/beta-lactamase inhibitor was associated with decreased mortality and reduced LOS (66). Houck et al. (67) examined the risk for mortality during the 30 days after admission to the hospital of 10,069 Medicare patients in three time periods: 1993, 1995, and 1997. In 1993, therapy with a macrolide plus a beta-lactam was associated with significantly lower mortality than therapy with either a beta-lactam alone or other regimens that did not include a macrolide, beta-lactam, or fluoroquinolone. This association was not observed in 1995 or 1997. The authors speculated that this may have been a result of a temporal variation in the incidence of atypical pathogen pneumonia.

EDUCATIONAL STRATEGIES TO PROMOTE RATIONAL ANTIBIOTIC USE

Issuing guidelines on appropriate antibiotic use for treatment of different types of infections is only the first step in ensuring that rational principles are adopted and followed in clinical practice. Educational strategies aimed at enhancing clinician awareness of guidelines and encouraging their implementation is necessary. Educational materials promoting the implementation of practice guidelines and emphasizing their benefits could be developed and provided to clinicians. Translation of guidelines into practice also must involve educational efforts geared toward patients. Patients need to understand that antibiotics are not appropriate for the treatment of viral infections. They also must be educated about the need to take antibiotics as directed and for the entire duration prescribed. Public health campaigns can help to spread the word, and traditional print and audiovisual patient education materials may also be useful.

Educational efforts aimed at providers and patients already have proven successful in promoting the rational use of antibiotics in upper RTIs. In a study in rural Alaska, the education of health care workers and the community concerning appropriate antimicrobial use in children with upper RTIs was associated with a 22% reduction in the number of antibiotic prescriptions in children younger than 5 years, and a 28% decrease in penicillin-resistant pneumococcal nasopharyngeal isolates compared with the two control regions not provided with the educational intervention (35). In a National Ambulatory Medical Care Survey, McCaig et al. (69) observed a decease in antimicrobial prescribing for RTIs among children and adolescents from 838 per 1,000 population in 1989 to 1990 to 503 in 1999 to 2000. The authors of the study attributed this decrease in part to the educational efforts of various professionals and public health organizations to promote appropriate antimicrobial prescribing.

In addition to educational campaigns, there is no substitute for the few moments taken by the treating clinician to explain fully why antibiotics are not necessary or why they are being prescribed. This approach helps patients realize that their condition is being taken seriously. The investment in time and personal attention can increase patient satisfaction with the selected treatment and can help ensure that patients comply with therapy.

CONCLUSION

The widespread morbidity caused by RTIs is a serious problem for society in general and clinicians in particular. The appropriate management of RTIs poses multiple challenges for the clinician. Inappropriate prescribing practices (e.g., selecting agents with insufficient antimicrobial activity and treating viral infections with antibiotics) have contributed to the development of drug resistance among common respiratory pathogens (e.g., *S. pneumoniae, H. influenzae*, and *M. catarrhalis*). Factors contributing to inappropriate antimicrobial use include patient expectations, clinician time constraints, and the practice of defensive medicine. Antibiotic therapy with the appropriate agent shortens the course of the illness, lowers the risk of complications due to untreated disease, helps to prevent disease progression and airway impairment, and avoids the added cost of multiple courses of antibiotics.

Clinicians are now presented with several sets of guidelines for the care of RTIs. These guidelines are intended to provide clinicians with general principles of disease management, and it is envisaged that these will be adapted to suit regional circumstances, local health care practices, and individual patient characteristics. All the guideline statements reflect thoughtful consideration by a panel of experts and should be viewed as recommendations for strategies of care and not definite stepwise rules of care. Indeed, clinicians must interpret such statements in the context that these recommendations cannot apply to all hypothetical settings. Rather, these statements represent general state-of-the-art documents, which require continuing change because of the changes in our understanding of these important infections. Educational efforts targeted toward clinicians as well as patients are necessary to encourage the implementation of guidelines, to avoid misuse of antibiotics for viral infections, and to prevent the prescription of antibiotics that are ineffective for treating the most likely respiratory pathogens. The judicious and rational use of appropriate antibiotic agents in the treatment of RTIs can help to improve the care of patients and reduce the complexities, costs, and disease complications that currently burden the management of these common conditions.

REFERENCES

1. File TF Jr. The epidemiology of respiratory tract infections Semin Respir Infect; 2000; 15:184–194.

2. Armstrong GL, Pinner RW. Outpatient visits for infectious diseases in the United States, 1980 through 1996 Arch Intern Med 1999; 159:2531–2536.

3. Wenzel RP, Edmond MB. Managing antibiotic resistance N Engl J Med; 2001; 343:1961–1962.

4. File TM Jr. Appropriate use of antimicrobials for drug-resistant pneumonia: focus on the significance of beta-lactam–resistant *S. pneumoniae* Clin Infect Dis; 2002; 34(Suppl 1):S17–S26.

5. Campbell GD Jr, Silberman R. Drug-resistant *Streptococcus pneumoniae* Clin Infect Dis; 1998; 26:1188–1195.

6. Leclercq R, Courvalin P. Resistance to macrolides and related antibiotics in *Streptococcus pneumoniae* Antimicrob Agents Chemother; 2002; 46:2727–2734.

7. Amsden GW. Pneumococcal macrolide resistance—myth or reality? J Antimicrob Chemother; 1999; 44:1–6.

8. Bishai W. The *in vivo-in vitro* paradox in pneumococcal respiratory tract infections J Antimicrob Chemother; 2002; 49: 433–436.

9. Lynch JP 3d, Martinez FJ. Clinical relevance of macrolide-resistant *Streptococcus pneumoniae* for community-acquired pneumonia Clin Infect Dis; 2002; 34(Suppl 1):S27–S46.

10. Siegel RE. The significance of serum vs tissue levels of antibiotics in the treatment of penicillin-resistant *Streptococcus pneumoniae* and community-acquired pneumonia. Are we looking in the wrong place? Chest; 1999; 116:535–538.

11. Rodvold KA, Gotfried MH, Danziger LH, Servi RJ. Intrapulmonary steady-state concentrations of clarithromycin and azithromycin in healthy adult volunteers Antimicrob Agents Chemother; 1997; 41:1399–1402.

12. Hyde TB, Gay K, Stephens DS, Vugia DJ, Pass M, Johnson S, Barrett NL, Schaffner W, Cieslak PR, Maupin PS, Zell ER, Jorgensen JH, Facklam RR, Whitney CG; Active Bacterial Core Surveillance/Emerging Infections Program Network. Macrolide resistance among invasive *Streptococcus pneumoniae* isolates JAMA;. Vol. 286, 2001:1857–1862.

13. Fogarty C, Goldschmidt R, Bush K. Bacteremic pneumonia due to multidrug-resistant pneumococci in 3 patients treated un-

successfully with azithromycin and successfully with levofloxacin Clin Infect Dis; 2000; 31:613–615.

14. Kelley MA, Weber DJ, Gilligan P, Cohen MS. Breakthrough pneumococcal bacteremia in patients being treated with azithromycin and clarithromycin Clin Infect Dis; 2000; 31: 1008–1011.

15. Musher DM, Dowell ME, Shortridge VD, Flamm RK, Jorgensen JH, Le Magueres P, Krause KL. Emergence of macrolide resistance during treatment of pneumococcal pneumonia N Engl J Med; 2002; 346:630–631.

16. Lonks JR, Garau J, Gomez L, Xercavins M, Ochoa de Echaguen A, Gareen IF, Reiss PT, Medeiros AA. Failure of macrolide antibiotic treatment in patients with bacteremia due to erythromycin-resistant Streptococcus pneumoniae Clin Infect Dis; 2002; 35:556–559.

17. Chen D, McGeer A, deAzavedo JC, Low DE, Low DE. Decreased susceptibility of Streptococcus pneumoniae to fluoroquinolones in Canada N Engl J Med; 1999; 341:233–239.

18. Ho PL, Yung RW, Tsang DN, Que TL, Ho M, Seto WH, Ng TK, Yam WC, Ng WW. Increasing resistance of Streptococcus pneumoniae to fluoroquinolones: results of a Hong Kong multicentre study in 2000 J Antimicrob Chemother; 2002; 49: 173–176.

19. McGee L, Goldsmith CE, Klugman KP. Fluoroquinolone resistance among clinical isolates of Streptococcus pneumoniae belonging to international multi-resistant clones J Antimicrob Chemother; 2002; 49:173–176.

20. Davidson R, Cavalcanti R, Brunton JL, Bast DJ, de Azavedo JC, Kibsey P, Fleming C, Low DE. Levofloxacin treatment failures of pneumococcal pneumonia in association with resistance N Engl J Med; 2002; 346:747–750.

21. Kays NB, Smith DW. Levofloxacin treatment failure in a patient with fluoroquinolone resistant Streptococcus pneumoniae pneumonia Pharmacotherapy; 2002; 22:395–399.

22. Ho PL, Tse WS, Tsang KW, Kwok TK, Ng TK, Cheng VC, Chan RM. Risk factors for acquisition of levofloxacin-resistant Streptococcus pneumoniae: a case-control study Clin Infect Dis; 2001; 32:701–707.

23. Interagency Task Force on Antimicrobial Resistance. Public Health Action Plan to Combat Antimicrobial Resistance. Atlanta: Centers for Disease Control and Prevention, 2001. Available at: www.cdc.gov/drugresistance/actionplan/.

24. Alliance for the Prudent Use of Antibiotics. Available at www.apua.org.

25. World Health Organization. Global Strategy for the Containment of Antimicrobial Resistance. Geneva: World Health Organization, 2001. Available at: www.who.international.

26. The European Commission. Communication from the Commission on a Community Strategy against Antimicrobial Resistance. Brussels: Commission of the European Communities, 2001:333. Available at: www.europa.eu.int.

27. Ball P, Baquero F, Cars O, File T, Garau J, Klugman K, Low DE, Rubinstein E, Wise R; Consensus Group on Resistance and Prescribing in Respiratory Tract Infection. Antibiotic therapy of community respiratory tract infection: strategies for optimal outcomes and minimized resistance emergence J Antimicrob Chemother; 2002; 49:31–40.

28. Hamm RM, Hicks RJ, Bemben DA. Antibiotics and respiratory infections: are patients more satisfied when expectations are met? J Fam Pract; 1996; 43:56–62.

29. Kristinsson KG, Hjalmarsdottir MA, Gudnason T. Continued decline in the incidence of penicillin non-susceptible pneumococci in Iceland, 38th Interscience Conference of Antimicrobial Agents and Chemotherapy, San Diego, September, 1998.

30. Seppala H, Klaukka T, Vuopio-Varkila J, Muotiala A, Helenius H, Lager K, Huovinen P. The effects of changes in the consumption of macrolide antibiotics on erythromycin resistance in group A streptococci in Finland N Engl J Med; 1997; 337: 441–446.

31. Pestotnik SL, Classen DC, Evans S, Burke JP. Implementing antibiotic practice guidelines through computer-assisted decision support: clinical and financial outcomes Ann Intern Med; 1996; 124:884–890.

32. Petersen KL, Hennessy TW, Parkinson AJ, Bruden D, Chiou L. Provider and community education decreases antimicrobial

use and carriages of penicillin-resistant *S. pneumoniae* in rural Alaska communities, 37th Annual Meeting of Infectious Diseases Society of America, Philadelphia, Nov 18–21, 1999.

33. Gonzales R, Steiner JF, Lum A, Barrett PH Jr. Decreasing antibiotic use in ambulatory practice: impact of a multidimensional intervention in the treatment of uncomplicated acute bronchitis in adults JAMA; 1999; 281:1512–1519.

34. Guillemot D, Henriet L, Lecoeur H, Weber P, Carbon C. Optimization of antibiotic rapidly decreases penicillin resistant *Streptococcus pneumoniae* carriage: the Aubeppin Study, 41st Interscience Congress on Antimicrobial Agents and Chemotherapy, Chicago, December 2001.

35. Dowell SF, Marcy SM, Phillips WR. Otitis media—principles of judicious use of antimicrobial agents Pediatrics; 1998; 101: 165–171.

36. Christenson B, Lunberg P, Hedlund J, Ortqvist A. Effects of a large-scale intervention with influenza and 23-pneumococcal vaccines in adults aged 65 years or older: a prospective study Lancet; 2001; 357:1008–1011.

37. Grimshaw JM, Russell IT. Effect of clinical guidelines on medical practice: a systematic review of rigorous evaluations Lancet; 1993; 342:1317–1322.

38. Beilby J, Marley J, Walder D. The impact of changes in antibiotic prescribing on patient outcomes in a community setting: a natural experiment in Australia, 37th Annual Meeting of the Infectious Diseases Society of America, Philadelphia, Nov 18–21, 1999.

39. Cabana MD, Rand CS, Powe NR, Wu AW, Wilson MH, Abboud PA, Rubin HR. Why don't physicians follow clinical practice guidelines? A framework for improvement JAMA; 1999; 282: 1458–1465.

40. Dowell SF, Butler JC, Giebink GS, Jacobs MR, Jernigan D, Musher DM, Rakowsky A, Schwartz B. Acute otitis media: management and surveillance in an era of pneumococcal resistance. A report from the Drug-Resistant *Streptococcus pneumoniae* Therapeutic Working Group Pediatr Infect Dis J; 1999; 18:1–9.

41. Varsano I, Volovitz B, Horev Z, Robinson J, Laks Y, Rosenbaum I, Cohen A, Eilam N, Jaber L, Fuchs C, Amir J. Intramuscular

ceftriaxone compared with oral amoxicillin-clavulanate for treatment of acute otitis media in children Eur J Pediatr; 1997; 156:858–863.

42. Amir J. Antimicrobial treatment guidelines for acute bacterial rhinosinusitis Otolaryngol Head Neck Surg; 2000; 123(Suppl): S1–S32.

43. Bisno AL. Acute pharyngitis N Engl J Med; 2001; 344:205–211.

44. Snow V, Mottur-Pilson C, Cooper RJ, Hoffman JR. Principles of appropriate antibiotic use for acute pharyngitis in adults Ann Intern Med; 2001; 134:506–508.

45. Hoffman JR. WHO Model Prescribing Information. Drugs Used in the Treatment of Streptococcal Pharyngitis and Prevention of Rheumatic Fever. Geneva: World Health Organization, 1999.

46. Bisno AL, Gerber MA, Gwaltney Jr, Kaplan EL, Schwartz RH. Practice guideline for the diagnosis and management of group A streptococcal pharyngitis Clin Infect Dis; 2002; 35:113–125.

47. Schwartz RH. Group A streptococcal infections Pickering LK, Ed Red Book 2000: Report on the Committee on Infectious Diseases. Elk Grove Village. IL: American Academy of Pediatrics, 2000:526–536.

48. Martin JM, Green M, Barbadora KA, Wald ER. Erythromycin-resistant group A streptococci in schoolchildren in Pittsburgh N Engl J Med; 2002; 346:1200–1206.

49. Niederman MS. Acute exacerbations of chronic bronchitis: The role of infection and the selection of appropriate therapy Pulm Crit Care Update; 1996; 27:1–8.

50. Bach PB, Brown C, Gelfand SE, McGory DC. Management of acute exacerbations of chronic obstructive pulmonary disease: a summary and appraisal of published evidence Ann Intern Med; 2001; 134:600–620.

51. Anthonisen NR, Manfreda J, Warren CPW, Hershfield ES, Harding GKM, Nelson NA. Antibiotic therapy in exacerbations of chronic obstructive pulmonary disease Ann Intern Med; 1987; 106:196–204.

52. Saint S, Bent S, Vittinghoff E, Grady D. Antibiotics in chronic obstructive pulmonary disease exacerbations: a meta-analysis JAMA; 1995; 273:957–960.

53. Snow V, Lascher S, Mottur-Pilson C. for the Joint Expert Panel on Chronic Obstructive Pulmonary Disease of the American College of Chest Physicians and the American College of Physicians–American Society of Internal Medicine. Evidence base for management of acute exacerbations of chronic obstructive pulmonary disease Ann Intern Med; 2001; 134:595–599.

54. Adams SG, Anzueto A. Antibiotic therapy in acute exacerbations of chronic bronchitis Semin Respir Infect; 2000; 15: 234–247.

55. Heffelfinger JD, Dowell SF, Jorgensen JH, Klugman KP, Mabry LR, Musher DM, Plouffe JF, Rakowsky A, Schuchat A, Whitney CG. Management of community-acquired pneumonia in the era of pneumococcal resistance: a report from the Drug-Resistant *Streptococcus pneumoniae* Therapeutic Working Group Arch Intern Med; 2000; 160:1399–1408.

56. Bartlett JG, Dowell SF, Mandell La, File Jr TM, Musher DM, Fine MJ. Guidelines from the Infectious Diseases Society of America. Practice guidelines for the management of community-acquired pneumonia in adults Clin Infect Dis; 2000; 31: 347–382.

57. Mandell LA, Marrie TJ, Grossman RF, Chow AW, Hyland RH. Canadian guidelines for the initial management of community-acquired pneumonia: an evidence-based update by the Canadian Infectious Diseases Society and the Canadian Thoracic Society Clin Infect Dis; 2000; 31:383–421.

58. Niederman MS, Mandell LA, Anzueto A, Bass JB, Broughton WA, Campbell GD, Dean N, File T, Fine MJ, Gross PA, Martinez F, Marrie TJ, Plouffe JF, Ramirez J, Sarosi GA, Torres A, Wilson R, Yu VL, Yu VL. Guidelines for the management of adults with community-acquired pneumonia Am J Respir Crit Care Med; 2001; 163:1730–1754.

59. Meehan TP, Fine MJ, Krumholz HM, Scinto JD, Galusha DH, Mockalis JT, Weber GF, Petrillo MK, Houck PM, Fine JM. Quality of care, process, and outcomes in elderly patients with pneumonia JAMA; 1997; 278:2080–2084.

60. Bratzler DW, Houck PM, Nsa W. Initial processes of care and outcomes in elderly patients with pneumonia Ann Emerg Med; 2001; 38(Suppl):S36.

61. Gleason PP, Kapoor WN, Stone RA, Lave JR, Obrosky DS, Schulz R, Singer DE, Coley CM, Marrie TJ, Fine MJ. Medical outcomes and antimicrobial costs with the use of the American Thoracic Society guidelines for outpatients with community-acquired pneumonia JAMA; 1997; 278:32–39.

62. Gordon GS, Throop D, Berberian L, Niederman M, Bass J. Validation of the therapeutic recommendations of the American Thoracic Society (ATS) guidelines for community-acquired pneumonia in hospitalized patients Chest; 1996; 110:55S.

63. Menendez R, Ferrando D, Valles D, Vallterra J. Influence of deviation from guidelines on the outcome of community-acquired pneumonia Chest; 2002; 122:612–617.

64. Stahl JE, Barza M, DesJardin J, Martin R, Eckman MH. Effect of macrolides as part of initial empiric therapy on length of stay in patients hospitalized with community-acquired pneumonia Arch Intern Med; 1999; 159:2576–2580.

65. Gleason PP, Meehan TP, Fine JM, Galusha DH, Fine MJ. Association between initial antimicrobial therapy and medical outcomes for hospitalized elderly patients with pneumonia Arch Intern Med; 1999; 159:2562–2572.

66. Dudas V, Hopefl A, Jacobs R, Guglielmo BJ. Antimicrobial selection for hospitalized patients with presumed community-acquired pneumonia: a survey of nonteaching US community hospitals Ann Pharmacother; 2000; 34:446–452.

67. Houck PM, MacLehose RF, Niederman MS, Lowery JK. Empiric antibiotic therapy and mortality among Medicare pneumonia inpatients in 10 Western states: 1993, 1995, and 1997 Chest; 2001; 119:1420–1426.

68. Jencks SF, Cuerdon T, Burwen DR, Fleming B, Houck PM, Kussmaul AE, Nilasena DS, Ordin DL, Arday DR. Quality of medical care delivered to Medicare beneficiaries JAMA; 2000; 284:1670–1676.

69. McCaig LF, Besser RE, Hughes JM. Trends in antimicrobial prescribing rates for children and adolescents JAMA; 2002; 287: 3133–3135.

16

Abbreviated Courses of Antibacterial Therapy

DEBBY BEN DAVID, GILI REGEV-YOCHAY, and ETHAN RUBINSTEIN

Infectious Diseases Unit, Sheba Medical Center,
Tel Aviv University School of Medicine,
Tel Hashomer, Israel

The length of antibiotic courses of therapy has rarely been rigorously studied, despite its apparent importance as a driver of microbial resistance in humans. Studies that were performed in the past have mainly concentrated on outpatient infections such as tuberculosis, malaria, and venereal diseases, with the main aim to keep compliance as high as possible and cost as low as possible. On the other hand, these issues in hospitalized patients were less relevant. The relevance and importance of bacterial resistance only started to be realized and seriously appreciated some 20 years ago, stressing the importance of the effect of antibiotic therapy on the development and spread of resistant microorganisms within hospitalized patients and individuals in the community. The introduction of new bactericidal agents with a rapid onset of action (particularly the carbapenems and fluoroquinolones), a deeper understanding of pharmacodynamics of antibacterial agents, and a better definition of patient populations have also contributed to the rationalization of antibiotic dosing and the ability to shorten antibiotic therapy courses. In this respect, one example is single-dose therapy for gonorrhea with ceftriaxone, cefixime, ciprofloxacin, ofloxacin, azithromycin, or doxycycline; therapy that previously lasted about 1 week. Very long courses of tuberculosis treatment have been reduced from around 18 to 24 months to much shorter periods—4 to 6 months in immunocompetent hosts (1)—as a result of the introduction of rifampin (a highly bactericidal agent) and directly observed therapy (DOT), which assures better compliance and therefore a lower rate of resistance development. The ability to treat meningococcal meningitis in children with 4 days of ceftriaxone therapy, or even a single administration of long-acting penicillin (2), or in adults with 2 days of ceftriaxone or 4 days of penicillin G also demonstrate the change occurring in our understanding of the necessary therapeutic period. In hospitals, the reduction of presurgical prophylaxis to a single dose (3) with no untoward effect on wound infection but with a significant reduction in resistant gram-negative wound isolates demonstrates the utility of short and ultra-short therapy and prophylaxis.

A course of therapy is conventionally defined as the time period during which an antimicrobial is administered. Because of the presence of counterfeit agents with decreased activity, irregular absorption, and other uncontrolled parameters, a better definition may be the period during which therapeutic concentrations are maintained at the site of infection.

The advantages of a short therapy (or prophylaxis) period include improved compliance of the patient with the reduction of the number of dosages and the period necessary for a full treatment course (4), reduced cost due to a decrease in the amount of drugs used and decreased cost of medical personnel and laboratory tests, and less waste of unused antibiotics. Obviously, when fewer antibiotics are prescribed, the risk for adverse events and drug–drug interaction is smaller. There is less risk for bacterial resistance development as well as of commensals if therapy is short. This has been shown to be true in the community (5), where therapy of upper respiratory tract infections in children for more than 7 days increased the risk of selection of penicillin-resistant *Streptococcus pneumoniae* (PRSP) (odds ratio [OR] = 5, 95% CI 1.3-9.8) compared with shorter treatment courses, as well as in the hospital, where prophylaxis for more than 48 hours increased the risk of acquired antibiotic resistance of Enterobacteriaceae and enterococci (OR 1.6 , CI 1.1-2.6) compared with prophylaxis for less than 48 hours (3). There is potentially less harm done to the ecology in the immediate vicinity of the patient and less risk of family members becoming carriers of resistant bacteria if fewer antibiotics are excreted and secreted from the patient into his or her immediate surroundings.

Evidently, there is a lower limit under which short therapy becomes ineffective. For example, for uncomplicated cystitis in women, short therapy of 3 days was as effective as 5-day and 7-day therapy. Nevertheless, reduction of the therapy course to less than 3 days was associated with an increasing rate of relapses and thus is not recommended (6). In addition, reducing the duration of therapy to less than 28 days in aortic valve endocarditis was associated with unsatisfactory results compared with a conventional duration of therapy. In another study, treating staphylococcal bacteremia for less than 10 days was associated with a high relapse rate (7). Similarly, in catheter-related *Staphylococcus aureus* bacteremia, therapy for more than 14 days was associated (albeit not significantly) with favorable outcomes, fewer complications, and a lower mortality rate (8).

A successful abbreviated treatment course depends on several mandatory factors, such as the patient, pathogen, infection site, and therapeutic agent (Table1), as well as the requirement that the host be fully immunocompetent so he or she can be cured with short courses of therapy. The host is required to have the full number of active leukocytes and macrophages, which are capable of killing bacteria. The host

Table 1   Features Necessary for a Successful Abbreviated Course of Therapy

Host factors	Pathogen factors	Infection factors	Antibiotic factors
Immuno-competent	Susceptible to antibiotics	At an easily accessible site	Bactericidal
Adequate white blood cell count	Low spontaneous mutation rate	Not as a biofilm	Rapid onset of action
Normal albumin level	Extracellular	Lack of foreign body	Lack of propensity to induce mutants
Adequately hydrated	Rapid multipli-cation rate	Not life threatening	Easy penetration into tissues
Adequately compliant		Caused by a single pathogen	Active against nondividing bacteria
		Not a closed space infection	Not affected by adverse conditions
		No adverse environmental factors	
		Early infectious state	

needs to be able to produce an adequate amount of antibodies and to be able to mount a satisfactory cell-mediated immune response. The patient (host) needs to have adequate concentrations of albumin to carry the antibiotic in the circulation and to have an adequate distribution of intra- and extracellular fluid to allow the agent to penetrate or diffuse to the sites of infection. The pathogen involved must be highly susceptible to the administered agent and must not have the tendency to develop resistance to the agent used (low spontaneous mutation rate). The pathogen should preferably be extracellular and divide frequently enough to allow for prolonged antibiotic-vulnerable periods. The infection should be at a site that is easily accessible to antibiotics; thus infections in sanctuaries such as the brain, prostate, and eye are not good candidates for abbreviated therapy courses. The pathogen, at the site of infection, should preferably be in a planktonic form and not adherent to solid phases such as bone and cartilage. The infection should not be life threatening nor should it be localized in or around foreign bodies to which the pathogen is adherent and at which it forms a biofilm. The infection should be caused by a single pathogen and should not be an abscess, empyema, or granuloma that does not allow antibiotics to penetrate or has conditions of low pH, acidity, white blood cell debris, or any other factor that inhibits antibiotic action. Experience has shown that infections on mucosal surfaces (e.g., upper and lower respiratory tract infections, intestinal infections, genitourinary infections) are best suited for abbreviated courses of therapy, whereas infections in the bones, joints or intracellular infections are not suited for such a treatment modality. The requirements for the agent to be successful in an abbreviated mode of therapy are that it must be bactericidal and must act rapidly—fulfilling Ehrlich's criteria: "Hit them early, hit them hard"—it must be associated with the lowest rate of resistance induction, and it must be able to penetrate easily into tissues and body fluids (requiring low molecular weight, low protein binding, and lipophilia). Agents with concentration-dependent bacteria-killing properties (e.g., aminoglycosides, fluoroquinolones, imidazoles) must be present at the site of infection in the highest concentrations possible. Agents with time-dependent bacteria-killing properties (e.g., beta-lactams, macrolides, glycopeptides) must be at the site of infection in concentrations above the minimum inhibitory concentration (MIC) for the required period of time (9).

GROUP A STREPTOCOCCAL PHARYNGITIS

Therapy of group A streptococcal (GAS) pharyngitis is intended to prevent both suppurative and nonsuppurative complications (rheumatic fever and perhaps poststreptococcal glomerulonephritis). To date, the treatment recommended by the American Heart Association, Infectious Diseases Society of America, and other organizations is 10 days of penicillin (10). Prevention of acute rheumatic fever is believed to require eradication of the infecting streptococci from the pharynx, an effect that depends on prolonged rather than high-dose penicillin therapy.

The efficacy of 10-day treatment with penicillin was first documented in the early 1950s. By 1953, the American Heart Association recommended treatment of GAS pharyngitis with oral penicillin for 10 days (11). In 1981, Schwartz et al. (12) reevaluated the duration of treatment in a study comparing patients with proven GAS infection treated for 7 or 10 days with penicillin V three times daily. The investigators concluded that the 10-day regimen was more effective than the 7-day regimen in eradicating GAS, but also concluded that persistence of GAS after adequate therapy may be common. It is now accepted that approximately 15% of patients continue to harbor the original infecting GAS serotype in their pharynx after completing a course of oral penicillin (10).

Gerber et al. (13), in a randomized, controlled trial, compared 5 versus 10 days of penicillin V treatment. Patients in the two treatment groups were comparable with respect to clinical findings, compliance, and serologic response to GAS. The same serotype of GAS was present at follow-up in 18% of the seventy-three patients treated for 5 days versus 6% of ninety-nine patients treated for 10 days. Thus, the need for 10 days of penicillin V treatment was confirmed.

Macrolides are an alternative choice, especially for penicillin-allergic patients. Several studies have examined short courses of various macrolides as an optional treatment for GAS pharyngitis. McCarty et al. (14) compared clarithromycin with penicillin V and demonstrated comparable rates of clinical success and a higher eradication rate with clarithromycin (94% vs. 78%). Boccazzi et al. (15) compared a 3-day azithromycin regimen to a 5-day ceftibuten regimen. They showed a somewhat higher eradication rate after ceftibuten than after azithromycin treatment. Yet, the widespread use of macrolides has been associated with the development of resistance by GAS, and this should limit the use of macrolides for GAS pharyngitis only to penicillin-allergic patients.

Oral cephalosporins are also highly effective in treating streptococcal pharyngitis. A meta-analysis of nineteen studies suggested that streptococcal eradication rates and clinical cure rates attained with these agents are even slightly higher than those achieved with penicillin (16). Since the mid-1990s, several randomized, controlled studies were carried out to compare shorter therapeutic courses (4 to 5 days of treatment) of cephalosporins with either the standard 10-day penicillin V regimen or with a 10-day treatment of cephalosporins. These studies demonstrated that the shorter treatments were equivalent or superior in bacteriologic eradication and clinical response. However, none of these studies evaluated the incidence of poststreptococcal sequelae. The general concern that shorter treatment courses might lead to an increased incidence of poststreptococcal sequelae was increased by clusters of rheumatic fever that occurred in the United States in the late 1980s.

Two recent European large-scale studies were performed by Adam et al. (17) to compare short-course treatments with the standard 10-day penicillin treatment. They evaluated 4,782 culture-proven cases of GAS pharyngitis and also measured the incidence of poststreptococcal sequelae at a follow-up of 1 year. They examined 5-day regimens with six antibiotics that had been shown effective in previous trials: amoxicillin-clavulanate, ceftibuten, cefuroxime axetil, loracarbef, clarithromycin, and erythromycin estolate. The 5-day regimens were as effective as the 10-day penicillin treatment. Both bacteriologic eradication and clinical success rates were equivalent. However, among patients treated with the short course, there were four cases of poststreptococcal late sequelae (three cases of rheumatic fever and one of glomerulonephritis), whereas only one patient in the 10-day penicillin group developed glomerulonephritis. The authors claimed that the poststreptococcal sequelae in these cases could not be definitely related to the streptococcal episode treated in the study according to their histories. A separate evaluation for cefuroxime axetil(5 days) versus penicillin (10 days) showed equivalence, with no streptococcal sequelae.

In summary, abbreviated courses (less than 10 days) of penicillin V were unsuccessful. Short courses of macrolide drugs have led to equivalent clinical and bacterial eradication results, but the concern of resistance development in GAS should limit these drugs to the treatment of penicillin-allergic patients only. Short courses of cephalosporins were equivalent or slightly better in clinical and bacterial eradication, but it is difficult to prove that poststreptococcal sequelae will not increase with these treatments, and the concern about antibiotic resistance should probably limit these drugs to the treatment of special cases. In addition, most of these agents are more expensive than penicillin, even when administered for short courses. Therefore, perhaps the best choice is still penicillin.

OTITIS MEDIA

Acute otitis media (AOM) remains one of the most common bacterial infections in childhood and the leading indication for antimicrobial use in this population. The objective of treating AOM is achieving rapid clinical relief and preventing complications such as mastoiditis, meningitis, and jugular vein thrombosis. Failure to eradicate the causative pathogens in the middle ear was shown to lead to a higher risk of relapse and long-term sequelae. Thus, most expert panels have recommended treating children with AOM. However, other studies demonstrated that even among bacterial infections, the majority will resolve spontaneously, with only a minor advantage of antibiotic treatment over nontreatment, and thus have recommended withholding antimicrobial treatment entirely in some or all cases of AOM unless symptoms persist or worsen (18).

Most clinical guidelines and expert panels still recommend 10 days of beta-lactams (drug of choice: amoxicillin) for most patients, some limiting this treatment to children younger than 2 years and allowing a shorter course of treatment (5 days) for older children (19).

Recently, interest in shortening the course of antibiotic therapy from the traditional 10 days to 5 days has emerged for reasons previously mentioned. Cefpodoxime, cefdinir, and azithromycin are the only oral antibiotics currently approved by the U.S. Food and Drug Administration for a 5-day short course of therapy for AOM.

A meta-analysis of randomized, controlled trials of shortened antibiotic therapy in AOM suggested that a 5-day course of a short-acting antibiotic was an effective treatment (20). However, patient subgroup sizes were too small to provide a reliable estimate of the risk of treatment failure in children younger than 2 years. Yet, it is precisely children in this age group who gain the greatest benefit from treatment and who have the highest risk of treatment failure.

When evaluating the results of AOM studies, it is particularly important to critically review the criteria used for diagnosis and for assessing outcome. In some of the previous trials, a combination of middle ear effusion and one or more nonspecific signs or symptoms has been considered sufficient. Outcomes in some of the studies have been based on symptomatic response alone, without regard to specific tympanic membrane findings, thus permitting inclusion of patients who do not actually have AOM but have otitis media with effusion (OME), a condition that is self-limited and has minor symptoms.

In summary, abbreviated 5-day courses have been shown to be equivalent to standard therapies in children older than 2 years and may be equivalent in those younger than 2 years who do not attend day care. Children younger than 2 years who attend day care should continue to receive the standard 10-day treatment in order to achieve good clinical success and prevent relapses.

ACUTE BACTERIAL SINUSITIS

Acute bacterial sinusitis is a common upper respiratory tract infection, with an estimated 20 million cases reported in the United States annually. There are no specific clinical features to distinguish between bacterial and viral etiologies. It is however accepted that patients who have symptoms of rhinosinusitis (purulent nasal secretions and maxillary facial pain) for less than 7 days are unlikely to have bacterial infection. The presence of symptoms for more than 7 days is a sensitive but nonspecific predictor of bacterial sinusitis. Two recent meta-analyses have concluded that antibiotics are statistically more efficacious than placebo in reducing symptoms, although their benefit is relatively small (21,22). It is generally recommended to initiate treatment with a narrow-spectrum agent, such as amoxicillin, doxycycline, or trimethoprim-sulfamethoxazole (TMP-SMX); however, these recommendations do not consider the increasing incidence of PRSP as a causative pathogen. The Sinus and Allergy Health Partnership published guidelines for treatment of bacterial rhinosinusitis recommending the stratification of patients according to severity of disease, rate of progression, recent antibiotic exposure, and local resistance data (23). Recommendations for initial therapy for adults with mild disease who have not received antibiotics include amoxicillin-clavulanate, amoxicillin (1.5 to 3 g/day), cefpodoxime proxetil, or cefuroxime axetil. However, the duration of therapy is not indicated in these guidelines.

As the optimal duration of antimicrobial treatment for acute sinusitis has not been adequately studied until recently, the duration of treatment was not well defined and was therefore generally based on physician preference. The standard duration of antibiotic treatment for acute bacterial sinusitis ranges between 7 and 14 days.

All the controlled comparative studies published between 1990 and 2002 that compared the efficacy of short-course treatment (fewer than 7 days) with that of a long course (more than 7 days) showed equivalent clinical and bacteriologic efficacy results for 3 to 5 days compared with 8 to 14 days of therapy with all agents studied. A single randomized, double-blind, placebo-controlled study compared amoxicillin-clavulanate administrated for 5 days versus a 10-day course (24). Risk factors of failure in the abbreviated course were a history of more than four bouts of sinusitis during the 2 years prior to therapy or a history of surgical drainage. Thus, longer treatment courses might be indicated for certain risk groups. Further studies are needed to resolve this question.

Azithromycin has a prolonged half-life, ranging between 2 and 5 days, and a slow release from tissues. These properties suggest that a short course of azithromycin could be comparable to prolonged antimicrobial therapy. Several studies demonstrated high efficacy of azithromycin in acute sinusitis when administered for 3 to 5 days. The response rates are comparable to those of prolonged therapy.

In summary, several studies have demonstrated similar efficacy of a short antimicrobial course compared with 8 to 14 days of antimicrobial treatment. Nevertheless, most studies included patients with maxillary sinusitis, and the results cannot be implicated for patients with frontal, methodical, or ethmoid sinusitis.

It is important to emphasize that most studies did not use sinus punctures to verify the bacterial etiology of sinusitis. As most cases of acute rhinosinusitis are caused by viruses and less than 2% are complicated by bacterial infection and there are no specific clinical features to distinguish between bacterial and viral etiologies, the true efficacy of prolonged antibiotic therapy compared with short-course therapy is difficult to assess.

COMMUNITY-ACQUIRED PNEUMONIA

The Infectious Diseases Society of America recommends treating pneumonia caused by *S. pneumoniae* until the patient is afebrile for 72 hours (25). Pneumonia due to bacteria that can cause necrosis of pulmonary parenchyma (e.g., *Staphylococcus aureus* or *Pseudomonas aeruginosa*) should be treated for longer than 2 weeks, and pneumonia due to atypical pathogens (e.g., *Mycoplasma pneumoniae* or *Chlamydia pneumoniae*) should be treated for at least 2 weeks. However, these recommendations are not based on randomized clinical trials and are supported by expert opinion only.

A recent study compared levofloxacin 750 mg/day administered once daily for 5 days with a course of levofloxacin 500 mg/day for 10 days in 530 patients with community-acquired pneumonia (CAP) (25a). Clinical success rates were 92.4% and

91.1% for the short and conventional therapy groups, respectively (95% CI -7.0-4.4), and microbiologic eradication rates were 93.2% and 92.4%, respectively. In the more severely ill patients (Pneumonia Severity Index class III, IV, and V), the clinical success rates were 90.8% and 84.9% for the short and conventional duration of therapy groups, respectively. Fourteen patients with pneumococcal bacteremia were identified, seven in each group. In the short-course therapy group all seven were cured, and in the conventional-duration group, one bacteremia persisted with a levofloxacin-susceptible *S. pneumoniae* strain. This study, which took advantage of the higher angle under the curve (AUC) obtained by the larger levofloxacin dose and higher concentrations of the drug in the various lung compartments, proved the ' "hit them early, hit them hard' " concept of Ehrlich and translated the pharmacodynamic advantages of levofloxacin into a clinically important achievement.

ACUTE EXACERBATION OF CHRONIC OBSTRUCTIVE PULMONARY DISEASE

Approximately 5% of Americans in their middle and late years have chronic bronchitis, which predisposes them to frequent episodes of bronchitis. Acute infectious exacerbation of chronic obstructive broncho-pulmonary disease (AE-COPD) contributes considerably to morbidity and mortality in this population. The benefit of antibiotics in AE-COPD in reducing mortality and morbidity has been demonstrated in several randomized, placebo-controlled studies. A meta-analysis demonstrated a small but statistically significant improvement due to antibiotic therapy in AE-COPD (26).

The optimal duration of antibiotic treatment has not been well defined and is generally based on physician preference. The administration of 10 to 14 days of treatment has been the standard. During the past few years, a large number of studies have been published supporting the use of short-course antimicrobial therapy in AE-COPD. Most studies used different antibiotic regimens that compared the efficacy of a short course (fewer than 7 days) with that of a long course (more than 7 days). All trials enrolled patients with a clinical diagnosis of AE-COPD. Across studies involving 6,629 patients published between 1988 and 2001, clinical and bacteriologic efficacy of various classes of antibiotics were equivalent for 3 to 5 days, compared with 8 to 14 days of therapy.

The new fluoroquinolones have a wide antimicrobial activity (including PRSP, *Haemophilus influenzae*, and atypical pathogens) and favorable pharmacokinetics and pharmacodynamics, including high bioavailability, extensive distribution into respiratory fluids, long elimination half-life, and potent and rapid killing. Based on their pharmacokinetic and pharmacodynamic profile, a shorter course of fluoroquinolones could have an efficacy equivalent to the traditional 10 to 14 days of therapy for AE-COPD. Several randomized trials have demonstrated high efficacy of the new fluoroquinolones in the treatment of AE-COPD. Abbreviated courses of various fluoroquinolones had similar efficacy compared with standard-duration therapy.

In summary, most studies have demonstrated similar efficacy of a short course of antimicrobial therapy in AE-COPD compared with standard-duration therapy. Therefore, abbreviated therapy should be considered for AE-COPD.

URINARY TRACT INFECTIONS

When considering treatment for urinary tract infections (UTIs), the prognosis of the untreated infection and the long-term results to be expected from therapy should be measured and compared with the side effects, cost, and inconvenience of different therapeutic regimens. As the prognosis of UTI in nonpregnant adult women is excellent and reinfection is common, therapy probably makes little contribution to the patient's well-being other than alleviating the symptoms. Hundreds of patients have been followed for years with persistent or recurrent infections without documenting progression of renal disease caused by the infection. Bacteriuria in the elderly is associated with degenerative and debilitating diseases but does not seem to aggravate the underlying condition. Thus, most experts do not recommend routine treatment of asymptomatic bacteriuria in the elderly.

Asymptomatic as well as symptomatic bacteriuria in preschool children with vesicouretheral reflux may result in stunted growth of the kidney, scar formation, and, rarely, renal failure. Bacteriuria in pregnancy may also have serious implications, such as preterm delivery, delivery of newborn with reduced body weight, and others. Thus, treatment of children and pregnant women is most likely to be beneficial.

Symptomatic patients, regardless of age, should be adequately treated, even when infection is likely to recur.

In the past, 7 to 10 days of therapy were routinely recommended for patients with lower-tract symptoms. However, in recent years, it has become apparent that most women with lower UTI have only a superficial mucosal infection that can be cured with much shorter courses of therapy, even with a single dose of an antimicrobial agent.

Short-course therapy with sulfonamides for UTI has been intensively studied, and more than seventy reports have been published. A meta-analysis of these trials revealed that single-dose therapy was less effective than longer-duration regimens (87% vs. 94% eradication), but 3-day regimens were equivalent to longer-duration treatments and were associated with a lower rate of adverse events (6).

Several trials have demonstrated the efficacy of a single dose of ciprofloxacin; however, this drug, like most agents studied, appeared to be more effective when given as a 3-day regimen (27). Since 1995, several randomized, controlled studies have confirmed that short courses of therapy (3 days) for fluoroquinolones and TMP-SMX are superior to 7-day treatments with the same drugs, mainly because of the lower rate of adverse events. McCarty et al. (28) showed equivalent efficacy of a 3-day course of ofloxacin, ciprofloxacin, and TMP-SMX. Iravani et al. (29) showed that in a 4- to 6-week follow-up, 100 mg of ciprofloxacin twice daily for 3 days had a higher bacteriologic eradication rate than 7-day TMP-SMX or nitrofurantoin (91% vs. 79% and 82%, respectively). The short-course ciprofloxacin therapy also resulted in fewer adverse events and similar clinical efficacy. Resistance has been increasing to the quinolones among strains of *Escherichia coli*, thus low doses should be avoided.

Nitrofurantoin short courses had a significantly lower eradication rate than TMP-SMX and should therefore be administered for a minimum of 7 days (30). Beta-lactam short-course therapy studies revealed that all beta-lactam regimens (e.g., amoxicillin, pivmecillinam, cefadroxil) were less effective when given in a regimen shorter than 7 days, demonstrating higher recurrence and lower eradication rates with the short courses. Several studies have compared a single dose of fosfomycin with longer-duration regimens. However, single-dose fosfomycin has not been compared with longer-duration treatments with the same drug. Many of the randomized, controlled trials examining fosfomycin were small, thus had only moderate power. Studies comparing single-dose fosfomycin to single-dose fluoroquinolone regimens had inconsistent results, some showing fosfomycin to be less effective, others showing it to have slightly higher or similar eradication rates.

To summarize: Beta-lactam and nitrofurantoin short-course regimens have failed and are less effective than the standard 7-day regimens. Three-day regimens of TMP-SMZ are equivalent to longer-duration treatments and may be the drug of choice in areas in which the resistance rate to this drug is low. Three-day regimens of fluoroquinolones are equivalent to longer-duration regimens and may be more effective than 3-day regimens of TMP-SMZ in areas where resistance to the latter is high. The data regarding single-dose fosfomycin are still not empowered enough to recommend it as first-line therapy. However, increasing resistance rates to fluoroquinolones in some areas may drive experts to recommend fosfomycin single-dose therapy as the preferable drug of choice.

INTESTINAL INFECTIONS

Intestinal infections are the most amenable to abbreviated courses of therapy because, in most instances, the pathogen is located on the epithelial surface or has penetrated the intestinal epithelial cell but has not invaded other tissues. The pathogen is classically a rapidly dividing bacterium, there is no foreign body, and the peristalsis of the intestine inhibits biofilm formation. The major obstacles to abbreviated therapy in this setting are the penetration of the antibiotic into the intestinal lumen and epithelial cells, the adverse effect of fecal material on the antibacterial activity of the agent (binding to fecal material), and the inactivation of the antimicrobial agent by neighboring bacteria that may produce extracellular enzymes, e.g., beta-lactamases, aminoglycoside-inactivating enzymes.

A randomized, double-blind, controlled trial compared 5-day ciprofloxacin with 5-day azithromycin therapy in seventy adult hospitalized men with shigellosis in Bangladesh (31). Clinical success (determined as disappearance of loose stools on day 5 and temperature below 37.8°C [100°F] on day 3) and bacteriologic eradication rates were equal in both groups. A study of 135 Vietnamese children with bacillary dysentery in a region with a high rate of multidrug-resistant shigellosis (of sixty-three isolates, 62% were multidrug resistant) compared the conventional therapy of nalidixic acid (55 mg/kg for 5 days) with two doses of ofloxacin (total 15 mg/kg). Resolution time for fever and diarrhea were similar; excretion time for stool pathogens was longer in the nalidixic acid group. The rate of treatment failure was 25% in the nalidixic acid group compared with 10% in the ofloxacin group ($p > 0.1$). The authors concluded that the two regimens were equally effective, thus a preference for the shorter therapy was obvious (32).

TYPHOID FEVER

Typhoid fever has traditionally been treated with 10 to 14 days of therapy with chloramphenicol and ceftriaxone. Attempts have been made to shorten the treatment period of ceftriaxone from 10 to 14 days to 5 to 7 days, but the long-term relapse rate has remained undefined (33). The current practice is to administer systemic antibiotic until the patient's fever is reduced and to continue with an oral cephalosporin for a total of 10 to 14 days. The fluoroquinolones, because of their *in vitro* activity against Salmonelleae, intracellular penetration, and transepithelial intestinal elimination reaching high intraepithelial concentrations, were considered attractive for shorter treatments of typhoid fever and other systemic salmonellosis (34). Seven-day treatment with ciprofloxacin 500 mg twice daily was compared with azithromycin 1 g initial oral dose followed by 500 mg once daily for 6 additional days in 123 Egyptian patients. Cure was similar in the two groups, with similar time to defervescence in both groups and no relapse in either group (35). When a 5-day course of ofloxacin 200 mg twice daily was compared with a 3-day course of ceftriaxone 3 g once daily, ofloxacin cured 100% of patients (twenty-two of twenty-two) whereas ceftriaxone cured eighteen of twenty-five patients (72%, $p = 0.01$), with defervescence in the ofloxacin group occurring far earlier than in the ceftriaxone group (36). In a study that compared ofloxacin 3 days to 5 days in multidrug-resistant typhoid fever in 438 patients in Vietnam, both regimens were equally effective (37). For fluoroquinolone-resistant and nalidixic acid–resistant *Salmonella typhi* (NARST), patients were treated with ofloxacin and the time for blood clearance was double (156 hours) for susceptible strains. A third of the NARST patients required retreatment (compared with 0.4% of those with susceptible strains). NARST-infected patients were, however, effectively treated with short-course (5-day) azithromycin therapy, with rapid defervescence, sterilization of stool cultures, and no relapses (38).

COMPLICATED INTRA-ABDOMINAL INFECTIONS

Because of the wide variety of organism combinations that are their etiologic agents and because they occur both in the community and hospital settings, complicated intra-abdominal infections are difficult to bring under a common denominator. A large variety of antimicrobials have been used, as single drugs or as combinations. For example, severe infections have been treated with piperacillin-tazobactam, imipenem-cilastatin, meropenem, third- and fourth-generation cephalosporins plus metronidazole, ciprofloxacin plus metronidazole, and aztreonam plus metronidazole. The most important point is the timing of the start of antimicrobial therapy, 24 hours or less before spread has been established. Antimicrobial therapy should be continued until the resolution of clinical signs of infection, including the normalization of temperature. The risk of failure appears to be low in patients who do not have evidence of clinical infection at the time of antibiotic discontinuation (38a). If fever and other signs of infection persist or recur after 5 to 7 days of effective therapy, appropriate diagnostic evaluation should be initiated while the patient continues to receive therapy (38b).

ENDOCARDITIS

In the thirteenth edition of *Cecil-Loeb Textbook of Medicine* (1971), Paul Beeson (38c), one of the best-known physicians interested in endocarditis, wrote that in cases in which signs and symptoms were favorable, 2- or 3-week therapy was sufficient, whereas in abacteremic patients or in those with long-standing disease, large vegetations, or relatively resistant organisms, it was wiser to continue therapy for 6 to 10 weeks. Today, infections with penicillin-susceptible streptococci and *Streptococcus bovis* (having penicillin MIC of 0.1 µg/mL or less) require a 2-week regimen of ceftriaxone or penicillin G combined with gentamicin, as long as the patient does not have extracardiac foci of infection, myocardial abscess, or prosthetic valve endocarditis. When the pathogen is relatively resistant to penicillin (MIC 0.1 to 0.5 µg/mL), penicillin (or ceftriaxone) for 4 weeks is required, accompanied in the first 2 weeks by gentamicin. In right-sided staphylococcal endocarditis in intravenous drug abusers, 2-week therapy with methicillin (or nafcillin) combined with gentamicin is necessary (39,40). The reason for shortening the therapy duration may be greater awareness of the possibility of endocarditis—which is now supported by heart echocardiography, allowing for earlier diagnosis—and a

deeper understanding of the pharmacokinetics and pharmacodynamics of the antibiotics used for treating this infection.

NOSOCOMIAL INFECTIONS

The widespread use of antibiotics in hospitals has a substantial impact on the cost of care, side effects, and spread of resistant microorganisms. Generally, nosocomial infections are
treated for 10 to 14 days. However, there are no randomized
clinical studies evaluating the optimal duration of antimicrobial treatment in most nosocomial infections. As the majority
of the hospitalized patients who develop infections are critical
patients who are immunocompromised, patients who have
undergone surgery, elderly patients, and patients with foreign
bodies, an abbreviated antimicrobial course could lead to therapeutic failure or relapse. On the other hand, prolonged antimicrobial therapy exposes these patients to drug toxicity and
the emergence of resistant microorganisms on an individual
level as well as affecting the ecology of the hospital or unit.

Nosocomial Pneumonia

Respiratory tract infections account for approximately 50% of
all antibiotics prescribed in intensive care units (ICUs). The
optimal duration of antimicrobial treatment in nosocomial
pneumonia has not been well defined. A short course of antimicrobial therapy has the potential disadvantage of therapeutic
failure or relapse. The American Thoracic Society recommends
that the duration be adapted to the severity of the disease,
time to clinical response, and microorganism involved (41).
Prolonged antimicrobial treatment is recommended for mul-
tilobar involvement, cavitation and isolation of *P. aeruginosa*
or *Acinetobacter* spp, and pneumonia associated with bacteremia. A short antimicrobial treatment (7 to 10 days) is recommended for *S. aureus* and *H. influenzae* pneumonia.

   A prospective nonrandomized clinical study of ventilator-
associated pneumonia (VAP) evaluated the efficacy of a clinical
guideline restricting the total duration of antimicrobial therapy to 7 days (42). The mean duration of treatment in the first

period was 14.8 days compared with 8.6 days. No significant differences in hospital mortality or hospital length of stay were found between the two study groups. However, patients in the before-evaluation group were more likely to develop a second episode of VAP compared with those in the after-evaluation group (24.0% vs. 7.7%, p = 0.030). In a French study conducted in 51 ICU during 1999–2002. 401 patients were included, 197 were randomized to receive an 8 days course and 204 patients were randomized to received a 15 days course of antibiotic therapy. The demographic characteristics of the two groups were similar with a mean age of 60 years, the majority being males, with 60–70% being medical admission to an ICU, with an average SOFA grade of 7.3–7.4 with half the patients having ARDS.

In a recent study from France (42a), 401 patients were randomly assigned to receive 8 days or 15 days of antibiotic therapy, the regimen having been selected by the treating physician. Patients treated for 8 days had neither excess mortality (18.8% vs. 17.2%; difference, 1.6%; 90% CI -3.7-6.9) nor more-recurrent infections (28.9% vs. 26.0%; difference, 2.9%; 90% CI -3.2-9.1), but they had more antibiotic-free days (13.1 ± 7.4 vs. 8.7 ± 5.2, p < .001). The number of mechanical ventilation–free days, number of organ failure–free days, and length of ICU stay, as well as mortality rates on day 60 for the two groups, did not differ. Patients with VAP caused by nonfermenting gram-negative bacilli, including *P. aeruginosa*, did not have more unfavorable outcomes when antimicrobial therapy lasted only 8 days, although they did have a higher pulmonary infection-recurrence rate compared with those receiving 15 days of treatment (40.6% vs. 25.4%; difference, 15.2%; 90% CI 3.9-26.6). Among patients who developed recurrent infections, multiresistant pathogens emerged less frequently in those who had received 8 days of antibiotics (42.1% vs. 62.0% of pulmonary recurrences, p = .04).

These two studies suggest that even VAP and nosocomial pneumonia can be treated for shorter periods of time if caused by nonfermenting gram-negative bacteria. Such a treatment reduction may accelerate discharge from the ICU, have a strong cost-saving effect, and, most importantly, minimize the development of multidrug-resistant organisms causing pneumonia.

Because VAP in the ICU has a high attributable mortality, empiric antimicrobial treatment is prescribed when new pulmonary infiltrates appear, despite a low likelihood of infection. In a randomized clinical study (43), patients with a low likelihood of nosocomial pneumonia (clinical pulmonary infection score [CPIS] <6) were randomized to receive ciprofloxacin (experimental group) for 3 days or standard therapy (choice and duration of antibiotics at the discretion of physician). Antibiotics were continued beyond 3 days in 90% of patients in the standard–therapy group compared with 28% in the ciprofloxacin group. The duration of antibiotics in patients with CPIS <6 and no other documented infection was 3 days, compared with 9.8 days for the standard-therapy group. Mortality and length of hospital stay did not differ between the two groups. Nevertheless, antimicrobial resistance or superinfection was documented in 15% of patients in the ciprofloxacin group, compared with 35% in the control group. Antimicrobial cost was significantly lower in the ciprofloxacin group. Such an approach in patients with mild-to-moderate nosocomial pneumonia, including VAP, may lead to significantly lower antimicrobial therapy costs, antimicrobial resistance rates, and superinfections.

Catheter-Related Bloodstream Infections

Currently, there are no randomized, controlled clinical trials evaluating the optimal duration of therapy for bloodstream infection. Patients with catheter-related bacteremia are separated into those with complicated infections (e.g., endocarditis, septic thrombosis) and those with uncomplicated infections. Patients with an uncomplicated infection should receive 10 to 14 days of antimicrobial therapy. Patients with complicated bacteremia should receive a prolonged course of antimicrobial therapy (4 to 6 weeks). There are no randomized trials evaluating the efficacy of abbreviated courses.

Nosocomial *S. aureus* bacteremia is a serious and common disease often associated with serious complications, including septic thrombosis, infective endocarditis, osteomyelitis, and metastatic abscesses. Despite several studies, the optimal duration of antimicrobial treatment for catheter-related *S. aureus* bacteremia (CRSAB) remains unknown. In the past, CRSAB was treated for 4 to 6 weeks, but recent studies have reported a low complication rate when the duration of treatment was 10 to 14 days. In several retrospective studies among patients with CRSAB and no early complications, a 10- to 15-day course of parenteral antibiotics was equivalent to longer courses of therapy (44). However, treatment with antimicrobial agents for less than 10 days appeared to be inadequate because of a high rate of relapse. Delayed removal of the catheter is associated with a high rate of relapse. A meta-analysis of studies reporting outcomes for patients with *S. aureus* bacteremia treated with short-course therapy (2 weeks or less) identified eleven studies (45). Late-complication rate ranged from 0% to 29%, and the relapse rate was 6.1%. However, most of the studies were uncontrolled.

No controlled trials have assessed the optimal duration of antibiotic treatment of catheter-related bloodstream infection due to gram-negative bacilli. Randomized trials are necessary to determine the optimalduration of treatment for bloodstream infection caused by various microorganisms.

SUMMARY

In summary, there is good evidence for shortening antibiotic therapy, provided the correct treatment is applied to the appropriate patient in a well-defined patient population for a clearly defined infection caused by a known pathogen with known antibiotic susceptibilities. Most efforts in this field have been dedicated to infections that can be treated on an outpatient basis; for severe infections, determining the appropriate length of therapy still needs additional data.

Antibiotic courses can probably be shortened in streptococcal pharyngitis if newer agents are used. The therapy course for otitis media in children older than 2 years can probably also be shortened, whereas in younger children attending day care, therapy should last longer. In women with uncomplicated cystitis, there is little justification to extend therapy beyond 3 days. Surgical prophylaxis is best conducted with a single antibiotic administration, provided the procedure will not take longer than 4 to 6 hours.

Duration of therapy for AE-COPD can be limited to 5 days with the new fluoroquinolones and other newer agents. In uncomplicated sinusitis, duration of therapy usually may also be shortened. Duration of therapy for endocarditis in intravenous drug abusers and in left-sided endocarditis caused by highly penicillin-susceptible streptococci may also be shortened considerably with adequate laboratory and clinical follow-up. In CAP, the treatment period can be shortened provided the most effective therapy is used at the maximum tolerable dose. In nosocomial pneumonia and many other severe infections, duration of therapy is probably too long. For VAP therapy, it has been shown convincingly that shortening the duration of therapy to 8 days is acceptable, provided nonfermenting bacteria are not the etiologic agents.

Evidently, with the antibiotics used presently, there is a limit to how short therapy can be. Available data suggest that shortening the duration of therapy to less than 3 days in uncomplicated cystitis is inappropriate and treating staphylococcal bacteremia for less than 10 days is associated with a higher failure rate and relapse. Treating streptococcal pharyngitis with penicillin requires 10 days of therapy if sequelae need to be eliminated.

REFERENCES

1. Cohn DL, Catlin BJ, Peterson KL, Judson FN, Sbarbaro JA. A 62-dose, 6-month therapy for pulmonary and extrapulmonary tuberculosis: a twice-weekly, directly observed, and cost-effective regimen Ann Intern Med; 1990; 112:407–415.

2. Macfarlane JT, Anjorin FI, Cleland PG, Hassan-King M, Tor-Agbidye S, Wali SS, Weir WR, Whittle HC, Yahaya HN, Greenwood BM. Single injection treatment of meningococcal meningitis. 1. Long-acting penicillin Trans R Soc Trop Med Hyg; 1979; 73:693–697.

3. Habarth S, Samore NH, Lichtenberg D, Carmeli Y. Prolonged antibiotic prophylaxis after cardiovascular surgery and its ef-

fect on surgical site infection and antimicrobial resistance Circulation; 2000; 101:2916–2922.

4. Kardas P. Patient compliance in antibiotic treatment for respiratory tract infections J Antimicrob Chemother; 2002; 49: 897–903.

5. Guillemot D, Carbon C, Balkau B, Geslin P, Lecoeur H, Vauzelle-Kervroedan F, Bouvenot G, Eschwege E. Low dosage and long treatment duration of beta-lactam: risk factors for carriage of penicillin-resistant *Streptococcus pneumoniae* JAMA; 1998; 279:365–370.

6. Warren JW, Abrutyn E, Hebel JR, Johnson JR, Schaeffer AJ, Stamm WE. Guidelines for antimicrobial treatment of uncomplicated acute bacterial cystitis in women. Infectious Diseases Society of America Clin Infect Dis; 1999; 29:745–758.

7. Iannini P, Crossley K. Therapy of *Staphylococcus aureus* bacteremia associated with a removable focus of infection Ann Int Med; 1976; 84:558–560.

8. Zeylemaker MM, Jaspers CA, van Kraaij MG, Visser MR, Hoepelman IM. Long-term infectious complications and their relation to treatment duration in catheter-related *Staphylococcus aureus* bacteremia Eur J Clin Microbiol Infect Dis; 2001; 20:380–384.

9. Craig WA. Does the dose matter? Clin Infect Dis; 2001; 15(Suppl 3):S233–S237.

10. Bisno AL, Gerber MA, Gwaltney JM Jr, Kaplan EL, Schwartz RH. Diagnosis and management of group A streptococcal pharyngitis: a practice guideline Clin Infect Dis; 1997; 25:574–583.

11. Breese BB, Bellows MT, Fischel EE, Kuttner A, Maesell BF, Rammelkamp HJ. Prevention of rheumatic fever; statements of American Heart Association Council on rheumatic fever and congenital heart disease JAMA; 1953; 151:141–143.

12. Schwartz RH, Wientzen RL, Pedreira F, Feroli EJ, Mella GW, Guandolo VL. Penicillin V for group A streptococcal pharyngotonsilitis—a randomized trial of seven vs. ten days therapy JAMA; 1981; 246:1790–1795.

13. Gerber MA, Randolph MF, Chanatry J, Wright LL, DeMeo K, Kaplan EL. Five vs. ten days of penicillin V therapy for streptococcal pharyngitis Am J Dis Child; 1987; 141:224–227.

14. McCarty J, Hedrick JA, Gooch WM. Clarithromycin suspension vs. penicillin V suspension in children with streptococcal pharyngitis Adv Ther; 2000; 17:14–26.

15. Boccazzi A, Tonelli P, Angelis M, Bellussi L, Passali D, Careddu P. Short course therapy with ceftibuten vs. azithromycin in pediatric streptococcal pharyngitis Ped Infect Dis J; 2000; 19: 963–967.

16. Pichichero ME, Margolis PA. A comparison of cephalosporins and penicillins in the treatment of group A streptococcal pharyngitis: a meta-analysis supporting the concept of microbial co-pathogenicity Pediatr Infect Dis J; 1991; 10:275–281.

17. Adam D, Scholz H, Helmerking M. Short-course antibiotic treatment of 4782 culture proven cases of group A streptococcal tonsillopharyngitis and incidence of poststreptococcal sequelae J Infect Dis; 2000; 182:509–516.

18. Van Buchem FL, Dunk JH, van' Hof MA. Therapy of acute otitis media: myringotomy, antibiotics or either? A double-blind study in children Lancet; 1981; 2:883–887.

19. Dowell SF, Butler JC, Giebink GS, Jacobs MR, Jernigan D, Musher DM, Rakowsky A, Schwartz B. Acute otitis media: management and surveillance in an era of pneumococcal resistance—a report from the drug-resistant *Streptococcus pneumoniae* Therapeutic Working Group Pediatr Infect Dis J; 1999; 18:1–9.

20. Kozyrskyj AL, Hildes-Ripstein GE, Longstaffe SE, Wincott JL, Sitar DS, Klassen TP, Moffatt ME. Treatment of acute otitis media with shortened course of antibiotics: a meta-analysis JAMA; 1998; 279:1738–1742.

21. Williams JW Jr, Aguilar C, Makela M, Cornell J, Holleman DR, Chiquette E, Simel DL. Antibiotic therapy for acute sinusitis: a systematic literature review Cochrane Database Syst Rev; 2000:CD000243.

22. Zucher DR, Balk E, Engels E. Agency for Health Care Policy and Research Publication No. 99-E016: Evidence Report/Technology Assessment Number 9. Diagnosis and Treatment of Acute Bacterial Rhinosinusitis. Available at: www.ahrq.gov/clinic/sinussum.htm.

23. Engels E. Antimicrobial treatment guidelines for acute bacterial rhinosinusits Otolaryngol Head Neck Surg; 2000; 123(Suppl 1):4–32.

24. Gehanno P, Beauvillain C, Bobin S, Chobaut JC, Desaulty A, Dubreuil C, Klossek JM, Pessey JJ, Peyramond D, Strunski A, Chastang C. Short therapy with amoxicillin/clavulanate and corticosteroids in acute sinusitis: results of a multicentere study in adults Scand J Infect Dis; 2000; 32:679–684.

25. Bartlett JG, Dowell SF, Mandell LA, File Jr TM, Musher DM, Fine MJ. Practice guidelines for the management of community acquired pneumonia in adults Clin Infect Dis; 2000; 31: 347–382.

25a. Dunbar LM, Wunderink RG, Habib MP, Smith LG, Tennenberg AM, Khashab MM, Wiesinger BA, Xiang JX, Zadeikis N, Kahn JB. High-dose, short-course levofloxacin for community-acquired pneumonia: a new treatment paradigm Clin Inf Dis; 2003; 37:752–760.

26. Saint S, Bent S, Vittinghoff E, Grady D. Antibiotics in chronic obstructive pulmonary disease exacerbations. A meta-analysis JAMA; 1995; 273:957–960.

27. Iravani A, Tice AD, McCarty J, Sikes DH, Nolen T, Gallis HA, Whalen EP, Tosiello RL, Heyd A, Kowalsky SF. Short-course ciprofloxacin treatment of acute uncomplicated urinary tract infection in women; the minimum effective dose Arch Intern Med; 1995; 155:485–494.

28. McCarty JM, Richard G, Huck W, Tucker RM, Tosiello RL, Shan M, Heyd A, Echols RM. A Randomized trial of short-course ciprofloxacin, ofloxacin, or trimethoprim/sulfamethoxazole for the treatment of acute urinary tract infection in women. Ciprofloxacin Urinary Tract Infection Group Am J Med; 1999; 106: 292–299.

29. Iravani A, Klimberg I, Briefer C, Munera C, Kowalsky SF, Echols RM, Echols RM. A trial comparing low-dose, short-course ciprofloxacin and standard 7-day therapy with co-trimoxazole or nitrofurantoin in the treatment of uncomplicated urinary tract infections J Antimicrob Chemother; 1999; 43(Suppl A):67–75.

30. Hooton TM, Winter C, Tiu F, Stamm WE. Randomized comparative trial and cost analysis of 3-day antimicrobial regimens for treatment of acute cystitis in women JAMA; 1995; 273:41–45.

31. Khan WA, Seas C, Dhar U, Salam MA, Bennish ML. Treatment of shigellosis: a comparison of azithromycin and ciprofloxacin.

A double randomized controlled trial Ann Intern Med; 1997; 126:697–703.

32. Vinh H, Wain J, Chinh MT, Tam CT, Trang PT, Nga D, Echeverria P, Diep TS, White NJ, Parry CM. Treatment of bacillary dysentery in Vietnamese children: two doses of ofloxacin versus 5-day nalidixic acid Trans R Soc Trop Med Hyg; 2000; 94: 323–326.

33. Moosa A, Rubidge CJ. Once daily ceftriaxone vs. chloramphenicol for treatment of typhoid fever in children Pediatr Infect Dis J; 1989; 8:696–699.

34. Alam MN, Haq SA, Das KK, Baral PK, Mazid MN, Siddique RU, Rahman KM, Hasan Z, Khan MA, Dutta P. Efficacy of ciprofloxacin in enteric fever: comparison of treatment durations in sensitive and multidrug- resistant *Salmonella* Am J Trop Med Hyg; 1995; 53:306–311.

35. Girgis NI, Butler T, Frenck RW, Sultan Y, Brown FM, Tribble D, Khakhria R. Azithromycin versus ciprofloxacin for treatment of uncomplicated typhoid fever in a randomized trial in Egypt that included patients with multidrug resistance Antimicrob Agents Chemother; 1999; 43:1441–1444.

36. Smith MD, Duong NM, Hoa NT, Wain J, Ha HD, Diep TS, Day NP, Hien TT, White NJ. Comparison of ofloxacin and ceftriaxone for short-course treatment of enteric fever Antimicrob Agents Chemother; 1994; 38:1716–1720.

37. Tran TH, Bethell DB, Nguyen TT, Wain J, To SD, Le TP, Bui MC, Nguyen MD, Pham TT, Walsh AL. Short-course of ofloxacin for treatment of multidrug-resistant typhoid Clin Infect Dis; 1995; 20:917–923.

38. Chinh NT, Parry CM, Thi Ly N, Duy Ha M, Xuan Tong M, Song Diep T, Wain J, White NJ, Farrar JJ. A randomized controlled comparison of azithromycin and ofloxacin for treatment of multidrug-resistant or nalidixic-acid resistant enteric fever Antimicrob Agents Chemother; 2000; 44:1855–1859.

38a. Lennard ES, Dellinger EP, Wertz MJ, Minshaw BH. Implication of leucocytosis and fever at conclusion of antibiotic therapy for intra-abdominal sepsis Ann Surg; 1982; 195:19–24.

38b. Solomkin JS, Mazuski JE, Baron EJ, Sawyer RG, Nathens AB, DiPiro JT, Buchman T, Dellinger EP, Jernigan J, Gorbach S,

Chow AW, Bartlett J. Infectious Diseases Society of America. Guidelines for the selection of anti-infective agents for complicated intra-abdominal infections Clin Infect Dis; 2003; 37: 997–1005.

38c. Paul B. Beeson, Bacterial Endocarditis (p 1098–1106) in: Cecil Loeb Textbook of Medicine, 13th edition. Editors: Beeson & McDermott. W.B. Saunders 1971.

39. Mylonakis E, Calderwood SB. Infective endocarditis in adults N Engl J Med; 2001; 345:1318–1330.

40. Calderwood SB. Antibiotic treatment of streptococcal, enterococcal, and staphylococcal endocarditis Heart; 1998; 79: 207–210.

41. Calderwood SB. Hospital-acquired pneumonia in adults: diagnosis, assessment of severity, initial antimicrobial therapy, and preventive strategies. A consensus statement, American Thoracic Society, November 1995 Am J Respir Crit Care Med; 1996; 53:1711–1725.

42. Ibrahim EH, Ward S, Sherman G, Schaiff R, Fraser VJ, Kollef MH. Experience with a clinical guideline for the treatment of ventilator-associated pneumonia Crit Care Med; 2001; 29: 1109–1115.

42a. Chastre J, Wolff M, Fagon JY, Chevret S, Thomas F, Wermert D, Clementi E, Gonzalez J, Jusserand D, Asfar P, Perrin D, Fieux F, Aubas S;, Pneum A, Pneum A. Comparison of 8 vs 15 days of antibiotic therapy for ventilator-associated pneumonia in adults: a randomized trial JAMA; 2003; 290:2588–2598.

43. Singh N, Rogers P, Atwood CW, Wagener MM, Yu VL. Short-course empiric antibiotic therapy for patients with pulmonary infiltrates in the intensive care unit Am J Respir Crit Care Med; 2000; 165:505–511.

44. Malanoski GJ, Samore MH, Pefanis A, Karchmer AW. *Staphylococcus aureus* catheter-associated bacteremia. Minimal effective therapy and unusual infectious complications associated with arterial sheath catheters Arch Intern Med; 1995; 155: 1161–1166.

45. Fowler VG Jr, Sanders RS, Corey GR, Sexton DJ, Kong L, Marr KA, Gopal AK, Gottlieb G, McClelland RS, Corey GR. Outcome of *Staphylococcus aureus* bacteremia according to compliance with recommendations of infectious diseases specialists: experience with 244 patients Clin Infect Dis; 1998; 27:478–486.

17

Antibiotic Cycling Strategies

LOU ANN BRUNO-MURTHA

Cambridge Health Alliance, Cambridge,
and Harvard Medical School,
Boston, Massachusetts, U.S.A.

During the past three decades, it has become evident that the increasing prevalence of antibiotic resistance is directly related to antibiotic use (1). Although the Centers for Disease Control and Prevention (CDC) and professional societies have embarked on initiatives to curb the inappropriate use of antibiotics (2–5), there is a lack of consensus regarding optimal antimicrobial strategies for the empiric treatment of infection. Antibiotic control programs were initially developed as a cost containment mechanism. Some programs have been successful in managing nosocomial outbreaks, at least in the short term, without adverse patient outcomes (6–10). Future antibiotic management efforts must attempt to reduce antibiotic selective pressures, promote infection control practices to prevent cross-transmission of resistant organisms, and be cost effective. Cycling or rotating antibiotics has been proposed as a potential strategy to limit antibiotic pressure as a stimulus for resistance (4). This chapter examines the definition of antibiotic cycling, the evidence to support this intervention, and the potential limitations. Implementation of an antibiotic cycling program is discussed, and considerations for future studies are explored.

DEFINITION AND RATIONALE

Presently, there is no consensus definition of antibiotic cycling. The concept has been loosely thought of as a periodic substitution of a new member of a drug class for one previously in use (11) (e.g., substitution of amikacin for gentamicin or tobramycin) or withdrawal of an antibiotic class from use in an attempt to limit selective pressures and later reintroducing it (12). Gerding (13) defined cycling as a premeditated cyclic introduction and removal of antimicrobial agents with the goal of preventing and reducing resistance. Others have defined cycling as the use of different antibiotics based on the site of infection to reduce the density of antibiotic pressure from a single agent during a given period (Table 1) (14). This conditional approach differs from single-agent cycling in that selective pressures are not maximized in a given time period and complete withdrawal of a drug from use is less frequent. Despite the differences, the theoretic premise of all cycling protocols remains the same: antimicrobial prescribing practices that are based heavily on one class of antibiotics may contribute to the emergence of antimicrobial resistance by imposing excessive selective pressures on the population and the microbial ecology in a given environment. Therefore, a more precise definition for prospective cycling would be the sequential use and withdrawal of an antibiotic(s) with a unique site of action and/or mechanism of resistance for a predetermined period, with an eventual return to the initial sequence.

Table 1 Antibiotic Rotation Schedule Representing Conditional Cycling

Quarter	Pneumonia	Peritonitis or sepsis of unknown origin
Jan–Mar	A	C
Apr–Jun	B	D
Jul–Sep	C	A
Oct–Dec	D	B

A, ciprofloxacin with or without clindamycin (add clindamycin for pneumonia if aspiration suspected; add ampicillin or vancomycin if *Enterococcus* spp. is suspected); B, piperacillin-tazobactam; C, carbapenem (imipenem or meropenem); D, cefepime with or without clindamycin or metronidazole (add clindamycin for pneumonia if aspiration suspected, metronidazole for peritonitis; add ampicillin or vancomycin if *Enterococcus* spp. is suspected).
Adopted from 14. Raymond DP, Pelletier SJ, Crabtree TD, Gleason TG, Hamm LL, Pruett TL, Sawyer RG. Impact of a rotating empiric antibiotic schedule on infectious mortality in an intensive care unit. Crit Care Med 2001; 29:1101–1108.

In the hospital setting, the colonization or infection of any individual affects the risk of colonization or infection of others; hence, antibiotic use in some patients may increase the risk of colonization/infection with resistant organisms, even in people who have not received antibiotics (15). It is for this reason that Dr. Stuart Levy, founder and president of the Alliance for the Prudent Use of Antibiotics, refers to antibiotics as *societal drugs*. He demonstrated that tetracycline-resistant coliforms appeared in farm family members after their chickens received tetracycline, and returned to baseline after tetracycline was withdrawn from the feed (16). In addition, mathematical modeling suggests that the strategy of withdrawing an antibiotic from use may reduce resistance in a population in weeks to months (17). In a Finnish clinical study, there was a significant decline in streptococcal resistance to macrolides associated with reduced macrolide consumption (18).These data support the theory that resistant bacterial subpopulations diminish as antibiotic selective pressures are removed from the individual or environment. Some experts theorize that cycling should not be used to reverse established resistance (19). However, much of the supporting data for this concept originated in response to endemic resistance and did not represent a proactive attempt to prevent resistance.

The most appropriate duration of a cycling interval in a clinical setting has yet to be determined. It is likely that this will vary depending on the density of antibiotic use in a given environment, the ability of the cycled drug to select for resistant organisms, the inherent potency of the antibiotic against the infecting organism, the immune status of the host, and the prevalence of resistance genes to the cycled antibiotic in the population or environment. Short cycles (1 month) are desirable for reducing selective pressures, but the frequent practice changes necessitated by such a schedule would be logistically difficult to implement. Furthermore, there would be substantial antibiotic carryover utilizing a monthly cycle (13). Intervals of longer duration (6 to 12 months) would make implementation easier, but this may lead to increasing acquisition of resistance, influence dormant resistance, or select drug-resistant mutants. From a purely empiric perspective, a 3- to 4-month cycling interval will be more conducive to maximizing clinician compliance and may provide a reasonable compromise, pending additional scientific data.

The antibiotics utilized in a cycling program should be guided by the hospital antibiogram, local surveillance data, and known efficacy of a particular antibiotic for common infections encountered in the population. If antimicrobial options appear equal, it is recommended to initiate a cycling program with an antibiotic that was minimally or not previously utilized and to delay the use of agents that had been frequently prescribed. There is no data to guide the order in which the antibiotics are cycled. However, it may be prudent to avoid the sequential use of fluoroquinolones and carbapenems in a cycling protocol if *Pseudomonas aeruginosa* is frequently encountered given that cross-resistance due to up-regulated efflux has been described (20).

It has been speculated that antibiotic cycling could potentially foster resistance by co-selecting linked resistance determinants by sequential antibiotic exposures. Some suggest that this strategy will likely fail in institutions where integrons (transposons that may contain several resistance gene cassettes) and insertion sequences are already established (21). Therefore, cycling may be most efficacious in environments in which resistance determinants have not yet become established because organisms that are resistant to one drug are more likely to become resistant to others (22). Similarly, it has not been proven whether there can be a sustained decline in resistance among important clinical pathogens once it becomes established. The outcome may vary according to the organism, drug, level of resistance, type of resistance determinant, antibiotic pressure, environment, cost to the organism in maintaining resistance, or existence of other selecting factors. There is reason to be skeptical about the utility of this intervention after resistance appears, based on the persistent resistance to streptomycin and chloramphenicol among gram-negative bacteria despite infrequent use of these antibiotics or recognized co-selecting agents (23). Indeed, a cycling program may have the most potential prior to the establishment of resistance in a given environment, or after the introduction of a new antibiotic class to the market (24).

EVIDENCE

Theoretically, the persistence of resistance determinants will have shorter half-lives if they confer a disadvantage in the presence of a new antibiotic pressure (21), thus providing a conceptual basis supporting the concept of antibiotic cycling. Clinical evidence to support this theory is discussed.

Aminoglycoside Cycling

Optimism about cycling originated from the experience of Gerding et al. (25), who rotated aminoglycosides over a 10-year period, depending on resistance in their facility, using amikacin when gentamicin resistance increased. The rationale was based on the fact that aminoglycoside-modifying enzymes that alter gentamicin and tobramycin are unlikely to modify amikacin. A significant reduction of resistance to gentamicin occurred on two separate occasions, and no significant increase in resistance to amikacin was reported. However, the first reintroduction of gentamicin resulted in a rapid increase in gentamicin resistance, indicating the persistence of aminoglycoside-modifying enzymes. Subsequently, a second and more gradual reintroduction of gentamicin was not associated with an increase in resistance because the original gentamicin resistance plasmid was no longer present (Table 2).

Data from two similar aminoglycoside cycling studies are less supportive of this approach. Aminoglycoside cycling was one of several control measures instituted by Saravolatz et al. (26) to combat an outbreak of gentamicin-resistant *Klebsiella pneumoniae* (GRK) in a neonatal intensive care unit (ICU). Amikacin replaced gentamicin and was followed by a significant reduction of rectal colonization with GRK from 77.8% to

Table 2 Aminoglycoside Resistance and Utilization during Five Aminoglycoside Cycles over 10 Years at the Minneapolis Veterans Affairs Medical Center

Study period	Months	Isolates			Resistance (%)	Relative use (%)		
		Amik	Gent	Tobra	(patient-days/mo)	Amik	Gent	Tobra
One (base-line)	3	950	3.8	12.0	9.5	496	1.2	76.6	22.2
Two (first amik)	26	6,235	3.2	6.4*	4.8*	705	92.3*	5.3*	2.4*
Three (first gent)	12	2,849	3.9	9.2*	6.0†	777	31.5*	66.5*	2.1
Four (second amik)	27	6,115	3.1	5.8*	4.0*	934	97.5*	0.9*	1.6
Five (second gent)	51	12,333	2.9	5.7	4.2	908	29.8*	68.2*	2.0

*$p < 0.001$.
†$p < 0.05$.
amik, amikacin; gent, gentamicin; tobra, tobramycin.
Data from Gerding DN, Larson TA, Hughes RA, Weiler M, Shanholtzer C, Pererson, LR. Aminoglycoside resistance and aminoglycoside usage: ten years experience in one hospital. Antimicrob Agents Chemother 1991; 35:1284–1290.

an average of 31.2% in 5 months ($p < 0.001$). Gentamicin was subsequently reintroduced, and rectal colonization with GRK promptly returned to 83.3% within 1 month. In another study, Young et al. (27) restricted gentamicin for 15 months and substituted amikacin as the principle aminoglycoside. Gentamicin resistance declined from 14% to 9.2% ($p < 0.0005$), but returned to baseline after a 21-month period of no restrictions. Amikacin resistance also increased significantly from 2.2% to 4% during the unrestricted period. In these two studies, alternating aminoglycosides reduced but did not eliminate resistance. Gerding's experience suggests that serial rotations may be needed prior to elimination of the resistance determinant and before a sustained effect can be realized (25).

Class Switching

The concept of class switching was summarized in a recent comprehensive review (28). Highlights of selected studies are instructional and worthy of comment here. Kollef et al. (29) observed a reduced incidence in pneumonia secondary to resistant, gram-negative organisms by a scheduled change in empiric antibiotic therapy for nosocomial infections in a cardiac surgical ICU. In this study, the investigators used ceftazidime for the empiric therapy of gram-negative sepsis in the first 6 months, followed by ciprofloxacin in the subsequent 6-month period. The incidence of ventilator-associated pneumonia (VAP) was reduced from 11.6% to 6.7%, and the incidence of VAP due to resistant gram-negative bacteria was reduced from 4% to 0.9% ($p = 0.013$).

Other reports suggested that alternating antibiotics may be an effective means of reducing resistance. Rahal et al. (8) published a study in which class restriction of cephalosporin use was associated with a 44% reduction of ceftazidime-resistant *Klebsiella* infection and colonization. Unfortunately, this beneficial effect was offset by an increase in imipenem resistance among *P. aeruginosa*, undoubtedly a response to the increased use of imipenem during the intervention period. In a similar study, restriction of third-generation cephalosporins increased imipenem use and resulted in the emergence of imipenem-resistant *Acinetobacter* (30). This emergence of resistance related to a change in antibiotic use has been referred to as *squeezing the balloon* (31). Piperacillin-tazobactam use associated with a reduction of ceftazidime administration was effective in reducing an outbreak of ceftazidime-resistant *K. pneumoniae* (32). Others have had success in reducing infection due to vancomycin-resistant enterococci (VRE) and *Clostridium difficile* by restricting third-generation cephalosporins, vancomycin, and clindamycin and using beta-lactamase inhibitor drug combinations (ampicillin-sulbactam and piperacillin-tazobactam) (33). Fecal colonization with VRE decreased from 47% to 15% ($p < 0.001$) and the incidence of *C. difficile* colitis declined by more than 50%. To date, the class-switching studies seem to be effective in reducing endemic resistance over finite periods of time, but an ongoing, dynamic program of antibiotic management will potentially be more effective in preventing the appearance of new resistance determinants.

Cycling Studies

There have been three published studies of antibiotic cycling (a predefined cycling interval with a return to the original antibiotic) (14,34,35). The salient features of these reports are summarized in Table 3. The study by Bradley et al. (34) was motivated by an increase in glycopeptide-resistant enterococci (GRE) in a hematology-oncology unit. The acquisition rate of GRE was determined by rectal swab over 4 months in period 1 (baseline). In phase 2, routine treatment for febrile neutropenia was changed from ceftazidime to piperacillin-tazobactam and improved hand hygiene was stressed for an 8-month interval. In the final 4 months (phase 3), ceftazidime was reintroduced and improved hand hygiene was continuously encouraged. Surveillance rectal swabs were done weekly to ascertain GRE acquisition rates. In phase 1, 57% of patients acquired GRE and five nosocomial GRE infections occurred. There was a significant decline in GRE acquisition during phase 2 (19%), especially apparent in the latter 4 months of the piperacillin-tazobactam period. A return toward baseline GRE acquisition occurred in phase 3

Table 3 Antibiotic Cycling Studies

Study (reference)	Duration	Site/country	Cycled drugs/interval (mo)	Objective	Intervention	Outcomes Microbiologic	Outcomes Clinical	Outcomes Costs
Bradley et al. (34)	16 mo	Hematology-oncology unit/UK	Ceftazidime (4/16, baseline) Piperacillin-tazobactam (8/16) Ceftazidime (4/16)	↓ GRE	Rotate treatment for febrile neutropenia Improve infection control	↓ GRE colonization in period 2, return toward baseline in period 3	Period 1, 5 GRE infxn Period 2, 0 GRE infxn Period 3, 3 GRE infxn	NR
Raymond et al. (14)	2 y	Surgical ICU/U.S.	Ciprofloxacin ± clindamycin (3/12) Piperacillin-tazobactam (3/12) Carbapenem* (3/12) Cefepime ± clindamycin (3/12)	↓ Infectious complications and mortality	Conditional cycling over 1 y (see Table 1 and text)		↓ Infections due to resistant GNs and GPs, Improved survival	NC
Moss et al. (35)	21 mo	Pediatric ICU/U.S.	Imipenem (3/9) Piperacillin-tazobactam (3/9) Ceftazidime† + clindamycin (3/9)	↓ Colonization and infection due to resistant bacteria	3 classes were systematically cycled every 3 mo over 1.5 y	Nonsignificant ↓ in colonization with resistant bacteria	Safe, nonsignificant ↓ resistant bloodstream infections	NR

(continued)

Table 3 *(continued)*

Study (reference)	Duration	Site/country	Cycled drugs/interval (mo)	Objective	Intervention	Outcomes	
						Microbiologic	Clinical
Gruson et al. (36)	24 mo	Medical ICU/ France	**Late VAP** Cefepime + AG (1/4) Piperacillin-tazobactam + AG (1/4) Imipenem + AG (1/4) Ticarcillin-clavulanate + AG (1/4) **Early VAP** Amoxicillin-clavulanate + AG (1/4) Cefotaxime + AG (1/4) Ceftriaxone + AG (1/4) Cefpirome + AG (1/4)	↓ Resistance to ceftazidime and ciprofloxacin, ↓ VAP due to resistant bacteria	Restricted ceftazidime and ciprofloxacin Supervised monthly antibiotic rotations for VAP	Improved susceptibilities of potentially resistant GNs and *S. aureus*	↓ VAP NR

* Imipenem or meropenem.

† Later changed to cefepime.

AG, aminoglycoside (cycled amikacin, tobramycin, netilmicin, and isepamycin sequentially); GNs, gram-negative organisms (*Pseudomonas aeruginosa*, *Burkholderia cepacia*, *Stenotrophomonas maltophilia*, *Acinetobacter baumannii*); GPs, gram-positive organisms; GRE, glycopeptide-resistant enterococci; ICU, intensive care unit; infnx, infections; NC, no change; NR, not reported; VAP, ventilator-associated pneumonia.

despite continued emphasis on hand hygiene and infection control measures. There was no change in glycopeptide utilization during the study. No GRE infections were reported in phase 2, but three nosocomial infections were encountered in phase 3. These findings suggest that the ceftazidime may have been responsible for GRE acquisition at a time when the prevalence of these organisms were at the lowest they had been in more than 2 years.

In an attempt to decrease infectious complications in a surgical ICU, Raymond et al. (14) treated patients according to a rotating empiric assignment (see Table 1). The protocol antibiotic(s) varied according to whether the patient had pneumonia versus peritonitis or sepsis of unknown origin (conditional cycling). The investigators chose different drug classes to improve compliance and diminish the density of antibiotic pressure in any given quarter. The percentage of infections caused by resistant gram-positive (17.9% vs. 25.4%, $p = 0.015$) and gram-negative (5.8% vs. 13.4%, $p = 0.0006$) bacteria was significantly less during the antibiotic rotation. Infections due to oxacillin-resistant staphylococci and gentamicin-resistant enterococci, *Pseudomonas* species, and *Acinetobacter* species declined significantly. Although the incidence of VAP was unchanged, antibiotic rotation was associated with fewer ventilator days and lower VAP mortality. Crude mortality rates following infection, attributable mortality (death during antibiotic treatment), and infectious mortality (2.9 deaths per 100 admits vs. 9.6 per 100 admits, $p < 0.0001$) declined significantly. Logistic regression identified antibiotic rotation as an independent predictor of survival (odds ratio [OR] 6.27, 95% CI 2.78-14.16). Antibiotic costs and length of stay (LOS) were not significantly different when comparing the 1-year study period to the prospective control period.

The most recent study was undertaken in a pediatric ICU to assess the safety and impact of antibiotic cycling on colonization and infection with resistant bacteria (35). Three antimicrobial classes were systematically cycled every 3 months over 18 months for empiric treatment. Imipenem, piperacillin-tazobactam, and ceftazidime (later changed to cefepime) plus clindamycin were selected to cover community-acquired and nosocomial pathogens. The regimen was subsequently continued if the bacterial isolate was susceptible. Biweekly nasopharyngeal and rectal swabs were obtained from all patients in the unit to determine colonization with antibiotic-resistant bacteria. Admission and discharge surveillance cultures were also obtained from all patients for 1 month prior to and every 6th month during the study. After adjustment, there was a nonsignificant decline (29.3% to 23.9%) in the prevalence of colonization with any resistant organism, defined as methicillin-resistant *Staphylococcus aureus* (MRSA), VRE, or a gram-negative organism resistant to ticarcillin, piperacillin, cefotaxime, ceftazidime, gentamicin, tobramycin, or imipenem. There were no detectable differences in the prevalence of resistance among admission surveillance cultures over the study period. Importantly, the study did not generate increased resistance or increased infections, despite the use of broad-spectrum antibiotics.

An alternative approach combining restriction of ceftazidime and ciprofloxacin with a monthly rotation of a beta-lactam antibiotic (cefepime, piperacillin-tazobactam, imipenem, or ticarcillin-clavulanate for late VAP [defined as occurring on or after day 7 of mechanical ventilation], or amoxicillin-clavulanate, cefotaxime, ceftriaxone, or cefpirome for early VAP) in conjunction with an aminoglycoside for the initial 5 days was evaluated by Gruson et al. (36) in a French medical ICU. Investigators based their antibiotic selection on the preceding month's antibiogram. The number of patients with microbiologically confirmed VAP decreased significantly (22.1% to 17.7%, $p < 0.01$) during the 2-year rotation period. The mortality rate in patients with VAP, however, was not significantly different. Methicillin-susceptible *S. aureus* infections increased significantly following the intervention (40% to 63%, $p < 0.05$), and susceptibilities among nosocomial gram-negative organisms improved. A significant reduction in the administration of inadequate empiric antibiotic therapy was realized following the intervention (32% vs. 20%, $p < 0.05$). This study differs from the three preceding reports in several ways: the investigators narrowed antibiotic therapy based on bacteriologic results, combination treatment with an aminoglycoside was used for initial therapy, ceftazidime and ciprofloxacin were restricted for the entire duration of the intervention because of the high prevalence of resistance in the baseline period, the study was limited to patients with VAP, and different antibiotics were designated for patients with early versus late disease. This study design does not meet the definition of antibiotic cycling as proposed earlier because neither ceftazidime nor ciprofloxacin were reintroduced after their use had been restricted. However, this same group of investigators recently published a 3-year follow-up study reporting a sustained decline in VAP (largely due to a decrease in early VAP) and improved susceptibilities among gram-negative nosocomial pathogens (37). The authors reported good compliance despite not enforcing the rotation schedule in their "closed" unit. Perhaps the most noteworthy finding was that reintroduction of ciprofloxacin and ceftazidime was not associated with a return of resistant *P. aeruginosa* to baseline rates.

In summary, the patient populations, inclusion criteria, study objectives, and interventions differed among the published studies. Two studies performed surveillance cultures to determine colonization rates (34,35). The surveillance methods of Moss et al. (35) were the most comprehensive in that admission and discharge cultures were obtained during defined periods. Design limitations, however, may have contributed to the lack of a significant reduction in colonization with resistant organisms. A significant decrease in clinical infections due to resistant bacteria was observed in two studies, and a significant reduction in mortality was reported by Raymond et al. (14,36). There was no significant difference in antibiotic expenditures in the one study investigating cost (14). Importantly, no increased resistance or adverse patient outcomes were identified in the published reports. All used historical controls and are therefore subject to confounding factors and study bias. For example, the introduction of alcohol handwash dispensers and an antibiotic surveillance team occurred prior to implementing one study, raising the possibility that these factors were responsible for reducing resistance or improving survival (14).

EXPERIENCE IN COMMUNITY HOSPITALS

Rationale and Cycling Guideline

There is a need to optimize antimicrobial therapy and minimize the emergence of resistance in community hospitals
(38). In an effort to improve patient care by providing more
appropriate antibiotic therapy, two community hospitals in
northeastern Massachusetts assessed the feasibility and
safety of an antibiotic cycling program for the empiric treatment of infection in medical and surgical inpatients from
July 2000 to June 2002 (39). The infectious disease physicians designed a cycling schedule, taking into account likely
pathogens, mechanisms of resistance, and local susceptibility
data. Fluoroquinolones, penicillin–beta-lactamase inhibitor
drug combinations (BLI), another fluoroquinolone period, and
cephalosporins were systematically cycled on a quarterly
basis (Table 4). This strategy intentionally de-emphasized
the use of the second- and third-generation cephalosporins,
which had been preferentially used prior to the study. Fluoroquinolones were used as the drug of choice for two cycles
because of their desirable acquisition cost, convenience of
once-daily dosing, suitability for prompt oral transition therapy, and ample clinical experience supporting efficacy for
the infections commonly encountered in our facilities. BLIs
were cycled for one quarter in hopes of preventing the emergence of extended-spectrum beta-lactamases (ESBLs), which
have recently become problematic in many medical centers.
Amikacin and gentamicin were also cycled in alternate quarters. Addition of an aminoglycoside to the quarterly empiric
treatment regimen was at the discretion of the attending
physician, primarily for occasions of neutropenic fever and
P. aeruginosa infection. Metronidazole was added for anaerobic organisms (intra-abdominal and diabetic foot infections)
in the two fluoroquinolone quarters and one cephalosporin
quarter. Doxycycline was encouraged for atypical organisms
associated with pneumonia in the two beta-lactam quarters.
Alternate suggestions for patients with drug allergies were
delineated, as were suggestions for oral transition therapy.
Patients on antibiotics during the transition to a new quarter

Table 4 Rotation of Empiric Antibiotics

Infection	July–September (Q3)*	October–December (Q4)†	January–March (Q1)*	April–June (Q2)‡
Lower respiratory	Quinolone	Penicillin-inhibitor ± doxycycline	Quinolone	3rd-gen. cephalosporin ± doxycycline
Pyelonephritis/UTI	Quinolone	Penicillin-inhibitor or ampicillin + gentamicin	Quinolone	3rd-gen. cephalosporin
Cellulitis	Quinolone	Oxacillin	Quinolone	Cefazolin
Diabetic ulcer	Quinolone + metronidazole	Penicillin-inhibitor	Quinolone + metronidazole	3rd-gen. cephalosporin + clindamycin or metronidazole
Intra-abdominal	Quinolone + metronidazole	Penicillin-inhibitor or ampicillin/ gentamicin/ metronidazole	Quinolone + metronidazole	3rd-gen. cephalosporin + metronidazole
Neutropenic fever	Ciprofloxacin ± amikacin	Penicillin-inhibitor ± gentamicin	Ciprofloxacin ± amikacin	Cefepime ± gentamicin
Alternative if allergy to FQ or beta-lactams	Non–beta-lactam ± amikacin	Vancomycin ± gentamicin ± metronidazole	Non—beta-lactam + amikacin	Vancomycin ± gentamicin ± metronidazole
Documented *P. aeruginosa*, add a second agent	Amikacin	Gentamicin	Amikacin	Gentamicin
Oral alternatives	Quinolone	Amoxicillin-clavulanate, a penicillin, or trimethoprim-sulfamethoxazole	Quinolone	Cephalosporin or trimethoprim-sulfamethoxazole

* Gatifloxacin or levofloxacin in year 1, gatifloxacin in year 2.
† Ticarcillin-clavulanate in year 1, piperacillin-tazobactam in year 2; ampicillin and gentamicin, ampicillin, gentamicin, and metronidazole were permitted for pyelonephritis/UTI and intra-abdominal infections, respectively, in year 1.
‡ Cefotaxime in year 1, ceftriaxone in year 2.
FQ, fluoroquinolone; UTI, urinary tract infection.

remained on their original regimen. Selection of a specific agent within a class was based on *in vitro* activity against inpatient clinical isolates and cost considerations. The treatment guideline facilitated prompt initiation of empiric antibiotic therapy directed against the likely pathogens according to the site of infection. It was endorsed by the pharmacy and therapeutics and infection control committees, and the feasibility study was approved by the Cambridge Health Alliance Institutional Review Board.

Implementation

A comprehensive educational effort was undertaken before implementation to inform the medical staff of our intention to optimize initial antibiotic treatment, reduce antibiotic selective pressures by periodically altering antibiotic use patterns, and review infection control measures designed to reduce cross-transmission of resistant organisms. The rationale behind the treatment guideline was presented at medical and surgical grand rounds, and pharmacy in-services were conducted at both hospitals before implementation to encourage staff support and cooperation. In addition, the treatment guideline was distributed quarterly by e-mail to the medical, pharmacy, and house staffs and posted on the hospital intranet and at selected nursing stations.

The guideline was applicable to all adult medical and surgical inpatients who required empiric antibiotic therapy, except those with meningitis, endocarditis, knowledge or concern of a resistant pathogen, or a sexually transmitted disease. Deviation from the schedule beyond the exclusion criteria required approval of an infectious diseases physician. Approval was usually obtained by phone and documented on the antibiotic order form or communicated to the hospital pharmacy. The pharmacists facilitated compliance and worked closely with the principal investigator to resolve concerns or disputes. During the hours of 10 p.m. to 8 a.m., no more than two doses of another antibiotic were permitted.

Antibiotic logs were maintained by the hospital's pharmacy in the first year of the study. Antibiotic order forms were implemented in year 2. The order form provided standardized dosing regimens based on the site of infection and served to alert the physician to adjust the dose when necessary, according to the patient's renal function. The form also suggested acceptable alternate antibiotics for drug allergies and oral transition therapy (Fig. 1). For transition to oral antibiotic therapy, an agent in the same class as the parenteral antibiotic was encouraged for continued treatment unless culture data revealed that the pathogen was resistant. Trimethoprimsulfamethoxazole was an oral alternative in the quarters in which beta-lactams were used. Antibiotic prescription at discharge was at the discretion of the attending physician.

The guideline was implemented at one teaching hospital (The Cambridge Hospital, Harvard-affiliated residency programs) and one nonteaching community hospital (Somerville Hospital). Infection control practices and guidelines for surgical prophylaxis were standardized at both hospitals given that they belonged to the same health care network (Cambridge Health Alliance).

The main purpose of this pilot study was to assess the feasibility of implementing a cycling program in the community hospital setting and to evaluate clinician compliance. We also had an obligation to ensure that the cycling program did not compromise patient care. For the purposes of this study, safety was evaluated by comparing targeted nosocomial infection rates in the 2-year cycling period with two preceding quarters of control data. These targeted nosocomial infections included *C. difficile* colitis (cases per 1,000 patient days) and, among ICU patients, VAP, indwelling catheter–related urinary tract infections (UTIs), and central line–associated sepsis (cases per 1,000 device days). Adverse drug events (ADEs) in the 2-year cycling period were compared with one retrospective control quarter. ADEs were captured by calls to the ADE hotline and/or medical record review by trained coders, and subsequently verified by a pharmacist or the principal investigator. Compliance was measured as the proportion of physician orders adhering to the guideline for patients who met inclusion criteria. Patients who received approval from an infectious diseases physician to deviate from the guideline were

CAMBRIDGE HEALTH ALLIANCE
ANTIBIOTIC ORDER FORM

1st Quarter (Jan.-Feb.-Mar.) FLUOROQUINOLONE QTR*   Allergies:
3rd Quarter (July-Aug.-Sept.)   Pt. Wt.:

Select both the infection and appropriate route of antibiotic administration.

INFECTION	INTRAVENOUS	ORAL
☐ Lower Respiratory	☐ Gatifloxacin 400mg IV q24hr**	☐ Gatifloxacin 400mg PO q24hr**
☐ Urosepsis	☐ Gatifloxacin 400mg IV q24hr**	☐ Gatifloxacin 400mg PO q24hr**
☐ UTI	☐ Gatifloxacin 200mg IV q24hr**	☐ Gatifloxacin 200mg PO q24hr**
☐ Cellulitis	☐ Gatifloxacin 400mg IV q24hr**	☐ Gatifloxacin 400mg PO q24hr**
☐ Diabetic Ulcer	☐ Gatifloxacin 400mg IV q24hr** ☐ AND Metronidazole 500mg IV q8hr	☐ Gatifloxacin 400mg PO q24hr** & ☐ Metronidazole 500mg PO q8hr
☐ Intra-Abdominal	☐ Gatifloxacin 400mg IV q24hr** ☐ AND Metronidazole 500mg IV q8hr	☐ Gatifloxacin 400mg PO q24hr** & ☐ Metronidazole 500mg PO q8hr
☐ Neutropenic Fever	☐ Ciprofloxacin 400mg IV q8hr** OR ☐ Ciprofloxacin 400mg IV q12hr** ☐ AND Amikacin 7.5mg/kg q12hr***	
☐ Quinolone Allergic	☐ Vancomycin 1Gm IV q12hr*** AND/OR ☐ Amikacin 7.5mg/kg q12hr***	☐ Azithromycin 500mg PO qd x 1 then 250mg PO qd x 4 days OR ☐ Clindamycin 300mg PO q6hr
☐ Documented *P. aeruginosa*	☐ Ciprofloxacin 400mg IV q8hr** OR ☐ Ciprofloxacin 400mg IV q12hr** ☐ AND Amikacin 7.5mg/kg IV q12hr***	☐ Ciprofloxacin 500mg PO BID** OR ☐ Ciprofloxacin 750mg PO BID**

*Patients with known prolongation of the QTc interval, patients with uncorrected hypokalemia, and
patients receiving class IA (e.g., quinidine, procainamide) or class III (e.g., amiodarone, sotalol)
antiarrhythmic agents should not receive fluoroquinolones
**Clcr ≥ 40ml/min for gatifloxacin and Clcr ≥ 50ml/min for ciprofloxacin
***Normal renal function

EXCLUSION CRITERIA (choose one):   **Write below the antibiotic of choice:**
☐ Resistant organism(s) (specify): _____
☐ Meningitis
☐ Endocarditis
☐ Surgical prophylaxis (guidelines on intranet/inf.cont/policies)
Deviation from above protocol; ID consulted, Dr. _____
  State reason: _____

TIME:_____ DATE: _____ SIGNATURE _____
BEEPER #: _____

Figure 1

considered to be acceptable exclusions. Antibiotic utilization was expressed in defined daily doses (DDDs), defined as the ratio of total grams of an antibiotic administered over the usual daily dose given to a patient with normal renal function. The method was adopted from the National Nosocomial Infectious Surveillance (NNIS) System–Intensive Care Antimicrobial Resistance Epidemiology project (40), although the usual daily dose was internally defined. Antibiotic acquisition costs for administered antibiotics (standardized for 1,000 patient days) and patients' LOS for the study period were compared with a 1-year retrospective control period.

The appropriateness of empiric therapy was determined by monitoring resistance among combined gram-negative clinical isolates to cycled agents and ceftazidime. The prevalence of VRE and MRSA were also assessed. Quarterly antibiogram data excluded screening cultures and duplicate specimens from the same site with a similar susceptibility profile.

Results

At Somerville Hospital (nonteaching facility), 1,430 patients (83%) were included in the 2-year study, 248 (15%) met exclusion criteria or received approval from an infectious diseases physician to deviate from the protocol, and thirty-seven (2%) protocol violations were encountered. At Cambridge Hospital (teaching facility), 969 patients (78%) were included, 216 (17%) were excluded, and there were fifty-eight (5%) protocol violations. Compliance with the protocol exceeded 97.5% at Somerville Hospital and 94.8% at Cambridge Hospital. The incidence rate ratios for the targeted nosocomial infections and adverse drug events were not significantly different at either site or between the two hospitals; data for the Cambridge Health Alliance is presented in Table 5. No significant change in incidence rates for safety outcomes was identified. Broad-spectrum cephalosporin use decreased and quinolone and BLI drug use increased at each hospital over the study period. Table 6 shows all the antibiotics administered to medical and surgical patients (including surgical prophylaxis) over the 2-year study period compared with 1 year of retrospective data from each

Table 5 Incidence Rate for Safety Outcomes at the Cambridge
Health Alliance

Safety outcome	Period	Event	Total	IR (95% CI) × 1,000	IRR (95% CI) × 1,000	p-Value
Adverse drug event	Control*	3	559	5 (1, 16)		
Adverse drug event	Cycle	17	2,399	7 (4, 11)	1.32 (0.38, 4.51)	0.66
C. difficile	Control†	9	12,591	1 (0, 1)		
C. difficile	Cycle	36	46,010	1 (1, 1)	1.09 (0.53, 2.27)	0.80
Central line sepsis	Control†	0	491	0 (0, 8)		
Central line sepsis	Cycle	3	1,658	2 (0, 5)	Infinite‡	1.0
Indwelling catheter—UTI	Control†	3	1,040	3 (1, 8)		
Indwelling catheter—UTI	Cycle	8	3,814	2 (1, 4)	0.73 (0.19, 2.74)	0.64
VAP	Control†	4	520	8 (2, 20)		
VAP	Cycle	5	1,430	3 (1, 8)	0.45 (0.12, 1.69)	0.24

* Control period was quarter 1, 2000.
† Control period was quarters 1 and 2, 2000.
‡ Infinite-control IR was zero.
CI, confidence interval; IR, incidence rate; IRR, incidence rate ratio; UTI, urinary tract infection; VAP, ventilator-associated pneumonia.

hospital. The preferred antibiotic class accounted for 57% (quarterly range, 46% to 64%) of all antibiotics (including surgical prophylaxis) administered to patients at Somerville Hospital and 48% (quarterly range, 35% to 62%) at Cambridge Hospital. Overall antibiotic use, standardized for patient days, was greater at Cambridge than at Somerville in both periods (45% and 19% higher in the control and study periods, respectively). Antibiotic costs increased $2,602.99 at Somerville and $2,146.82 at Cambridge per 1,000 patient days during the study period, attributable to the higher costs for the BLIs and an increase in overall antibiotic use during the study period (29% at Somerville, 6% at Cambridge). These cost figures do

Table 6 Quarterly Antibiotic Utilization in Defined Daily Doses at Somerville and Cambridge Hospitals

	Q3 '99	Q4 '99	Q1 '00	Q2 '00	Q3 '00	Q4 '00	Q1 '01	Q2 '01	Q3 '01	Q4 '01	Q1 '02	Q2 '02
Somerville												
FQ	115.3	127.8	426.8	130.8	1,393.9	157	1,553.3	140.73	1,127.6	53.9	995.5	74.9
BLI	109.1	67.8	101.3	13	18.8	920.5	53.8	2.3	21.3	795	27.13	6.1
3 CF	184	299.6	447.9	191	45.3	40	18	671.5	62.3	8	67	559.3
Other*	1,108	818.7	1,060.5	597.3	854.6	884.8	645.2	1,292.9	812.8	871.4	359.1	767.4
DDD/1,000 px days	576	424	534	272	658	608	608	560	556	551	500	602
Cambridge												
FQ	203.4	346.8	258.5	300.7	508.6	129.3	1,096.5	195.2	764.9	152.7	853.2	140.7
BLI	268.4	124.8	122.6	137.4	1.3	524.8	15.5	28.8	30.6	535.9	75.1	35.1
3 CF	274.3	306.1	384	356.6	15.7	11	141.9	624.5	59.2	5	151.9	1,142.2
Other*	1,315.7	1,357.9	770.5	1,147.9	340.4	814.3	508.5	981.4	474.1	840.1	1,013.8	1,304.2
DDD/1,000 px days	668.5	727.1	472.9	747.4	423.8	658.1	757.7	763.7	582.3	683.5	770	887

* All other antibiotics.

3 CF, third-generation cephalosporins; BLI, beta-lactam-inhibitor drug combinations; DDD/1,000 px days, defined daily doses per 1,000 patient days FQ, fluoroquinolones; Q, quarter.

not reflect rebates or take into account inflation rates. Average LOS declined by 1 day during the study at both study sites. The incidence rate ratios of antibiotic resistance among clinical isolates at Somerville and Cambridge were not significantly different. Therefore, data from both hospitals were combined and analyzed (Table 7). Resistance of combined gram-negative clinical isolates to ceftazidime declined significantly at the Cambridge Health Alliance. A similar trend was seen for cefotaxime. Fluoroquinolone resistance increased nonsignificantly during the 2-year cycle period. A nonsignificant decrease in resistance to piperacillin-tazobactam and a nonsignificant increase in resistance to ticarcillin-clavulanate occurred over the study period at the Cambridge Health Alliance. There was a nonsignificant decrease in VRE and a nonsignificant

Table 7   Resistance Rates in the Study and Control Periods at the Cambridge Health Alliance

	Period	IR/1,000 (95% CI)	IRR (95% CI)	*p*-Value
Resistance of gram-negatives				
Ceftazidime	Control	114 (69, 179)		
	Study	58 (43, 77)	0.5 (0.3, 0.9)	0.01
Cefotaxime	Control	175 (117, 251)		
	Study	124 (102, 150)	0.7 (0.5, 1.1)	0.11
Levofloxacin	Control	48 (21, 95)		
	Study	93 (74, 116)	1.9 (0.9, 4.0)	0.08
Ciprofloxacin	Control	72 (37, 126)		
	Study	120 (98, 145)	1.7 (0.9, 3.1)	0.10
Piperacillin-	Control	74 (38, 129)		
tazobactam	Study	48 (34, 65)	0.7 (0.3, 1.2)	0.18
Ticarcillin-	Control	91 (51, 151)		
clavulanate	Study	135 (112, 162)	1.5 (0.9, 2.5)	0.16
VRE	Control	130 (48, 284)		
	Study	62 (31, 111)	0.5 (0.2, 1.3)	0.05
MRSA	Control	393 (274, 547)		
	Study	559 (491, 633)	1.4 (1.0, 2.0)	0.05

CI, confidence interval; IR, incidence rate; IRR, incidence rate ratio of study to control period; MRSA, methicillin-resistant *Staphylococcus aureus*; VRE, vancomycin-resistant enterococci.

GNR-Ceftaz

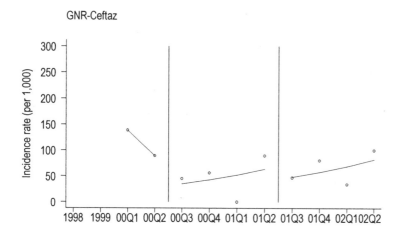

Figure 2 Quarterly resistance rate among gram-negatives to ceftazidime (GNR-Ceftaz) at the Cambridge Health Alliance.

VRE Resistence

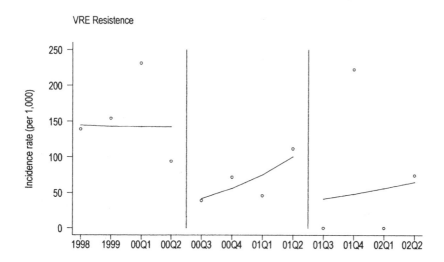

Figure 3 Quarterly resistance among enterococci at the Cambridge Health Alliance. Duplicate specimens were excluded from 1998 to 1999 data for this observation. VRE, vancomycin-resistant enterococci.

increase in MRSA at the Cambridge Health Alliance. Although an inadequate number of clinical isolates precluded quarterly statistical analysis, two alternating patterns became apparent over the study period. Quarterly resistance rates to ceftazidime (Fig. 2) were consistently higher and VRE were more prevalent during the beta-lactam drug quarters. Additional data sets were included in the VRE analysis, after excluding duplicates from 1998 to 1999 (Fig. 3). No other patterns were evident after plotting quarterly resistance rates for several antibiotics.

Discussion

Our initial experience demonstrates that excellent compliance with an antimicrobial cycling program is achievable in the community hospital setting. We were able to achieve this in both a teaching and nonteaching hospital. Multidisciplinary cooperation among physician leaders (infectious diseases physicians and department chiefs), infection control practitioners, pharmacy services, and clinical microbiology was instrumental to its success. Education and a clinical guideline for empiric therapy based on local surveillance and acceptable practice as well as dispensing procedures were critical in achieving excellent compliance. The preferred antibiotic class accounted, on average, for 57% and 48% of all antibiotic use over the 2-year study period at Somerville Hospital and Cambridge Hospital, respectively. This is superior to the experience reported from other cycling studies in ICUs with smaller patient populations (14,36). Quarterly variation was expected because of the inherent guideline flexibility and frequency of purported beta-lactam allergy. The pharmacy at Cambridge Hospital was unable to enter all antibiotic orders on the antibiotic log or completely enforce the use of the antibiotic order form that was used to determine the number of patients who met inclusion and exclusion criteria. Hence, this hospital appeared to have fewer study patients than Somerville Hospital when, in fact, Cambridge Hospital had a higher density of antibiotic use. This partly reflects a more proactive pharmacy at Somerville, where the pharmacists routinely remind physicians to reassess the need for continued antibiotic treatment, enforce discontinuation of preoperative antibiotic prophylaxis 24 hours after surgery, and encourage streamlining and transition to oral treatment when patients meet established criteria. Nonetheless, we believe we were able to determine the relative proportion of patients who met criteria at Cambridge Hospital, as the forms reviewed likely reflected a representative sample of the medical and surgical patient population. We did not assess for severity of illness or comorbidities in this pilot study; therefore, we cannot exclude these factors as contributing to the higher density of antibiotic use at Cambridge.

Before the study, monotherapy with a cephalosporin was commonly used for empiric therapy. The cycling protocol encouraged the use of metronidazole to optimize coverage for anaerobes in three of four annual cycles for patients with intra-abdominal and diabetic foot infections, and doxycycline for atypical pathogens associated with pneumonia in the two beta-lactam quarters. In addition, clinicians were encouraged to consider the addition of empiric vancomycin when patients presented with a potential staphylococcal infection and had risk factors for MRSA (prior history of MRSA colonization or infection, residence in a long-term care facility, and antibiotic exposure or recent hospitalization within the preceding 2 months) (41). Recent literature supports the initiation of appropriate initial antibiotic therapy, as inadequate treatment has been associated with increased morbidity, mortality, LOS, and health care costs (42). Hence, using more DDDs to optimize empiric therapy, as our cycling protocol encouraged, may be desirable. There must be efforts, nonetheless, to discourage initiating antibiotics when bacterial infection is unlikely, to streamline therapy once culture data becomes available, and to encourage reassessing the need for antibiotics when cultures remain negative and bacterial infection appears less likely.

Given the higher antibiotic costs, the economic impact of this strategy needs to be explored. Had rebates and inflation been considered, actual cost differences would have been much less. Cycling may prove to be cost effective if more appropriate empiric therapy is administered, resistance acquisition can be prevented, or nosocomial infections can be reduced. Although LOS declined, we did not adjust for the increasing role of hospitalists and the additional emphasis on care management; hence, other factors may have contributed to this observation.

Importantly, no increases in nosocomial infections or adverse drug events were attributed to the cycling protocol at either site. Like other investigators, we found antibiotic cycling to be a safe modality (14,34–37). We reviewed the hospital-specific antibiogram quarterly to ensure the appropriateness of the empiric therapy. Because of limited resources and personnel, we did not separate community, health care–associated, or nosocomial isolates. Although a limitation of this study, cumulative susceptibility data from inpatients have been shown to reflect susceptibility patterns among isolates associated with nosocomial infections (43). In quarter 4 of 2001 (a nonfluoroquinolone quarter), nine of the sixteen levofloxacin-resistant isolates were *Escherichia coli*, eight of which originated from urine specimens. Only one of the nine cultures was obtained 72 hours after hospital admission, suggesting that the overwhelming majority of patients presented to the hospital with the resistant isolate. Residence in an extended-care facility was a common feature among this cohort. The increase in fluoroquinolone resistance is not unexpected given the recent increase in fluoroquinolone prescriptions in the outpatient setting (38). In the future, hospitals may need to de-emphasize the use of fluoroquinolones in empiric treatment regimens when gram-negative organisms are potential pathogens because of this emerging problem. The observed decline in resistance among gram-negatives to ceftazidime at the Cambridge Health Alliance, at a time when the NNIS System was reporting an increase in ESBLs is interesting (44). The alternating quarterly pattern of ceftazidime resistance suggests that antibiotic cycling may have had an impact on ESBLs and AmpC beta-lactamases (Fig. 2). It is curious that the prevalence of VRE at Cambridge Hospital (17.4% to 3.4%, $p = 0.03$) fell below what was reported from Project ICARE (Intensive Care Antimicrobial Resistance Epidemiology) in 1998 to 1999, in which 11.3% and 15% of enterococcal isolates were resistant to vancomycin in non-ICUs and ICUs, respectively

(38). Again, the alternating quarterly pattern over the study period at the Cambridge Health Alliance suggests that the nonfluoroquinolone quarters may have increased the selection pressures for VRE (Fig. 3). Although intriguing, it is important to emphasize that these patterns are simply observations and should not be construed as scientific proof.

DIRECTIONS FOR FUTURE STUDIES

Antibiotic use is one of several factors contributing to the development of antimicrobial resistance (45). Changes in the patient population, dictated by several forces (economics, immigration, demographic shifts, increased severity of illness among hospitalized patients), and infection control practices affect resistance prevalence. Ongoing technologic advancements, as well as nearly universal implementation of alcohol-based hand disinfectants, have improved standards of practice but serve to confound studies attempting to determine the effect of altered antibiotic use on resistance. Future investigative efforts should be of sufficient size to control for these confounding factors and include baseline and follow-up surveillance cultures and a matched control group targeting clinically important antibiotic–organism pairs for the population of interest.

Based on limited and preliminary experience with antibiotic cycling, there is some optimism that cycling may prove to be an effective strategy for preventing resistance. A proactive cycling program, combined with meticulous infection control practices, may be a useful modality as hospitals strive to avoid "squeezing the balloon". With the increased availability of drugs active against gram-positive organisms (linezolid, daptomycin), future studies should evaluate their role in reducing selection of glycopeptide resistance among staphylococci and enterococci. A preemptive cycling approach may prove to increase the clinical longevity of these new products.

Cycling may also be a way to provide more appropriate empiric treatment regimens in a hospital setting (46). An institution deciding to implement an antibiotic cycling program should have infectious disease physician and/or infectious disease pharmacy leadership willing to lead the effort and promote this modality as a potential means of preventing resistance. Antibiotic cycling requires a multidisciplinary effort involving the medical staff, pharmacy (to track total antibiotic use, costs, and adverse reactions), infection control (to ensure adherence to infection control policies and procedures and to monitor nosocomial infection rates), and microbiology (to make available timely inpatient antibiograms). Education is fundamental to achieving cooperation, but a system to enforce the scheduled rotation is essential for compliance. As with any good antimicrobial stewardship program, there should also be guidelines in place for preoperative surgical prophylaxis and a means of encouraging de-escalation from the broad empiric regimen once culture data become available. An attempt to maintain the scheduled antibiotic class is desirable for de-escalation or streamlining, if clinically appropriate. Suggested performance indicators for a cycling program may include:

Inclusion rate; strive for 80% of the patient population

Antibiotic utilization (in DDDs per 1,000 patient days); the majority of antibiotic use should conform to the rotation schedule

Targeted nosocomial infection rates; rates should not exceed benchmarking standards and/or historical control data

Antibiotic susceptibility among inpatient isolates; significant increases in resistance should prompt an investigation to assess the adequacy of the infection control program

Results from the CDC-sponsored, multicenter antibiotic cycling study conducted in ICUs are eagerly anticipated.

I am indebted to Dr. Philip Carling for his comments and suggestions, and to Dr. Timothy Murtha for his support.

Unrestricted support was provided by Abbott, Bristol-Myers Squibb, GlaxoSmithKline, Roche, and Wyeth Pharmaceuticals for the study of antibiotic cycling at the Cambridge Health Alliance.

REFERENCES

1. Gaynes R. The impact of antimicrobial use on the emergence of antimicrobial-resistant bacteria in hospitals Infect Dis Clin North Am; 1997; 11:757–765.

2. www.cdc.gov/drugresistance/actionplan/html/index.htm (accessed April 2, 2002).

3. Gaynes R. Report of the ASM task force on antimicrobial resistance Antimicrob Agents Chemother 1995; 39(Suppl):2–23.

4. Shlaes DM, Gerding DN, John JF, Craig WA, Bornstein DL, Duncan RA, Echman MR, Farrer WE, Greene WH, Lorian V, Levy S, McGowan JE, Paul SM, Ruskin J, Tenover FC, Watanakunakorn C. Society for Healthcare Epidemiology of America and Infectious Diseases Society of America Joint Committee on the Prevention of Antimicrobial Resistance: guidelines for the prevention of antimicrobial resistance in hospitals Infect Control Hosp Epidemiol; 1997; 18:275–291.

5. Goldmann DA, Weinstein RA, Wenzel RP, Tablan OC, Duma RJ, Gaynes RP, Schlosser J, Martone WJ. Strategies to prevent and control the emergence and spread of antimicrobial-resistant microorganisms in hospitals JAMA; 1996; 275:234–240.

6. White AC, Atmar R, Wilson J, Cate TR, Stager CE, Greenburg SB. Effects of requiring prior authorization for selected antimicrobials: expenditures, susceptibilities, and clinical outcomes Clin Infect Dis; 1997; 25:230–239.

7. Frank MO, Batteiger BE, Sorensen SJ, Hartstein AI, Carr JA, McComb JS, Clark CD, Abel SR, Mikuta JM, Jones RB. Decrease in expenditures and selected nosocomial infections following implementation of an antimicrobial-prescribing improvement program Clin Perform Qual Health Care; 1997; 5: 180–188.

8. Rahal JJ, Urban C, Horn D, Freeman K, Segal-Maurer S, Maurer J, Mariano N, Marks S, Burns J, Dominick D, Lim M. Class restriction of cephalosporin use to control total cephalosporin resistance in nosocomial *Klebsiella* JAMA; 1998; 280: 1233–1237.

9. Rice LB, Eckstein EC, DeVente J, Shlaes DM. Ceftazidime-resistant *Klebsiella pneumoniae* isolates recovered at the Cleve-

land Department of Veterans Affairs Medical Center Clin Infect Dis; 1996; 23:118–124.

10. Meyer KS, Urban C, Eagan JA, Berger BJ, Rahal JJ. Nosocomial outbreak of *Klebsiella* infection resistant to late-generation cephalosporins Ann Intern Med; 1993; 119:353–358.

11. McGowan JE. Minimizing antimicrobial resistance in hospital bacteria: can switching or cycling drugs help? Infect Control; 1986; 7:573–576.

12. Kollef MH. Is there a role for antibiotic cycling in the intensive care unit? Crit Care Med; 2001; 29:N135–N142.

13. Gerding DN. Antimicrobial cycling: lessons learned from the aminoglycoside experience Infect Control Hosp Epidemiol; 2000; 21(Suppl):S12–S17.

14. Raymond DP, Pelletier SJ, Crabtree TD, Gleason TG, Hamm LL, Pruett TL, Sawyer RG. Impact of a rotating empiric antibiotic schedule on infectious mortality in an intensive care unit Crit Care Med; 2001; 29:1101–1108.

15. Lipsitch M, Samore MH. Antimicrobial use and antimicrobial resistance: a population perspective Emerg Infect Dis; 2002; 8: 347–354.

16. Levy S, Fitzgerald G, Macone A. Changes in intestinal flora of farm personnel after introduction of a tetracycline-supplemented feed on a farm N Engl J Med; 1976; 295:583–588.

17. Lipsitch M, Bergstrom CT, Levin BR. The epidemiology of antibiotic resistance in hospitals: paradoxes and prescriptions Proc Natl Acad Sci U S A; 2000; 97:1938–1943.

18. Seppala H, Klaukka T, Vuopio-Varkila J, Muotiala A, Helenius H, Lager K, Huovinen P. The effect of changes in the consumption of macrolide antibiotics on erythromycin resistance in group A streptococci in Finland N Engl J Med; 1997; 337: 441–446.

19. Rapp RP, Empey KM. Antimicrobial cycling to control bacterial resistance Ann Pharmacother; 2001; 35:1289–1290.

20. Livermore DM. Multiple mechanisms of antimicrobial resistance in *Pseudomonas aeruginosa*: our worst nightmare? Clin Infect Dis; 2002; 34:634–640.

21. John JF, Rice LB. The microbial genetics of antibiotic cycling Infect Control Hosp Epidemiol; 2000; 21(Suppl):S22–S31.

22. Levy SB. Multidrug resistance—a sign of the times N Engl J Med; 1998; 338:1376–1378.

23. Chiew YF, Yeo SF, Hall LM, Livermore DM. Can susceptibility to an antimicrobial be restored by halting its use? The case of streptomycin vs. Enterobacteriaceae J Antimicrob Chemother; 1998; 41:247–251.

24. Lavin BS. Antibiotic cycling and marketing into the 21st century: a perspective from the pharmaceutical industry Infect Control Hosp Epidemiol; 2000; 21(Suppl):S22–S31.

25. Gerding DN, Larson TA, Hughes RA, Weiler M, Shanholtzer C, Pererson LR. Aminoglycoside resistance and aminoglycoside usage: ten years experience in one hospital Antimicrob Agents Chemother; 1991; 35:1284–1290.

26. Saravolatz LD, Arking L, Pohlod D, Fisher EJ, Borer R. An outbreak of gentamicin-resistant *Klebsiella pneumoniae*: analysis of control measures Infect Control; 1984; 5:79–84.

27. Young EJ, Sewell M, Koza MA, Clarridge JE. Antibiotic resistance patterns during aminoglycoside restriction Am J Med Sci; 1985; 290:223–227.

28. Hodges BM, White RL. Antibiotic cycling: the future or a fad? Ann Pharmacother; 2001; 35:1224–1232.

29. Kollef MH, Vlasnik J, Sharpless L, Pasque C, Murphy D, Fraser V. Scheduled change of antibiotic class: a strategy to decrease the incidence of ventilator-associated pneumonia Am J Respir Crit Care Med; 1997; 156:1040–1048.

30. Go E, Urban C, Burns J, Kreiswirth B, Eisner W, Mariano N, Mosinka-Snipas K, Rahal J. Clinical and molecular epidemiology of *Acinetobacter* infections sensitive only to polymyxin B and sulbactam Lancet; 1994; 344:1329–1332.

31. Burke JP. Antibiotic resistance—squeezing the balloon? JAMA; 1998; 280:1270–1271.

32. Rice LB, Eckstein EC, DeVente J, Shlaes DM. Ceftazidime-resistant *Klebsiella pneumoniae* isolates recovered at the Cleve-

land Department of Veterans Affairs Medical Center Clin Infect Dis; 1996; 23:118–124.

33. Quale J, Landman D, Saurina G, Atwood E, DiTore V, Patel K. Manipulation of a hospital antimicrobial formulary to control an outbreak of vancomycin-resistant enterococci Clin Infect Dis; 1996; 23:1020–1025.

34. Bradley SJ, Wilson ALT, Allen MC, Sher HA, Goldstone AH, Scott GM. The control of hyperendemic glycopeptide-resistant *Enterococcus* spp. on a haematology unit by changing antibiotic usage J Antimicrob Chemo; 1999; 43:261–265.

35. Moss WJ, Beers MC, Johnson E, Nichols DG, Perl TM, Dick JD, Veltri MA, Willoughby RE Jr. Pilot study of antibiotic cycling in a pediatric intensive care unit Crit Care Med; 2002; 30: 1877–1882.

36. Gruson D, Hilbert G, Vargas F, Valentino R, Bebear C, Allery A, Bebear C, Gbikpi-Benissan G, Cardinaud JP. Rotation and restricted use of antibiotics in a medical intensive care unit: impact on the incidence of ventilator-associated pneumonia caused by antibiotic-resistant Gram-negative bacteria Am J Respir Crit Care Med; 2000; 162:837–843.

37. Gruson D, Hilbert G, Vargas F, Valentino R, Bui N, Pereyre S, Bebear C, Bebear CM, Gbikpi-Benissan G. Strategy of antibiotic rotation: Long-term effect on incidence and susceptibilities of Gram-negative bacilli responsible for ventilator-associated pneumonia Crit Care Med; 2003; 31:1908–1914.

38. Fridkin SK, Hill HA, Volkova NV, Edwards JR, Lawton RM, Gaynes RP, McGowan JE Jr. Temporal changes in prevalence of antimicrobial resistance in 23 U.S. hospitals Emerg Infect Dis; 2002; 8:697–701.

39. Bruno-Murtha LA, Brusch J, Bor D, Li W, Zucker D. A pilot study of antibiotic cycling in the community hospital setting. Manuscript accepted for publication. Infect Control Hosp Epidemiol. Accepted on Feb. 12, 2004.

40. Fridkin SK, Steward CD, Edwards JR, Pryor ER, McGowan JE, Archibald LK, Gaynes RP, Tenover FC, Tenover FC. Surveillance of antimicrobial use and antimicrobial resistance in US hospitals: Project ICARE phase 2 Clin Infect Dis; 1999; 29: 245–252.

41. Maranan MC, Moreira B, Boyle-Vavra S, Daum RS. Antimicrobial resistance in staphylococci Infect Dis Clin North Am; 1997; 11:813–849.

42. Livermore DM. Bacterial resistance: origins, epidemiology, and impact Clin Infect Dis; 2003; 36(Suppl 1):S11–S23. .

43. Fridkin SK, Edwards JR, Tenover FC, Gaynes RP, McGowan JE. Antimicrobial resistance prevalence rates in hospital antibiograms reflect prevalence rates among pathogens associated with hospital-acquired infections Clin Infect Dis; 2001; 33: 324–330.

44. www.cdc.gov/drugresistance/healthcare/ha/HASlideSet.pdf (accessed April 30, 2003).

45. McGowan JE. Do intensive hospital antibiotic control programs prevent the spread of antibiotic resistance? Infect Control Hosp Epidemiol; 1994; 15:478–483.

46. Fridkin SK. Routine cycling of antimicrobial agents as an infection-control measure Clin Infect Dis; 2003; 36:1438–1444.

18

Outpatient Parenteral Antimicrobial Therapy: Role in Optimizing Length of Hospital Stay

ALAN D. TICE

Section of Infectious Diseases,
John A Burns School of Medicine,
University of Hawaii at Manoa,
Honolulu, Hawaii, U.S.A.

JETAHN KELLEY

Consultants in Infectious Diseases, LLP,
and Texas Tech University,
Lubbock, Texas, U.S.A.

Outpatient parenteral antimicrobial therapy (OPAT) offers a number of opportunities to improve patient care, avoid the development of antimicrobial resistance, and save health care dollars. Most communities are now able to provide OPAT; however, the operating base, models used, and leadership vary greatly. In general, the role of the pharmacist is a key one in terms of safety, quality improvement, patient education, practical applications, and information management. This chapter explores some of the aspects of OPAT from a pharmacy perspective. Additional resources that may be helpful include the first four references (1–4).

HISTORY OF OUTPATIENT PARENTERAL ANTIMICROBIAL THERAPY

Outpatient parenteral antimicrobial therapy is a relatively new concept in health care. Until the 1980s, patients needing infusion therapy had no option but to remain in an inpatient setting until the completion of their therapy (5,6). OPAT programs have since evolved in the search for an effective, safe, and less expensive alternative to inpatient care. When these programs first began, patients were discharged to their homes with 24-hour-a-day, 7-day-a-week nursing care, not only for the administration of intravenous (IV) medication, but also to monitor clinical status and maintain venous access—a virtual hospital-in-the-home approach.

It soon became obvious that many of these patients could be managed safely with only intermittent nurse visits, in which the nurse came to the home only when needed to administer the IV medication or perform other procedures that required skilled nursing care. From this point, it was only a short step to teaching patients or family members how to administer the IV therapy on their own, with the home nursing visits focused on supervision and support. Today, a once-weekly nurse visit may be sufficient for some patients—unless the patient is unstable or requires additional home care services or monitoring related to his or her drug therapy or disease process (7).

In addition to traditional home care, other models have evolved (2,8). The ambulatory infusion center (AIC) model can provide infusions or may simply provide education, medication, supplies, and support for the patient as he or she self-administers his or her therapy at home. It typically functions as an added service from a physician's office, hospital, or outpatient clinic. This model provides more supervision of the patient than does home care and may be less expensive. The AIC is also a method to generate additional revenue for health care providers as they expand and diversify their services in ambulatory care.

The first infections reported to be treated with OPAT were recurrent chest infections in children with cystic fibrosis (9). Other infections that required prolonged courses of IV therapy in otherwise relatively normal hosts followed. These included osteomyelitis and endocarditis (10,11). Since then, successful treatment has been reported with almost every serious infection (2).

Outpatient parenteral antimicrobial therapy has continued to grow over the last several decades and is now an integral part of therapy for patients with serious infections. The expanding use of this cost-effective form of treatment has been possible through the growth of available home care services, long-acting antimicrobials, and improved technology in vascular access as well as infusion devices. Leadership and creativity on the part of pharmacists, nurses, and physicians have also been a critical factor in exploring and developing this form of therapy in a safe and effective manner.

OUTPATIENT PARENTERAL ANTIMICROBIAL THERAPY VERSUS HOSPITALIZATION

Outpatient parenteral antimicrobial therapy requires a multidisciplinary approach with input from physicians, pharmacists, nurses, and often social workers and administrators (12,13). The goal is to provide patient-focused care with a team that can provide care planning, coordinated care, sterile product preparation and distribution, clinical monitoring, patient education, documentation of activities, and on-call responsibilities (14).

Following proper diagnosis of the infection, stabilization of the patient's condition, and patient education, most of the antimicrobials that have traditionally been administered in the inpatient setting can now be managed with OPAT. Patients generally prefer OPAT to hospital care. The incidence of health care–related infections may also be reduced. The disruption of a normal lifestyle may be minimal with OPAT, and many patients are able to go to work while on therapy. OPAT also allows patients to become more involved in their own care, giving them a sense of empowerment and responsibility for the success of their treatment—in contrast to the hospital, where they lie passively in a hospital bed and learn little about their disease or therapy. Unlike in the inpatient setting, however, the patient must be capable and interested in the additional responsibilities that come with self-care and personal responsibility. They must be educated about their diseases and their medications and how to deal with any problems or adverse events that may arise. The cost of care is also far less with OPAT, as only a limited portion of hospital expenses is for medication and administration of medication (15).

CONSIDERATION FOR SELECTION OF OUTPATIENT PARENTERAL ANTIMICROBIAL THERAPY PATIENTS

Selection of patients for OPAT involves many variables not usually considered with hospital care (16). Patients must be carefully evaluated and selected for OPAT, as their responsibilities are quite different. The medical staff, facilities, equipment, and safeguards of the hospital are not immediately available. Patients must be willing to be treated as outpatients and be reliable and compliant. Family support and help are important considerations. The patient or caregiver must be evaluated for resources, abilities, and skills as outlined in Table 1 (17).

The first consideration should be whether the patient is able to self-administer therapy. If the patient is not independent, he or she must have a support system and a caregiver capable of providing OPAT. The patient and caregiver must be motivated and willing to learn the necessary procedures for

Table 1 Home Infusion Assessment Considerations

	Data	Assessment considerations
Demographics	Patient's service address—this may be different from the patient's permanent address	Is the patient within the pharmacy's service area? Which home care nursing services are in the area? What are the response and delivery times to the service address? How far is the nearest emergency facility?
	Patient's age	Does the patient belong to a special population, e.g., pediatrics, elderly?
Clinical	Medication regimen	Is it safe to give at home? How has patient responded to medication? What is the goal of therapy? What is the anticipated duration of OPAT?
	Tolerance to medication—first dose	Was the first dose given in a controlled setting? Were there adverse effects?
	Allergy history	Is there a potential allergy to the medication ordered?
	All diagnoses, clinical condition (identify diagnosis related to infusion)	Are there medication–disease interactions? Is the treatment regimen appropriate? Is the dose appropriate? Is the patient clinically stable? Are there significant vascular diseases? Are there drug or alcohol problems?
	Laboratory studies (as applicable)— electrolytes, renal function, hepatic function, CBC, drug levels	Baseline laboratory studies for monitoring (usually for hematology, renal, or liver disease) Were antimicrobial levels done? Are antimicrobial levels needed?
	Vascular Access Device	Is the device appropriate for medication, duration? What care will be needed? Is patient capable of self-care of catheter?

(continued)

Table 1 *Continued*

	Data	Assessment considerations
	Drainage tubes	Are there drainage tubes? What are the type and amount of drainage? Is fluid and electrolyte loss significant?
	Patient mobility, skills	How much is patient/caregiver able to learn? Is ambulatory or stationary system to be used? Can patient see, hear, communicate?
	Complete medication profile	Are there any potential drug interactions? Is the diagnosis listed in the database?
	Therapeutic goals	What are the goals? Is patient/family in agreement?
Psychosocial	Motivation	Are patient and family motivated and willing to learn for safe home infusion?
	Risk factors	Does patient have a history of drug abuse?
	Support system	Who will provide care, or is patient independent?
	Home situation	Does patient have a home situation that is safe and appropriate for home infusion? Does patient have utilities, a telephone, and a refrigerator?
Reimbursement	Insurance eligibility and benefits	Does patient have insurance coverage for home infusion? If Medicare—is this medication a covered service? If covered, does patient meet clinical criteria for coverage and is this documented? Is patient aware of possible costs?
	Authorization	Is preauthorization required? Does the pharmacy have the clinical information needed for authorization?

CBC, complete blood count; OPAT, outpatient parenteral antibiotic therapy; VAD, vascular access device.

Adapted from Wilder GL. Home Infusion Pharmacy Certificate Program. Module I: Introduction to Home Infusion Practice. Alexandria, VA: National Home Infusion Association, 2004.

safe home infusion. They must also commit to completing the regimen as ordered.

The provider should assess the patient's mobility and skills. Is the patient or caregiver able to learn the techniques and safeguards necessary for home care? Can the patient see, hear, read written instructions, and communicate? Will family members be available? Will an interpreter be needed? The patient or caregiver will require some degree of dexterity and strength in order to administer the prescribed therapy. The exact amount of strength and dexterity required will vary based on the regimen delivery method and equipment involved.

ANTIMICROBIAL REGIMEN

As drug regimens become increasingly complicated, the possibility of errors and poor outcomes also increases. Not only is this true in the inpatient setting, but also for OPAT. Regimens that require multiple doses per day or multiple medications lend themselves to error and require diligent teaching, follow-up, and support. The clinical team must consider medication compatibilities, especially if the patient has a single-lumen vascular access device. Antimicrobial regimens that can be administered once daily lend themselves easily to any OPAT model and are also the most cost effective. Special consideration of the pharmacokinetic, pharmacodynamic, and pharmacoeconomic issues apply to OPAT (18,19).

As in the acute care setting, pharmacists are responsible for the sterile admixture of infusion medications. It is important to point out, however, that the conditions under which the medication is prepared and stored are rarely comparable to those of the hospital, and should be closely monitored by pharmacy staff. Drug stability is a more important factor with OPAT than with hospital care.

Outpatient parenteral antimicrobial therapy may require consideration of extended dating issues and the specialized products used to infuse medications on an outpatient basis. Essential considerations include the stability of compounded admixtures at room temperature and body temperature as well as refrigerated temperature. Table 2 lists the stability properties of antimicrobials that are commonly used in OPAT (2,18,19). With outpatient therapy, antimicrobials are often mixed days, if not a week, before administration. They may be frozen or refrigerated, depending on their stability. This may create a problem for the patient in regard to the time it takes to warm the infusion before it is given, especially if the treatments are given more than once daily. It may also be a problem with continuous infusions if a medication is to be given over 24 hours and is in a reservoir carried at essentially body temperature. Some medications with limited stability can be mixed by the patient immediately prior to administration, such as with the ADD-Vantage system (Abbott Laboratories, Abbott Park, IL)™. With this system, the patient simply breaks a barrier between the solution and the powder, mixes them, and then administers them. This also reduces pharmacist time and avoids the problem of waiting for the medication solutions to warm up. The clinician is encouraged to consult current references for stability information, extended stability information, recommended concentrations, and storage conditions.

DRUG SAFETY—ADVERSE EVENTS

The safety of medications is always of paramount importance, particularly when the infusion will be outside of a controlled environment, i.e., in the patient's home. The clinician must carefully select the agents to be given, with due diligence afforded the side-effect profile.

Antimicrobials are commonly considered to be safe drugs, but some are not safe, and the consequences of a reaction or adverse event may be severe and sometimes fatal. The OPAT Outcomes Registry (www.OPAT.com) has been collecting information about patients treated with OPAT through a network of twenty or more sites over the past 5 years. From data gathered from more than 12,000 courses of therapy, it appears there are significant differences among antibiotics, as indi-

Table 2 Antimicrobials Commonly Used in Outpatient Parenteral
Antibiotic Therapy and Their Properties at Various Temperatures

Drug	Half-life (h)	Dilution (mg/mL)	Duration of stability§		
			−20°C	5°C	25°C
Acyclovir*	2–3.5	5		37 d	37 d
Amphotericin B†	24–360	0.1		35 d	5 d
Liposomal amphotericin B†	24–360	4		24 h	5 d
Amphotericin B lipid complex†	24–360	1		48 h	6 h
Ampicillin	1	30		48 h	8 h
Ampicillin-sulbactam	1	20		48 h	8 h
Caspofungin	>48	0.2–0.3		24 h	1 d
Cefazolin	1–2	10–20	30 d	10 d	1 d
Cefoperazone	1.5–25	40	96 d	80 d	80 d
Ceftazidime	1.4–2	1–40	90 d	21 d	2 d
Ceftriaxone	5.4–10.9	10–40	180 d	10 d	3 d
Cefuroxime	1–2	5–10	30 d	180 d	1 d
Chloramphenicol	1.5–4	10–20	180 d	30 d	30 d
Clindamycin	2–3	6–12	56 d	32 d	16 d
Daptomycin	8.1–9.0	—	—	48 h	12 h
Doxycycline†	22–24	0.1–1	56 d	48 h	3 d
Erythromycin lactobionate	1.5–2	0.1–0.2	30 d	14 d	1 d
Ertapenem	4	20		24 h	6 h
Ganciclovir	2.5–3.5	5	364 d	35 d	5 d
Gentamicin	2–3	0.6–1	30 d	30 d	30 d
Imipenem-cilastatin	0.8–1.3	2.5–5		2 d	10 h
Linezolid	4.5	2		24 h	4 h
Meropenem	1.5	5–20		24 h	4 h
Nafcillin	0.5–1.5	2–40	90 d	3 d	1 d
Oxacillin	0.3–0.3	10–100	30 d	7 d	1 d
Penicillin G‡	0.4–0.9	0.2 mu/mL‖	84 d	14 d	2 d
Quinupristin-dalfopristin	3/1	2		54 h	5 h
Trimethoprim-sulfamethoxazole*	8–11/10–13	8		6 h	
Tobramycin	2–3	0.2–3.2	30 d	4 d	2 d
Vancomycin	4–6	5	63 d	63 d	7 d

* Should not be refrigerated.
† Protect from sunlight.
‡ Degradation products may form after a few hours.
§ If space left blank, data not available.
‖ mu = million units
Optimal solutions may vary from saline to 5% dextrose, depending on the antibiotic.
Adapted from Tice AD, Rehn SJ, Dalorisio JR, Bradley JS, Martinelli LP, Graham DR, et al. Practice Guidelines for Outpatient Parenteral Antimicrobial Therapy. Clin Infect Dis 2004;38:1651-72.

Table 3 Frequency of Adverse Effects from Intravenous Antimicrobials with Outpatient Parenteral Antibiotic Therapy*

	CZ	CTZ	CTRX	CL	GENT	OX	NAF	VC	Total
Antimicrobial Courses	781	456	4,670	442	327	479	266	2881	10,302
Stopped early (no.)	32	16	136	34	26	40	26	144	454
Stopped early (%)	4.1	3.5	2.9	7.7	8.0	8.4	9.8	5.0	4.4
Rash (%)	1.92	2.19	1.39	5.43	0.61	3.55	4.51	2.29	2.05
Diarrhea (%)	0.38	0.00	0.45	0.90	0.00	0.63	0.38	0.07	0.33
Nausea (%)	0.77	0.22	0.36	0.90	0.92	1.88	1.50	0.24	0.50
Renal (%)	0.13	0.22	0.00	0.00	2.75	0.21	0.75	0.42	0.25
Leukopenia (%)	0.26	0.22	0.09	0.23	0.00	0.42	2.26	0.21	0.21
Urticaria (%)	0.51	0.00	0.19	0.45	0.00	0.21	0.00	0.49	0.29
Fever (%)	0.00	0.44	0.41	0.45	0.00	0.42	0.75	1.18	0.59
Vestibular (%)	0.00	0.00	0.00	0.00	3.06	0.00	0.00	0.10	0.13
Hepatic (%)	0.13	0.00	0.04	0.00	0.00	1.04	0.38	0.00	0.09
Anaphylaxis (%)	0.26	0.00	0.04	0.00	0.31	0.21	0.00	0.14	0.10
Anaphylactoid (%)	0.26	0.00	0.02	0.00	0.00	0.00	0.00	0.07	0.05
Anemia (%)	0.00	0.22	0.00	0.00	0.00	0.21	0.75	0.00	0.04

* Information gathered from the Outpatient Parenteral Antibiotic Therapy Outcomes Registry as of October 2002. Reactions recorded were only those serious enough to stop therapy with that antimicrobial. More than one reason for stopping therapy was noted in 20.1% of cases.
CZ, cefazolin; CTZ, ceftazidime; CTRX, ceftriaxone; CL, clindamycin; NAF, nafcillin; OX, oxacillin; GENT, gentamicin; VC, vancomycin.
From Poole SM, Nowobilski-Vasilios A, Free F. Intravenous push medications in the home [abstract]. J Intraven Nurs 1999, 22:209–215.

cated in Table 3 (20). Some parenteral antimicrobials, such as gentamicin and oxacillin, are stopped early because of an adverse event in nearly one in ten cases. Other antibiotics, such as the cephalosporins, have to be stopped early in only about 3% of cases.

SAFETY AND EFFECTIVENESS OF OUTPATIENT PARENTERAL ANTIMICROBIAL THERAPY

The safety of OPAT has been well documented by the OPAT Outcomes Registry. Bacterial and clinical outcomes indicate a success rate of more than 95% in the twenty OPAT centers over the past 5 years. This is generally considered a good outcome, but there is little basis for comparison. Complications or problems with OPAT were also assessed and found to be consistent and low in frequency (21,22).

The specific antibiotic to be administered is a significant factor in the decision to treat a patient outside the hospital setting. Drugs administered once daily are most desirable because they result in minimal lifestyle disruption and higher potential for compliance. In addition, minimal manipulation of the IV site reduces the potential of catheter-associated complications (2). Before home therapy begins, the first dose of an antimicrobial should be given in an inpatient setting, with ready access to physicians, nurses, and emergency intervention medications and supplies in case of anaphylaxis (2).

SPECIAL CONSIDERATIONS

Unlike in an inpatient setting, an evaluation of the patient's home environment is important for positive OPAT outcomes. A home visit is helpful but usually not necessary. The home should have basic utilities and be a safe environment. Supportive family and neighbors are important considerations. In many cases, refrigeration of the medication is required in the patient's home. In some cases, a thermometer may need to be provided for monitoring refrigerator temperatures. Telephone access is also important, so the patient can contact providers to report adverse events, ask questions, or receive general support. A patient must have access to reliable transportation for follow-up appointments with physicians, or, if an AIC is utilized, to present to the facility for scheduled infusions. Weather may be a consideration. Emergency services must be readily available.

A patient's history of compliance is important and can often be obtained from the primary care physician. Drug or alcohol problems should be specifically evaluated before therapy is initiated. Injection drug users who may abuse a vascular access system are poor candidates for OPAT (2,24); a skilled nursing facility may be more appropriate. Placement then removal of an infusion device each day may be reasonable for some patients (18).

INFECTION CONTROL

Considerations are also different in the home care setting. The resources for hand washing, basic sanitation, sterile technique, and waste disposal are limited. Medical knowledge and common sense should lead to optimal use of available facilities. There are, however, a number of regulations that may apply, and these vary from state to state (26,27).

DRUG DELIVERY METHODS

Specialized delivery methods are often employed in OPAT. The clinician's role in the regimen design is to provide the therapy with as little inconvenience as possible so that the patient can return to normal life activities. A variety of systems and devices may be used to provide therapy (28–30).

Gravity Infusions

Many antimicrobial agents can be safely administered using a gravity drip system. In most cases, this method is also the least expensive. Using the gravity drip system, a bag or bottle is hung on a hook or pole above the patient, and fluid flows down the line and into the catheter. The rate of flow in a simple gravity drip system is controlled primarily by a special clamp or valve on the line that can be adjusted to permit the prescribed amount of fluid to flow through. This method of infusion works well for antimicrobials that are to be administered one to two times per day.

If there is concern about limiting or controlling the rate of infusion, a flow regulator may be added to the gravity infusion system. A flow regulator usually consists of a device attached to or incorporated into the tubing, with a dial that can be preset by the clinician to automatically deliver the prescribed amount of fluid over the appropriate time frame. Most flow regulators have settings from 5 to 250 mg/mL and are manufactured in such a way as to prevent accidental adjustment. This infusion method is appropriate for antimicrobials such as vancomycin or amphotericin, which have a high incidence of adverse events resulting from rapid administration.

ELASTOMERIC DEVICES

An elastomeric infusion device is a disposable plastic container. It contains an internal elastic bladder that is filled with medication. Although the cost of these devices can be substantial, so can the benefits. These are convenient and safe storage devices that can be easily used by patients. The patient simply attaches the device to his or her indwelling catheter and releases the clamps. The infusion rate is predetermined by the narrow rate-limiting bore, so no adjustments are necessary. These devices are commercially available in a variety of sizes and infusion rates. Benefits of this administration method include ease of administration, the ability of the patient to be ambulatory during the infusion, and controlled rate of infusion. Disadvantages include the cost of purchasing these devices, plus the increased labor costs involved in filling them.

STATIONARY ELECTRONIC PUMP

A stationary infusion pump, similar to those employed in the inpatient setting, may also be used in the home or AIC setting. However, in most instances, this can be avoided, especially when dealing with antimicrobials. Although this is a proven, trusted, and effective delivery route, problems do exist. First, there is the acquisition cost of the device and specialized tubing. The patient must also be educated in operating and troubleshooting the device. The pump is often cumbersome, and the patient's activities are limited because the device is electrically powered, hence the patient must remain near an electrical outlet throughout the infusion.

Ambulatory Infusion Pump

Although expensive to acquire and maintain, the ambulatory infusion pump is often the most desirable infusion method available. This method allows for either intermittent or continuous infusion of medication. The pump is programmed by clinicians, and the medication reservoirs are disposable. Ambulatory infusion pumps are ideal for medications with an extended stability rating (at least 24 hours at room temperature) and for those that need to be administered several times a day. These pumps allow the patient to change the disposable reservoir usually once per day. The programmed pump will deliver the prescribed dose of medication at the ordered frequency and rate without the patient's intervention. The continuous infusion of medication may reduce the management time and incidence of phlebitis from intermittent flow. Ambulatory pumps allow the patient to quickly resume the activities of a normal lifestyle and assure compliance with the prescribed regimen, as dosing intervals and rate of infusion are no longer concerns for the patient. Newer pump models also offer clinician intervention via computers and telephone if the patient reports a problem with the pump or if the clinician suspects noncompliance.

Because of the highly concentrated medications in the reservoir, ambulatory infusion pumps are usually not recommended with a peripheral vascular access device. Infiltration of the medication may be a problem, as the device will continue pumping even if the peripheral vascular device becomes dislodged. These highly concentrated solutions may be caustic and cause tissue necrosis. Therefore, ambulatory infusion pumps are generally only considered when the patient has a central catheter.

Intravenous Push

Before the 1970s, many IV medications, including antimicrobials, were given by direct injection over 1 to 5 minutes (IV push). In the 1970s, IV admixtures were generally moved from the nursing station to the pharmacy and antimicrobials were administered after mixing the dose in 50 to 100 mL of diluent.

Infusions were then given with an administration set over 20 to 60 minutes (IV piggyback). Today, with incentives to decrease the cost of care, home infusion providers are looking to the past with a view to reviving older, more cost-efficient technologies (31,32). Although the safety and adverse effects of rapid infusions have not been evaluated thoroughly, studies are in progress to do so.

VASCULAR ACCESS DEVICES

Today, more than 5 million vascular access devices (VADs) are placed in patients in the United States every year (14). With a growing number of outpatient and alternate-site therapy applications, it is critical that OPAT clinicians be familiar

Table 4 Vascular Access Devices

Catheter type	Dwell time	Advantages	Disadvantages
Peripheral	72–96 h	Convenient	Infiltration Site rotation needed Infection rate
Peripherally inserted central catheter	Several months	Centrally placed tip	Position must be confirmed.
Nontunneled central venous catheter	Short term	Can be placed quickly	Infection rate Dislodgement risk
Tunneled central venous catheter	Long term	Lower infection rate	Surgical placement Surgical removal
Implanted port	Long term	Usually visibly undetectable Simple care and maintenance	Infiltration if not accessed properly
Midline catheter	1–2 wk	Usually upper arm catheter into axillary vein	Does not need radiology check; inexpensive

with the selection, care, and maintenance of VADs as noted in Table 4 (28–30).

Vascular access devices may be divided into two broad categories: peripheral VADs and central VADs. If the terminal tip of the VAD enters the superior vena cava, the VAD is categorized as a central venous catheter (CVC). All other VADs with tips terminating in the veins distal to the superior vena cava are categorized as peripheral catheters.

Peripheral Intravenous Devices

Short peripheral catheters provide convenient short-term venous access for a few days of therapy. Some OPAT programs leave them in place for up to a week, but that is not consistent with hospital policies (14). Complications common to peripheral IV devices include infiltration of infusate into surrounding tissue, infections at the site where the catheter exits the skin (site infections), phlebitis, and bloodstream infections (19,33).

New practice guidelines published by the U.S. Centers for Disease Control and Prevention (CDC) in August 2002 recommend that peripheral IV sites be rotated every 72 to 96 hours (14). This may not be practical for the OPAT patient, and careful consideration should be given to the insertion of a longer-term or central venous catheter.

Peripherally Inserted Central Catheters

Peripherally inserted central catheter (PICC) lines are usually inserted in an antecubital vein and threaded into the superior vena cava or right atrium. Before use, the position of the catheter must be confirmed by fluoroscopy, radiography, or ultrasound (33). PICCs have become popular devices for OPAT patients. The appropriate duration of use is unclear. It is common to use them for several months, and some have been left in place for considerably longer without apparent adverse effects (14).

Complications associated with PICCs may vary from phlebitis to bloodstream infections. Published studies show lower rates of infection for PICC and midline access compared with other CVCs (14).

Central Venous Catheters

Central venous catheters include both tunneled and nontunneled types. Nontunneled CVCs are percutaneously placed into the central venous system via the subclavian, jugular, or femoral veins. These catheters are secured by sutures and require diligent care to maintain. Nontunneled catheters are commonly multiple lumen, with staggered lumen lengths that allow for the concurrent infusion of several incompatible medications. They typically exit under the midclavicular area of the chest (29).

Tunneled catheters are typically long silicone or polyurethane catheters that are secured to the body tissue through tissue adhesion to a catheter cuff located near the exit site of the catheter. These catheters are surgically placed into the distal subclavian or proximal axillary vein and are advanced into the superior vena cava. They are then tunneled subcutaneously from the exit site on the distal chest wall. Tunneled catheters are often inserted with a cuff placed near or at the exit site and along the tunnel, allowing the catheter to adhere to the chest wall and potentially prevent bacteria migration into the central venous system. These catheters are sutured in place initially to allow adherence of the cuff to the chest wall. When the site is well healed, the sutures may be removed (29). The costs of surgery and operating room time make CVCs considerably more expensive than PICC lines, which are commonly placed by a nurse at the bedside.

Implanted Vascular Access Devices (Ports)

Implanted VADs, also known as ports, are placed in a subcutaneous pocket near the midclavicular area, chest area, abdomen, or, less commonly, in the femoral vein. A silicone or polyurethane catheter extending from the superior vena cava is attached to a metal or plastic reservoir that is sutured into place in a small pocket under the skin. IV access requires a special right-angle Huber needle with a beveled end. The device is completely covered by the skin so it is waterproof when not accessed and may be much more acceptable from a cosmetic standpoint (29).

The maintenance of an implanted port may also be simpler than that of other VADs. When the port is not being used, the patient is free from a regimen of dressing changes or daily flushing, thus making a port a good option for children who require long-term OPAT or chemotherapy.

ECONOMIC CONSIDERATIONS

Outpatient parenteral antibiotic therapy has a remarkable economic advantage over hospitalization in that the overhead costs of a facility, staffing, and feeding can be averted. Most of the costs of hospital care do not go to medicines or medical therapies. Estimates are that an average day in the hospital costs more than $1,000, whereas OPAT may cost only a few hundred dollars (2). There are, however, many factors that must be weighed with OPAT, including transportation, home care, and child care (2,34). Managed care perspectives on OPAT vary with the payer and the model of delivery to be used (35,36). The potential for cost savings for Medicare patients is also apparent, but regulatory issues prevent compensation for the home infusion model at this time (37).

ACCREDITATION AND REGULATION

As the OPAT sector has evolved, so has the regulatory infrastructure surrounding it. In the 1980s, any pharmacy with a laminar and/or vertical flow hood could compound complex IV therapies to provide to patients in their homes, with virtually no requirements other than a retail pharmacy license. Regulatory requirements have increased as OPAT has become recognized as a growing practice that involves a number of potentially high-risk services provided in a potentially high-risk environment (7).

State Boards of Pharmacy

State boards of pharmacy have gradually increased their requirements for home infusion providers, although many still ask only that pharmacies maintain a traditional retail pharmacy license. Because of an increasing focus on medication safety issues, other states may seek to develop additional regulations; for example, the California legislature passed a bill in 2001 addressing mandatory guidelines for sterile product preparation to be implemented by the California Board of Pharmacy in 2003 (38). Because regulations and requirements vary among states, it is imperative that pharmacists check with their state board of pharmacy when considering the development of an OPAT program.

National Professional Practice Standards

In addition to state regulations, national professional practice standards have emerged over the past decade to address sterile drug compounding (7). The American Society of Health-System Pharmacists (ASHP) has published guidelines that provide detailed recommendations for sterile product preparation based on the "risk level" associated with the compounded products. Most apply to home care as well. The United States Pharmacopoeia (USP), Chapter 797, also provides detailed requirements for sterile product preparation (39).

U.S. Drug Enforcement Administration

The use and recordkeeping of controlled substances is regulated by the Drug Enforcement Administration (DEA) and requires a current, valid DEA license and adherence to applicable DEA regulations.

Occupational Safety and Health Administration

Occupational Safety and Health Administration (OSHA) regulations have a significant impact on the provision of OPAT. Providers must be in compliance with OSHA regulations in terms of safety, protection, education of both staff and patients, and handling and disposing of biohazardous waste.

Guidelines for Outpatient Parenteral Antibiotic Therapy

The Infectious Diseases Society of America published guidelines for OPAT in 1997 (2). They provide a review of OPAT plus information on some of the pharmacy aspects as well as advice on quality improvement and outcomes measures. They are presently under revision and should be published this year. The CDC has developed guidelines addressing the prevention of infection related to the use of VADs. They have addressed such issues as the frequency of administration tubing and IV line changes as well as flushing guidelines and other protocols for reducing the potential for catheter infections (14).

Medicare Standards and Other Applicable Regulations

Organizations providing services to Medicare and Medicaid patients must be aware of and compliant with the standards, requirements, and regulatory activities of the U.S. Department of Health and Human Services (HHS). Within HHS, the agencies most applicable to home infusion practice are the Centers for Medicare and Medicaid Services (CMS) and the HHS Office of the Inspector General (OIG), the investigative arm of the department. In addition, HHS has jurisdiction over other regulations that affect the private health insurance markets, the most significant of which is the Health Insurance Portability and Accountability Act (HIPAA) of 1996 (7).

CONCLUSION

In summary, OPAT offers a safe and cost-effective method of providing essential parenteral antimicrobials without the inconvenience, risks, and expense of hospitalization. Selection of patients appropriate for OPAT requires a team approach, with knowledge of the pharmacology of the medications and their use essential. Multiple factors must be considered, including mixing, sterility, stability, interactions, dispensing, and storage, as well as potential adverse effects and drug interactions. Insight and understanding of these factors and communication with other members of the OPAT team can bring benefits to patients as well as savings of valuable health care dollars.

REFERENCES

1. Tice AD. Handbook of Outpatient Parenteral Therapy for Infectious Diseases. New York: Scientific American Inc., 1997.

2. Tice AD, Rehn SJ, Dalorisio JR, Bradley JS, Martinelli LP, Graham DR. et al. Practice Guidelines for Outpatient Parenteral Antimicrobial Therapy. Clin Infect Dis 2004; 38:1651–72.

3. Tice AD. Infect Dis Clin North Am 1998; No.4.

4. Tice AD. Outpatient intravenous antibiotic therapy. In: Mandell GA, Bennett JE, Dolin R, Eds Principles and Practices of Infectious Diseases. Philadelphia: Churchill Livingstone, 2000: 546–550.

5. Dolin R. Why Are Infusion Therapies Performed at Home? Available at: http://www.nhianet.org (accessed October 7, 2003).

6. Nolet BR. Outpatient parenteral antibiotic (OPAT) therapy in ambulatory infusion centers: opportunities and management issues Infusion 2002; 1:26–33.

7. Flores K, Wilder G. Home Infusion Pharmacy Certificate Program. Module I: Introduction to Home Infusion Practice 1–22. Alexandria. VA: National Home Infusion Association, 2004.

8. Tice AD. Outpatient parenteral antibiotic therapy (OPAT) in the United States: delivery models and indications for use Can J Infect Dis 2000; 11(suppl A):17A–21A.

9. Rucker RW, Harrison GM. Outpatient intravenous medications in the management of cystic fibrosis Pediatrics 1974; 54: 358–360.

10. Rehm SJ. Outpatient parenteral antimicrobial therapy for endocarditis Infect Dis Clin North Am 1998; 12:879–902.

11. Tice AD. Outpatient parenteral antimicrobial therapy for osteomyelitis Infect Dis Clin North Am 1998; 12:903–920.

12. Tice AD. Outpatient parenteral antimicrobial therapy as an alternative to hospitalization Int J Clin Pract Suppl 1998; 95: 4–8.

13. Rehm SJ, Weinstein AJ. Home intravenous antibiotic therapy: a team approach Ann Intern Med 1983; 99:388–392.

14. Weinstein AJ. Guidelines for prevention of intravascular device–related infections MMWR Morb Mortal Wkly Rep 2002; 51(RR-10).

15. Tice AD. Pharmacoeconomic considerations in the ambulatory use of parenteral cephalosporins Drugs 2000; 59(suppl 3): 29–35.

16. Nolet BR. Patient selection in outpatient parenteral antimicrobial therapy Infect Dis Clin North Am 1998; 12:835–849.

17. Wilder GL. Home Infusion Pharmacy Certificate Program. Module I: Introduction to Home Infusion Practice. Alexandria. VA: National Home Infusion Association, 2004.

18. Andes D, Craig WA. Pharmacokinetics and pharmacodynamics of outpatient intravenous antimicrobial therapy Infect Dis Clin North Am 1998; 12:849–860.

19. Phillips LD. Manual of IV Therapeutics. 3d ed. Philadelphia: FA Davis Co, 2001.

20. Tice AD, Seibold GL, Martinelli LP. Adverse effects from intravenous antibiotics with OPAT, 40th Annual Meeting of the Infectious Diseases Society of America, Chicago, October 2002.

21. Kunkel MJ. Quality assurance and outcomes in outpatient parenteral antibiotic therapy Infect Dis Clin North Am 1998; 12: 1023–1034.

22. Tice AD, Seibold GL, Martinelli LP. Reasons for failures with OPAT, 41st Annual Meeting of the Infectious Diseases Society of America, San Diego, October 2003.

23. Nathwani D, Tice A. Ambulatory antimicrobial use: the value of an outcomes registry J Antimicrob Chemother 2002; 49: 149–154.

24. Williams D. Home intravenous antibiotic therapy (HIVAT): indications, patients and antimicrobial agents Int J Antimicrob Agents 1995; 5:3–8.

25. Poretz DM. Home management of antibiotic therapy Curr Clin Top Infect Dis 1989; 10:27–42.

26. Wade BH, Bush SE. Infection control and outpatient parenteral antibiotic therapy Infect Dis Clin North Am 1998; 12:979–994.

27. Tice AD. Home health care. In: Abrutyn E, Goldmann DA, Scheckler WE, Eds Saunders Infection Control Reference Service. 2d ed: WB Saunders, 2000 14:151–154.

28. Mortlock NJ, Schleis T. Outpatient parenteral antimicrobial therapy technology Infect Dis Clin North Am 1998; 12:861–878.

29. Cain D, Kelley HL. Home Infusion Pharmacy Certificate Program Module 3: Overview of Infusion Devices, Vascular Access Devices, and Ancillary Supplies. Alexandria. VA: National Home Infusion Association, 2004.

30. www.opitsourcebook.com (accessed Aug 2004).

31. Poole SM, Nowobilski-Vasilios A, Free F. Intravenous push medications in the home [abstract] J Intraven Nurs 1999; 22: 209–215.

32. Nowobilski-Vasilios A, Poole SM. Development and preliminary outcomes of a program for administering antimicrobials by i.v. push in home care Am J Health Syst Pharm 1999; 56: 76–79.

33. Masoorli S. Extravasation injuries associated with the use of central vascular access devices J Vasc Access Devices 2003; 8: 21–23.

34. Tice AD, Hoaglund PA, Nolet B, McKinnon PS, Mozaffari E. Cost perspectives for outpatient intravenous antimicrobial therapy Pharmacotherapy 2002; 22(2 pt 2):63S–70S.

35. Hindes R, Winkler C, Kane P, Kunkel MJ. Outpatient intravenous antibiotic therapy in Medicare patients: cost-savings analysis Infect Dis Clin Pract 1995; 4:211–217.

36. Tice AD. Medicare coverage of outpatient ambulatory intravenous antibiotic therapy: a program that pays for itself Clin Inf Dis 1998; 27:1415–1421.

37. California State Board of Pharmacy. Proposed regulations for sterile compounding, 2001 (CA Bill # SB 293).

38. Tice AD. United States Pharmacopoeia XXIV. National Formulary 19. Rockville. MD: U.S. Pharmacopeial Convention, Inc, 1999:2130–2143.

39. U.S. Pharmacopoeia. USP General Chapter ⟨797⟩ Pharmaceutical Compounding—Sterile Preparations. January 1, 2004.

19

Rational Use of Antifungals for Invasive Fungal Infections in the Institutional Setting

RICHARD H. DREW, MELISSA D. JOHNSON, and ELIZABETH DODDS ASHLEY

Infectious Diseases Clinical Pharmacy, Duke University Medical Center, and Duke University School of Medicine, Durham, and Campbell University School of Pharmacy, Buies Creek, North Carolina, U.S.A.

JOHN R. PERFECT

Division of Infectious Diseases, Duke University School of Medicine, Durham, North Carolina, U.S.A.

The incidence of invasive fungal infections (IFIs) is increasing at an alarming rate. In the past decade alone, *Candida* spp.

577

have become the fourth leading cause of nosocomial blood-stream infections in the United States (1). The incidence of *Aspergillus* infections is also increasing (2,3). Much of this increase is thought to be a consequence of the growing numbers of patients at risk. With the expanded use of bone marrow and solid organ transplantation as life-saving therapies for malignancies and end-stage organ failure, the medical community is faced with a growing number of immunosuppressed patients. Furthermore, advances in the care of these patients are now sustaining them through the initial treatment phase, when bacterial infections were previously fatal, and into the time frame for increased risk from fungal pathogens.

In addition to the increased incidence of IFIs, there have been some significant changes in the fungal pathogens causing these infections. For example, non-*albicans Candida* species are isolated with increasing frequency in both invasive (1,4) and vaginal (5) candidiasis. Moulds such as *Aspergillus spp* and *Fusarium spp* have been reported with increasing frequency (3,6). Finally, *Scedosporium* and *Paecilomyces* species are among the emerging pathogens causing invasive disease in immuncompromised patients (7).

Until the early 1990s, therapeutic options for treating invasive fungal infections were limited to a few agents with significant treatment-limiting toxicities. Fortunately, the past decade has seen the introduction of a new class of antifungal agents (the echinocandins) as well as expanded options within the azole and polyene classes. However, these new therapies have come with significant increases in institutional expenditures and, in some instances, drug-related toxicities. Considering these issues, as well as the complexity of the population at risk and severity of these diseases, there is a well-established need for both disease- and drug-specific treatment guidelines for the optimal management of IFIs.

CHALLENGES IN EVALUATING AGENTS TO TREAT INVASIVE FUNGAL INFECTIONS

Impact of Host Factors on Treatment Outcomes

Perhaps the most significant influence on treatment outcomes in IFIs is the impact of host factors, such as resolution of neutropenia, graft-versus-host disease (GVHD), return of graft function from bone or solid organ transplantation, and control of the underlying disease. This is most critically evident in invasive aspergillosis in the immunocompromised host, in which response rates remain less than 30% despite the availability of agents with potent *in vitro* activity against this pathogen (8,9). In contrast, success rates for treatment may approach 70% in certain risk groups that are less immunocompromised (10). Although recent data (which included a diverse population of patients with aspergillosis) showed that a complete or partial response rates with a new treatment option (voriconazole) was approximately 50% (11), it is sobering to note that 3-month survival for patients with invasive asperillosis is only 30% to 40% (12).

Lack of Routine In Vitro Susceptibility Testing

In contrast to bacteria, antifungal susceptibility testing for pathogens causing IFIs is not routinely performed at most institutions. This is due to multiple factors, including lack of standardized methodology, lack of available laboratory resources, and lack of data correlating microbiologic resistance or susceptibility and patient outcomes.

The currently approved *in vitro* susceptibility testing methodologies are limited to the testing of *Candida* spp for itraconazole, fluconazole, and flucytosine (13). Newly proposed methods for disk diffusion apply only to fluconazole and voriconazole, although these methods may enable application with other antifungal agents in the future (14). There are no currently approved standards for testing of yeast against polyenes such as amphotericin B, or echinocandins such as caspofungin.

In vitro susceptibility testing of *Candida* spp has had limited application in routine clinical practice, which likely relates to issues regarding the need for timely accessibility to these test results. The lack of automated testing methods makes these processes extremely labor intensive, time consuming, and costly. Therefore, many institutions limit susceptibility testing of *Candida* spp. to specific circumstances in which there is a high suspicion of resistance and often rely on reference laboratories for these services. Specific indications for which-susceptibility testing may be routinely performed include non-*albicans Candida* bloodstream isolates with unpredictable susceptibility to azoles (such as *Candida glabrata*), isolates from patients with increased risk of resistance (such as those receiving prior antifungal therapy), and yeast isolates obtained from patients with relapsed infection. Because *Candida krusei* is inherently resistant to fluconazole, susceptibility testing for organisms to this agent is not recommended and resistance can be presumed. Newly proposed guidelines for disk diffusion testing methods for yeasts may facilitate testing procedures to allow more rapid availability of these test results (14). An automated panel for susceptibility testing of yeasts was recently approved by the Food and Drug Administration, but has not yet been widely implemented in clinical laboratories. In time, these advances may permit routine testing of all isolates and allow more widespread application of susceptibility test results to patient care.

In addition to methodologic concerns, another factor contributing to the lack of widespread use of susceptibility testing is the general lack of clinical studies correlating *in vitro* susceptibilities to clinical outcomes for patients with fungal infections. The current interpretive standards for *Candida* spp. were based on outcomes in immunocompetent patients with invasive disease, consisting primarily of candidemia, and in patients with oropharyngeal and esophageal candidiasis treated with either fluconazole or itraconazole (15). There are limited data, however, that demonstrate a correlation between minimum inhibitory concentrations (MICs) for *Candida* spp and clinical outcomes with amphotericin B therapy among patients with candidemia (16). Although not directly evaluated, the currently approved interpretive standards do appear to be reasonable for use in select patients with more invasive disease as well (17). What is not known is the ability to directly apply these data to severely immunocompromised patients with IFIs. In addition, clinical experience in the treatment of IFIs with select agents demonstrating *in vitro* activity may be limited. For example, whereas azoles such as itraconazole and voriconazole may have activity *in vitro* against *C. krusei*, clinical correlates of this activity are limited mostly to oropharyngeal or esophageal candidiasis. Because data demonstrating efficacy of these azoles in the setting of more invasive candidial infections with fluconazole-resistant species are generally lacking, alternative treatment approaches should be considered.

Standardization of *in vitro* antifungal susceptibility testing for moulds is still in evolution. In 2002, the National Committee for Clinical Laboratory Standards approved metholodogies for susceptibility testing of filamentous moulds; however, they have several limitations in common with the currently approved standards for testing of yeasts as described above (18). As with yeast infections, data are sparse regarding correlations of *in vitro* susceptibility testing results to patient outcomes for most mould infections, except perhaps for one study that suggested a correlation between MICs and outcome of patients with invasive aspergillosis receiving amphotericin B (19). Several issues hinder the potential clinical utility of *in vitro* mould susceptibility testing. Technical variability can greatly influence end points that are already difficult to measure. Furthermore, predictive ability of these tests is complicated by host factors, which strongly influence treatment outcomes. Occasionally, *in vitro* testing may be helpful in the setting of relapsed infection, unusual moulds, or for certain fungal strains with unpredictable response to antifungals.

Determining the Standard of Care

Since its availability in 1959, amphotericin B deoxycholate (AmBd) was the standard of care to treat most serious invasive fungal infections, including aspergillosis, cryptococcosis, candidiasis, blastomycosis, histoplasmosis, and zygomycosis (20,21). Its established role, however, was based largely on noncomparative trials during an era in which treatment options were extremely limited (20,21). Despite the introduction of newer agents, AmBd continued to be identified as the treatment of choice for many invasive fungal infections because of its broad spectrum of antifungal activity, proven efficacy, and low rates of fungal resistance (20,21).

Recent studies have suggested that newer agents may provide comparable or superior efficacy with significant reductions in toxicity (21). Evidence-based studies in aspergillosis and candidiasis have demonstrated that triazoles (11) or echinocandins (22) are equivalent or superior to AmBd, but with significantly less toxicity. Emerging data also suggest potential differences in therapeutic outcome between the lipid-based formulations of amphotericin B as empiric therapy for IFIs in febrile, neutropenic patients (21,23,24)

Recently published clinical treatment guidelines help establish the new standard of care (8,25–31). However, even published guidelines may not be able to keep pace with emerging data that reflect developments with newer agents, and therefore need constant revision. One example is the use of voriconazole for the treatment of invasive aspergillosis. A recent study established the superiority of this agent over amphotericin B for the management of invasive disease (11). This trial was completed after the Infectious Diseases Society of America (IDSA) guidelines for management of invasive aspergillosis were published. Therefore, although most would agree that voriconazole represents the new "gold standard" for treatment of invasive aspergillosis, it is not reflected in the initial published treatment strategies (8).

Diagnostic Uncertainty

For some invasive fungal infections, a certain amount of diagnostic uncertainty exists in establishing both the presence of infection and determining the level of host invasion (32). Many of the clinical findings in infected patients are both insensitive and nonspecific; therefore, risk factor assessment has become a critical feature of clinical decisions. In addition, many fungal pathogens, such as *Aspergillus* spp and *Candida* spp, are ubiquitous in nature and frequent colonizers of the human host. Therefore, isolation of these organisms from nonsterile body sites, such as the respiratory tract, may not necessarily represent invasive disease. However, isolation of a fungal pathogen in the setting of supporting clinical, radiologic, and laboratory evidence, along with the presence of specific host risk factors, may enable the clinician to better predict the likelihood of infection. An example would be in establishing a diagnosis of invasive aspergillosis (8). Although isolation of *Aspergillus* species from sputum or nares would be insufficient to establish a diagnosis of aspergillosis, the positive predictive value of this finding is greater among patients with risk factors for IFIs, such as aggressively-treated leukemia patients or those who have recently undergone bone marrow transplantation (33,34).

Guidelines have been published by the Mycoses Study Group (MSG) in collaboration with the European Organization for Research and Treatment of Cancer (EORTC) to assist clinicians in diagnosing invasive fungal infections (35). These criteria are based primarily on laboratory, clinical, radiologic, and microbiologic findings, recognizing that rapid and reliable non–culture-based methods for diagnosis of most invasive fungal infections are still lacking. They rate diagnosis according to likelihood of infection: definite, probable, or possible. The *definite* classification of disease is relatively well-defined by histopathology and cultures. In contrast, the definition of *possible* disease is a weaker diagnosis, and lends itself to empiric studies that are much less robust in their conclusions. The *probable* disease category is the crucial group to define for studies, and its accuracy tends to lend credibility and accuracy to conclusions of any study. Although currently applied to various patient populations, these definitions were originally developed to specifically identify fungal infections in the neutropenic oncology patient and address nuances encountered in this patient population. Regardless of definitions used for purposes of clinical research, it may be difficult to apply study definitions to clinical decisions regarding the treatment of an individual patient. This separation is important to note. For instance, diagnostic criteria, such as "halo" or "crescent sign" for aspergillosis, may be masked in patients with suppressed immune systems. Therefore, development of this sign may only signify return of immune function in a patient with established infection. At this point, it may be too late to effectively initiate therapy (8). In routine clinical practice, the decision to initiate empiric antifungal therapy may be based more on patient risk factors and clinical course rather than these specific diagnostic criteria that have been used in clinical trials.

Serologic testing is a minimally invasive approach to survey for fungal disease when lack of a competent immune system may mask clinical signs and symptoms of infection. One very successful serologic test is the latex agglutination test for cryptococcal antigen that can approach 100% sensitivity and specificity for this disease (36). Further advances in laboratory techniques to diagnose fungal infections include the use of *Aspergillus* galactomannan assays (37,38) and glucan and polymerase chain reaction tests (39,40). These tests may aid in establishing a more rapid detection of infection, but they are presently under study or only recently released in the United States and require further clinical experience to determine their value.

Preemptive Treatment Strategies

In addition to prophylactic and treatment strategies for the management of invasive fungal infections, improvements in diagnostic techniques may enable the use of early, preemptive antifungal therapy before the onset of clinical infection (29). Similar strategies have been employed in the treatment of cytomegalovirus (CMV) infections in patients undergoing solid organ and hematopoietic stem cell transplantation (HSCT) (41). This strategy is based on the reasonable assumption that therapeutic outcome has a better chance of a positive result when the burden of fungal organisms is substantially less. These strategies may often be considered prophylactic, but with more objective data for evidence of disease. For instance, "preemptive" therapy among select surgical intensive care unit (ICU) patients with multiple risk factors for infection is another approach that has potential merit. This is largely because IFIs are often undiagnosed premortem in this patient population (42–45).

Emerging Role of Combination Therapy

Although combination therapy is frequently employed for the treatment of serious bacterial infections, tuberculosis, and

HIV, the role of combination therapy for the treatment of invasive fungal infections is less clear. *In vitro* and animal model data are available for most common fungal pathogens, whereas clinical data in humans are less abundant (14,46). In general, limited clinical data have been published to document that outcomes are improved with combinations relative to single-agent therapy. One exception is the combination of amphotericin B and flucytosine for the treatment of cryptococcal meningitis (30), in which the addition of flucytosine has clearly been associated with faster clearance of yeasts from the cerebrospinal fluid and fewer relapses. In contrast, a recent trial documented similar overall efficacy of the combination of amphotericin B and fluconazole for the treatment of candidemia compared with fluconazole alone (47). Therefore, the role of combination therapy in candidemic patients remains unclear. To date, only limited studies have reported efficacy of antifungal combinations in the management of patients with invasive aspergillosis, and large comparative studies have not been performed. Two comparative pilot studies with the combination of echinocandins and liposomal amphotericin B were recently performed, but the number of patients included overall was small, and results have not yet been published. Experience is even more limited for the more rare fungal infections. Additional studies are necessary to help define the role of this treatment approach, but the expense and time involved in performing such trials makes these kinds of investigations particularly challenging.

Antifungal Drug Resistance

Some fungal pathogens may be inherently resistant to an antifungal agent. Examples include *C. krusei* to fluconazole, *Candida lusitaniae* to amphotericin B, and *Scedosporium prolificans* to all available antifungal agents (17). However, most failures or relapses occur with apparently susceptible strains. Although resistance with *C. glabrata*, *C. krusei* and *C. albicans* during treatment with amphotericin B and fluconazole has been reported (48), treatment-emergent resistance from isolates initially susceptible to azoles and polyene antifungals remains uncommon. Less is known regarding treatment-emergent resistance with the echinocandins, but to date, it has not been reported from clinical trials or other published experience.

Because there are several mechanisms for drug resistance, cross-resistance within a class of agents, such as the azoles, is not always certain. An example of this is the efficacy of itraconazole in treating oropharyngeal and esophageal candidiasis due to fluconazole-resistant *Candida* spp (49). Clinical experience is helpful in guiding selection of therapy in situations in which data may be lacking. In some situations, *in vitro* susceptibility testing may be helpful in deciding whether there is cross-resistance, but the limitations of such testing should be considered.

In contrast to antibacterial agents, the potential development of specific direct drug resistance has rarely limited the use of antifungals (17,50). However, it is possible that frequent antifungal drug use (such as routine antifungal prophylaxis) will change the epidemiology of fungal infections observed within a hospital. An example of this potential is the increased isolation of *C. krusei* in centers utilizing fluconazole prophylaxis or therapy (50–53). With the widespread use of extended-spectrum azoles (e.g., voriconazole), the potential exists for a shift toward more azole-resistant mould and yeast infections.

ASSESSING UNIQUE INSTITUTIONAL NEEDS FOR SELECT ANTIFUNGAL AGENTS

As a consequence of the unique patient populations cared for at each medical facility, the needs for specific antifungal agents may vary substantially between institutions. Identification of the patient populations most likely to receive antifungal therapy and the types of indications for which these drugs may be employed is helpful in designing and implementing antifungal clinical programs. Periodic reassessment is required to ensure that available drugs are meeting the needs of the institution and providing state-of-the-art care for patients.

Population-Specific Needs

Several studies have indicated that certain patient subgroups are at higher risk of invasive fungal infections. For example, total parenteral nutrition, central venous catheter use, and abdominal surgery have been identified as risk factors for candidemia (29). Similarly, cancer chemotherapy, transplantation, and other immunosuppressive treatments have been associated with an increased risk of aspergillosis (8) and other invasive fungal infections. These infections and their treatment are part of the cost of care in medical centers that treat these seriously ill patients.

Patients with Malignancies

Patients with prolonged neutropenia following chemotherapy are at increased risk for developing fungal infections. Although bloodstream infections due to *Candida* spp and invasive mould infections due to *Aspergillus* spp are the most common fungal pathogens seen, there has recently been an increase in more rare and difficult-to-treat fungi (54–57). Among those with hematologic malignancies, principal risk factors include neutropenia, mucotoxicity, T cell depression related to corticosteroid use, underlying disease and GVHD disease in patients who ultimately require transplantation (58,59). The duration and degree of neutropenia have been established as significant risk factors for development of invasive aspergillosis in this patient population, and the correlation with GVHD and its treatment with corticosteroids with aspergillosis is (2,59–61). Loss of mucosal immunity appears to be a risk factor for development of invasive candidiasis, and many times this occurs concurrently with neutropenia (60,62–64).

Patients with untreated Hodgkin's disease, acute lymphocytic leukemia, chronic lymphocytic and hairy cell leukemia, and multiple myeloma have defects in T cell–related immunity as a results of their underlying disease or receipt of corticosteroid therapy (63,65–67) These patients are at increased risk of fungal infections from a broad array of opportunistic fungal pathogens, including *Cryptococcus neoformans*,

Aspergillus spp, filamentous fungi, and *Pneumocystis carinii* (6,67). Lymphopenia has been suggested as a risk factor for developing fungal infections in this population and is commonly associated with agents that target lymphocytes, such as fludarabine, and the recent use of monoclonal antibodies such as alemtuzumab (Campath; Berlex Laboratories, Richmond, CA)™ (63,68–70).

Hematopoietic Stem Cell Transplant Recipients

Patients undergoing HSCT are at extremely high risk for IFIs. In recent series, IFIs were documented in 15% of HSCT patients (71). *Aspergillus* spp are often the predominant pathogen isolated in IFIs among HSCT recipients. Overall, the incidence of invasive aspergillosis in this patient population varies and ranges from 3% to 15% in most published series (71–76). In more recent studies, *Candida* spp and other less common fungi, such as *Fusarium*, *Scedosporium*, and *Zygomycetes*, have been increasingly isolated (66,71). Invasive candidiasis was reported in more than 10% of patients (60,77–80) but has decreased substantially with implementation of effective fluconazole prophylactic regimens (61,71,81,82). Breakthrough candidal infections have been reported, however, in the setting of prophylaxis and seem to be increasingly problematic (83–85). In some series of HSCT recipients, 60% of patients who died as the result of infection had invasive aspergillosis or invasive candidiasis (80,86). These findings have been similar among both adult and pediatric bone marrow transplant recipients (80,86).

Traditionally, most fungal infections have been diagnosed during the period before engraftment, but recent reports in allogeneic HSCT recipients describe a much longer period of risk for this population (87). This may, in part, result from the increased risk for GVHD following allogeneic transplantation, which necessitates use of high-dose corticosteroids and other immunosuppressants. In this population, diagnosis of IFIs commonly occurs more than 3 months post-transplantation and (increasingly) more than 6 months after transplantation (66,71,76). Among pediatric HSCT recipients, those with autologous HSCT typically experienced IFIs within the first month after transplantation, during the neutropenic phase, whereas allogeneic HSCT recipients had IFIs diagnosed most often 1 or more months after transplantation (86).

When compared with autologous HSCT recipients, allogeneic HSCT patients appear to exhibit both a higher incidence (76,80,86) and mortality (80) due to fungal infections. In one series, the incidence of IFI following nonmyeloablative allogeneic HSCT was reported to be as high as 23%, with 80% attributable mortality (88). The majority of these infections were invasive aspergillosis, with a median time to infection of 81 days (range, 11 to 175 days) (88). Recipients of cord blood and T cell–depleted or CD34-selected stem cells also appear to be at higher risk of developing invasive aspergillosis, both early (within 40 days) and late (41 to 180 days) following transplantation (66).

In addition to the type of transplant, other risk factors in HSCT recipients for IFI include increased age of the recipient, severity and prolonged duration of neutropenia, donor mismatch, seropositivity for CMV in the recipient, and development of acute GVHD (60,66,77,78,80,86,89). Transplantations for myelodysplastic syndrome, high-risk acute leukemia, and use of a human leukocyte antigen–matched unrelated donor have also been implicated as significant risk factors for IFI in this patient population (66,71). Multiple myeloma has also been implicated as a risk factor for development of invasive aspergillosis in the late post-transplantation period (41 to 180 days post-transplantation) (66). In the post-transplantation phase, specific risk factors include delayed engraftment, development of acute or chronic GVHD, treatment of GVHD, and ongoing viral infection including CMV or respiratory viruses (66,71). Finally, cumulative doses of steroids are a significant risk factor for development of invasive aspergillosis in this patient population (76).

In institutions providing care for HSCT recipients, it must be emphasized that many antifungal agents lack relevant activity or treatment experience against the less common mould infections (such as *Fusarium, Scedosporium, Paecilomyces, Zygomycetes*, and some black moulds). These moulds may be particularly important in the bone marrow transplantation setting and are associated with high rates of mortality (3).

Solid Organ Transplant Recipients

Patients receiving solid organ transplants are at significant risk of invasive fungal infections owing to a number of factors, and the risk of these infections varies according time after transplantation (90). In the first month after transplantation, patients are primarily at risk for invasive candidiasis, with risk factors similar to those of patients undergoing other surgical procedures (90). These risk factors include use of vascular access devices, intubation, presence of foreign bodies, and tissue and/or fluid collections that are poorly perfused. Less frequently, transmission of *Candida* spp and subsequent infection occurs through the allograft. During the period 1 to 6 months after tranplantation, the duration and severity of immunosuppression increases and correspondingly, the risk of IFIs such as aspergillosis, cryptococcosis, and endemic mycoses rises (90). The presence of ongoing viral infections such as CMV, HIV, hepatitis B, Epstein-Barr virus (EBV), and other human herpesviruses also increases the risk for IFIs during this time period (90–92). After 6 months, 5% to 10% of patients experience graft rejection, which significantly increases the risk of fungal opportunists such as *Pneumocystis jiroveci* (formerly *P. carinii*), *C. neoformans*, and *Aspergillus* spp (93–95).

Surgical Intensive Care Unit Patients

A number of epidemiologic surveillance studies have documented the risk of developing invasive candidiasis among surgical ICU populations (96–98). Although the overall incidence of infection is low, a subset of patients at increased risk has been identified. Risk factors in this population include use of broad-spectrum antibiotics, acute renal failure, central catheterization, receipt of total parenteral nutrition, presence of *Candida* spp colonization, diabetes mellitus, gastrointestinal disease or recent abdominal surgery, transfer from another hospital, bladder catheterizaton, hemodialysis, diarrhea, and increasing duration of ICU stay (96–98). These risk factors may evolve during the hospitalization. A recent study suggested that within the first 3 days of ICU admission, independent predictors of *Candida* spp colonization or infection include diarrhea, central catheterization for longer than 72 hours, and receipt of multiple surgical procedures (97). As the length of ICU hospitalization increases, predictors of *Candida* spp colonization or infection change somewhat, and by 6 to 8 days include multiple surgical procedures, central catheterization, mechanical ventilation, hemodialysis, white blood cell count greater than 10,000 cells/mcL, broad-spectrum antibiotics, presence of solid tumor, and lack of enteral or parenteral nutrition (97). In addition, patients who develop local colonization or infection have an average of eight to nine risk factors, whereas those who remain noncolonized with *Candida* spp typically have fewer than seven risk factors present (97).

Burn Patients

Few studies have examined the specific risk factors for IFIs among burn patients, but this population appears to be at increased risk of bloodstream infections due to *Candida* spp (99). This risk is related to compromise of the epidermis, frequent acidosis, and routine use of central venous catheters. In particular, those receiving longer courses of broad-spectrum antibiotics may be at increased risk for developing invasive candidiasis (99).

Elderly

Limited data are available specifically evaluating risks for invasive fungal infections among the elderly, but elderly patients frequently experience these infections in the setting of other underlying diseases. Surveillance studies for *Candida* spp have suggested that non-*albicans Candida* infections, such as *C. glabrata*, occur more frequently in the elderly and that mortality among this population may be higher than that of their younger counterparts (100,101). Older patients often require urinary catheterization, especially in the nursing home setting, which increases the risk for *Candida* spp colonization and infection (102). Oropharyngeal and esophageal candidiasis may also be particularly frequent among the elderly, and prosthetic devices such as dentures may foster development and persistence of *Candida* spp colonization in the orophaynx (103).

HIV-Infected Patients

Defects in T cell–mediated immunity among patients with HIV infection make these patients particularly susceptible to cryptococcal infection, especially when CD4+ T cell counts are below 50 cells/mm^3 (104). Oropharyngeal and esophageal candidiasis are also common, typically occurring when CD4+ T cell counts are less than 250 cells/mm^3 (104). Many of these infections are caused by *C. albicans*, but non-*albicans* or mixed infections with more than one *Candida* species are not uncommon. The endemic mycoses, such as histoplasmosis, blastomycosis, and coccidioidomycosis, may also occur with increased frequency in this population, especially as reactivation of old disease as CD4+ T cells decline with advancing HIV infection. Furthermore, sporotrichosis may occur in these patients by direct inoculation from an environmental source, such as rose thorns or soil. Mould infections, however, are not typically observed with increased frequency in this patient population in the absence of other risk factors, such as chemotherapy or immunosuppressive drug therapy. With the advent of the era of highly-active antiretroviral therapy (HAART), mortality rates among HIV patients due to opportunistic infections such as cryptococcosis have declined dramatically (105–107). Some studies suggest that increases in CD4+ T cell count with HAART reduce the incidence of primary fungal infections and rates of subsequent relapse (107,108). In addition, the need for lifelong secondary prophylaxis following treatment of cryptococcal meningitis may be reduced in the setting of immunologic response to antiretroviral therapy, particularly when CD4+ T cells increase to more than 100 cells/mm^3 (109–111). Likewise, control of virologic replication may reduce the risk of developing oropharyngeal and esophageal candidiasis (112,113).

FORMULATING ANTIFUNGAL TREATMENT STRATEGIES

Justification for Prevention and Treatment Guidelines

The juxtaposition of increasing incidence of invasive fungal infections, the high cost of new treatment options, and the complexity of the underlying patient population infected with these pathogens supports the need for judicious use of the antifungal armamentarium. One strategy addressing all these issues is to manage infected patients and the formulary through development of guidelines for appropriate usage within a specific medical center.

Control Treatment-Related Costs

Budgetary considerations with antifungal agents are paramount given that many of these agents have high acquisition costs (Table 1). As is often seen with many other therapeutic classes, the primary motivating force for initiating guidelines for antifungal therapy is often to control drug expenditures and associated costs. This was initially demonstrated with the first triazole antifungal, fluconazole, which was available in both intravenous and oral formulations. The cost disparity between these preparations prompted the establishment of programs which prompted conversion from parenteral to oral administration at many institutions (114–116). High acquisition costs are also associated with lipid-based formulations of amphotericin B, which can cost up to 100 times more than AmBd (Table 1). However, the reduction in nephrotoxic effects afforded by these lipid formulations could result in overall cost savings to the health system. Unfortunately in most health systems, pharmacy departments are charged with controlling the expanding drug budget and do not reap the benefit from cost-avoidance of nephrotoxicity and requirement for dialysis (117). Similarly, newer drugs such as caspofungin and voriconazole have substantially higher acquisition costs relative to that of AmBd and oral azole therapy but offer improved toxicity profiles over AmBd. Use of combination antifungal therapy, which has little evidence-based support for serious invasive

Table 1 Average Wholesale Prices of Selected Antifungals

Price	Price per unit (unit size)	Comparison dose	Acquisition cost for daily dose of therapy in a 70-kg patient (nonloading doses)*
Amphotericin B deoxycholate (AmBd, Fungizone™)	$20.54 (50 mg)	0.7 mg/kg qd	$20.54
Amphotericin B colloidal dispersion (ABCD, Amphotec™)	$160.00 (100 mg)	5 mg/kg qd	$560.00
Amphotericin B lipid complex (ABLC, Abelcet™)	$230.00 (100 mg)	5 mg/kg qd	$805.00
Liposomal amphotericin B (L-AmB, AmBisome™)	$188.40 (50 mg)	5 mg/kg qd	$1,318.80
Voriconazole injection (Vfend™)	$106.00 (200 mg)	6 mg/kg q12h × 2 doses, then 4 mg/kg q12h	$148.75
Voriconazole tablets (Vfend™)	$937.50 for 30 tablets (200 mg; $25.00 per tab)	200 mg q12h	$62.50
Itraconazole injection (Sporanox™)	$193.93 (250 mg IV kit)	200 mg q12h × 4 doses, then 200 mg qd	$193.93
Itraconazole oral solution (Sporanox™)	$128.28 (1,500 mg bottle)	200 mg q12h × 4 doses, then 200 mg qd	$17.10
Itraconazole capsules (Sporanox™)	$189.09 for 30 100 mg capsules	200 mg q12h × 4 doses, then 200 mg qd	$12.61
Fluconazole injection (Diflucan™)	$147.58 (400 mg IV)	Systemic infection: 400 mg IV qd	$147.58
Fluconazole tablets (Diflucan™)	$13.98 for one 200 mg capsule	Systemic infection: 400 mg qd	$27.96
Caspofungin injection (Cancidas™)	$485.54 (70 mg) $376.91 (50 mg)	70 mg × 1 dose, then 50 mg qd	$376.91

* Daily price assumes no organ dysfunction or pharmacy wastage.
IV, intravenous; qd, daily.
Modified from Gallagher JC, Dodds Ashley ES, Drew RH, Perfect. JR. Antifungal pharmacotherapy for invasive mould infections. Expert Opin Pharmacother 2003;4:147–164, used with permission.

infections, can further escalate treatment costs. The high acquisition costs, use of combination therapy, and prolonged durations of treatment have pushed antifungals to the top of antimicrobial drug expenditures at many institutions.

Assure Safe Administration

Assurance of safe administration of antifungals requires that procedures are in place to prevent drug-related toxicities whenever possible, detect treatment-related adverse effects, and minimize the potential for drug–drug interactions. Expanded discussions of drug-specific strategies are found elsewhere in this chapter.

Because some of the toxicities secondary to antifungal therapy cannot always be prevented, it is important to ensure that they are recognized as early in the treatment course as possible, to facilitate positive outcomes. Therefore, specific guidelines may also be used to ensure appropriate detection and management of the serious toxicities associated with each of the antifungal agents. In addition, treatment courses for invasive fungal infections may range from weeks to years. Therefore, it is essential to perform routine monitoring so that therapy may be altered by either substitution of another agent or alteration in dose. Finally, nearly all of the antifungal agents, especially the azole antifungals, interact with other commonly prescribed medications. This is especially true in the immunocompromised patient population who are also at increased risk for developing invasive fungal infections. Comprehensive guidelines should include recommendations for practitioners to carefully evaluate patient regimens for the presence of interacting medications and to consider modifications of therapy when necessary.

Educational Benefits

Guidelines may also have an educational impact, particularly within teaching institutions. Recent discussion has brought attention to the fact that U.S. medical school curricula dedicated to treatment of invasive fungal infections are increasingly sparse. Programs typically focus on basic microbiology and diagnosis of these infections, leaving minimal time for pharmacotherapy of these diseases. This also means that clinicians receive most of their training about antifungal pharmacotherapy from their postgraduate medical education (ie in internships, residencies, and fellowships). By training physicians to follow specific treatment algorithms, guidelines can teach the decision processes behind management of IFIs. If guidelines are comprehensive enough to include dosing, monitoring parameters, and toxicity management, the practitioner is also exposed to important information regarding the individual pharmacologic agents.

Process of Formulating Antifungal Guidelines

The process for developing guidelines for antifungal agents is similar to that for antibacterials and is discussed elsewhere within this text. There are, however, some unique characteristics of the antifungal armamentarium and the patient populations in which it is most likely to be employed that are worth noting.

Sources of Information Unique to Antifungal
Agents

As with other therapeutic areas in which information changes rapidly, it would be insufficient to rely solely on routine published sources (such as product package inserts). Professional meetings, published guidelines, and Internet resources can provide valuable supplemental information. Major national and international meetings that specifically focus on the area of antifungal agents include the Interscience Conference on Antimicrobial Agents and Chemotherapy (ICAAC–American Society of Microbiology; www.icaac.com), IDSA (www.idsociety.org), and Focus on Fungal Infections (www.imedex.com). In addition, conferences devoted to specific patient populations, such as those presented by transplantation and hematology/oncology societies, often include data regarding fungal infections in these specific patient groups. Program proceedings from these conferences may serve as an invaluable source of new and emerging information.

National guidelines and consensus statements for the management of invasive fungal infections have been published. Those prepared by IDSA include guidelines for treatment and management of cryptococcosis (30), aspergillosis (8), candidiasis (29), coccidioidomycosis (26), blastomycosis (25), sporotrichosis (27), and histoplasmosis (31). These may be freely accessed at the IDSA website (www.IDSociety.org). Consensus guidelines for the management of candidiasis have also been published by the Europeans (118). For HIV-infected persons, the U.S. Public Health Service/IDSA guidelines address appropriate measures for both primary and secondary prophylaxis of fungal infections (119). These guidelines are frequently updated and available on the web (http://www.aidsinfo.nih.gov). Finally, guidelines that address the prevention and treatment of IFIs in patients with malignancy have also been published, including the appropriate management of fever in the neutropenic patient (98) and prophylaxis of invasive fungal infections in the setting of bone marrow transplantation (120); these guidelines are available at www.IDSociety.org and http://www.cdc.gov/mmwr/preview/mmwrhtml/rr4910a1.htm, respectively.

In addition to reference texts and consensus guidelines, there are some comprehensive sites available through the Internet that contain a vast amount of information about fungi and invasive fungal infections. One such site is http://www.doctorfungus.org, which covers human, animal, and laboratory mycoses. This site also includes a data bank for trends in antifungal resistance. A comprehensive site devoted to *Aspergillus* spp infections is http://www.aspergillus.man.ac.uk. This site also includes expert commentary on invasive fungal infections and an area where users can submit questions to be answered by expert panel members.

CLASS-SPECIFIC GUIDELINES

Polyenes

Amphotericin B

Amphotericin B deoxycholate revolutionized the treatment of fungal infections when it was introduced in 1956 (20). To provide effective treatment for previously fatal infections, clinicians were forced to accept the risk of significant organ toxicities, most notably infusion-related side effects and nephrotoxicity. However, as scientific knowledge surrounding this agent grew and the mechanisms of common toxicities were elucidated, guidelines began to have an essential role in ensuring safe and effective administration of this polyene.

Currently there are four marketed formulations of amphotericin B in the United States: AmBd, liposomal amphotericin B (L-AmB [AmBisome™; Fujisawa Healthcare, Inc., Deerfield, IL]), amphotericin B lipid complex (ABLC [Abelcet™; Enzon Inc., Piscataway, NJ]) and amphotericin B colloidal dispersion (ABCD [Amphotec™; InterMune, Inc., Brisbane, CA]). Comprehensive reviews for both AmBd (20) and the lipid-based formulations (21,121) have been published previously.

Because amphotericin B has the broadest spectrum and is the most consistently fungicidal antifungal agent currently available, it is often the preferred empiric agent in situations in which the patient is at high risk for serious invasive fungal infections with rapid clinical deterioration but the diagnosis is not clear. AmBd has proven effective as empiric therapy in high-risk populations, including febrile neutropenic patients, and is currently recommended for neutropenic patients with persistent fever after 3 to 5 days of antibiotic treatment (98). Other studies demonstrate comparable activity of fluconazole (122,123), itraconazole (124) and liposomal amphotericin B (125) in this high-risk patient population.

Numerous randomized, comparative, controlled clinical trials have been published to evaluate lipid-based formulations of amphotericin B (125–133). Data from these trials have been extensively reviewed elsewhere (21). To briefly summarize, most of these trials compared different formulations of amphotericin B in the empiric treatment of neutropenic patients with fever (125,131–133). Other indications included neutropenia with suspected or documented invasive fungal infection (127,130), cryptococcal infections in patients with AIDS (128,130), histoplasmosis (129), and aspergillosis (126). In general, these trials did not establish superior clinical or mycologic efficacy of the lipid-based formulation over AmBd (21). Therefore, guidelines published by IDSA clearly outline an appropriate place for therapy with AmBd. Arguably, this formulation is still considered to be the gold standard for initial treatment of many invasive mycotic diseases (8,25–31), although there is a recent call to adopt lipid-based formulations of amphotericin B in place of AmBd for many situations in routine clinical practice (21). Once a lipid-based formulation is determined to be required (because of safety issues relative to AmBd), situations in which one lipid-based formulation is preferred over others (based on efficacy) may be based more on the predominance of published clinical experience than on true superiority. Such is probably the case for the use of L-AmB in the treatment of cryptococcal meningitis (30).

Infusion-related reactions such as fever, chills, rigors, nausea, vomiting, and headache are common and irritating clinical complications related to amphotericin B therapy (20). These effects are often transient, occur during or immediately following the infusion, and seem to cause no long-term effects. However, the impact on patient comfort may be profound. In some cases, these reactions will necessitate a discontinuation of therapy or conversion to a different amphotericin B formulation. The best strategy to minimize infusion-related toxicities is to include recommendations regarding premedications in any amphotericin B administration guidelines. It is common practice in many institutions to administer acetaminophen and diphenhydramine before all amphotericin B infusions (134). Nonsteroidal anti-inflammatory agents such as ibuprofen have also been used in lieu of acetaminophen but may be less desirable because of the potential for nephrotoxicity. Meperidine or morphine sulfate have been reserved for more severe cases of rigors (135). In addition, corticosteroids such as methylprednisolone have also been employed but generally are not recommended because of their immunosuppressive effects (20).

Comparisons among the various amphotericin B formulations regarding infusion-related reactions have produced mixed results. It appears that L-Amb may reduce the incidence of infusional toxicities when compared with AmBd (125). The reductions in infusion-related reactions associated with ABLC are less clear, and this agent does not appear to decrease the requirement for premedications, when compared with AmBd (121). ABCD may actually have increased infusion-related reactions compared with AmBd (21,121,132). The nature and severity of these reactions have limited the routine use of ABCD in clinical practice (21). As with other comparisons among amphotericin B formulations, it is important to include a critical evaluation of the published literature. In the case of infusional toxicities, the one major caveat is that premedications, an important preventative strategy, are typically not allowed during the first day of treatment. Therefore, when assessing toxicities in clinical trials, practitioners must be sure to determine whether or not premedications were allowed at the time of comparison, as differences among agents maybe nullified when premedications are allowed. This strategy may effectively reduce infusion-related fever and chills and has only minimal impact on institutional costs.

A triad of symptoms including (i) chest pain, dyspnea, and hypoxia; (ii) abdominal pain, leg pain, and/or flank pain; and/or (iii) flushing and/or urticaria have been reported with lipid-based amphotericin B preparations and in particular, L-AmB (136,137). These reactions occur during the drug infusion and can mimic symptoms of myocardial infarction or pulmonary embolism. The severe nature of these symptoms may prompt a costly medical workup to rule out other causes of chest pain and, in severe cases, initiate admission or transfer to the ICU. Although this reaction has been reported with all the formulations of amphotericin B, hypoxia seems to occur more frequently with ABCD than with any of the other agents, including AmBd (132). In fact, clinical trials with ABCD have been halted because of this effect (128). It appears that this reaction may be related to the lipid component, as it has been reported more frequently with the liposomal preparation than with the lipid complex (136).

Electrolyte imbalances (most notably potassium and magnesium wasting) have been associated with the administration of amphotericin B in various formulations (20). In many cases, such needs are confounded by comorbidities in the seriously ill patients being treated. Although amiloride and spironolactone have been proposed as methods to decrease potassium requirements among patients receiving AmBd, these approaches have not been widely implemented in the clinical setting (138,139).

Perhaps the most serious and costly toxicity caused by amphotericin B therapy is nephrotoxicity, which is characterized as nonoliguric acute renal failure secondary to tubular necrosis (131,140–142). The extent of toxicity can range from self-limiting elevations in laboratory parameters to renal failure that requires renal replacement therapies. This complication may or may not be reversible. Its occurrence is relatively common, with a reported incidence ranging from 49% to 65%, depending on the definition used (140,141). Ultimately, up to 15% of some populations of treated individuals require hemodialysis following therapy with the deoxycholate formulation (140,141). There are significant consequences associated with development of amphotericin B–induced nephrotoxicity, including increased mortality (54% vs. 16%; odds ratio [OR], 6.6), length of hospitalization (8.2 days), and cost ($29,823 per case) (143).

Several strategies may be employed to avoid or minimize amphotericin B–related nephrotoxicity. The first is to identify alternative treatment options (Table 2). If amphotericin B therapy is required, the least expensive option is to assure that patients receive adequate hydration with 1 L of 0.9% normal saline prior to AmBd administration, a strategy known as "saline loading" (144,145). This approach appears to decrease toxicity without affecting efficacy. Although administering AmBd via 24-hour continuous infusion has been shown to decrease the incidence of nephrotoxicity (146,147), the efficacy of this approach in patients with documented severe invasive fungal infections has not yet been established. This strategy also has potential drawbacks in that it requires a dedicated intravenous line. Finally, amphotericin B is known to exhibit concentration-dependent pharmacodynamic activity, which would be compromised by such an administration method.

Lipid-based formulations of amphotericin B are associated with a significantly lower incidence of nephrotoxicity

Table 2 Common Challenges and Potential Solutions Regarding
Administration and Monitoring of Systemic Antifungal Therapy

Drug	Problem	Potential solution(s)	Source (reference)
Amphotericin B			
All formulations	Infusion-related reactions (fever, chills, rigors)	Premedications (e.g., diphenhydramine, acetaminophen) Liposomal amphotericin B may decrease occurrence relative to amphotericin B deoxycholate	(20), (133)
	Nephrotoxicity	Saline loading Reduced incidence with lipid-based preparations*†	(21), (121), (144), (145)
Liposomal amphotericin B and amphotericin B colloidal dispersion	Infusion-related "acute chest syndrome"	Switch to alternate formulation	(136), (137)
Itraconazole			
All formulations	Drug interactions	Careful monitoring	(222)
	Congestive heart failure (CHF)	Use alternate therapy and/or discontinue itraconazole use if symptoms of CHF develop on therapy	(223)
Capsule	Erratic bioavailability	Switch to oral solution Administer with acidic beverage (such as cola)	(223), (224), (225)

(continued)

Table 2 *Continued*

Drug	Problem	Potential solution(s)	Source (reference)
Intravenous	Vehicle may accumulate in patients with renal dysfunction—labeling information includes precaution against use in patients with CrCl <30 mL/min	Seek out alternative therapies; use oral formulation if possible.	(226)
Oral solution	Diarrhea associated with vehicle	Carefully monitor; switch to alternative agent	(223)
Voriconazole			
All formulations	Hepatitis	Monitor	(227)
	Visual hallucinations	Careful patient counseling; Will usually abate after approximately 1 wk	(227)
	Photosensitivity	Counsel patients to remain out of the sun Sunscreen will not prevent symptoms	(227)
Intravenous	Avoid use in patients with CrCl <50 mL/min.	Consider using oral formulation (excellent oral bioavailability)	(227)
Caspofungin	Contraindication when used in combination with cyclosporine	Data based on healthy volunteers. Increasing data are available that the combination may be safe; however, most practitioners would switch to tacrolimus	(170)

* Liposomal amphotericin B, amphotericin B lipid complex, amphotericin B colloidal dispersion.
† Continuous infusion (i.e., 24 h) and combination of amphotericin B and intralipids have been suggested to reduce nephrotoxicity. However, insufficient efficacy data exist with these strategies.
CrCl, Creatinine clearance.
With permission from Gallagher JC, Dodds Ashley ES, Drew RH, Perfect JR. Antifungal pharmacotherapy for invasive mould infections. Expert Opin Pharmacother 2003; 4:147–164.

compared with AmBd (125,131,132,142,148–150). Although their higher acquisition costs may prohibit routine use of lipid-based products in all patients who require amphotericin B therapy, the significant morbidity and costs associated with end-stage renal disease requiring hemodialysis justifies use of a lipid-based formulation in select patients to minimize this complication. Identification of appropriate candidates, therefore, is essential. Criteria used in clinical studies to identify patients experiencing amphotericin B nephrotoxicity include 1.5- to two-fold elevations in serum creatinine from baseline values (133). These patients may benefit from a change in therapy to a lipid-based product if continued amphotericin B–based therapy is necessary. The population of patients at increased risk of nephrotoxicity, without current laboratory evidence of reduced renal function, may also benefit. Identification of risk factors may be useful in predicting a patient's likelihood of developing nephrotoxicity, either before or after initiation of therapy (151). These factors include patient care setting (ICU or intermediate care), concurrent therapy with nephrotoxins (e.g., cyclosporine, tacrolimus, aminoglycosides), baseline renal dysfunction, and high daily amphotericin B dose (with greatest risk when receiving more than 60 mg of AmBd per day) (53,151,152). Additional risk factors may include HSCT as well as prolonged amphotericin B exposure, such as is required with invasive mould infections (141). Although these predictive strategies need to be validated on a broader basis, they may be used as a starting point for clinicians in assessing overall patient risk.

Controversy remains regarding which of the lipid-based formulations has the greatest impact on reducing nephrotoxicity. In one comparative trial, L-AmB had a much lower incidence than ABLC (14.1 vs. 42.3%, $p = 0.001$) (133). The rate of nephrotoxicity with ABLC reported in this study, however, was much higher than that reported in other clinical trials. In contrast, other data suggest that there is actually no clinical difference in nephrotoxicity among the lipid formulations (132,149,153,154). It is important to note, however, that none of these agents eliminate amphotericin B–induced nephrotoxicity entirely. Therefore, patients must still be closely monitored for this adverse effect.

Although there are published guidelines for the use of lipid-based amphotericin B formulations in stem cell transplant recipients (28), these were prepared before the release of voriconazole and caspofungin. Many institutions attempt to limit the use of lipid-based amphotericin B formulations to patients who are either experiencing AmBd-induced nephrotoxicity or who are at highest risk for developing amphotericin B–induced nephrotoxicity. It is generally accepted that any of the lipid-based formulations are effective in attaining this goal. Although controversy remains over the best formulation (23,24), many practitioners consider either ABLC or L-AmB to be interchangeable from a therapeutic standpoint (21). The ultimate decision about which agent to include on a hospital formulary is often driven by contract-specific pricing and anticipated volume of use.

Restriction and dosing guidelines may have a further influence on the use of lipid-based formulations of amphotericin B. The impact of pharmacy- and/or infectious diseases–based programs on restricting the use of lipid-based formulations of amphotericin B have been reported in the literature (155,156). These programs often include either telephone or formal consultation from an infectious diseases consultant. Each institution would have to evaluate the available resources and scope of use for these agents to determine the potential benefit from any restriction program. In order to minimize waste associated with the weight-based dosing of these agents, dosing guidelines have been established by some institutions. An example of dosing guidelines used by Duke University Medical Center for amphotericin B lipid complex is found in Table 3.

Flucytosine

Flucytosine has been extensively reviewed elsewhere (157). In brief, the clinical application of flucytosine is limited because of issues of toxicity, rapid development of resistance (when used as monotherapy), and lack of parenteral formulation. Combination therapy with amphotericin B has proven to im-

Table 3 Dosing Guidelines for Amphotericin B Lipid
Complex at Duke University Medical Center

Total body weight (kg)	Dosage (mg)
45	200 q.d.
46–54	300 q.o.d, alternating with 200 q.o.d.
55–65	300 q.d.
66–74	400 q.o.d., alternating with 300 q.o.d.
75–85	400 q.d.
86–94	500 q.o.d., alternating with 400 q.o.d.
95–105	500 q.d.
106–114	600 q.o.d., alternating with 500 q.o.d.
115–120	600 q.d.
121–134	700 q.o.d., alternating with 600 q.o.d.
135–145	700 q.d.

q.d., daily; q.o.d., every other day.
With permission from Gallagher JC, Dodds Ashley ES, Drew RH,
Perfect JR. Antifungal pharmacotherapy for invasive mould infec-
tions. Expert Opin Pharmacother 2003;4:147–164.

prove outcome in patients with cryptococcal meningitis when
given as initial therapy, and is therefore used as part of combination therapy for patients with severe infection (30). Other
clinical applications may include combinations with amphotericin B for the treatment of severe or refractory invasive
candidiasis (29) or aspergillosis (8). Administration may be
complicated by side effects such as gastrointestinal intolerance
and rash. Hematologic toxicities (including myelosupression)
are thought to be related to serum concentration.

Guidelines for flucytosine use generally center around
serum concentration monitoring. The pharmacokinetics of flucytosine have been extensively summarized elsewhere (157).
Data are lacking to correlate flucytosine serum concentrations
to efficacy. In contrast, clinical studies have correlated the increased risk of flucytosine toxicity with peak (2-hour postdose)
serum flucytosine levels of 100 µg/mL or more during 2 or
more weeks of therapy (158,159). Flucytosine assays may not
be routinely available in some institutions. Therefore, serum
concentration monitoring may not be performed in all patients
and frequent white blood cell counts must be performed. How-

ever, patients receiving high doses of drug for prolonged periods of time should be initially monitored. A 2-hour postdose serum concentration of flucytosine should be determined after three to five doses have been administered. Recent consensus guidelines for the treatment of cryptococcal infections recommend optimal serum concentrations between 30 and 80 µg/mL for this infection (30). Similar guidelines for the treatment of candidal meningitis state target concentrations of 40 to 60 µg/mL (29). In any case, a reasonable goal is to avoid levels below 25 µg/mL and above 100 µg/mL.

In lieu of the availability of serum concentration monitoring, periodic determinations of blood counts may be a more practical way to predict excessive flucytosine concentrations. In addition, because of renal drug elimination, renal function should also be monitored frequently to assess the potential need to modify the dose (160).

Echinocandins

Caspofungin is the first echinocandin approved for use in the treatment of invasive aspergillosis in patients refractory or intolerant to other therapies (161–163). Studies have demonstrated efficacy in the treatment of oropharyngeal candidiasis refractory to prior therapy (164–166). In addition, a recent study established efficacy of caspofungin in the treatment of invasive candidiasis, including in patients with candidemia (22). Caspofungin is not active *in vitro* against *C. neoformans* or several filamentous fungi (163,167). It demonstrates some *in vitro* activity against dimorphic fungi such as *Histoplasma capsulatum* and *Coccidioides immitis*, but no published clinical data are available for treatment of these infections (163,167).

Caspofungin appears to have a favorable toxicity profile (168,169). Rates of discontinuation due to drug toxicity are substantially less than those seen with AmBd (168). Adverse effects in clinical trials are infrequent and include nausea, thrombophlebitis, headache, fever, and elevations in hepatic enzymes (168,169). Data are lacking regarding safety in long-term use. Although not metabolized by the cytochrome P-450 system, concomitant administration of caspofungin with tacrolimus has resulted in reductions in tacrolimus serum concentration (170). In addition, caspofungin administered concomintantly with cyclosporin A resulted in elevations of liver enzymes and caspofungin serum concentrations by an unknown mechanism (170). Therefore, concomitant use of cyclosporin A and caspofungin should be used with caution until further data are available.

Because of the toxicities associated with the use of amphotericin B formulations and its lack of cross-resistance to polyenes and azoles, caspofungin has emerged as a viable treatment option for invasive candidiasis and refractory *Aspergillus* infections. One of the growing areas of interest for use of caspofungin would be as part of combination therapy for severe, refractory, invasive fungal infections such as aspergillosis (171,172). *In vitro* studies and small case series indicate that caspofungin does not appear to be antagonistic when combined with other antifungals, such as itraconazole, voriconazole, or amphotericin B, against *Aspergillus* spp (167). In addition, its excellent tolerability, broad spectrum of candidal activity, fungicidal nature, and activity against *Candida* spp biofilms lend support to a prominent role in management of candidal infections. However, experience with this agent in the neutropenic patient population is generally lacking (22).

As a result of the high cost of therapy and availability only in intravenous formulation, caspofungin is usually restricted to use in patients with either documented or probable fungal infections in two populations. The first is in patients with invasive aspergillosis refractory to or intolerant of other therapies. Those with invasive candidiasis who are failing treatment with azoles and unable to receive amphotericin B formulations either because of intolerance or are at high risk of amphotericin-B nephrotoxicity may also be considered for caspofungin therapy. Patients receiving cyclosporin A may be candidates for changing the immunosupressive regimen to tacrolimus, although tacrolimus serum concentrations may decrease and should be monitored.

Azoles

Because common issues relating to spectrum of activity, toxicities, drug interactions, and dosage/availability exist among the azoles, there is a need for careful monitoring and/or practice guidelines for utilization of these antifungal agents in the clinical setting. All of the azoles have potential drug–drug interactions with other agents via CYP 450 isoenzyme–mediated interactions (Table 4), whereby increased or decreased concentrations of azole or concomitantly administered drug may be experienced. In addition, intravenous formulations of azoles are substantially more expensive than their oral formulations, supporting the need for active "IV-to-oral" switch programs in the health care setting. Optimal selection of individual agents within the azole class requires knowledge of agent-specific spectrum of activity, efficacy data, pharmacokinetic profile, dosage forms, and safety, as well as cost.

Ketoconazole

Although ketoconazole was one of the first azoles available orally for the treatment of invasive mycoses (primarily candidiasis), it has largely been replaced by newer, safer azoles. Side effects such as dose-related hepatotoxicity, gastrointestinal effects, and endocrine suppression (both cortisol and testosterone) have been problematic (173). Ketoconazole is highly dependent on gastric acid for absorption, and bioavailability is significantly reduced among patients with pharmacologically- or pathologically-induced achlorhydria (174–176). Its lack of significant penetration into the central nervous system (CNS) and urine has also limited its clinical utility. Unlike fluconazole and itraconazole which can be given intravenously, ketoconazole lacks an injectable preparation. Drug–drug interactions with this agent have also been problematic, requiring careful monitoring or use of alternate agents (177). Therefore, ketoconazole's current place in the treatment of IFIs is uncertain. Its current clinical use is more commonly for noninfectious diseases such as prostate cancer (178). In light of these limitations and the availability of more effective and/or less toxic agents, guidelines published by IDSA include ketoconazole on a limited basis for certain situations. These include use as an alternate agent in the manage-

Table 4 Selected Antifungal Drug Interactions

Antifungal	Interacting drug(s)	Result	Action
Amphotericin B	Aminoglycosides, CSA, TAC	Increased nephotoxicity	Cautiously monitor renal function use LFABs as indicated
Caspofungin	CSA	Caspofungin concentrations increased	Monitor liver function tests
	TAC	TAC concentrations decreased	Monitor TAC levels
Itraconazole	Dofetilide, quinidine, pimozide	Increased concentrations of these drugs; potential torsades de pointes	Concurrent use contraindicated
	Simvastatin, lovastatin	Increased concentrations of these drugs; potential rhabdomyolysis	Concurrent use contraindicated
	CSA, TAC, oral hypoglycemics, protease inhibitors, benzodiazepines, calcium channel blockers, carbamazepine, atorvastatin	Increased concentrations of these drugs	Monitor for adverse effects; follow serum concentrations for CSA, TAC, carbamazepine
	Phenytoin, carbamazepine, phenobarbital, rifampin, isoniazid, nevirapine	Decreased concentrations of itraconazole	Monitor effectiveness of therapy
	Antacids, proton pump inhibitors, H_2-receptor antagonists, grapefruit juice	Decreased absorption of oral itraconazole	Avoid concurrent use
Voriconazole	Sirolimus	Increased concentrations of sirolimus (seven- to eleven-fold)	Concurrent use contraindicated
	Quinidine, pimozide	Increased concentrations of these drugs; potential torsades de pointes	Concurrent use contraindicated

(continued)

Table 4 *Continued*

Antifungal	Interacting drug(s)	Result	Action
	Rifabutin	Decreased voriconazole concentrations increased rifabutin concentrations	Concurrent use contraindicated
	TAC	Increased TAC levels	Decrease TAC dose 67%, and monitor concentrations
	Warfarin	Increased PT/INR	Monitor INR carefully
	Oral hypoglycemics, benzodiazepines, calcium channel blockers, HMG-CoA-reductase inhibitors	Possible increased concentrations of these drugs	Monitor for adverse effects
	Phenytoin	Decreased voriconazole levels; increased phenytoin concentrations	Increase voriconazole dose from 4 mg/kg to 5 mg/kg IV, or from 200 mg to 400 mg PO; carefully monitor phenytoin concentrations
	Omeprazole	Increased omeprazole concentrations	Decrease omeprazole dose 50%
	Protease inhibitors	Increased voriconazole and protease inhibitor concentrations	Monitor for adverse effects
	NNRTIs	Mixed effects on NNRTI levels, decreased voriconazole concentrations	Monitor for adverse effects

CSA, cyclosporine; H_2, histamine; HMG-CoA, hydroxy-methylglutaryl coenzyme A; INR, International Normalized Ratio; IV, intravenously; LFAB, lipid formulation of amphotericin B; NNRTI, non-nucleoside reverse transcriptase inhibitor; PO, by mouth; PT, prothrombin time; TAC, tacrolimus.
Modified from Gallagher JC, Dodds Ashley ES, Drew RH, Perfect JR. Antifungal pharmacotherapy for invasive mould infections. Expert Opin Pharmacother 2003; 4:147–164, used with permission.

ment of coccidioidomycosis (26), chronic mucocutaneous candidiasis (29), recurrent azole-susceptible *C. albicans* vaginitis (29), mild-to-moderate non-CNS or pulmonary blastomycosis in the nonimmunocompromised host (25), chronic pulmonary histoplasmosis (31), and disseminated histoplasmosis in immunocompetent adults when other agents (including itraconazole) are contraindicated (31).

Itraconazole

Like ketoconazole, itraconazole possesses *in vitro* activity against the endemic mycoses and moulds in addition to most *Candida* spp (179). Because of its activity against *Aspergillus* spp, itraconazole has often been employed as both prophylaxis and treatment of invasive aspergillosis (180–182). In addition to more invasive disease, itraconazole may be used in HIV-infected patients with esophageal candidiasis and has demonstrated activity against fluconazole-resistant infections (183). It is also the drug of choice for non–life-threatening histoplasmosis and blastomycosis, dematiaceous fungal infections, and sporotrichosis (25,27,31). In contrast to fluconazole, absorption following oral administration of itraconazole capsules may be erratic (184–187). This is due in part, to its dependency on a low pH for dissolution. Gastric pH may be elevated in patients receiving concomitant histamine$_2$-antagonists or proton pump inhibitors. Erratic absorption has also been demonstrated in both granulocytopenic cancer patients and HIV-infected patients with achlorhydria. Although itraconazole oral solution has demonstrated improved bioavailability, it also exhibits wide interpatient variability (188,189) and may cause gastrointestinal disturbances such as diarrhea (190–192). An intravenous preparation of itraconazole has been approved for use. In this formulation, solubilization of the drug in cyclodextrin affords excellent bioavailability, and target serum concentrations can be rapidly achieved (193).

Guidelines for the use of itraconazole in routine clinical practice have usually focused on issues of cost and safety, including methods for appropriate serum concentration monitoring and identifying patients eligible to receive the intravenous formulation. For example, administration of the intravenous formulation is not recommended in patients with severe renal dysfunction because of safety concerns with the cyclodextrin vehicle in this patient population (194). In addition, serum concentration monitoring is usually established to document adequate absorption following oral administration for treatment of serious IFIs. Although a specific therapeutic range has not been defined, maintenance of serum concentrations above 0.25 to 0.5 µg/mL has been associated with therapeutic success as prophylaxis in neutropenic patients and among patients with oropharyngeal candidiasis (15,180–182,195). The need for serum itraconazole concentration monitoring to document adequate drug absorption is reflected in the recent guidelines for the treatment of aspergillosis published by IDSA (8). A common clinical practice for such invasive infections has been to determine serum concentrations 2 to 4 hours after oral dosing to document that sufficient absorption has occurred. More recent data suggest that trough concentrations of at least 0.25 to 0.5 µg/mL may be important for success in the clinical setting (181).

Fluconazole

The spectrum of activity, pharmacokinetics, safety, and clinical applications of fluconazole have been reviewed extensively elsewhere (196). Unlike ketoconazole and itraconazole, fluconazole lacks activity against moulds, but it does posess *in vitro* activity against most *Candida* spp, *C. neoformans, Blastomyces dermatitidis, C. immitis,* and *H. capsulatum* (196). Fluconazole is highly active *in vitro* against *C. albicans* (196). However, activity against non-*albicans Candida* (such as *C. glabrata*) is less predictable, and *C. krusei* is intrinsically resistant (197,198).

Guidelines for the use of fluconazole have generally focused on the conversion of intravenous therapy to oral administration, appropriate use in selected patients with invasive candidiasis, and identification of high-risk surgical patients who may be qualified for preemptive therapy (114–116,199). Because of fluconazole's excellent oral bioavailability and the significant cost reduction of the oral dose form (when compared with intravenous therapy), many institutions have established criteria to convert patients from intravenous to oral formulations (114,115). It has been estimated that as many as half of fluconazole-treated patients could benefit from intravenous-to-oral conversion (116). These kinds of interventional programs can be extremely effective, as demonstrated in one hospital, where nearly 99% of patients received fluconazole via the institution-defined appropriate route after implementation of a restriction program (200). Concerns regarding the potential for decreased absorption following oral administration prompted investigations in special populations, such as HIV-infected (201), postsurgical (202,203), malignancy (204,205), burn (206,207), obese (206), and HSCT (208) patient populations. Although some variability does exist, exclusion of these patients as candidates for oral therapy is not justified. In addition, routine assessment of fluconazole serum concentrations is not justified and is not available in most institutions.

Guidelines for the use of fluconazole may also include its use in the treatment of invasive candidiasis. Because dose-dependent susceptibility may occur for many non-*albicans* *Candida* spp, infections with these species may respond to higher doses of fluconazole (12 mg/kg in adults) (15,209–212). Therefore, for patients with severe or life-threatening candidiasis, use of alternative agents (such as amphotericin B or caspofungin) or higher doses of fluconazole should be considered until speciation is known or susceptibility test results are available (15). In randomized, controlled trials performed in non-neutropenic patients with candidemia, fluconazole has resulted in similar clinical efficacy with reduced toxicity when compared with AmBd (213,214). However, data supporting use of fluconazole for invasive candidiasis among neutropenic patients are generally lacking. In this population, non-*albicans* *Candida* spp may be observed more frequently and host immunosuppression plays a critical role in clinical outcomes (29).

As previously reviewed, a subset of surgical patients at high risk for invasive fungal infections may be considered for fluconazole therapy as part of a prophylactic or preemptive treatment strategy. Broad-spectrum antibiotics, acute renal failure, central catheterization, receipt of total parenteral nutrition, presence of *Candida* spp colonization, diabetes mellitus, gastrointestinal disease or recent abdominal surgery, transfer from another hospital, bladder catheterizaton, hemodialysis, diarrhea, and duration of ICU stay have been associated with increased risk of invasive fungal infections (96–98). Therefore, appropariate use of fluconazole in these patients should be part of an effort to stratify patients according to risk, but the precision of risk stratification still requires further studies.

Among the azoles, fluconazole is the preferred agent in the maintenance phase of treatment for cryptococcal meningitis, typically following "induction" with amphotericin B plus flucytosine (30). Fluconazole is preferred over itraconazole during the maintenance phase because it was associated with fewer relapses in a randomized, controlled clinical trial (215). Finally, fluconazole has recently been employed as preemptive treatment in surgical patients at high risk for invasive fungal infections (42).

Voriconazole

Voriconazole, like itraconazole and ketoconazole, demonstrates activity *in vitro* against *Aspergillus* spp and has also demonstrated activity in the clinical setting against *Candida* spp, *Fusarium* spp, and *Scedosporium apiospermum* infections (101,216–218). Voriconazole is now considered by most to be the preferred first-line agent for invasive aspergillosis, based on a clinical trial demonstrating superiority of voriconazole over amphotericin B as primary therapy (11). The role of voriconazole in empiric therapy of fever in neutropenic patients remains to be determined because of the failure of voriconazole to establish noninferiority when compared with L-AmB (219). Notably, voriconazole lacks activity against Zygomycetes infections, and it is important to consider this when employing voriconazole as empiric or prophylactic therapy. Infections due to organisms such as *Rhizopus* and other Zygomycetes have emerged during voriconazole therapy (219). In contrast to other azoles, voriconazole has a unique adverse event profile, with visual disturbances, hallucinations, and phototoxicity reported (217,219).

Voriconazole guidelines include conversions of the intravenous to oral formulations, identification of patient populations in which voriconazole would be the preferred agent, and monitoring guidelines to minimize the potential for adverse drug events and drug interactions. Because of voriconazole's high oral bioavailability (217,220), use of intravenous voriconazole is generally restricted to patients unable to receive oral therapy. Because injectable voriconazole is solubilized in cyclodextrin, it is not recommended for patients with creatinine clearances less than 50 mL/minute (217). Drug–drug interactions are well described for voriconazole and include a long list of agents that are contraindicated for concomitant use (217). Dosage modifications may be necessary for either voriconazole or the object drug, and dosages of agents such as cyclosporin A or tacrolimus may also need to be adjusted again after voriconazole therapy is completed. In addition, adverse events such as elevations in liver enzymes may be associated with higher plasma concentrations of voriconazole (221). Higher plasma concentrations of this agent may be particularly problematic among individuals who are poor metabolizers of voriconazole, because of genetic mutations in CYP 2C19. In the future, these individuals, (typically those of Asian descent) may be potential candidates for more intensive monitoring of voriconazole plasma concentrations (217). However, routine monitoring of voriconazole plasma concentrations in the clinical setting is not recommended at this time. Finally, the lack of microbiologic activity of voriconazole against certain pathogens, such as Zygomyecetes, cannot be overlooked, and it is important to utilize clinical guidelines to ensure that patients at risk for these pathogens are not empirically treated with voriconazole.

ANTIFUNGAL PROGRAM SURVEILLANCE AND BENCHMARKING

End points such as expenditures, physician compliance with prescribing guidelines, adverse events, and patient outcomes are the "traditional" measures of an antimicrobial intervention program's impact. However, in contrast to antibacterial susceptibilities, epidemiologic surveillance of fungal pathogens is less frequently employed.

As in other therapeutic areas, expenditures for antifungal drugs may be significantly influenced by the introduction of new therapeutic options, a change in the institution's patient population, or drug availability. For example, during the 2001 fiscal year, hospitals saw the introduction of caspofungin (Cancidas℗; Merck & Co., Inc., Whitehouse Station, NJ). Despite a relatively high acquisition cost, it made little impact on antifungal drug use at the end of the fiscal year, primarily because a shortage occurred shortly after its approval. As a consequence, many institutions significantly underestimated the impact of this agent on the antifungal drug budget. Changing treatment paradigms may also significantly affect antifungal utilization. For example, data supporting the efficacy of caspofungin in the treatment of invasive candidiasis (22) significantly expanded the patient population eligible to receive the drug. Therefore, increases or decreases in antifungal drug use may be no reflection on the guideline program, but rather may be the result of changes in the standard of care. Evolving data on the use of this agent as part of combination regimens may also have a significant impact on utilization. Finally, changes in success rates may also affect cost indicators. For patients with a favorable clinical response, long-term therapy may ensue. Therefore, the "consequence" of successful therapy may actually increase drug acquisition costs.

Endpoints such as prescriber compliance with antifungal guidelines and patient outcomes are generally more difficult to assess. Assessment of prescriber compliance with the guideline or restriction program allows determination of antifungal use in populations other than those targeted. If drug restriction is a major component of the program, it might also be useful to determine the number of times the drug was requested but not approved.

Although the most important endpoint to antifungal therapy is treatment outcome, it is the most difficult to assess. Criteria used to determine the efficacy of fungal infections may vary widely among studies. As previously stated, diagnostic criteria may be difficult to apply to nononcologic patients. In addition, recovery from underlying disease states (such as malignancy) may have a significant impact on treatment outcome, making morbidity and mortality attributable to the invasive fungal infection difficult to determine. A more difficult, but perhaps more applicable, endpoint in assessing antifungal efficacy is death with or without invasive fungal infection. Because patients at greatest risk for invasive fungal infections have high mortality rates owing to comorbidities, it is probably more important for clinicians to determine the portion of patients succumbing to fungal infections. Finally, treatment courses for many invasive fungal infections are often prolonged and, if successful, often extend beyond the hospital admission.

Another manner to assess the potential impact of antifungal use is surveillance of the epidemiology of fungal infections at a particular institution. This practice, commonly employed for bacterial infections, is readily available at many institutions in the form of an antibiogram. Microbiology laboratories that are equipped with the appropriate technology can provide data on the pattern of fungal infections on given wards and the susceptibilities of those pathogens. Tracking trends in antifungal resistance, especially among *Candida* spp, may aid in the selection of appropriate empiric therapies and potentially affect patient outcomes.

CONCLUSION

The use of systemic antifungals for the treatment of invasive fungal infections produces challenges unique to this therapeutic class of antibiotics. The appropriate selection and monitoring of such therapy may have a significant impact on both patient outcome and treatment costs. Institutional strategies to promote optimal use of these agents generally require the production of both drug- and patient-specific prescribing guidelines. These are best produced by input from pharmacy, infectious disease specialists, microbiology, infection control practitioners, and clinicians experienced in the treatment of immunocompromised patients.

REFERENCES

1. Trick WE, Fridkin SK, Edwards JR, Hajjeh RA, Gaynes RP, Gaynes RP. Secular trend of hospital-acquired candidemia among intensive care unit patients in the United States during 1989–1999. Clin Infect Dis 2002; 35:627–630.

2. Marr KA, Carter RA, Boeckh M, Martin P, Corey L. Invasive aspergillosis in allogeneic stem cell transplant recipients: changes in epidemiology and risk factors. Blood 2002; 100: 4358–4366.

3. Marr KA, Carter RA, Crippa F, Wald A, Corey L. Epidemiology and outcome of mould infections in hematopoietic stem cell transplant recipients. Clin Infect Dis 2002; 34:909–917.

4. Pfaller MA, Jones RN, Doern GV, Sader HS, Hollis RJ, Messer SA. International surveillance of bloodstream infections due to *Candida* species: frequency of occurrence and antifungal susceptibilities of isolates collected in 1997 in the United States, Canada, and South America for the SENTRY Program. The SENTRY Participant Group. J Clin Microbiol 1998; 36: 1886–1889.

5. Sobel JD. Vaginitis. N Engl J Med 1997; 337:1896–1903.

6. Boutati EI, Anaissie EJ. *Fusarium*, a significant emerging pathogen in patients with hematologic malignancy: ten years' experience at a cancer center and implications for management. Blood 1997; 90:999–1008.

7. Perfect JR, Schell WA. The new fungal opportunists are coming. Clin Infect Dis 1996; 22(suppl 2):S112–S118.

8. Stevens DA, Kan VL, Judson MA, Morrison VA, Dummer S, Denning DW, Bennett JE, Walsh TJ, Patterson TF, Pankey

GA. Practice guidelines for diseases caused by *Aspergillus*. Infectious Diseases Society of America. Clin Infect Dis 2000; 30:696–709.

9. Denning DW, Lee JY, Hostetler JS, Pappas P, Kauffman CA, Dewsnup DH, Galgiani JN, Graybill JR, Sugar AM, Catanzaro A. NIAID Mycoses Study Group multicenter trial of oral itraconazole therapy for invasive aspergillosis. Am J Med 1994; 97:135–144.

10. Herbrecht R. Improving the outcome of invasive aspergillosis: new diagnostic tools and new therapeutic strategies. Ann Hematol 2002; 81(suppl 2):S52–S53.

11. Herbrecht R, Denning DW, Patterson TF, Bennett JE, Greene RE, Oestmann JW, Kern WV, Marr KA, Ribaud P, Lortholary O, Sylvester R, Rubin RH, Wingard JR, Stark P, Durand C, Caillot D, Thiel E, Chandrasekar PH, Hodges MR, Schlamm HT, Troke PF, de Pauw B, de Pauw B. Voriconazole versus amphotericin B for primary therapy of invasive aspergillosis. N Engl J Med 2002; 347:408–415.

12. Perfect JR, Cox GM, Lee JY, Kauffman CA, de Repentigny L, Chapman SW, Morrison VA, Pappas P, Hiemenz JW, Stevens DA; Mycoses Study Group. The impact of culture isolation of *Aspergillus* species: a hospital-based survey of aspergillosis. Clin Infect Dis 2001; 33:1824–1833.

13. Stevens DA. Reference Method for Broth Dilution Antifungal Susceptibility Testing of Yeast: Approved Standard. 2d ed. NCCLS document M-27A2.. Wayne. PA: NCCLS, 2002.

14. Stevens DA. Method for Antifungal Disk Diffusion Susceptibility Testing of Yeasts; Proposed Guideline. NCCLS document M44-P.. Wayne. PA: NCCLS, 2003.

15. Rex JH, Pfaller MA, Galgiani JN, Bartlett MS, Espinel-Ingroff A, Ghannoum MA, Lancaster M, Odds FC, Rinaldi MG, Walsh TJ, Barry AL. Development of interpretive breakpoints for antifungal susceptibility testing: conceptual framework and analysis of *in vitro–in vivo* correlation data for fluconazole, itraconazole, and candida infections. Subcommittee on Antifungal Susceptibility Testing of the National Committee for Clinical Laboratory Standards. Clin Infect Dis 1997; 24:235–247.

16. Clancy CJ, Nguyen MH. Correlation between *in vitro* susceptibility determined by E test and response to therapy with amphotericin B: results from a multicenter prospective study of candidemia. Antimicrob Agents Chemother 1999; 43: 1289–1290.

17. Rex JH, Pfaller MA. Has antifungal susceptibility testing come of age? . Clin Infect Dis 2002; 35:982–989.

18. Pfaller MA. Reference Method for Broth Dilution Antifungal Susceptibility Testing of Filamentous Fungi: Approved Standard. NCCLS document M38-A.. Wayne. PA: NCCLS.

19. Lass-Florl C, Kofler G, Kropshofer G, Hermans J, Kreczy A, Dierich MP, Niederwieser D. *In-vitro* testing of susceptibility to amphotericin B is a reliable predictor of clinical outcome in invasive aspergillosis. J Antimicrob Chemother 1998; 42: 497–502.

20. Gallis HA, Drew RH, Pickard WW. Amphotericin B: 30 years of clinical experience. Rev Infect Dis 1990; 12:308–329.

21. Ostrosky-Zeichner LMK. Amphotericin B: time for a new 'gold standard.' . Clin Infect Dis 2003; 37:415–425.

22. Mora-Duarte J, Betts R, Rotstein C, Colombo AL, Thompson-Moya L, Smietana J, Lupinacci R, Sable C, Kartsonis N, Perfect J, Caspofungin Invasive Candidiasis Study Group. Comparison of caspofungin and amphotericin B for invasive candidiasis. N Engl J Med 2002; 347:2020–2029.

23. Frothingham R. Lipid formulations of amphotericin B for empirical treatment of fever and neutropenia. Clin Infect Dis 2002; 35:896–897.

24. Wingard JR. Lipid formulations of amphotericins: are you a lumper or a splitter? . Clin Infect Dis 2002; 35:891–895.

25. Chapman SW, Bradsher RW Jr, Campbell GD Jr, Pappas PG, Kauffman CA. Practice guidelines for the management of patients with blastomycosis. Infectious Diseases Society of America. Clin Infect Dis 2000; 30:679–683.

26. Galgiani JN, Ampel NM, Catanzaro A, Johnson RH, Stevens DA, Williams PL. Practice guideline for the treatment of coccidioidomycosis. Infectious Diseases Society of America. Clin Infect Dis 2000; 30:658–661.

27. Kauffman CA, Hajjeh R, Chapman SW. Practice guidelines for the management of patients with sporotrichosis. For the Mycoses Study Group. Infectious Diseases Society of America. Clin Infect Dis 2000; 30:684–687.

28. Quilitz RE, Arnold AD, Briones GR, Dix SP, Ippoliti C, Kennedy LD, Lucich JL, Mehta J, Peters BG, Tice DS;, Tice DS. Practice guidelines for lipid-based amphotericin B in stem cell transplant recipients. Ann Pharmacother 2001; 35:206–216.

29. Pappas PG, Rex, JH, Sobel JD, Filler SG, Dismukes WE, Walsh TJ, Edwards JE. Guidelines for treatment of candidiasis. Clin Infect Dis. 2004;38:161–189.

30. Saag MS, Graybill RJ, Larsen RA, Pappas PG, Perfect JR, Powderly WG, Sobel JD, Dismukes WE. Practice guidelines for the management of cryptococcal disease. Infectious Diseases Society of America. Clin Infect Dis 2000; 30:710–718.

31. Wheat J, Sarosi G, McKinsey D, Hamill R, Bradsher R, Johnson P, Loyd J, Kauffman C. Practice guidelines for the management of patients with histoplasmosis. Infectious Diseases Society of America. Clin Infect Dis 2000; 30:688–695.

32. Patterson TF. Approaches to fungal diagnosis in transplantation. Transpl Infect Dis 1999; 1:262–272.

33. Yu VL, Muder RR, Poorsattar A. Significance of isolation of *Aspergillus* from the respiratory tract in diagnosis of invasive pulmonary aspergillosis. Results from a three-year prospective study. Am J Med 1986; 81:249–254.

34. Horvath JA, Dummer S. The use of respiratory-tract cultures in the diagnosis of invasive pulmonary aspergillosis. Am J Med 1996; 100:171–178.

35. Ascioglu S, Rex JH, de Pauw B, Bennett JE, Bille J, Crokaert F, Denning DW, Donnelly JP, Edwards JE, Erjavec Z, Fiere D, Lortholary O, Maertens J, Meis JF, Patterson TF, Ritter J, Selleslag D, Shah PM, Stevens DA, Walsh TJ; Invasive Fungal Infections Cooperative Group of the European Organization for Research and Treatment of Cancer; Mycoses Study Group of the National Institute of Allergy and Infectious Diseases. Defining opportunistic invasive fungal infections in immunocompromised patients with cancer and hematopoietic stem

cell transplants: an international consensus. Clin Infect Dis 2002; 34:7–14.

36. Sekhon AS, Garg AK, Kaufman L, Kobayashi GS, Hamir Z, Jalbert M, Moledina N. Evaluation of a commercial enzyme immunoassay for the detection of cryptococcal antigen. Mycoses 1993; 36:31–34.

37. Maertens J, Van Eldere J, Verhaegen J, Verbeken E, Verschakelen J, Boogaerts M. Use of circulating galactomannan screening for early diagnosis of invasive aspergillosis in allogeneic stem cell transplant recipients. J Infect Dis 2002; 186: 1297–1306.

38. Herbrecht R, Letscher-Bru V, Oprea C, Lioure B, Waller J, Campos F, Villard O, Liu KL, Natarajan-Ame S, Lutz P, Dufour P, Bergerat JP, Candolfi E. *Aspergillus* galactomannan detection in the diagnosis of invasive aspergillosis in cancer patients. J Clin Oncol 2002; 20:1898–1906.

39. Kami M, Fukui T, Ogawa S, Kazuyama Y, Machida U, Tanaka Y, Kanda Y, Kashima T, Yamazaki Y, Hamaki T, Mori S, Akiyama H, Mutou Y, Sakamaki H, Osumi K, Kimura S, Hirai H. Use of real-time PCR on blood samples for diagnosis of invasive aspergillosis. Clin Infect Dis 2001; 33:1504–1512.

40. Buchheidt D, Baust C, Skladny H, Baldus M, Brauninger S, Hehlmann R. Clinical evaluation of a polymerase chain reaction assay to detect *Aspergillus* species in bronchoalveolar lavage samples of neutropenic patients. Br J Haematol 2002; 116:803–811.

41. Singh N. Preemptive therapy versus universal prophylaxis with ganciclovir for cytomegalovirus in solid organ transplant recipients. Clin Infect Dis 2001; 32:742–751.

42. Pelz RK, Hendrix CW, Swoboda SM, Diener-West M, Merz WG, Hammond J, Lipsett PA. Double-blind placebo-controlled trial of fluconazole to prevent candidal infections in critically ill surgical patients. Ann Surg 2001; 233:542–548.

43. Sypula WT, Kale-Pradhan PB. Therapeutic dilemma of fluconazole prophylaxis in intensive care. Ann Pharmacother 2002; 36:155–159.

44. Eggimann P, Francioli P, Bille J, Schneider R, Wu MM, Chapuis G, Chiolero R, Pannatier A, Schilling J, Geroulanos S,

Glauser MP, Calandra T. Fluconazole prophylaxis prevents intra-abdominal candidiasis in high-risk surgical patients. Crit Care Med 1999; 27:1066–1072.

45. Safran DB, Dawson E. The effect of empiric and prophylactic treatment with fluconazole on yeast isolates in a surgical trauma intensive care unit. Arch Surg 1997; 132:1184–1188.

46. Johnson MD, MacDougall C, Ostrosky-Zeichner L, Perfect JR, Rex JH. Combination antifungal therapy. Antimicrob Agents Chemother 2004; 48:693–715.

47. Rex JH, Pappas PG, Karchmer AW, Sobel J, Edwards JE, Hadley S, Brass C, Vazquez JA, Chapman SW, Horowitz HW, Zervos M, McKinsey D, Lee J, Babinchak T, Bradsher RW, Cleary JD, Cohen DM, Danziger L, Goldman M, Goodman J, Hilton E, Hyslop NE, Kett DH, Lutz J, Rubin RH, Scheld WM, Schuster M, Simmons B, Stein DK, Washburn RG, Mautner L, Chu TC, Panzer H, Rosenstein RB, Booth J;, Booth J. A randomized and blinded multicenter trial of high-dose fluconazole plus placebo versus fluconazole plus amphotericin B as therapy for candidemia and its consequences in nonneutropenic subjects. Clin Infect Dis 2003; 36:1221–1228.

48. White TC, Marr KA, Bowden RA. Clinical, cellular, and molecular factors that contribute to antifungal drug resistance. Clin Microbiol Rev 1998; 11:382–402.

49. Safdar A, Chaturvedi V, Koll BS, Larone DH, Perlin DS, Armstrong D. Prospective, multicenter surveillance study of *Candida glabrata*: fluconazole and itraconazole susceptibility profiles in bloodstream, invasive, and colonizing strains and differences between isolates from three urban teaching hospitals in New York City (Candida Susceptibility Trends Study, 1998 to 1999). Antimicrob Agents Chemother 2002; 46: 3268–3272.

50. Perea S, Patterson TF. Antifungal resistance in pathogenic fungi. Clin Infect Dis 2002; 35:1073–1080.

51. Wingard JR, Merz WG, Rinaldi MG, Johnson TR, Karp JE, Saral R. Increase in *Candida krusei* infection among patients with bone marrow transplantation and neutropenia treated prophylactically with fluconazole. N Engl J Med 1991; 325: 1274–1277.

52. Wingard JR, Merz WG, Rinaldi MG, Miller CB, Karp JE, Saral R. Association of *Torulopsis glabrata* infections with fluconazole prophylaxis in neutropenic bone marrow transplant patients. Antimicrob Agents Chemother 1993; 37:1847–1849.

53. Wingard JR. Importance of *Candida* species other than *C. albicans* as pathogens in oncology patients. Clin Infect Dis 1995; 20:115–125.

54. Groll AH, Shah PM, Mentzel C, Schneider M, Just-Nuebling G, Huebner K. Trends in the postmortem epidemiology of invasive fungal infections at a university hospital. J Infect 1996; 33:23–32.

55. Viscoli C, Girmenia C, Marinus A, Collette L, Martino P, Vandercam B, Doyen C, Lebeau B, Spence D, Krcmery V, De Pauw B, Meunier F. Candidemia in cancer patients: a prospective, multicenter surveillance study by the Invasive Fungal Infection Group (IFIG) of the European Organization for Research and Treatment of Cancer (EORTC). Clin Infect Dis 1999; 28:1071–1079.

56. Wald A, Leisenring W, van Burik JA, Bowden RA. Epidemiology of *Aspergillus* infections in a large cohort of patients undergoing bone marrow transplantation. J Infect Dis 1997; 175:1459–1466.

57. Groll AH, Walsh TJ. Uncommon opportunistic fungi: new nosocomial threats. Clin Microbiol Infect 2001; 7(suppl 2):8–24.

58. Segal BH, Bow EJ, Menichetti F. Fungal infections in nontransplant patients with hematologic malignancies. Infect Dis Clin North Am 2002; 16:935–964.

59. Gerson SL, Talbot GH, Hurwitz S, Strom BL, Lusk EJ, Cassileth PA. Prolonged granulocytopenia: the major risk factor for invasive pulmonary aspergillosis in patients with acute leukemia. Ann Intern Med 1984; 100:345–351.

60. Goodrich JM, Reed EC, Mori M, Fisher LD, Skerrett S, Dandliker PS, Klis B, Counts GW, Meyers JD. Clinical features and analysis of risk factors for invasive candidal infection after marrow transplantation. J Infect Dis 1991; 164: 731–740.

61. Goodman JL, Winston DJ, Greenfield RA, Chandrasekar PH, Fox B, Kaizer H, Shadduck RK, Shea TC, Stiff P, Friedman

DJ. A controlled trial of fluconazole to prevent fungal infections in patients undergoing bone marrow transplantation. N Engl J Med 1992; 326:845–851.

62. Blijlevens NM, Donnelly JP, de Pauw BE. Impaired gut function as risk factor for invasive candidiasis in neutropenic patients. Br J Haematol 2002; 117:259–264.

63. Bow EJ, Loewen R, Cheang MS, Shore TB, Rubinger M, Schacter B. Cytotoxic therapy-induced D-xylose malabsorption and invasive infection during remission-induction therapy for acute myeloid leukemia in adults. J Clin Oncol 1997; 15:2254–2261.

64. Rotstein C, Bow EJ, Laverdiere M, Ioannou S, Carr D, Moghaddam N. Randomized placebo-controlled trial of fluconazole prophylaxis for neutropenic cancer patients: benefit based on purpose and intensity of cytotoxic therapy. The Canadian Fluconazole Prophylaxis Study Group. Clin Infect Dis 1999; 28:331–340.

65. Karabinis A, Hill C, Leclercq B, Tancrede C, Baume D, Andremont A. Risk factors for candidemia in cancer patients: a case-control study. J Clin Microbiol 1988; 26:429–432.

66. Marr KA, Carter RA, Boeckh M, Martin P, Corey L. Invasive aspergillosis in allogeneic stem cell transplant recipients: changes in epidemiology and risk factors. Blood 2002; 100: 4358–4366.

67. Denning DW, Marinus A, Cohen J, Spence D, Herbrecht R, Pagano L, Kibbler C, Kcrmery V, Offner F, Cordonnier C, Jehn U, Ellis M, Collette L, Sylvester R. An EORTC multicentre prospective survey of invasive aspergillosis in haematological patients: diagnosis and therapeutic outcome. EORTC Invasive Fungal Infections Cooperative Group. J Infect 1998; 37: 173–180.

68. Prentice HG, Kibbler CC, Prentice AG. Towards a targeted, risk-based, antifungal strategy in neutropenic patients. Br J Haematol 2000; 110:273–284.

69. Anaissie EJ, Kontoyiannis DP, O'Brien S, Kantarjian H, Robertson L, Lerner S, Keating MJ. Infections in patients with chronic lymphocytic leukemia treated with fludarabine. Ann Intern Med 1998; 129:559–566.

70. Blay JY, Chauvin F, Le Cesne A, Anglaret B, Bouhour D, Lasset C, Freyer G, Philip T, Biron P. Early lymphopenia after cytotoxic chemotherapy as a risk factor for febrile neutropenia. J Clin Oncol 1996; 14:636–643.

71. Jantunen E, Ruutu P, Niskanen L, Volin L, Parkkali T, Koukila-Kahkola P, Ruutu T. Incidence and risk factors for invasive fungal infections in allogeneic BMT recipients. Bone Marrow Transplant 1997; 19:801–808.

72. Nosanchuk JD, Sepkowitz KA, Pearse RN, White MH, Nimer SD, Armstrong D. Infectious complications of autologous bone marrow and peripheral stem cell transplantation for refractory leukemia and lymphoma. Bone Marrow Transplant 1996; 18:355–359.

73. Kruger W, Sobottka I, Stockschlader M, Mross K, Hoffknecht M, Russmann B, Horstmann M, Betker R, Zander A. Fatal outcome of disseminated candidosis after allogeneic bone marrow transplantation under treatment with liposomal and conventional amphotericin-B. A report of 4 cases with determination of the MIC values. Scand J Infect Dis 1996; 28:313–316.

74. Meyers JD, Bowden RA, Counts GW. Infectious complications of marrow transplant: risk factors for infection. Prog Clin Biol Res 1989; 309:357–366.

75. Zander AR, Reuben JM, Johnston D, Vellekoop L, Dicke KA, Yau JC, Hersh EM. Immune recovery following allogeneic bone marrow transplantation. Transplantation 1985; 40: 177–183.

76. Grow WB, Moreb JS, Roque D, Manion K, Leather H, Reddy V, Khan SA, Finiewicz KJ, Nguyen H, Clancy CJ, Mehta PS, Wingard JR. Late onset of invasive aspergillus infection in bone marrow transplant patients at a university hospital. Bone Marrow Transplant 2002; 29:15–19.

77. Tollemar J, Ringden O, Bostrom L, Nilsson B, Sundberg B. Variables predicting deep fungal infections in bone marrow transplant recipients. Bone Marrow Transplant 1989; 4: 635–641.

78. Verfaillie C, Weisdorf D, Haake R, Hostetter M, Ramsay NK, McGlave P. *Candida* infections in bone marrow transplant recipients. Bone Marrow Transplant 1991; 8:177–184.

79. Meyers JD. Fungal infections in bone marrow transplant patients. Semin Oncol 1990; 17:10–13.

80. Kruger W, Russmann B, Kroger N, Salomon C, Ekopf N, Elsner HA, Kaulfers PM, Mack D, Fuchs N, Durken M, Kabisch H, Erttmann R, Zander AR. Early infections in patients undergoing bone marrow or blood stem cell transplantation—a 7 year single centre investigation of 409 cases. Bone Marrow Transplant 1999; 23:589–597.

81. Alangaden G, Chandrasekar PH, Bailey E, Khaliq Y. Antifungal prophylaxis with low-dose fluconazole during bone marrow transplantation. The Bone Marrow Transplantation Team. Bone Marrow Transplant 1994; 14:919–924.

82. Slavin MA, Osborne B, Adams R, Levenstein MJ, Schoch HG, Feldman AR, Meyers JD, Bowden RA. Efficacy and safety of fluconazole prophylaxis for fungal infections after marrow transplantation—a prospective, randomized, double-blind study. J Infect Dis 1995; 171:1545–1552.

83. Kontoyiannis DP, Reddy BT, Hanna H, Bodey GP, Tarrand J, Raad II. Breakthrough candidemia in patients with cancer differs from *de novo* candidemia in host factors and *Candida* species but not intensity. Infect Control Hosp Epidemiol 2002; 23:542–545.

84. Myoken Y, Kyo T, Kohara T, Fujihara M, Sugata T, Mikami Y. Breakthrough fungemia caused by azole-resistant *Candida albicans* in neutropenic patients with acute leukemia. Clin Infect Dis 2003; 36:1496–1497.

85. Uzun O, Ascioglu S, Anaissie EJ, Rex JH. Risk factors and predictors of outcome in patients with cancer and breakthrough candidemia. Clin Infect Dis 2001; 32:1713–1717.

86. Hovi L, Saarinen-Pihkala UM, Vettenranta K, Saxen H. Invasive fungal infections in pediatric bone marrow transplant recipients: single center experience of 10 years. Bone Marrow Transplant 2000; 26:999–1004.

87. Morrison VA, Haake RJ, Weisdorf DJ. Non-*Candida* fungal infections after bone marrow transplantation: risk factors and outcome. Am J Med 1994; 96:497–503.

88. Hagen EA, Stern H, Porter D, Duffy K, Foley K, Luger S, Schuster SJ, Stadtmauer EA, Schuster MG. High rate of inva-

sive fungal infections following nonmyeloablative allogeneic transplantation. Clin Infect Dis 2003; 36:9–15.

89. Wingard JR, Beals SU, Santos GW, Merz WG, Saral R. *Aspergillus* infections in bone marrow transplant recipients. Bone Marrow Transplant 1987; 2:175–181.

90. Fishman JA, Rubin RH. Infection in organ-transplant recipients. N Engl J Med 1998; 338:1741–1751.

91. George MJ, Snydman DR, Werner BG, Griffith J, Falagas ME, Dougherty NN, Rubin RH. The independent role of cytomegalovirus as a risk factor for invasive fungal disease in orthotopic liver transplant recipients. Boston Center for Liver Transplantation CMVIG-Study Group. Am J Med 1997; 103: 106–113.

92. Fortun J, Martin-Davila P, Moreno S, De Vicente E, Nuno J, Candelas A, Barcena R, Garcia M. Risk factors for invasive aspergillosis in liver transplant recipients. Liver Transplant 2002; 8:1065–1070.

93. Fishman JA. *Pneumocystis carinii* and parasitic infections in transplantation. Infect Dis Clin North Am 1995; 9:1005–1044.

94. Hadley S, Karchmer AW. Fungal infections in solid organ transplant recipients. Infect Dis Clin North Am 1995; 9: 1045–1074.

95. Rubin RH, Wolfson JS, Cosimi AB, Tolkoff-Rubin NE. Infection in the renal transplant recipient. Am J Med 1981; 70: 405–411.

96. Blumberg HM, Jarvis WR, Soucie JM, Edwards JE, Patterson JE, Pfaller MA, Rangel-Frausto MS, Rinaldi MG, Saiman L, Wiblin RT, Wenzel RP;, Wenzel RP. Risk factors for candidal bloodstream infections in surgical intensive care unit patients: the NEMIS prospective multicenter study. The National Epidemiology of Mycosis Survey. Clin Infect Dis 2001; 33: 177–186.

97. McKinnon PS, Goff DA, Kern JW, Devlin JW, Barletta JF, Sierawski SJ, Mosenthal AC, Gore P, Ambegaonkar AJ, Lubowski TJ. Temporal assessment of *Candida* risk factors in the surgical intensive care unit. Arch Surg 2001; 136: 1401–1408.

98. Hughes WT, Armstrong D, Bodey GP, Bow EJ, Brown AE, Calandra T, Feld R, Pizzo PA, Rolston KV, Shenep JL, Young LS. 2002 guidelines for the use of antimicrobial agents in neutropenic patients with cancer. Clin Infect Dis 2002; 34: 730–751.

99. Cochran A, Morris SE, Edelman LS, Saffle JR. Systemic *Candida* infection in burn patients: a case-control study of management patterns and outcomes. Surg Infect 2002; 3:367–374.

100. Diekema DJ, Messer SA, Brueggemann AB, Coffman SL, Doern GV, Herwaldt LA, Pfaller MA. Epidemiology of candidemia: 3-year results from the emerging infections and the epidemiology of Iowa organisms study. J Clin Microbiol 2002; 40: 1298–1302.

101. Pfaller MA, Diekema DJ, Jones RN, Sader HS, Fluit AC, Hollis RJ, Messer SA;, Messer SA. International surveillance of bloodstream infections due to *Candida* species: frequency of occurrence and *in vitro* susceptibilities to fluconazole, ravuconazole, and voriconazole of isolates collected from 1997 through 1999 in the SENTRY antimicrobial surveillance program. J Clin Microbiol 2001; 39:3254–3259.

102. Kauffman CA, Vazquez JA, Sobel JD, Gallis HA, McKinsey DS, Karchmer AW, Sugar AM, Sharkey PK, Wise GJ, Mangi R, Mosher A, Lee JY, Dismukes WE. Prospective multicenter surveillance study of funguria in hospitalized patients. The National Institute for Allergy and Infectious Diseases (NIAID) Mycoses Study Group. Clin Infect Dis 2000; 30:14–18.

103. Rothan-Tondeur M, Lancien E, Pialleport T, Meaume S, Moulias R, Marzais M, Cambau E, Le Blanche AF. Prevalence of oropharyngeal candidiasis in geriatric inpatients. J Am Geriatr Soc 2001; 49:1741–1742.

104. Marty F, Mylonakis E. Antifungal use in HIV infection. Expert Opin Pharmacother 2002; 3:91–102.

105. Kaplan JE, Hanson D, Dworkin MS, Frederick T, Bertolli J, Lindegren ML, Holmberg S, Jones JL. Epidemiology of human immunodeficiency virus-associated opportunistic infections in the United States in the era of highly active antiretroviral therapy. Clin Infect Dis 2000; 30(suppl 1):S5–S14.

106. Mocroft A, Vella S, Benfield TL, Chiesi A, Miller V, Gargalianos P, d'Arminio Monforte A, Yust I, Bruun JN, Phil-

lips AN, Lundgren JD. Changing patterns of mortality across Europe in patients infected with HIV-1. EuroSIDA Study Group. Lancet 1998; 352:1725–1730.

107. Palella FJ Jr, Delaney KM, Moorman AC, Loveless MO, Fuhrer J, Satten GA, Aschman DJ, Holmberg SD. Declining morbidity and mortality among patients with advanced human immunodeficiency virus infection. HIV Outpatient Study Investigators. N Engl J Med 1998; 338:853–860.

108. Kovacs JA, Masur H. Prophylaxis against opportunistic infections in patients with human immunodeficiency virus infection. N Engl J Med 2000; 342:1416–1429.

109. Vibhagool A, Sungkanuparph S, Mootsikapun P, Chetchotisakd P, Tansuphaswaswadikul S, Bowonwatanuwong C, Ingsathit A. Discontinuation of secondary prophylaxis for cryptococcal meningitis in human immunodeficiency virus-infected patients treated with highly active antiretroviral therapy: a prospective, multicenter, randomized study. Clin Infect Dis 2003; 36:1329–1331.

110. Martinez E, Garcia-Viejo MA, Marcos MA, Perez-Cuevas JB, Blanco JL, Mallolas J, Miro JM, Gatell JM. Discontinuation of secondary prophylaxis for cryptococcal meningitis in HIV-infected patients responding to highly active antiretroviral therapy. AIDS 2000; 14:2615–2617.

111. Rollot F, Bossi P, Tubiana R, Caumes E, Zeller V, Katlama C, Bricaire F. Discontinuation of secondary prophylaxis against cryptococcosis in patients with AIDS receiving highly active antiretroviral therapy. AIDS 2001; 15:1448–1449.

112. Arribas JR, Hernandez-Albujar S, Gonzalez-Garcia JJ, Pena JM, Gonzalez A, Canedo T, Madero R, Vazquez JJ, Powderly WG. Impact of protease inhibitor therapy on HIV-related oropharyngeal candidiasis. AIDS 2000; 14:979–985.

113. Hoegl L, Thoma-Greber E, Rocken M, Korting HC. Persistent oral candidosis by non-albicans *Candida* strains including *Candida glabrata* in a human immunodeficiency virus-infected patient observed over a period of 6 years. Mycoses 1998; 41:335–338.

114. Gianarkis D. Drug use evaluation and successful therapeutic interchange of IV to oral fluconazole. J Clin Pharm 1996; 21: 327–350.

115. Lambert JE. Outcomes associated with an antibiotic/antifungal IV to oral switch program [abstract]., 33rd ASHP Midyear Clinical Meeting American Society of Health-Systems Pharmacists, Las Vegas, December 1998.

116. Schachtner JM, Guharoy R, Medicis JJ. Drug utilization evaluation of fluconazole at a university hospital [abstract]., 35th ASHP Midyear Clinical Meeting American Society of Health-Systems Pharmacists, Las Vegas, Dec 2–6, 2000.

117. Rex JH, Walsh TJ. Estimating the true cost of amphotericin B. Clin Infect Dis 1999; 29:1408–1410.

118. Buchner T, Fegeler W, Bernhardt H, Brockmeyer N, Duswald KH, Herrmann M, Heuser D, Jehn U, Just-Nubling G, Karthaus M, Maschmeyer G, Muller FM, Muller J, Ritter J, Roos N, Ruhnke M, Schmalreck A, Schwarze R, Schwesinger G, Silling G;, Silling G. Treatment of severe *Candida* infections in high-risk patients in Germany: consensus formed by a panel of interdisciplinary investigators. Eur J Clin Microbiol Infect Dis 2002; 21:337–352.

119. Masur H, Kaplan JE, Holmes KK, Holmes KK, Holmes KK. Guidelines for preventing opportunistic infections among HIV-infected persons—2002. Recommendations of the U.S. Public Health Service and the Infectious Diseases Society of America. Ann Intern Med 2002; 137:435–478.

120. Dykewicz CA. Guidelines for preventing opportunistic infections among hematopoietic stem cell transplant recipients: focus on community respiratory virus infections. Biol Blood Marrow Transplant 2001; 7(suppl):19S–22S.

121. Wong-Beringer A, Jacobs RA, Guglielmo BJ. Lipid formulations of amphotericin B: clinical efficacy and toxicities. Clin Infect Dis 1998; 27:603–618.

122. Winston DJ, Hathorn JW, Schuster MG, Schiller GJ, Territo MC. A multicenter, randomized trial of fluconazole versus amphotericin B for empiric antifungal therapy of febrile neutropenic patients with cancer. Am J Med 2000; 108:282–289.

123. Viscoli C, Castagnola E, Van Lint MT, Moroni C, Garaventa A, Rossi MR, Fanci R, Menichetti F, Caselli D, Giacchino M, Congiu M. Fluconazole versus amphotericin B as empirical antifungal therapy of unexplained fever in granulocytopenic

cancer patients: a pragmatic, multicentre, prospective and randomised clinical trial. Eur J Cancer 1996; 32A:814–820.

124. Boogaerts M, Winston DJ, Bow EJ, Garber G, Reboli AC, Schwarer AP, Novitzky N, Boehme A, Chwetzoff E, De Beule K;, De Beule K. Intravenous and oral itraconazole versus intravenous amphotericin B deoxycholate as empirical antifungal therapy for persistent fever in neutropenic patients with cancer who are receiving broad-spectrum antibacterial therapy. A randomized, controlled trial. Ann Intern Med 2001; 135:412–422.

125. Walsh TJ, Finberg RW, Arndt C, Hiemenz J, Schwartz C, Bodensteiner D, Pappas P, Seibel N, Greenberg RN, Dummer S, Schuster M, Holcenberg JS. Liposomal amphotericin B for empirical therapy in patients with persistent fever and neutropenia. National Institute of Allergy and Infectious Diseases Mycoses Study Group. N Engl J Med 1999; 340:764–771.

126. Bowden R, Chandrasekar P, White MH, Li X, Pietrelli L, Gurwith M, van Burik JA, Laverdiere M, Safrin S, Wingard JR. A double-blind, randomized, controlled trial of amphotericin B colloidal dispersion versus amphotericin B for treatment of invasive aspergillosis in immunocompromised patients. Clin Infect Dis 2002; 35:359–366.

127. Ellis M, Spence D, de Pauw B, Meunier F, Marinus A, Collette L, Sylvester R, Meis J, Boogaerts M, Selleslag D, Krcmery V, von Sinner W, MacDonald P, Doyen C, Vandercam B. An EORTC international multicenter randomized trial (EORTC number 19923) comparing two dosages of liposomal amphotericin B for treatment of invasive aspergillosis. Clin Infect Dis 1998; 27:1406–1412.

128. Hamill R, Sobel J, El-Sadr W. Randomized, double-blind trial of AmBisome (liposomal amphotericin B) and amphotericin B in acute cryptococcal meningitis in AIDS patients [abstract]., 39th Interscience Conference on Antimicrobial Agents and Chemotherapy, San Francisco, Sept 26–29, 1999.

129. Johnson PC, Wheat LJ, Cloud GA, Goldman M, Lancaster D, Bamberger DM, Powderly WG, Hafner R, Kauffman CA, Dismukes WE;. Dismukes WE. Safety and efficacy of liposomal amphotericin B compared with conventional amphotericin B for induction therapy of histoplasmosis in patients with AIDS. Ann Intern Med 2002; 137:105–109.

130. Leenders AC, Reiss P, Portegies P, Clezy K, Hop WC, Hoy J, Borleffs JC, Allworth T, Kauffmann RH, Jones P, Kroon FP, Verbrugh HA, de Marie S. Liposomal amphotericin B (AmBisome) compared with amphotericin B both followed by oral fluconazole in the treatment of AIDS-associated cryptococcal meningitis. AIDS 1997; 11:1463–1471.

131. Prentice HG, Hann IM, Herbrecht R, Aoun M, Kvaloy S, Catovsky D, Pinkerton CR, Schey SA, Jacobs F, Oakhill A, Stevens RF, Darbyshire PJ, Gibson BE. A randomized comparison of liposomal versus conventional amphotericin B for the treatment of pyrexia of unknown origin in neutropenic patients. Br J Haematol 1997; 98:711–718.

132. White MH, Bowden RA, Sandler ES, Graham ML, Noskin GA, Wingard JR, Goldman M, van Burik JA, McCabe A, Lin JS, Gurwith M, Miller CB. Randomized, double-blind clinical trial of amphotericin B colloidal dispersion vs. amphotericin B in the empirical treatment of fever and neutropenia. Clin Infect Dis 1998; 27:296–302.

133. Wingard JR, White MH, Anaissie E, Raffalli J, Goodman J, Arrieta A;/, Arrieta A. A randomized, double-blind comparative trial evaluating the safety of liposomal amphotericin B versus amphotericin B lipid complex in the empirical treatment of febrile neutropenia. L Amph/ABLC Collaborative Study Group. Clin Infect Dis 2000; 31:1155–1163.

134. Belden T, Drew RH, Perfect JR. Predicting subsequent infusion-related reactions from responses to initial doses of amphotericin b lipid complex [abstract]., American College of Clinical Pharmacy 2002 Spring Practice and Research Forum, Savannah, GA, April 7–10, 2002.

135. Burks LC, Aisner J, Fortner CL, Wiernik PH. Meperidine for the treatment of shaking chills and fever. Arch Intern Med 1980; 140:483–484.

136. Johnson MD, Drew RH, Perfect JR. Chest discomfort associated with liposomal amphotericin B: report of three cases and review of the literature. Pharmacotherapy 1998; 18:1053–1061.

137. Roden MM, Nelson LD, Knudsen TA, Jarosinski PF, Starling JM, Shiflett SE, Calis K, DeChristoforo R, Donowitz GR, Buell

D, Walsh TJ. Triad of acute infusion-related reactions associated with liposomal amphotericin B: analysis of clinical and epidemiological characteristics. Clin Infect Dis 2003; 36: 1213–1220.

138. Ural AU, Avcu F, Cetin T, Beyan C, Kaptan K, Nazaroglu NK, Yalcin A. Spironolactone: is it a novel drug for the prevention of amphotericin B-related hypokalemia in cancer patients? . Eur J Clin Pharmacol 2002; 57:771–773.

139. Bearden DT, Muncey LA. The effect of amiloride on amphotericin B-induced hypokalaemia. J Antimicrob Chemother 2001; 48:109–111.

140. Deray G. Amphotericin B nephrotoxicity. J Antimicrob Chemother 2002; 49(suppl 1):37–41.

141. Wingard JR, Kubilis P, Lee L, Yee G, White M, Walshe L, Bowden R, Anaissie E, Hiemenz J, Lister J. Clinical significance of nephrotoxicity in patients treated with amphotericin B for suspected or proven aspergillosis. Clin Infect Dis 1999; 29:1402–1407.

142. Luke RG, Boyle JA. Renal effects of amphotericin B lipid complex. Am J Kidney Dis 1998; 31:780–785.

143. Bates DW, Su L, Yu DT, Chertow GM, Seger DL, Gomes DR, Dasbach EJ, Platt R. Mortality and costs of acute renal failure associated with amphotericin B therapy. Clin Infect Dis 2001; 32:686–693.

144. Anderson CM. Sodium chloride treatment of amphotericin B nephrotoxicity. Standard of care? . West J Med 1995; 162: 313–317.

145. Sawaya BP, Briggs JP, Schnermann J. Amphotericin B nephrotoxicity: the adverse consequences of altered membrane properties. J Am Soc Nephrol 1995; 6:154–164.

146. Imhof A, Walter RB, Schaffner A. Continuous infusion of escalated doses of amphotericin B deoxycholate: an open-label observational study. Clin Infect Dis 2003; 36:943–951.

147. Eriksson U, Seifert B, Schaffner A. Comparison of effects of amphotericin B deoxycholate infused over 4 or 24 hours: randomized controlled trial. BMJ 2001; 322:579–582.

148. Sharkey PK, Graybill JR, Johnson ES, Hausrath SG, Pollard RB, Kolokathis A, Mildvan D, Fan-Havard P, Eng RH, Patterson TF, Pottage JC Jr, Simberkoff MS, Wolf J, Meyer RD, Gupta R, Lee LW, Gordon DS. Amphotericin B lipid complex compared with amphotericin B in the treatment of cryptococcal meningitis in patients with AIDS. Clin Infect Dis 1996; 22:315–321.

149. White MH, Anaissie EJ, Kusne S, Wingard JR, Hiemenz JW, Cantor A, Gurwith M, Du Mond C, Mamelok RD, Bowden RA. Amphotericin B colloidal dispersion vs. amphotericin B as therapy for invasive aspergillosis. Clin Infect Dis 1997; 24: 635–642.

150. Walsh TJ, Seibel NL, Arndt C, Harris RE, Dinubile MJ, Reboli A, Hiemenz J, Chanock SJ. Amphotericin B lipid complex in pediatric patients with invasive fungal infections. Pediatr Infect Dis J 1999; 18:702–708.

151. Bates DW, Su L, Yu DT, Chertow GM, Seger DL, Gomes DR, Platt R. Correlates of acute renal failure in patients receiving parenteral amphotericin B. Kidney Int 2001; 60:1452–1459.

152. Fisher MA, Talbot GH, Maislin G, McKeon BP, Tynan KP, Strom BL. Risk factors for amphotericin B-associated nephrotoxicity. Am J Med 1989; 87:547–552.

153. Cannon JP, Garey KW, Danziger LH. A prospective and retrospective analysis of the nephrotoxicity and efficacy of lipid-based amphotericin B formulations. Pharmacotherapy 2001; 21:1107–1114.

154. Oravcova E, Mistrik M, Sakalova A, Drgona L, Kollar T, Helpianska L, Ilavska I, Sorkovska D, Spanik S, Kukuckova E. Amphotericin B lipid complex to treat invasive fungal infections in cancer patients: report of efficacy and safety in 20 patients. Chemotherapy 1995; 41:473–476.

155. Gibson G, Hundress J, Suh K. Assessment of compliance with established guidelines for the use of amphotericin B lipid complex at a large university teaching hospital [abstract]., 35th ASHP Midyear Clinical Meeting, Las Vegas, Dec 2–6, 2000.

156. Small F, Dinning RS, Campbell B, Churchill W. Impact of clinical pharmacists on the prescribing practices of liposomal amphotericin B (AmBisome) at a large teaching hospital [ab-

stract]., 35th ASHP Midyear Clinical Meeting, Las Vegas, Dec 2–6, 2000.

157. Drew RH, Perfect JR. Flucytosine. In: . Yu VL, Merigan TC, Barriere SL, Eds Antimicrobial Therapy and Vaccines. 1st ed. Baltimore: Williams & Wilkins, 1999:1170–1184.

158. Stamm AM, Diasio RB, Dismukes WE, Shadomy S, Cloud GA, Bowles CA, Karam GH, Espinel-Ingroff A. Toxicity of amphotericin B plus flucytosine in 194 patients with cryptococcal meningitis. Am J Med 1987; 83:236–242.

159. Vermes A, van Der SH, Guchelaar HJ. Flucytosine: correlation between toxicity and pharmacokinetic parameters. Chemotherapy 2000; 46:86–94.

160. Vermes A, Guchelaar HJ, Dankert J. Prediction of flucytosine-induced thrombocytopenia using creatinine clearance. Chemotherapy 2000; 46:335–341.

161. Pacetti SA, Gelone SP. Caspofungin acetate for treatment of invasive fungal infections. Ann Pharmacother 2003; 37:90–98.

162. Stone EA, Fung HB, Kirschenbaum HL. Caspofungin: an echinocandin antifungal agent. Clin Ther 2002; 24:351–377.

163. Johnson MDP. Caspofungin: first approved agent in a new class of antifungals. Expert Opin Pharmacother 2003; 4:807–823.

164. Garbino J, Lew D, Hirschel B, Rohner P. Caspofungin in the treatment of oropharyngeal candidiasis. Int J Clin Pract 2003; 57:143–144.

165. Kartsonis N, Dinubile MJ, Bartizal K, Hicks PS, Ryan D, Sable CA. Efficacy of caspofungin in the treatment of esophageal candidiasis resistant to fluconazole. J Acquir Immune Defic Syndr 2002; 31:183–187.

166. Sollima S, Corbellino M, Cicconi P, Piazza M, Vigano O, Antinori S. Resolution of multidrug-refractory oesophageal candidiasis in an AIDS patient after treatment with caspofungin. AIDS 2002; 16:1303–1304.

167. Deresinski SCS. Caspofungin. Clin Infect Dis 2003; 36:1445–1457.

168. Sable CA, Nguyen BY, Chodakewitz JA, Dinubile MJ. Safety and tolerability of caspofungin acetate in the treatment of fungal infections. Transplant Infect Dis 2002; 4:25–30.

169. Groll AH, Walsh TJ. Caspofungin: pharmacology, safety and therapeutic potential in superficial and invasive fungal infections. Expert Opin Investig Drugs 2001; 10:1545–1558.

170. &Walsh TJ. Cancidas (Caspofungin) for Injection, product information.. Whitehouse Station. NJ: : Merck & Co, 2003.

171. Aliff TB, Maslak PG, Jurcic JG, Heaney ML, Cathcart KN, Sepkowitz KA, Weiss MA. Refractory *Aspergillus* pneumonia in patients with acute leukemia: successful therapy with combination caspofungin and liposomal amphotericin. Cancer 2003; 97:1025–1032.

172. Roling EE, Klepser ME, Wasson A, Lewis RE, Ernst EJ, Pfaller MA. Antifungal activities of fluconazole, caspofungin (MK0991), and anidulafungin (LY 303366) alone and in combination against *Candida* spp. and *Crytococcus neoformans* via time-kill methods. Diagn Microbiol Infect Dis 2002; 43:13–17.

173. Terrell CL. Antifungal agents. Part II. The azoles. Mayo Clin Proc 1999; 74:78–100.

174. Piscitelli SC, Goss TF, Wilton JH, D'Andrea DT, Goldstein H, Schentag JJ. Effects of ranitidine and sucralfate on ketoconazole bioavailability. Antimicrob Agents Chemother 1991; 35:1765–1771.

175. Lake-Bakaar G, Tom W, Lake-Bakaar D, Gupta N, Beidas S, Elsakr M, Straus E. Gastropathy and ketoconazole malabsorption in the acquired immunodeficiency syndrome (AIDS). Ann Intern Med 1988; 109:471–473.

176. Lelawongs P, Barone JA, Colaizzi JL, Hsuan AT, Mechlinski W, Legendre R, Guarnieri J. Effect of food and gastric acidity on absorption of orally administered ketoconazole. Clin Pharm 1988; 7:228–235.

177. Chapman SA, Lake KD, Solbrack DF, Milfred SK, Marshall PS, Kamps MA. Considerations for using ketoconazole in solid organ transplant recipients receiving cyclosporine immunosuppression. J Transpl Coord 1996; 6:148–154.

178. Bare RL, Torti FM. Endocrine therapy of prostate cancer. Cancer Treat Res 1998; 94:69–87.

179. Carrillo-Munoz AJ, Ruesga M, Brio S, del Valle O, Rodriguez V, Santos P, Hernandez-Molina JM, Canton E, Peman J, Guarro J, Quindos G. Comparison of *in vitro* antifungal activities of amphotericin B lipid complex with itraconazole against 708 clinical yeast isolates and opportunistic moulds determined by National Committee for Clinical Laboratory Standards methods M27-A and M38-P. Chemotherapy 2002; 48: 224–231.

180. Harousseau JL, Dekker AW, Stamatoullas-Bastard A, Fassas A, Linkesch W, Gouveia J, De Bock R, Rovira M, Seifert WF, Joosen H, Peeters M, De Beule K. Itraconazole oral solution for primary prophylaxis of fungal infections in patients with hematological malignancy and profound neutropenia: a randomized, double-blind, double-placebo, multicenter trial comparing itraconazole and amphotericin B. Antimicrob Agents Chemother 2000; 44:1887–1893.

181. Boogaerts MA, Verhoef GE, Zachee P, Demuynck H, Verbist L, De Beule K. Antifungal prophylaxis with itraconazole in prolonged neutropenia: correlation with plasma levels. Mycoses 1989; 32:103–108.

182. Glasmacher A, Hahn C, Leutner C, Molitor E, Wardelmann E, Losem C, Sauerbruch T, Marklein G, Schmidt-Wolf IG. Breakthrough invasive fungal infections in neutropenic patients after prophylaxis with itraconazole. Mycoses 1999; 42: 443–451.

183. Koks CH, Meenhorst PL, Bult A, Beijnen JH. Itraconazole solution: summary of pharmacokinetic features and review of activity in the treatment of fluconazole-resistant oral candidosis in HIV-infected persons. Pharmacol Res 2002; 46: 195–201.

184. Vandewoude K, Vogelaers D, Decruyenaere J, Jaqmin P, De Beule K, Van Peer A, Woestenborghs R, Groen K, Colardyn F. Concentrations in plasma and safety of 7 days of intravenous itraconazole followed by 2 weeks of oral itraconazole solution in patients in intensive care units. Antimicrob Agents Chemother 1997; 41:2714–2718.

185. Glasmacher A, Molitor E, Mezger J, Marklein G. Antifungal prophylaxis with itraconazole in neutropenic patients: pharmacological, microbiological and clinical aspects. Mycoses 1996; 39:249–258.

186. Patterson TF, Peters J, Levine SM, Anzueto A, Bryan CL, Sako EY, Miller OL, Calhoon JH, Rinaldi MG. Systemic availability of itraconazole in lung transplantation. Antimicrob Agents Chemother 1996; 40:2217–2220.

187. Zhao Q, Zhou H, Pesco-Koplowitz L. Pharmacokinetics of intravenous itraconazole followed by itraconazole oral solution in patients with human immunodeficiency virus infection. J Clin Pharmacol 2001; 41:1319–1328.

188. Michallet M, Persat F, Kranzhofer N, Levron JC, Prat C, Belhabri A, Chwetzoff E, Le Moing JP, Fiere D, Piens MA. Pharmacokinetics of itraconazole oral solution in allogeneic bone marrow transplant patients receiving total body irradiation. Bone Marrow Transplant 1998; 21:1239–1243.

189. Menichetti F, Del Favero A, Martino P, Bucaneve G, Micozzi A, Girmenia C, Barbabietola G, Pagano L, Leoni P, Specchia G, Caiozzo A, Raimondi R, Mandelli F. Itraconazole oral solution as prophylaxis for fungal infections in neutropenic patients with hematologic malignancies: a randomized, placebo-controlled, double-blind, multicenter trial. GIMEMA Infection Program. Gruppo Italiano Malattie Ematologiche dell' Adulto. Clin Infect Dis 1999; 28:25.

190. Barone JA, Moskovitz BL, Guarnieri J, Hassell AE, Colaizzi JL, Bierman RH, Jessen L. Enhanced bioavailability of itraconazole in hydroxypropyl-beta-cyclodextrin solution versus capsules in healthy volunteers. Antimicrob Agents Chemother 1998; 42:1862–1865.

191. Prentice AG, Warnock DW. Itraconazole more bioavailable in solution. Blood 1996; 88:3662–3663.

192. Stevens DA. Itraconazole in cyclodextrin solution. Pharmacotherapy 1999; 19:603–611.

193. Boogaerts MA, Maertens J, Van Der Geest R, Bosly A, Michaux JM, Van Hoof A, Cleeren M, Wostenborghs R, De Beule K. Pharmacokinetics and safety of a 7-day administration of intravenous itraconazole followed by a 14-day administration of itraconazole oral solution in patients with hematologic malignancy. Antimicrob Agents Chemother 2001; 45: 981–985.

194. Slain D, Rogers PD, Cleary JD, Chapman SW. Intravenous itraconazole. Ann Pharmacother 2001; 35:720–729.

195. Poirier JM, Cheymol G. Optimization of itraconazole therapy using target drug concentrations. Clin Pharmacokinet 1998; 35:461–473.

196. Goa KL, Barradell LB. Fluconazole. An update of its pharmacodynamic and pharmacokinetic properties and therapeutic use in major superficial and systemic mycoses in immunocompromised patients. Drugs 1995; 50:658–690.

197. Fisher MA, Shen SH, Haddad J, Tarry WF. Comparison of *in vivo* activity of fluconazole with that of amphotericin B against *Candida tropicalis*, *Candida glabrata*, and *Candida krusei*. Antimicrob Agents Chemother 1989; 33:1443–1446.

198. Karyotakis NC, Anaissie EJ, Hachem R, Dignani MC, Samonis G. Comparison of the efficacy of polyenes and triazoles against hematogenous *Candida krusei* infection in neutropenic mice. J Infect Dis 1993; 168:1311–1313.

199. Anassi EO, Egbunike IG, Akpaffiong MJ, Ike EN, Cate TR. Developing and implementing guidelines to promote appropriate use of fluconazole therapy in an AIDS clinic. Hosp Pharm 581; 29:576–578.

200. Costantini MK, Goff DA, Fass RJ, Siegel J. Formulary addition of fluconazole with pre-approved guidelines for use: new approach to compliance management [abstract]., ASHP Midyear Clinical Meeting, New Orleans, LA, December 1991.

201. Tett S, Moore S, Ray J. Pharmacokinetics and bioavailability of fluconazole in two groups of males with human immunodeficiency virus (HIV) infection compared with those in a group of males without HIV infection. Antimicrob Agents Chemother 1995; 39:1835–1841.

202. Pelz RK, Lipsett PA, Swoboda SM, Merz W, Rinaldi MG, Hendrix CW. Enteral fluconazole is well absorbed in critically ill surgical patients. Surgery 2002; 131:534–540.

203. Rosemurgy AS, Markowsky S, Goode SE, Plastino K, Kearney RE. Bioavailability of fluconazole in surgical intensive care unit patients: a study comparing routes of administration. J Trauma 1995; 39:445–447.

204. Kami M, Sawada Y, Mori S, Hirate J, Kojima N, Kanda Y, Moriya A, Yuji K, Saito T, Chiba S, Hirai H. Serum levels of

fluconazole in patients after cytotoxic chemotherapy for hematological malignancy. Am J Hematol 2001; 66:85–91.

205. Ellis ME, Spence D, Ernst P, Greer W. Variability of plasma fluconazole levels in patients with hematologic malignancy. Clin Infect Dis 1997; 24:86–87.

206. Pittrow L, Penk A. Special pharmacokinetics of fluconazole in septic, obese and burn patients. Mycoses 1999; 42(suppl 2): 87–90.

207. Boucher BA, King SR, Wandschneider HL, Hickerson WL, Hanes SD, Herring VL, Canada TW, Hess MM. Fluconazole pharmacokinetics in burn patients. Antimicrob Agents Chemother 1998; 42:930–933.

208. el Yazigi A, Ellis M, Ernst P, Hussein R, Baillie FJ. Effect of repeated dosing on the pharmacokinetics of oral fluconazole in bone marrow transplant patients. J Clin Pharmacol 1997; 37:1031–1037.

209. Lee SC, Fung CP, Huang JS, Tsai CJ, Chen KS, Chen HY, Lee N, See LC, Shieh WB. Clinical correlates of antifungal macrodilution susceptibility test results for non-AIDS patients with severe *Candida* infections treated with fluconazole. Antimicrob Agents Chemother 2000; 44:2715–2718.

210. Revankar SG, Kirkpatrick WR, McAtee RK, Dib OP, Fothergill AW, Redding SW, Rinaldi MG, Hilsenbeck SG, Patterson TF. A randomized trial of continuous or intermittent therapy with fluconazole for oropharyngeal candidiasis in HIV-infected patients: clinical outcomes and development of fluconazole resistance. Am J Med 1998; 105:7–11.

211. Voss A, de Pauw BE. High-dose fluconazole therapy in patients with severe fungal infections. Eur J Clin Microbiol Infect Dis 1999; 18:165–174.

212. Duswald KH, Penk A, Pittrow L. High-dose therapy with fluconazole ≥ 800 mg day-1. Mycoses 1997; 40:267–277.

213. Rex JH, Bennett JE, Sugar AM, Pappas PG, van der Horst CM, Edwards JE, Washburn RG, Scheld WM, Karchmer AW, Dine AP. A randomized trial comparing fluconazole with amphotericin B for the treatment of candidemia in patients without neutropenia. Candidemia Study Group and the National Institute. N Engl J Med 1994; 331:1325–1330.

214. Phillips P, Shafran S, Garber G, Rotstein C, Smaill F, Fong I, Salit I, Miller M, Williams K, Conly JM, Singer J, Ioannou S. Multicenter randomized trial of fluconazole versus amphotericin B for treatment of candidemia in non-neutropenic patients. Canadian Candidemia Study Group. Eur J Clin Microbiol Infect Dis 1997; 16:337–345.

215. Saag MS, Cloud GA, Graybill JR, Sobel JD, Tuazon CU, Johnson PC, Fessel WJ, Moskovitz BL, Wiesinger B, Cosmatos D, Riser L, Thomas C, Hafner R, Dismukes WE. A comparison of itraconazole versus fluconazole as maintenance therapy for AIDS-associated cryptococcal meningitis. National Institute of Allergy and Infectious Diseases Mycoses Study Group. Clin Infect Dis 1999; 28:291–296.

216. Pearson MM, Rogers PD, Cleary JD, Chapman SW. Voriconazole: a new triazole antifungal agent. Ann Pharmacother 2003; 37:420–432.

217. Johnson LB, Kauffman CA. Voriconazole: a new triazole antifungal agent. Clin Infect Dis 2003; 36:630–637.

218. Espinel-Ingroff A. *In vitro* activity of the new triazole voriconazole (UK-109,496) against opportunistic filamentous and dimorphic fungi and common and emerging yeast pathogens. J Clin Microbiol 1998; 36:198–202.

219. Walsh TJ, Pappas P, Winston DJ, Lazarus HM, Petersen F, Raffalli J, Yanovich S, Stiff P, Greenberg R, Donowitz G, Schuster M, Reboli A, Wingard J, Arndt C, Reinhardt J, Hadley S, Finberg R, Laverdiere M, Perfect J, Garber G, Fioritoni G, Anaissie E, Lee J;, Lee J. Voriconazole compared with liposomal amphotericin B for empirical antifungal therapy in patients with neutropenia and persistent fever. N Engl J Med 2002; 346:225–234.

220. Lazarus HM, Blumer JL, Yanovich S, Schlamm H, Romero A. Safety and pharmacokinetics of oral voriconazole in patients at risk of fungal infection: a dose escalation study. J Clin Pharmacol 2002; 42:395–402.

221. Tan KKC, BN KKC, Oakes M. Investigation into the relationship between plasma voriconazole concentrations and liver function test abnormalities in therapeutic trials [abstract A18]., 41st Interscience Conference on Antimicrobial Agents and Chemotherapy, Chicago, Dec 16–19, 2001.

222. Boogaerts M, Maertens J. Clinical experience with itracona-
     zole in systemic fungal infections. Drugs 2001; 61(suppl 1):
     39–47.

223. Janssen Pharmaceutica. Sporanox™ (itraconazole) capsules,
     product information. Titusville, NJ: Janssen Pharmaceutica
     Products, LP., 2001.

224. Wimberley SL, Haug MT 3rd, Shermock KM, Qu A, Maurer
     JR, Mehta AC, Schilz RJ, Gordon SM. Enhanced cyclosporine-
     itraconazole interaction with cola in lung transplant recipi-
     ents. Clin Transplant 2001; 15:116–122.

225. Jaruratanasirikul S, Kleepkaew A. Influence of an acidic bev-
     erage (Coca-Cola) on the absorption of itraconazole. Eur J Clin
     Pharmacol 1997; 52:235–237.

226. Ortho Biotech Products. Sporanox™ (itraconazole) injection
     product information. Raritan, NJ: Ortho Biotech Products,
     LP., 2001.

227. Pfizer. Vfend™ (voriconazole) tablet and injection product in-
     formation. New York: Pfizer, Inc.., 2003.

228. Gallagher JC, Dodds Ashley ES, Drew RH, Perfect JR. Anti-
     fungal pharmacotherapy for invasive mould infections. Expert
     Opin Pharmacother 2003; 4:147–164.

Index